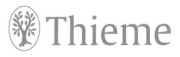

Histology

An Essential Textbook

D. J. Lowrie Jr., MS, PhD
Professor, Educator
Department of Medical Education
University of Cincinnati College of Medicine
Cincinnati, Ohio

846 illustrations

Thieme
New York • Stuttgart • Delhi • Rio de Janeiro

Library of Congress Cataloging-in-Publication Data

Names: Lowrie, D. J., Jr. (Donald James), 1965- author.

Title: Histology : an essential textbook / D.J. Lowrie Jr. Description: New York : Thieme, [2020]

Identifiers: LCCN 2019015004| ISBN 9781626234130 (softcover : alk. paper) |

 ISBN 9781626234147 (eISBN)

Subjects: | MESH: Histology | Programmed Instruction

Classification: LCC QM552 | NLM QS 518.2 | DDC 611/.018--dc23

 LC record available at https://lccn.loc.gov/2019015004

Important note: Medicine is an ever-changing science undergoing continual development. Research and clinical experience are continually expanding our knowledge, in particular our knowledge of proper treatment and drug therapy. Insofar as this book mentions any dosage or application, readers may rest assured that the authors, editors, and publishers have made every effort to ensure that such references are in accordance with **the state of knowledge at the time of production of the book.**

Nevertheless, this does not involve, imply, or express any guarantee or responsibility on the part of the publishers in respect to any dosage instructions and forms of applications stated in the book. **Every user is requested to examine carefully** the manufacturers' leaflets accompanying each drug and to check, if necessary in consultation with a physician or specialist, whether the dosage schedules mentioned therein or the contraindications stated by the manufacturers differ from the statements made in the present book. Such examination is particularly important with drugs that are either rarely used or have been newly released on the market. Every dosage schedule or every form of application used is entirely at the user's own risk and responsibility. The authors and publishers request every user to report to the publishers any discrepancies or inaccuracies noticed. If errors in this work are found after publication, errata will be posted at www.thieme. com on the product description page.

Some of the product names, patents, and registered designs referred to in this book are in fact registered trademarks or proprietary names even though specific reference to this fact is not always made in the text. Therefore, the appearance of a name without designation as proprietary is not to be construed as a representation by the publisher that it is in the public domain.

© 2020 Thieme Medical Publishers, Inc.
Thieme Publishers New York
333 Seventh Avenue, New York, NY 10001 USA
+1 800 782 3488, customerservice@thieme.com

Thieme Publishers Stuttgart
Rüdigerstrasse 14, 70469 Stuttgart, Germany
+49 [0]711 8931 421, customerservice@thieme.de

Thieme Publishers Delhi
A-12, Second Floor, Sector-2, Noida-201301
Uttar Pradesh, India
+91 120 45 566 00, customerservice@thieme.in

Thieme Publishers Rio de Janeiro, Thieme Publicações Ltda.
Edifício Rodolpho de Paoli, 25º andar
Av. Nilo Peçanha, 50 – Sala 2508
Rio de Janeiro 20020-906, Brasil
+55 21 3172 2297

Cover design: Thieme Publishing Group
Typesetting by Prairie Papers

Printed in the United States of America by King Printing Co., Inc.

ISBN 978-1-62623-413-0

Also available as an e-book:
eISBN 978-1-62623-414-7

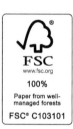

FSC
www.fsc.org
100%
Paper from well-managed forests
FSC® C103101

This book is dedicated to my wife, Jane Lowrie, whose love and infinite patience made this project possible.

Contents

Video Contents

Preface

Like many medical schools, the University of Cincinnati College of Medicine recently underwent a curriculum revision, which included changing from traditional basic science courses (histology, pathology) to integrated, organ-system–based courses (e.g. blood and cardiovascular). Previous to revision, histology and cell biology was a course that included approximately fifty hours of lecture and thirty-one laboratory sessions.

Curricular change created a need to streamline our histology content. This resulted in a reassessment of how we were teaching histology, particularly, the use of live laboratory sessions. The result was the creation of approximately fifty Power Point-based, self-study histology modules. These modules are designed to replace the live laboratory sessions, and, as such, have a main focus on structure identification at the light and electron microscopic levels. To accomplish this, a variety of teaching methods are used, including numerous images, short text, short videos, and quizzes. Although the main focus of the modules is on structure identification, appropriate connections to other disciplines are prominent, including references to gross anatomy, embryology, physiology, and pathology.

At the University of Cincinnati, these modules are assigned as homework to be completed the evening before didactic sessions on a particular topic. In most cases, live presentations that follow these modules begin with a short recapitulation of module content, followed by detailed discussion of appropriate physiology or pathology. Because the modules are focused and maintain student attention, they are completed faithfully by our students before live sessions, which is usually not the case for assigned reading from larger textbooks. Faculty appreciate that they are presenting their material to students who have acquired a foundational knowledge of the material before the live sessions.

This text is a modification of these modules to fit publication standards. Most of these changes relate to format, converting Power Point files with short bulleted text to chapters in prose. However, the main spirit of the modules is retained: shorter, targeted concepts accompanied by numerous illustrations, videos demonstrating key features of histological structures, correlations to other basic science disciplines, and self-assessment quizzes at the end of each chapter.

For the student, this text and accompanying videos are a useful aid in learning to identify histological structures. This is a crucial skill for doing well on practical exams and provides a foundation for other basic and clinical science disciplines. For faculty, this resource provides an opportunity to allow students to learn basic histology on their own, freeing up precious contact time with students to address more challenging topics in histology or other disciplines.

The slides used for most of the images in this book are derived from the University of Cincinnati. Also included are images obtained from the University of Michigan Virtual Microscope Slide collections, used with permission of the copyright holders. These slides, and other collections, can be accessed and downloaded for noncommercial use under a Creative Commons BY-NC-SA 4.0 license from the Virtual Microscopy Database (VMD) (http://virtualmicroscopydatabase.org/). The VMD is supported by the American Association of Anatomists and was developed for educators and researchers to share resources to advance histology education. The VMD is not designed for direct student access or as an unmodified course resource.

Some notes about the use of this text.

As described previously, *Histology, an Essential Textbook,* arose from Power Point-based, self-directed learning modules. As such, the user should view it as a step-by-step learning resource, as opposed to a "be-all, tell-all" reference text. Many complicated concepts are intentionally presented in a piecemeal fashion, so that the user can digest a single concept or overview first, before delving into more complicated details. Therefore, many figures and the accompanying text will only point out one or two features of each image, leaving the details for later discussion (where that same image will appear again). For example, in the hematopoiesis series, an initial chapter describes features of these developing cells without specifically identifying such cells. Specific cell identification is then addressed in subsequent chapters.

In addition, some discussions are intentionally left out or are simply presented as an overview. The most notable example is in the cell biology chapter, where detailed discussions on gene expression, cell regulation, and cell metabolism found in other histology texts are not presented. This text focuses on histology and the underlying relationship between structure and function. Therefore, most of the descriptions in this book are directly related to an image or figure. Hopefully, the result is that each chapter is of manageable size and maintains the reader's interest.

Student feedback on the original modules is that the associated videos are the most valuable part. These videos are mostly recapitulations of what is described in the print text, so it may be tempting for the reader to skip over them. However, keep in mind that, in histology and other visual disciplines, there is nothing better than an instructor actually pointing out and describing structures in a live setting, similar to a personal tutor. Furthermore, there are links throughout the text that indicate the proper placement of each video. It may be tempting to read an entire chapter first and then play all the videos from that chapter at the end, or vice-versa. However, as described above, the text introduces basic concepts first and then delves into details later. Therefore, I highly recommend that the user watch each video when prompted in the text, as they will solidify understanding of simpler concepts before more complicated structures are discussed.

Finally, each chapter has a quiz designed to reinforce material covered in that chapter. Since histology is a visual discipline, many of these questions are straight identification similar to what many readers will see on practical exams. Each quiz also includes several questions related to structure-function or may delve into other disciplines, such as basic physiology or pathology. These questions are designed to prepare the reader for image-based questions on written and board exams.

These chapter quizzes are online only and are hosted on Thieme's MedOne Education site: https://medone-education.thieme.com. Use the code on the media page at the front of this book to gain access. An institutional license to the site is required to access these questions in an interactive format, and individual users are required to register for an individual account to track results.

D. J. Lowrie Jr.

Acknowledgments

I would like to thank a number of people who have helped me in my career and have made this project possible:

- My lifelong mentor and Masters advisor, Bruce Giffin, PhD, who has always been a role model and colleague as I pursued a teaching career.
- My PhD advisor, Wally Ip, PhD, who supported and encouraged my interest in teaching while I worked in his laboratory.
- John Michaels, PhD and Emma Lou Cardell, PhD, for spending long hours patiently teaching me the nuances of histological structure and function.
- Other histology faculty at the University of Cincinnati who helped me along the way, most notably Bob Brackenbury, PhD, Linda Parysek, PhD, and Bob Cardell, PhD. Dr. Cardell also provided some of the images used in this text.
- Peter Stambrook, PhD and Rick Drake, PhD, for opening the door to my teaching career here at the University of Cincinnati.
- Jane Lowrie, who made beautiful color hand drawings that were used as templates for most of the illustrations in this text.
- Michael Hortsch, PhD, University of Michigan, for his help in obtaining valuable images from the University of Michigan, and for guidance as we set up our online digital slide system here at the University of Cincinnati.
- To members of UCIT, notably Greg Fish and Tim Thornton, who assisted in setting up our digital slide systems.
- To all my current and former students who have provided valuable feedback on the modules that led to this work.
- To the members at Thieme for their assistance in converting a PowerPoint-based set of modules into a publishable text. In particular, Kenny Chumbley was instrumental in providing insight and guidance in the editing process.
- And last but not least, to my mom and dad.

D. J. Lowrie Jr.

1 An Introduction to Light Microscopy and the Cell

After completing this chapter, you should be able to:
— Name the parts and describe the use of the light microscope
— Describe other types of microscopy, specifically digital microscopy and electron microscopy
— Recognize major features of a tissue in light microscopy
  • Cell
    ◦ Nucleus
    ◦ Cytosol (cytoplasm)
  • Extracellular matrix
— Briefly describe the procedures used to prepare a specimen for visualization with the light microscope
  • Recognize the most common histologic stains, including the basic principle of the stain, the colors of the stain, the cellular components that are stained, and how variations in staining can provide clues about the structure and function of cells and tissues
    ◦ Hematoxylin and eosin (H and E)
    ◦ Periodic acid–Schiff (PAS)
  • Provide examples of how tissue preparation affects the appearance of a tissue and how those features may provide clues to the structure and function of the cells or tissues in that specimen
— Propose a histologic technique (type of microscopy and stain) that would be ideal for a specific study

1.1 Microscopy

1.1.1 The Light Microscope

Samples too small to see with the naked eye are visualized with the aid of a **microscope**. Although digital slide technology is slowly replacing the traditional microscope as the preferred method to study histologic tissues, understanding how to use a traditional microscope is still a useful skill and will help in analyzing both glass and digitized slides. Note that the following is a brief overview, and that individual microscopes may be slightly different.

A light microscope is designed to magnify the image of a tissue mounted on a glass slide (**Fig. 1.1**). Light generated by a **light source** (bulb) is focused with **condensers**, passes through the tissue specimen mounted on a **stage**, and then passes through sets of lenses (the **objectives** and the **eyepiece**), which magnify the image.

In **Fig. 1.1**, the head (blue box) is oriented away from the user for storage. Loosening the **head locking screw** at the base of the head allows it to rotate. It is best to rotate the head 180° from its position in this image to use the microscope, and then rotate it back for storage.

A glass slide holding the specimen is placed on the stage, where it is held in place by a **specimen holder** or clip. The **X-Y translation mechanism** moves the stage forward and back or from side to side to allow the user to view different portions of the slide.

> **Helpful Hint**
>
> The image seen through the microscope is upside down and reversed left to right. This makes the image seen through the lenses move in the opposite direction from the actual movement of the specimen.

A bulb in the base of the microscope is the source of light. There is an on-off switch and an **illumination intensity control** to adjust the brightness.

A condenser focuses the light from the light source before it passes through the specimen. There is a **condenser adjustment knob** that can raise or lower the condenser. For most slides, the proper position of the condenser is 1 mm below the slide.

> **Helpful Hint**
>
> There will be some instances in which it is helpful to lower the condenser. For example, elastic fibers are more easily visualized with the condenser lowered.

After light passes through the specimen on the slide, the image is magnified by two objectives. There are usually three or four lower objectives on a revolving **nosepiece**, or **turret**, which can be rotated to select the desired magnification. The upper objective is the eyepiece (see below). The magnification stated results from the combination of the upper and lower objectives. For convenience, and to avoid damaging the objectives and slides, always start with the objective with the lowest magnification (usually 4X), focus the image, and then progress to higher magnifications (typically 10X, 40X, and 100X oil).

> **Helpful Hint**
>
> Most microscopes are parfocal, which means that, as objectives are changed, the image remains in focus (or at least close to it). This is quite helpful because the user can easily focus on a structure at 4X and then increase magnification, adjusting the focal plane as necessary. Higher-magnification lenses have a narrow focal plane; jumping straight to higher-magnification lenses without first progressing from lower-magnification lenses will make it difficult to find the focal plane.

The specimen is focused using knobs that raise or lower the stage. The **coarse focus knob** moves the stage more quickly and should be used only under low magnification. After an image is focused under low power, switch to higher magnifications and then use the **fine focus knob**.

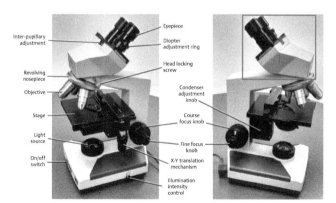

Fig. 1.1 **Typical light microscope.**

The higher-magnification lenses have longer tubes on the turret and, therefore, sit closer to the glass slides. Using the coarse focus knob with high-magnification lenses has the risk of driving the lens through and breaking the slide or, worse, damaging the objective lens.

Finally, the eyepieces, or oculars, also magnify the image (usually 10X). It is beneficial to use both eyes when looking at a specimen; this will save a lot of headaches. One important adjustment to the eyepieces is the interpupillary distance, which can be adjusted on the microscope to match the user's eyes. Note that some microscopes have an **interpupillary adjustment roller**, while others allow free movement of the eyepieces.

Another important adjustment of the eyepieces ensures that both eyes see the image in focus. One of the eyepieces has a **diopter adjustment ring**. This changes the focal plane for that eyepiece. To make this adjustment, start by closing the eye corresponding to the adjustable eyepiece (the left eye on the microscope in **Fig. 1.1**) and adjust the focus for the other eye (the "fixed" eyepiece) using the coarse and fine focus knobs until the image is sharp through that eyepiece. Then close that eye and adjust the focus on the other eyepiece with the diopter adjustment ring until the image is sharp through that eye as well.

1.1.2   Digital Microscopy

Traditional microscopes have been used for centuries to look at samples on glass slides and are still used today by many practitioners and researchers. However, digital slide technology is becoming more common and is the format that many schools utilize to study histologic specimens.

To create digital slides, glass slides are scanned in a slide scanner. There are several formats for the resulting data, but ultimately digital slides can be viewed using any computer (**Fig. 1.2**). Mouse controls are fairly intuitive. For example, dragging and dropping is used to move around the slide. The mouse may have a scroll wheel that can be used (sometimes with the Ctrl key) to change magnification, or magnification can be selected from a menu (**Fig. 1.2**, circle). The inset in the upper right shows a scanning view of the slide. The box in the inset shows the user where the view is on the slide, and it changes size depending on magnification. As mentioned, each digital slide platform is different, and functionality varies based on operating system, type of mouse, and other features of the computer system. The best way to learn is by experimentation.

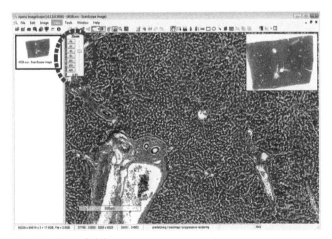

Fig. 1.2   **Digital slide.**

1.1.3   Traditional versus Digital Microscopy

When using a traditional light microscope, magnification is determined by multiplying the magnifications of the objective and ocular lenses. The magnification of the objective lens is selected by the user, while the eyepiece magnification is typically 10X. So, with the nosepiece set to the 40X objective, then the total magnification of the image is 400X (40 × 10).

When creating digital slides, only the objective lenses equivalent to the ones on a traditional microscope are used. Depending on the system, the digital slide view may include a zoom bar that shows the magnification of the image. The magnification can be changed by adjusting the cursor on the magnification bar or by zooming in and out using the mouse scroll wheel. Typically, the magnification bar goes only to 20X or 40X, so one would naturally think that the magnification of digital slides pales in comparison to traditional microscopes. However, remember that the traditional microscope image is projected through tiny eyepieces, while digital slides are projected on large computer screens at high resolution.

To approximate magnification on digital slides, users typically multiply the magnification in the zoom bar by 10. This isn't exact but close enough, and it compares quite well to what is seen in the traditional light microscope. In this publication, scale bars will be included in images as often as possible.

1.1.4   Other Types of Microscopy

There are other types of microscopy used to visualize cells and tissues (e.g., phase contrast, confocal), which are beyond the scope of this publication. One that needs to be mentioned here is transmission electron microscopy. The basic principles of transmission electron microscopy are quite similar to those of the light microscope, except that electrons are passed through a specimen instead of light. This provides greater magnification and resolution than light microscopy. The study of electron micrographs will be addressed in a subsequent chapter.

1.2   Basic Features of Cells and Tissues

Before delving into detailed histology, it's a good idea to start with a simple drawing of a single cell (**Fig. 1.3**). Although this book will not cover detailed cell biology (e.g., at the molecular level), the general structure and function of the cell's components will be described in subsequent chapters. For now, appreciate that:

— The outer membrane of the cell, the **plasma membrane**, separates the cell's contents from the extracellular matrix.
— The cell contains many **organelles**, of which the most prominent is the **nucleus**.
— The content of the cell other than the nucleus is referred to as the **cytoplasm** (or **cytosol**, though the two are not exactly the same).

Technically, the cytoplasm is everything in the cell other than the nucleus, whereas the cytosol is the liquid component of the cytoplasm—that is, the cytoplasm minus the organelles seen in the image (e.g., mitochondria, endoplasmic reticulum). However, these two terms are often used interchangeably.

Typical cell

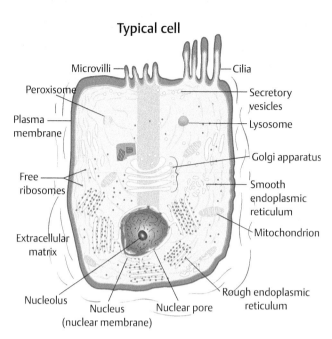

Fig. 1.3   **Simplified diagram of a typical cell.**

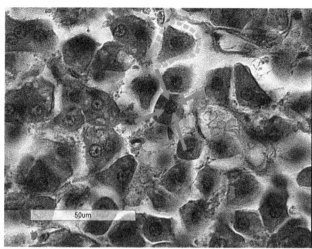

Fig. 1.4   **Liver, indicating cells (green outline) and nuclei (blue arrows).**

Fig. 1.4 is an image taken from a slide of the liver. The liver is a good place to start because the cells are clearly defined (one cell is outlined in green).

The most prominent organelle in the cell, and the only one easily seen in the light microscope, is the nucleus (**Fig. 1.4**, blue arrows), which appears blue on this slide. The remainder of the cell (pinkish-purple on this slide) is the cytoplasm; the organelles within the cytoplasm are too small to visualize at this resolution.

The material between the cells is the extracellular matrix. However, this is complicated somewhat in the liver (and other organs), since the paler pink tissue between the cells includes blood vessels, which are composed of some cells, and other connective tissue cells (more on this later).

Helpful Hint

There are some cells with two nuclei; this is not unusual for liver and other types of cells.

Video 1.1   Cells, nuclei, cytoplasm, and extracellular matrix

Be able to identify:
— Cells
   • Nuclei
   • Cytosol (cytoplasm)
— Extracellular matrix
https://www.thieme.de/de/q.htm?p=opn/tp/308390101/
978-1-62623-414-7_c001_v001&t=video

In the cells shown in **Fig. 1.4**, it is easy to pick out cell borders. However, this is the exception rather than the rule. The strip of tissue between the green brackets in **Fig. 1.5** contains approximately 30 to 50 cells, based on the number of nuclei in that region (one nucleus bounded by blue arrows). The pink region

around, but mostly above, the nucleus is the cytoplasm. The plasma membranes between the cells are, for the most part, not visible, though they are visible in some locations (black arrows).

Helpful Hint

When cell borders are not obvious, it helps to draw them in mentally to get a sense of the shape and size of the cells. For example, the mentally drawn outline of a single cell (**Fig. 1.5**, black dotted outline) indicates that these cells are columnar in shape (rectangular).

Video 1.2   Cells, nuclei, cytoplasm, and extracellular matrix

Be able to identify:
— Cells
   • Nuclei
   • Cytosol (cytoplasm)
— Extracellular matrix
https://www.thieme.de/de/q.htm?p=opn/tp/308390101/
978-1-62623-414-7_c001_v002&t=video

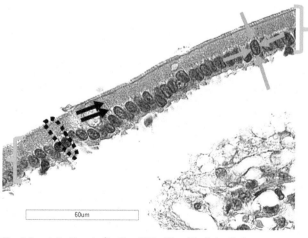

Fig. 1.5   **Intestine, indicating 30 to 50 epithelial cells (green brackets), a single cell (outlined), a border between two cells (black arrows), and nucleus (blue arrows).**

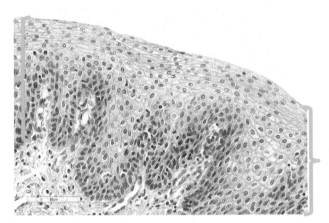

Fig. 1.6   **Pharynx, indicating epithelium (green brackets) and connective tissue cell (yellow arrow).**

Fig. 1.6 shows another image for practice. The region between the green brackets consists of over a hundred cells; most of them are cuboidal (square) or round. In most cases, the border between most cells is clearly visible, especially in the middle and upper regions. In places where the cell borders are not evident, they should be mentally drawn in.

The region in the bottom left in **Fig. 1.6**, below the tissue indicated by the green brackets, is slightly different. Here, the cells are smaller, with smaller nuclei; the nucleus of one cell is indicated by the yellow arrow. This type of tissue has more extracellular matrix than the tissue bounded by the green brackets. Therefore, the pink between the nuclei in this region includes both cytoplasm and extracellular matrix; the border between these is not visible. We'll look at why the tissues, cells, and nuclei are different in this region in subsequent chapters.

1.3   Slide Preparation

A complete understanding of the details of slide preparation is not necessary to study histology. However, understanding the procedure in general will make it easier to interpret histological slides.

The four major steps of slide preparation are:

1. Fixation
2. Embedding
3. Sectioning
4. Staining

1.3.1   Tissue Fixation

Tissue fixation terminates cell metabolism and prevents tissue degeneration. This can be accomplished with reagents that cross-link adjacent proteins (chemical fixation). **Fig. 1.7** shows a schematic representation of a heart in fixative solution.

Chemical fixation is time consuming and destroys protein structure. In some cases, if time or loss of enzymatic activity is a concern, tissues can be preserved by quick-freezing, a procedure in which the tissue is immersed in liquid nitrogen instead of a chemical fixative.

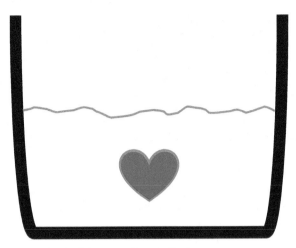

Fig. 1.7   **Sketch of tissue specimen in fixative.**

Surgeons can biopsy tissues and send them to the pathology lab for quick analysis. Quick-freezing enables the pathologist to return the results of that analysis rapidly, even while the patient is still on the operating table. Surgical options can then be selected based on the results.

1.3.2   Embedding

Since organs and other specimens come in all shapes and sizes, fixed tissues are embedded in a medium that allows easy handling and sectioning. The result is a specimen within a block of embedding medium, which is solid (**Fig. 1.8**).

Embedding is not simply coating the outside of the tissue (**Fig. 1.9a**), but actual perfusion of the embedding substance into the tissue so that the tissue becomes part of the embedded block (**Fig. 1.9b**) and is less likely to fall apart on sectioning.

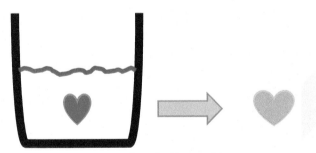

Fig. 1.8   **Tissue specimen in embedding media.**

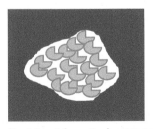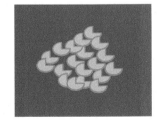

Fig. 1.9   **Schematic showing penetration of embedding media into tissue. (a) Medium does not embed into tissue. (b) Embedding media penetrating into the tissue.**

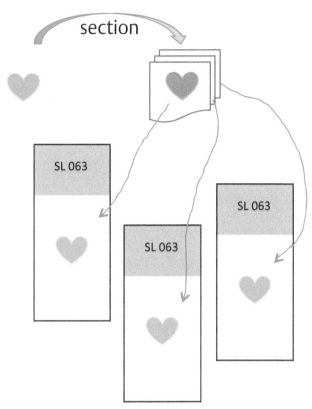

Fig. 1.10   **Tissue sectioning.**

Fig. 1.11   **Unstained tissue.**

The liver cells in **Fig. 1.12** were stained with H and E. Note that hematoxylin staining of the negatively charged DNA molecules gives the nucleus a blue color (arrows), while the red/pink eosin stains proteins in the cytoplasm. Proteins in the extracellular regions (outlined) also are eosinophilic.

Ribosomes are cellular structures in the cytoplasm that synthesize proteins. Because ribosomes contain RNA, which is negatively charged and, therefore, basophilic, cells actively synthesizing large amounts of protein will demonstrate some hematoxylin stain in portions of the cytoplasm. This adds blue to the typically pink cytoplasm, creating a darker or purple shade, a feature referred to as **cytoplasmic basophilia**.

Fig. 1.13 is an image taken from the pancreas stained with H and E. In the pancreas and other organs, clusters of several cells are organized into structures called acini (black outline, **Fig. 1.13**). Most of the cells in an acinus are pyramid-shaped (yellow outline). In this image, most of the cells demonstrate cytoplasmic basophilia, especially surrounding the nucleus. Two cells with intense cytoplasmic basophilia are indicated by the yellow arrows.

1.3.3   Sectioning

The embedded tissue is then sectioned into thin (5–15 μm thick) slices using a microtome; the slices are mounted on glass slides (**Fig. 1.10**). **Fig. 1.10** shows only three sections from the sample. Hundreds of sections can be obtained from a single specimen. This process is called serial sectioning, since all the slides are generated from the same tissue.

1.3.4   Staining

Stains are used to enhance the visualization of cellular components. There are a number of procedures that can help visualize components on a slide; each will highlight a different cellular structure. This can range from relatively nonselective staining based on charge to very specific staining based on antibody-antigen interaction.

Fig. 1.11 shows an intestinal slide that either is unstained or did not stain very well. This image provides an idea of what an unstained piece of tissue looks like.

In the following paragraphs, two very common staining techniques are presented:
— Hematoxylin and eosin (H and E)
— Periodic acid–Schiff (PAS)

Hematoxylin and Eosin

Hematoxylin is a blue dye that localizes to negatively charged cell structures (e.g., deoxyribonucleic acid [DNA], ribonucleic acid [RNA]). Structures that bind to hematoxylin are referred to as **basophilic**.

Eosin is a red/pink dye that localizes to positively charged cell structures (e.g. proteins, mitochondria). Structures that bind to eosin are commonly referred to as **eosinophilic** or, sometimes, **acidophilic**.

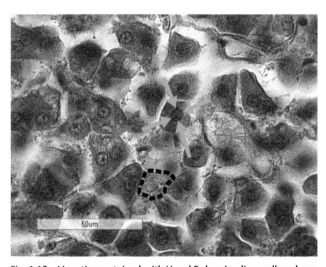

Fig. 1.12   **Liver tissue stained with H and E showing liver cell nucleus (blue arrows) and interstitial tissue (outlined).**

Video 1.3   H and E staining

Be able to identify:
— Hematoxylin and eosin (H and E) staining
  • Basophilic structures
  • Eosinophilic structures
https://www.thieme.de/de/q.htm?p=opn/
tp/308390101/978-1-62623-414-7_c001_v003&t=video

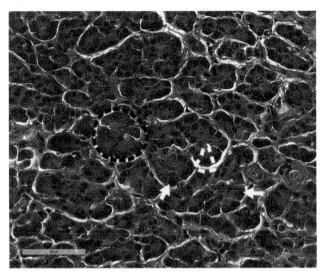

Fig. 1.13   **Pancreas stained with H and E, showing acinus (black outline), individual cell (yellow outline), and cytoplasmic basophilia (yellow arrows).**

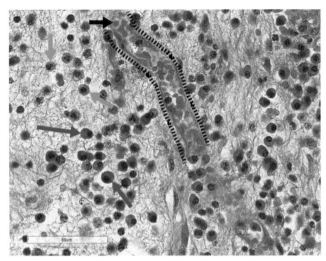

Fig. 1.14   **Inflamed tissue stained with H and E, showing cells with (blue arrows) and without (green arrows) cytoplasmic basophilia; this view also includes a blood vessel (dotted lines) with red blood cells (black arrow).**

Video 1.4   H and E staining with cytoplasmic basophilia

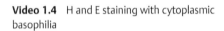

Be able to identify:
— H and E staining
  • Basophilic structures
    ◦ Cytoplasmic basophilia
  • Eosinophilic structures
https://www.thieme.de/de/q.htm?p=opn/tp/308390101/
978-1-62623-414-7_c001_v004&t=video

Fig. 1.14 shows another example of cells with cytoplasmic basophilia (blue arrows). Compare to cells with eosinophilic cytoplasm (green arrows).

Helpful Hint

While looking at **Fig. 1.14**, it's useful to point out the blood vessel located between the dotted lines. At the top and bottom, the vessel seems to disappear because it turns and leaves the plane of this section. Note the highly eosinophilic red blood cells, which lack nuclei (black arrow).

Cells with abundant cytoplasmic proteins show more intense eosinophilia. **Fig. 1.15a** shows cells with abundant mitochondria (black outline), while **Fig. 1.15b** is from skeletal muscle.

Just as the staining properties of the cytoplasm can provide clues to the function of a cell, the staining properties of the nucleus can also suggests a cell's relative activity. The genetic material in the nucleus, DNA, can be in a condensed (inactive) form called **heterochromatin** or in a decondensed (active) form called **euchromatin**. Condensed DNA in a cell will result in a smaller, more densely stained nucleus (black arrows, **Fig. 1.16**), whereas an active cell will have a larger, paler nucleus (yellow arrows).

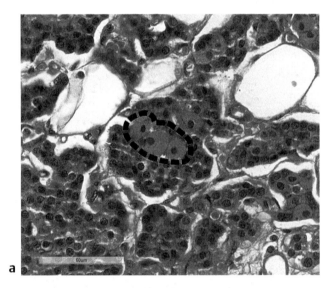

a

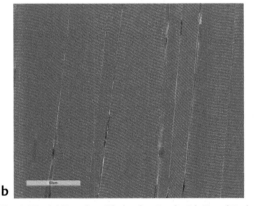

b

Fig. 1.15   **(a) Parathyroid gland stained with H and E, showing cells with intense cytoplasmic eosinophilia (outlined). (b) Skeletal muscle stained with H and E.**

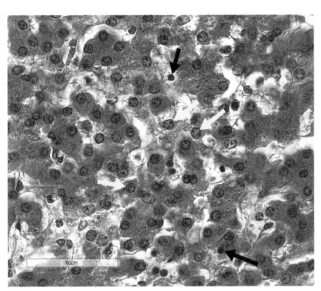

Fig. 1.16   **Liver, showing nuclei of active (yellow arrows) and inactive (black arrows) cells.**

Video 1.5: H and E nucleus

Be able to identify:
— A cell's activity based on its nuclear profile
https://www.thieme.de/de/q.htm?p=opn/tp/308390101/978-1-62623-414-7_c001_v005&t=video

Periodic Acid–Schiff (PAS)

Periodic acid–Schiff (PAS) is a staining technique that highlights carbohydrates. Structures that react with this procedure are referred to as **PAS positive (PAS+)** and show up as a bright magenta (purple). The tissue is typically counterstained with a basic dye to highlight the nucleus. PAS+ structures within the cell are the Golgi apparatus, plasma membrane, and the mucus-containing vesicles of goblet cells. These structures will be discussed in detail in subsequent chapters.

Fig. 1.17 is a tissue stained with PAS. The lipid bilayer of plasma membranes includes a carbohydrate component called the glycocalyx; therefore, cell borders are more clearly defined in tissue stained with PAS. The cells that stain intensely positive with PAS (black arrows) contain abundant secretory vesicles in the cytoplasm, which are filled with glycoproteins. In addition, other structures in the cells and the extracellular matrix are PAS+. More details about all these PAS+ structures will be discussed in upcoming chapters.

Video 1.6: PAS

Be able to identify:
— A tissue stained with PAS
https://www.thieme.de/de/q.htm?p=opn/tp/308390101/978-1-62623-414-7_c001_v006&t=video

1.3.5   Artifacts

A final topic regarding preparation of slides is **artifacts**. Artifacts are features of a prepared slide that are not present in the original sample but are introduced during tissue preparation.

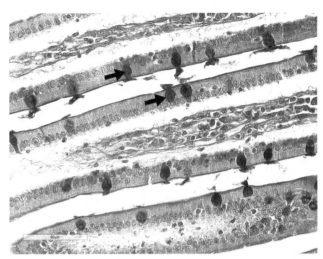

Fig. 1.17   **Jejunum stained with PAS. Cells rich in carbohydrate, called goblet cells, are indicated (black arrows).**

The absence of staining in the cytoplasm suggests the presence of specific molecules in the tissue. Some components of the cell do not take up a particular stain very well. For example, liver cells (hepatocytes) contain glycogen, which does not stain well in routine H and E tissue preparation. In **Fig. 1.18**, varying levels of glycogen in the hepatocytes results in slightly more or less staining in the cytoplasm. Although all the cells show some degree of lack of cytoplasmic staining, cells with more abundant clear areas, and thus more glycogen, are outlined.

Some cellular components also wash away from the sample during tissue fixation. This leaves a clear area that is a clue to what once existed in the original tissue. In the adrenal cortex, lipid droplets are stored in the cytoplasm of cells as precursors to the steroid hormones the cells produce. These lipid droplets wash away on routine tissue preparation. In **Fig. 1.19**, the degree of cytoplasmic staining varies in different regions; the cells with the most washed-out cytoplasm are in the center.

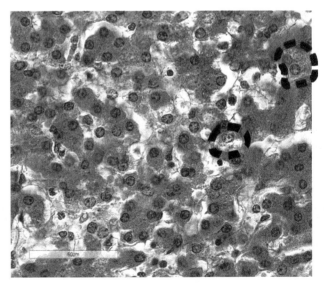

Fig. 1.18   **Liver, showing cells with pale-staining regions (outlined) due to abundant glycogen.**

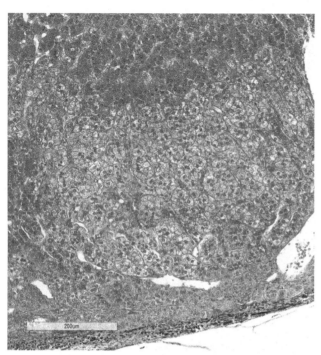

Fig. 1.19   **Adrenal gland, showing pale-staining region (center) due to abundant lipid droplets.**

Video 1.7   H and E liver

Video 1.8   H and E adrenal gland

Be able to identify:
— A cell's cytoplasmic contents based on appearance (for now, at least list possibilities of what could be there)
https://www.thieme.de/de/q.htm?p=opn/tp/308390101/
978-1-62623-414-7_c001_v007&t=video
https://www.thieme.de/de/q.htm?p=opn/tp/308390101/
978-1-62623-414-7_c001_v008&t=video

Helpful Hint

The preceding text states that glycogen is pale because it does not take up H and E stain well, while the video states that glycogen washes away during routine tissue preparation. Both explanations have been given to explain the pale appearance of glycogen-containing areas in liver cells, as well a similar appearance of carbohydrates in other cells (e.g., mucus, described in a later chapter). It's likely that the former explanation is correct, since similarly prepared slides stained with PAS demonstrate these carbohydrate components of the cell. For practical purposes, it makes no difference; understanding the significance of pale regions in cells stained with H and E (i.e., what they represent) is sufficient.

Another artifact of sample preparation is tissue shrinkage. This occurs in most routine preparations of tissue samples, though some fixation procedures minimize tissue shrinkage. Not all tissues in a sample shrink to the same extent. When one tissue shrinks more than an adjacent tissue, the tissues pull away from each other, creating spaces within the sample. For example, in the image of cartilage in **Fig. 1.20**, the extracellular

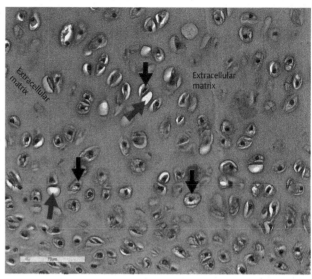

Fig. 1.20   **Hyaline cartilage, showing cells (black arrows) and empty lacuna (blue arrows), and extracellular matrix.**

matrix is semisolid, so it shrinks less than the cells (black arrows) that are embedded within it. This creates holes (called lacunae), in which the shrunken cells are located. In many places (blue arrows), the cells have fallen out of their lacuna during sectioning.

Video 1.9   Lacunae

Be able to identify:
— Cells in lacunae
https://www.thieme.de/de/q.htm?p=opn/tp/
308390101/978-1-62623-414-7_c001_
v009&t=video

Helpful Hint

Although artifacts are representations on slides that aren't really present in real tissues, in some cases, features created during tissue preparation can actually be helpful in tissue identification. In this example, since only cartilage and bone have shrunken cells within lacunae, recognizing this feature helps in identifying these tissues.

Fig. 1.21 shows two examples of artifacts that are not so helpful. **Fig. 1.21a** shows a cross section of an elastic artery. During tissue shrinkage, the vessel folded up on itself, creating dark bands (green arrows) that are not real structures but are simply areas of overlapped tissue. **Fig. 1.21b** features torn tissue (black arrow) and a piece of debris (blue arrow).

1.4   Chapter Review

Histology is the study of biologic structures too small to be visible with the naked eye. To study them, microscopes are used to magnify the image of a structure. Alternatively, tissues can be digitally scanned and presented to the user electronically (digital slides). To prepare a tissue for visualization, it must be fixed, embedded, sectioned, and stained. A wide

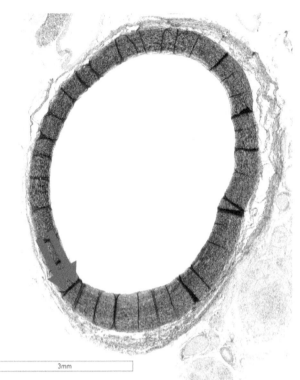

variety of stains can be used to highlight specific structures. The most commonly used histologic stain is hematoxylin and eosin (H and E). In H and E–stained slides, nuclei are blue and the cytoplasm and extracellular matrix are typically pink. However, cells synthesizing large amounts of proteins have abundant ribosomes in the cytoplasm and will demonstrate cytoplasmic basophilia on H and E staining. Another common histological stain is periodic acid–Schiff (PAS), which stains carbohydrates. Artifacts are features introduced during tissue preparation and include clear spaces due to lack of staining, washing out of tissue components, or tissue shrinkage. These artifacts may be useful in determining cellular function or in identifying tissue types.

Questions and Answers

An online-only section of questions and answers accompanying this chapter is hosted on Thieme's MedOne Education site: https://medone-education.thieme.com. Use the code on the media page at the front of this book to gain access. An institutional license to the site is required to access these questions in an interactive format, and individual users are required to register for an individual account to track results.

3mm

a

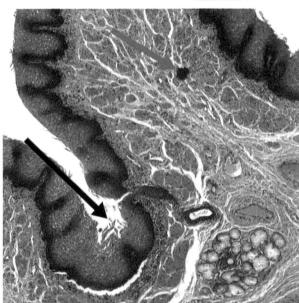

b

Fig. 1.21 (a) Aorta, showing folds in the tissue (green arrows). (b) Esophagus, showing tear (black arrow) and debris (blue arrow).

2 The Nucleus

After completing this chapter, you should be able to:
— Identify, at the light microscopic level, each of the following
  • Cell
    ○ Nucleus
    ○ Nuclear envelope (nuclear membrane)
    ○ Nucleolus
    ○ Euchromatin
    ○ Heterochromatin
  • Phases of the cell cycle
    ○ Interphase
    ○ Mitosis
      ▪ Prophase
      ▪ Metaphase
      ▪ Anaphase
      ▪ Telophase
— Identify, at the electron microscopic level, each of the following
  • Cell
    ○ Nucleus
    ○ Nuclear envelope (nuclear membrane)
    ○ Nuclear pores
    ○ Nucleolus
    ○ Euchromatin
    ○ Heterochromatin
— Evaluate the status (activity) of a cell based on the appearance of the nucleus
— Predict the effect of agents that interfere with the cell cycle
— Evaluate the activity of a tissue based on the presence of mitotic figures

2.1 Typical Nucleus

The previous chapter introduced the main features of the cell visible using light microscopy. In **Fig. 2.1**, an entire cell is outlined in green, and a **nucleus** from another cell is shown (blue arrows).

In H and E staining, nuclei are basophilic, while the eosinophilic **cytoplasm** includes everything in the cell except the nucleus.

That chapter focused on large nuclei for convenience. This chapter takes a more detailed look at the nucleus.

First off, note that nuclei come in different shapes and sizes (**Fig. 2.1**, black and blue arrows). In most cases, nuclear shape reflects the shape of the cell; for example, a round cell will have a round nucleus (blue arrows), while a spindle-shaped cell (yellow outline) has a longer, narrower nucleus.

Second, and maybe more importantly, the size of the nucleus typically reflects the activity level of the cell. Active cells are often involved in either DNA or RNA synthesis, which represent cell division or protein expression, respectively. Therefore, the nucleus provides a clue as to whether the cell is very active (blue arrows) or relatively inactive (black arrows).

To examine the **nucleus** in more detail, it helps to select a large nucleus (black arrows, **Fig. 2.2**). The outer border of the nucleus is the **nuclear envelope** (tips of the black arrows), which consists of two lipid bilayers that cannot be distinguished at the light microscopic level. The content of the nucleus is referred to as the **nucleoplasm**. In this cell, most of the nucleoplasm is pale; this color represents **euchromatin**, which is decondensed DNA involved in either DNA replication or RNA transcription. The large dark structure in the center of the nucleus is the **nucleolus**, which is the site of ribosome synthesis. The other smaller dark regions, and in particular the dark structures just under the nuclear envelope, represent **heterochromatin**, inactive condensed DNA.

Helpful Hint

Just as nuclear size provides a sense of the activity of the cell, the relative amount of euchromatin in the nucleus will indicate how active a cell is, because it represents DNA that is in the decondensed (active) state. Smaller nuclei (yellow arrow) are composed mostly of heterochromatin, suggesting a less active cell.

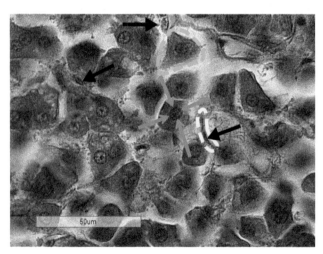

Fig. 2.1 **Liver, showing liver cell (green outline), an active nucleus (blue arrows), inactive nuclei (black arrows), and an inactive cell (yellow outline).**

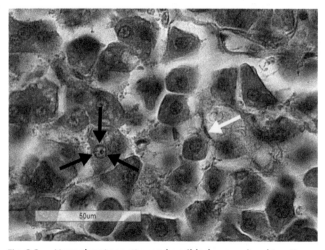

Fig. 2.2 **Liver, showing active nucleus (black arrows) and inactive nucleus (yellow arrow).**

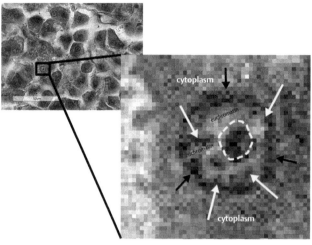

Fig. 2.3 Liver cell nucleus, showing cytoplasm, euchromatin, heterochromatin (yellow arrows), nucleolus (yellow outline), and nuclear envelope (black arrows).

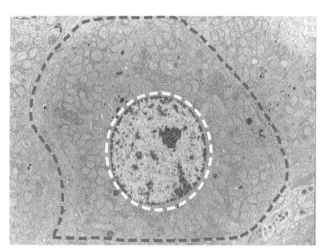

Fig. 2.4 Liver, electron micrograph, showing entire cell (red outline) and nucleus (yellow outline). Image courtesy of Robert and Emma Lou Cardell.

Fig. 2.3 shows a region from **Fig. 2.2** artificially enlarged. This enlarged image is pixelated but allows for more accurate labels to indicate the parts of the nucleus:
- Nuclear envelope: not visible; location is the tips of the black arrows
- Nucleolus: outlined in yellow
- Euchromatin: pale areas indicated by text
- Heterochromatin: yellow arrows

Video 2.1 Typical nucleus

Be able to identify:
— Nucleus
— Nuclear envelope
— Nucleolus
— Euchromatin
— Heterochromatin
https://www.thieme.de/de/q.htm?p=opn/tp/308390101/978-1-62623-414-7_c002_v001&t=video

Helpful Hint

Note that even though **Fig. 2.3** is enlarged and pixelated, it can be used as a reference to go back to **Fig. 2.2** or any other image of the nucleus and see its details.

2.2 Electron Microscopy of the Nucleus

As mentioned in **Chapter 1**, electron microscopy is an imaging technique similar to light microscopy, but it uses electrons instead of light to create the image, which provides greater magnification and resolution of the specimen.

In the electron micrograph (EM) shown in **Fig. 2.4**, the approximate border of a single cell is outlined in red, and its nucleus is outlined in yellow. Note that numerous structures within the cytoplasm that are not evident in light microscopy are readily evident in electron micrographs; these will be discussed in detail in the next chapter.

Fig. 2.5 shows an enlarged view of the nucleus from the cell in **Fig. 2.4**, revealing greater detail of structures that were seen in the light micrograph:
- Nuclear envelope: barely visible, location is the tips of the black arrows
- Nucleolus: outlined in yellow
- Euchromatin: pale areas indicated by text
- Heterochromatin: yellow arrows

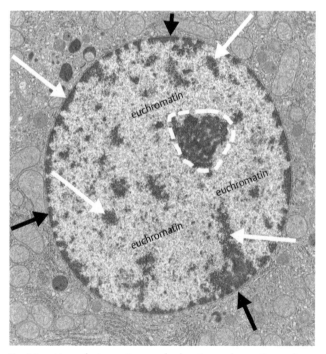

Fig. 2.5 Liver, electron micrograph, showing euchromatin, nuclear envelope (black arrows), heterochromatin (yellow arrows), nucleolus (yellow outline). Image courtesy of Robert and Emma Lou Cardell.

Note that in this EM the nuclear envelope can be seen a little more clearly (but not quite). Heterochromatin is scattered throughout this nucleus, but mostly against the inner part of the nuclear envelope. Abundant euchromatin suggests that the cell is either an active cell (expressing numerous genes) or undergoing DNA synthesis to prepare for cell division. This is a liver cell, so it is indeed very active metabolically. The nucleolus is prominent, suggesting assembly of ribosomes necessary for protein synthesis.

Fig. 2.6 shows a more detailed view of the edge of the nucleus. The **nuclear envelope** consists of two membranes (two lipid bilayers); each shows up as a linear structure at this magnification. The outer membrane is indicated by the series of red arrows and is studded with round structures (ribosomes). The inner membrane (yellow arrows) is less distinct due to the heterochromatin (labeled and at 3) adjacent to it. The space between the membranes is referred to as the perinuclear cisterna (1). The black arrows indicate **nuclear pores**, openings in the nuclear envelope that allow molecular trafficking between the nucleus and cytoplasm. The label 2 indicates rough endoplasmic reticulum in the cytoplasm, discussed in the next chapter.

2.3   The Cell Cycle

Many cells in a specimen are in the process of cell division. While part of this involves the physical division of one cell into two, a cell must spend significant time preparing for this division, including replication of organelles and, most importantly, the genetic material (DNA). Therefore, actively dividing cells are typically in one of four phases of the **cell cycle** (see **Fig. 2.7**):

- G_1 (growth phase): A cell that has just divided grows under the influence of resource availability and hormonal signals. During the G_1 phase, the cell assesses its environment and will divide if conditions are optimal. If the conditions are right, the cell will enter the S phase, at which time it will be committed to progress through the remainder of the cell cycle back to the G_1 phase.
- **S** (synthesis phase): This is the phase in which the genetic material is duplicated.
- G_2 (growth phase): Here the cell assesses the duplicated genetic material and prepares for cell division.
- **M** (mitosis): This is the visible manifestation of cell division, in which the single cell divides into two. **Mitosis** specifically consists of the division of the nucleus and itself has

phases, highlighted in the next section. Mitosis is capped by **cytokinesis**, which is the division of the cytoplasm.

Note that the first three phases of the cell cycle, G_1, S, and G_2, are collectively referred to as **interphase**; cells in these phases are indistinguishable by light microscopy.

Many of the cells in tissues such as the epidermis of the skin or the gut epithelium are continually regenerating to replace damaged cells and, therefore, are continuously progressing through the cell cycle. However, cells in many tissues stop dividing and may differentiate into specialized cell types. These cells leave the G_1 phase and enter a phase referred to as G_0. For example, after development is complete, neurons in the brain stop dividing and function to transmit action potentials; these cells are considered to be in the G_0 phase because they are no longer actively dividing. In other tissues, cells may enter the G_0 phase temporarily, returning to the cell cycle when necessary. For example, fibroblasts in the skin are relatively quiescent but can be stimulated to divide in order to regenerate damaged tissue.

2.3.1   Mitosis

Fig. 2.8a–h depict a cell proceeding through mitosis. **Fig. 2.8a** is a cell in interphase; recall that cells in G_1, G_0, S, and G_2 are all in interphase and will all appear similar in routine light microscopy. The oval structure is the nucleus, and the nuclear envelope is at the tips of the blue arrows. Note the nuclear material in interphase in this cell is largely euchromatin, so individual chromosomes are not seen. At least one or two of the visible structures in the nucleus are nucleoli. The cytoplasm is very poorly stained, but it is easiest to see in **Fig. 2.8h**.

The phases of mitosis are:
1. **Prophase** (**Fig. 2.8b**): The nuclear envelope breaks apart, and the chromatin condenses, forming visible chromosomes. Structures called centrioles that assemble the mitotic spindle that guides the chromosomes during mitosis move to opposite poles of the cell (in this image, top and bottom), but these are not visible in this image.

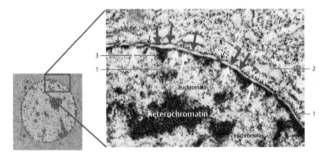

Fig. 2.6   **Nuclear envelope, showing inner (yellow arrows) and outer (red arrows) nuclear membranes, nuclear pores (black arrows), euchromatin, heterochromatin (3), perinuclear cisterna (1), and rough endoplasmic reticulum (2).**

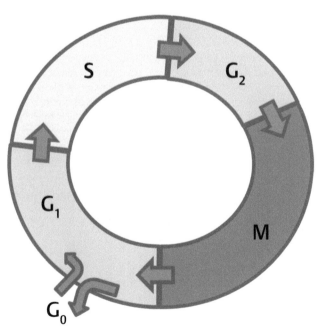

Fig. 2.7   **The cell cycle.**

Cell Division - Mitosis

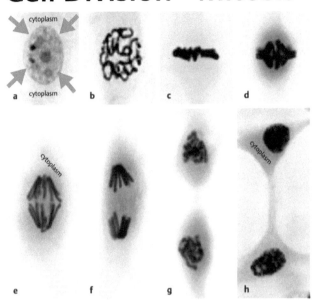

Fig. 2.8   Mitosis. (a) Interphase. (b) Prophase. (c) Metaphase. (d–f) Anaphase. (g–h) Telophase. The blue arrows in (a) indicate the nuclear envelope, which breaks down in prophase.

2. **Metaphase** (**Fig. 2.8c**): The chromosomes line up along the middle of the cell, called the equator.
3. **Anaphase** (**Fig. 2.8d–f**): The chromosomes are moved to opposite poles of the cell.
4. **Telophase** (**Fig. 2.8g–h**): The chromosomes have reached their respective poles; division of the cytoplasm (cytokinesis) occurs, the nuclear envelopes reform, and the chromatin decondenses.

Helpful Hint

Mitosis is a continuum, so many cells seen in tissue specimens are somewhere between the four phases outlined above.

To study the phases of mitosis, it is useful to select a specimen containing many rapidly dividing cells, such as embryonic tissue; the following figures show sections from whitefish embryos. Recall that, even in rapidly dividing tissues, many cells will be in interphase, not mitosis. In **Fig. 2.9**, most of the cells are in interphase. One cell in this image is outlined; the nucleus is the large, basophilic structure in the center of the cell. Note the distinct nuclear envelope; the chromatin is a mixture of euchromatin and heterochromatin (no visible chromosomes).

Helpful Hint

It might be tempting to think that many of the cells in this image that do not show nuclei are in some phase of mitosis. However, this is not the case because, as the next set of images will demonstrate, mitotic cells have distinct chromosomes.

The reason those cells lack a visible nucleus in this image is that the plane of section passed through a portion of the cell that did not include the nucleus.

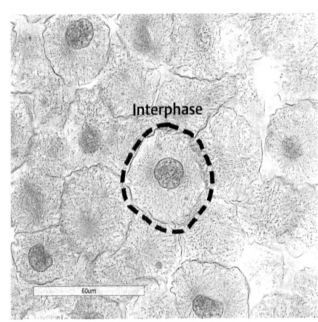

Fig. 2.9   Cells from whitefish embryo in interphase.

The first phase of mitosis is prophase (**Fig. 2.10a**). Here, the nuclear envelope breaks down, and the chromatin condenses to form visible chromosomes (purple speckles in the center of the cell).

Metaphase is highlighted by the alignment of the chromosomes along the equator (**Fig. 2.10b**). The cage-shaped structure is the **mitotic spindle** (black arrows), which is made up of **microtubules** and is responsible for movement of the chromosomes.

Anaphase, shown in **Fig. 2.11a**, is highlighted by movement of the chromosomes to opposite ends of the cell (poles).

Once the chromosomes reach the poles, telophase begins (**Fig. 2.11b,c**). During this phase, the cytoplasm of the cell divides (cytokinesis). Eventually, the nuclear envelope will reappear, and the chromatin will decondense. The resulting cells will enter interphase (G_1).

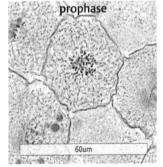
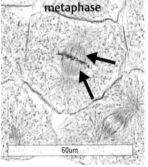

a   **b**

Fig. 2.10   Cells from whitefish embryo in (a) prophase and (b) metaphase.

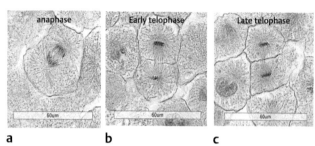

a   **b**   **c**

Fig. 2.11   Cells from whitefish embryo in (a) anaphase and (b,c) telophase.

Video 2.2   Phases of mitosis

Be able to identify:
— Interphase
— Prophase
— Metaphase
— Anaphase
— Telophase

https://www.thieme.de/de/q.htm?p=opn/tp/308390101/978-1-62623-414-7_c002_v002&t=video

2.4   Mitotic Figures in Tissues

In select tissues such as the whitefish embryo, it's easy to find cells in mitosis and to identify the specific phase of mitosis. However, in most other tissues, cells in mitosis are not as common, even in proliferative tissues such as the epidermis of the skin.

In **Fig. 2.12**, taken from the pharynx, most of the cells are in interphase (three cells in interphase are outlined in black). Note the nucleus and the cytoplasm of these cells.

Outlined in yellow is a cell in mitosis, characterized because it lacks a nuclear envelope and has visible dense chromosomes. It is likely that this cell is in late telophase or has just finished cytokinesis and the chromosomes of the progeny cells have yet to decondense. Because it is often difficult to determine a specific stage of mitosis for cells in tissues, they are often referred to as **mitotic figures**.

Clinical Correlate

In many histologic and pathologic specimens, recognizing mitotic figures is useful in determining tissue type or type of pathology.

Video 2.3   Mitotic figures

Be able to identify:
— Mitotic figures

https://www.thieme.de/de/q.htm?p=opn/tp/308390101/978-1-62623-414-7_c002_v003&t=video

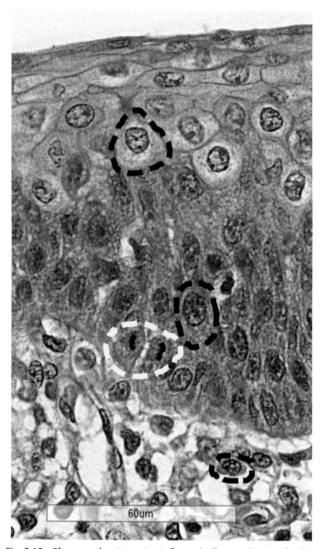

Fig. 2.12   Pharynx, showing mitotic figure (yellow outline) and cells in interphase (black outlines).

2.5   Chapter Review

The nucleus is typically the largest and most visible organelle in the cell. It houses the genetic material, DNA, in the form of chromosomes. Portions of these chromosomes are either in a decondensed or condensed form, seen in light and electron microscopy as euchromatin or heterochromatin, respectively. Nucleoli within the nucleus are the sites of ribosome assembly. Actively dividing cells progress through a cell cycle that is highlighted by phases of growth (G_1, G_2), DNA synthesis (S), and cell division (mitosis, M). The phases of mitosis are prophase, metaphase, anaphase, and telophase. Mitotic figures can be seen in tissue sections and underscore the mitotic activity of a normal or pathologic tissue.

Questions and Answers

An online-only section of questions and answers accompanying this chapter is hosted on Thieme's MedOne Education site: https://medone-education.thieme.com. Use the code on the media page at the front of this book to gain access. An institutional license to the site is required to access these questions in an interactive format, and individual users are required to register for an individual account to track results.

3   The Cytoplasm

After completing this chapter, you should be able to:
— Identify, at the light microscopic level, each of the following:
  - Cell
    - Plasma membrane
    - Cytoplasm
  - Cytoplasmic basophilia
— Identify, at the electron microscopic level, each of the following:
  - Cell
    - Plasma membrane
    - Cytoplasm
    - Mitochondria
    - Rough endoplasmic reticulum
    - Smooth endoplasmic reticulum
    - Golgi apparatus
    - Lysosomes
— Outline the function of the cellular structures listed
— Predict the organelles that would be prominent in a cell or tissue based on its function
— Predict the appearance of cells in light micrographs based on their appearance in electron micrographs, and vice versa

3.1   Cytoplasm

Fig. 3.1 shows a typical cell (liver cell). The arrows have been moved to indicate the **cytoplasm**, which is the main focus of this chapter. Recall that, due to high protein content, the cytoplasm in most cells is eosinophilic when stained with H and E. Cells that are actively synthesizing proteins, on the other hand, have cytoplasmic basophilia. In fact, certain regions in these liver cells have purple hues in the cytoplasm, reflecting active protein synthesis.

3.2   The Plasma Membrane

Recall that the outer structure of a cell is the **plasma membrane (cell membrane)**, which forms the boundary between the cell and its extracellular environment. The plasma membrane is composed of a lipid bilayer with associated proteins and a carbohydrate component on the external surface called the **glycocalyx**. In light micrographs, the plasma membrane is seen as a linear structure. In **Fig. 3.1**, the edge of the cell indicates the location of the plasma membrane, even though no obvious line is visible. In **Fig. 3.2**, the plasma membranes are seen as visible lines; these lines are, in fact, two plasma membranes (one from each cell) adjacent to each other. In many cases, such as the bottom left portion of **Fig. 3.2**, the plasma membrane is not clearly visible, so the cytoplasm of those cells cannot be distinguished from the extracellular matrix.

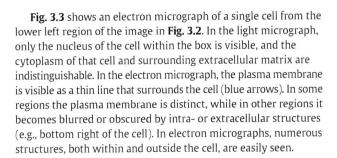

Video 3.1   Plasma membrane

Be able to identify:
— Cell (plasma) membrane
— Cytoplasm
— Extracellular matrix
https://www.thieme.de/de/q.htm?p=opn/
tp/308390101/978-1-62623-414-7_c003_v001&t=video

Fig. 3.3 shows an electron micrograph of a single cell from the lower left region of the image in **Fig. 3.2**. In the light micrograph, only the nucleus of the cell within the box is visible, and the cytoplasm of that cell and surrounding extracellular matrix are indistinguishable. In the electron micrograph, the plasma membrane is visible as a thin line that surrounds the cell (blue arrows). In some regions the plasma membrane is distinct, while in other regions it becomes blurred or obscured by intra- or extracellular structures (e.g., bottom right of the cell). In electron micrographs, numerous structures, both within and outside the cell, are easily seen.

3.3   Cytoplasmic Organelles

The basic structure of the cell was introduced in **Chapter 1**. The remainder of this chapter will focus on the major organelles found within the cytoplasm (mitochondria, ribosomes, rough

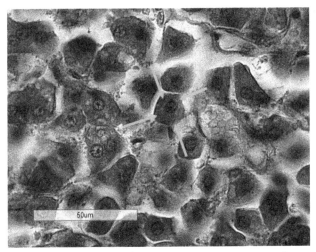

Fig. 3.1   **Typical cell from the liver. Blue arrows indicate cytoplasm.**

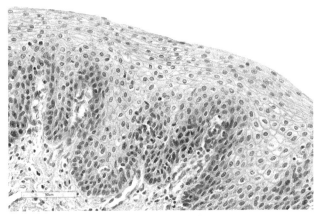

Fig. 3.2   **Typical cells from the stratified squamous epithelium of the pharynx. Note the plasma membranes visible in the upper layers.**

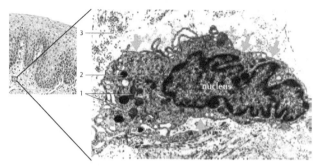

Fig. 3.3   Typical cell (electron micrograph), showing cell membrane (arrows) and nucleus (labeled). Mitochondria (1), secretory granules (2), collagen fibers (3).

and smooth endoplasmic reticulum, Golgi apparatus, lysosomes). Other organelles are mentioned here and discussed in more detail as they are encountered in subsequent chapters.

Many organelles in the cytoplasm are bounded by lipid bilayers with a composition similar to the plasma membrane. These membranes are shown in **Fig. 3.4** as thin lines and, like the plasma membrane, are visible on electron micrographs.

3.3.1   Nucleus

Before discussion of organelles in the cytoplasm, recall that the **nuclear envelope** is composed of two lipid bilayers (indicated by red and yellow arrows, respectively, in **Fig. 3.5**). Most cellular organelles are bounded by one lipid bilayer, the exceptions being the nucleus and mitochondria, which are bounded by two bilayers.

3.3.2   Mitochondria

Mitochondria are the powerhouses of the cell, responsible for oxidizing pyruvate and fatty acids to generate high energy bonds in the form of adenosine triphosphate (ATP).

Fig. 3.6 is a drawing of the membrane structure of a mitochondrion. Like the nucleus, mitochondria are bounded by two membranes (two lipid bilayers). These membranes are termed the **outer membrane**, which is the outer boundary of the mitochondrion, and the **inner membrane**, which is typically thrown up into folds (**cristae**) to increase surface area.

Outside the mitochondrion is the cytoplasm. The substance within the inner membrane is the **matrix**, while the

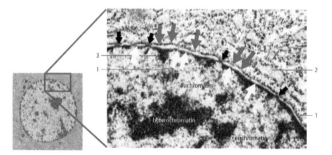

Fig. 3.5   (Left) Electron micrograph showing complete nucleus. Image courtesy of Robert and Emma Lou Cardell. (Right) More highly magnified electron micrograph of part of the nucleus corresponding to the inset region of the micrograph at left. Red and yellow arrows: outer and inner bilayers of nuclear envelope, respectively. Black arrows: nuclear pores. Perinuclear cisterna (1), rough ER (2), heterochromatin (3).

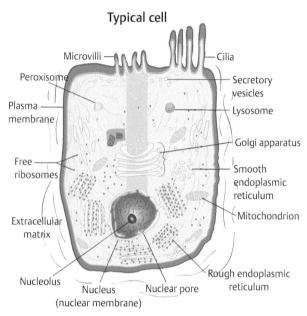

Fig. 3.4   **Illustration of a typical cell.**

intermembrane space is the thin region between the inner and outer membranes.

In electron micrographs, mitochondria are readily recognized as oval structures (**Fig. 3.7**), though some are more elongated, while others are seen in cross section and appear round. At this magnification it is challenging to differentiate the inner and outer membranes distinctly when they are adjacent to each other.

Fig. 3.8 shows a drawing of a mitochondrion (**Fig. 3.8a**) and a corresponding electron micrograph showing multiple mitochondria (**Fig. 3.8b**). The folds (cristae) of the inner membrane (blue arrows) appear as double lines because the inner membrane folds back on itself. In contrast, double lines at the outer edge of the mitochondria (red arrows) are adjacent inner and outer membranes.

The cristae of the inner membrane of many mitochondria are flattened, so they appear linear in electron micrographs. However, in some cells, the inner membrane has tubular cristae, as shown in **Fig. 3.9**. These mitochondria are typical of steroid-secreting cells and will be helpful in identifying such cells in later chapters.

When looking at electron micrographs, it is always useful to take a moment and consider the size of cellular structures to maintain perspective. In **Fig. 3.10** a single cell is outlined in red, and the nucleus is outlined in yellow. This cell has over 50 mitochondria visible here; a single mitochondrion is outlined in purple. Compare the size of a mitochondrion to the size of the nucleus, and to the size of the entire cell.

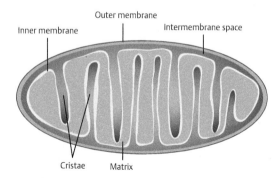

Fig. 3.6   **Illustration of mitochondrion.**

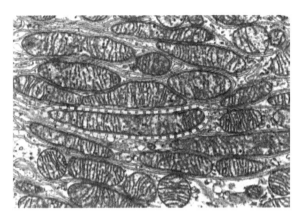

Fig. 3.7 Electron micrograph of a cell with multiple mitochondria; one is outlined in yellow.

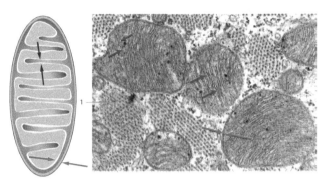

Fig. 3.8 (a) Drawing and (b) electron micrograph of mitochondria showing double lipid bilayers at cristae (blue arrows) and inner and outer membranes (red arrows). Myofilament bundles (1).

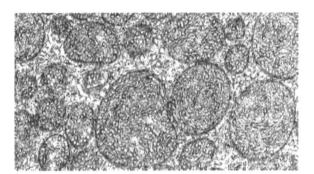

Fig. 3.9 Electron micrograph of mitochondria from a steroid-secreting cell showing tubular cristae.

3.3.3 Ribosomes

Ribosomes are the site of protein synthesis. In electron micrographs (**Fig. 3.11**), ribosomes appear as dense, round structures about 30 nanometers in diameter (indicated by 2 and 3 in the figure). Compare the size of ribosomes to the mitochondrion (1 in the figure). The ribosome at 3 in **Fig. 3.11** is a **free ribosome**,

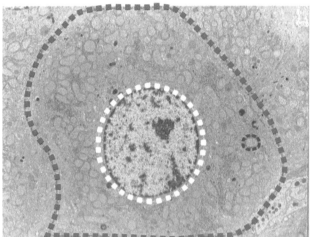

Fig. 3.10 Electron micrograph of liver cell, showing cell (red outline), nucleus (yellow outline), and one mitochondrion (purple outline). Image courtesy of Robert and Emma Lou Cardell.

which synthesizes proteins destined to reside in the cytoplasm (marked with a red X in the figure), nucleus, mitochondria, or peroxisomes. The ribosomes at 2 in the figure are attached to the **rough endoplasmic reticulum** (RER; see **Fig. 3.4**), which will be discussed in the next section.

> **Helpful Hint**
>
> Because they cover a wide range of sizes, nuclei, mitochondria, and ribosomes are helpful to determine the relative size of other structures in electron micrographs.

3.3.4 Rough Endoplasmic Reticulum

Proteins synthesized by ribosomes found on rough endoplasmic reticulum are either inserted into the membrane of the rough ER, or placed in the RER lumen during translation. From there, vesicles containing these proteins bud from the rough ER and fuse with the Golgi apparatus, which processes these proteins (e.g., adding carbohydrate). This post-translational modification is crucial for proper function of these proteins. After processing through the Golgi, these proteins are moved to their destination in the cell via vesicles that bud from the Golgi apparatus. The rough ER/Golgi synthesizes and processes proteins that are destined for the following locations: lysosomes, secretory vesicles, the plasma membrane, the extracellular space, and resident proteins of the rough ER and Golgi.

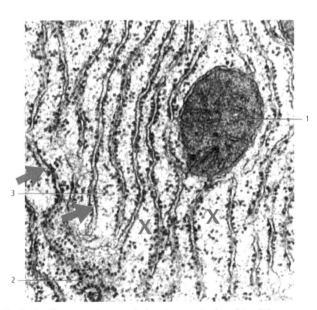

Fig. 3.11 Electron micrograph showing a mitochondrion (1), ribosomes attached to rough endoplasmic reticulum (RER) (2), free ribosomes (3). Arrows mark the lumen of RER, and cytoplasm is marked with Xs.

Observing RER in Electron Microscopy

In **Fig. 3.11**, the RER is best seen immediately to the left of the mito-chondrion (1), where the membranes of the RER are more distinct and clearly studded with ribosomes. The lumen of the RER is marked for orientation purposes by the tips of red arrows in the figure. Proteins translated by ribosomes on RER are inserted into the lumen or RER membrane as they are synthesized.

Helpful Hint

Note that ribosomes stud the outside of the RER membrane, which should provide orientation of this organelle relative to the cyto-plasm.

In **Fig. 3.12**, the RER is the major organelle in the outlined region. At this lower magnification, it is more challenging to see individual ribosomes clearly. However, note that RER typically forms stacks of membranes, making identification of RER possible even at lower magnifications in which ribosomes are not visible.

Helpful Hint

Histologists and pathologists often use food references to describe histological features of tissues and cellular structures. With respect to RER, a stack of pancakes may serve this purpose, maybe with chocolate chips on top and in between the pancakes.

RER is typically, but not always, seen as stacks of membranes in electron micrographs. In the cell shown in **Fig. 3.13,** the lumen of the RER (at 1) is dilated with proteins. Close examination shows ribo-somes studding the membranes of the RER. This dilation of the RER is characteristic of cells that are secreting large amounts of proteins.

Observing RER in Light Microscopy

Individual ribosomes and membranes of RER are not visible using light microscopy. However, clues to the amount of RER in the cell can be suggested by the staining properties of the cell. Cells actively synthesizing proteins contain numerous ribosomes. This is particularly true of cells secreting large amounts of proteins, which will have abundant rough endoplasmic reticulum, caus-ing **cytoplasmic basophilia**, discussed in **Chapter 1** (e.g., the

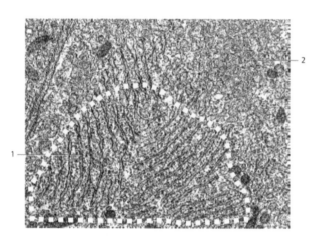

Fig. 3.12   **Rough endoplasmic reticulum outlined (and at 1) on electron micrograph. Smooth endoplasmic reticulum (2) also shown for comparison.**

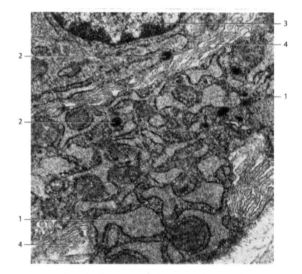

Fig. 3.13   **Rough endoplasmic reticulum in a cell actively secreting protein. Lumen of RER (1), secretory granules (2), nucleus (3), intercellular space (4).**

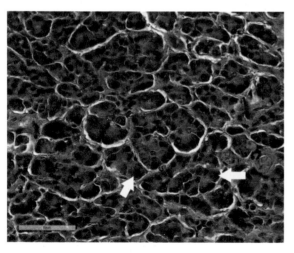

Fig. 3.14   **Exocrine pancreas, showing cytoplasmic basophilia (arrows).**

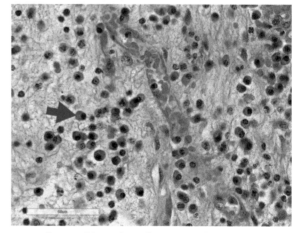

Fig. 3.15   **Plasma cell (arrow) in inflammation, showing cytoplasmic basophilia.**

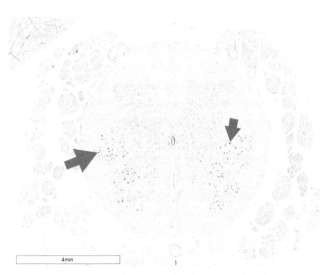

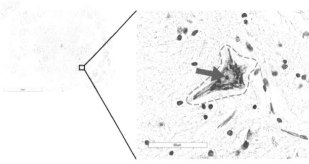

Fig. 3.17   (Left) Cross section of spinal cord under low magnification; (right) motor neuron at high magnification under Nissl stain, showing neuron (outlined) with RER-rich cytoplasm and active nucleolus (arrow).

Fig. 3.16   **Cross section of spinal cord under Nissl stain. Motor neurons are indicated by the arrows.**

pancreas cells secreting digestive enzymes in **Fig. 3.14** and the plasma cells secreting antibodies in **Fig. 3.15**).

Special stains other than H and E can help visualize the presence of RER. **Fig. 3.16** is a section of the spinal cord. For this discussion, it is not important to know the details of the spinal cord (**Chapter 15**); suffice it to say that motor neurons in the spinal cord are quite large. Even in this low-magnification image these motor neurons can be seen as small purple dots (red arrows). **Fig. 3.17** shows an expanded view of a region containing these motor neurons; one neuron is outlined in blue. The large, oval, pale region in the center of the cell is the nucleus, while the round, dark structure in the middle of the nucleus is the nucleolus (tip of the red arrow). This is a special stain (**Nissl stain**), which stains RNA, a major component of ribosomes. That is why it strongly stains the nucleolus (where ribosomes are made; **Chapter 2**) and RER. If the cytoplasm of a cell stains intensely with Nissl stain, it is because that cell has abundant RER for protein synthesis. The other strongly stained round structures in **Fig. 3.17** are nuclei of glial cells, which support the neuron. The pale, tubular structure just to the right of and below the motor neuron is a blood vessel.

Video 3.2   Nissl stain of motor neurons

Be able to identify:
— Nissl substance (RER)
— Nucleus (review)
— Nucleolus (review)
https://www.thieme.de/de/q.htm?p=opn/
tp/308390101/978-1-62623-414-7_c003_v002&t=video

3.3.5   Golgi Apparatus

Proteins synthesized by the RER undergo some additional processing (e.g., adding carbohydrate molecules). This **post-translational modification** is crucial for proper function of these proteins. This processing is performed by the **Golgi apparatus**, a complex of several stacked disk-shaped compartments called cisternae, enclosed by membranes similar to the ER. The typically three to eight cisternae of the Golgi complex work as a single unit. Vesicles containing newly synthesized proteins bud off from the RER and

fuse with the membranes of the first cisterna of the Golgi complex on one side, termed the **cis face**. Proteins progress through the Golgi apparatus via **transport vesicles** that bud off each cisterna and fuse with the next, undergoing chemical modifications along the way. Mature proteins in the last cisterna are finally released from the **trans face** of the Golgi apparatus in vesicles.

In **Fig. 3.18**, the Golgi apparatus is outlined. As mentioned, it is similar to RER in that it consists of stacks of flattened compartments enclosed by membranes. However, it is not studded with ribosomes. The cisternae typically bow slightly, so that the cis face is the convex side of the Golgi apparatus (2), while the trans face is the concave side (3). Transport vesicles are numerous (1), and a portion of the nucleus of this cell is indicated (4).

Helpful Hint

Looking for the absence of ribosomes to identify the Golgi apparatus (relative to RER) is a logical thing to do. However, it helps to have other features to differentiate these organelles in low-magnification images. As mentioned, note that the Golgi tends to bow (bend) slightly and has numerous vesicles at its periphery and trans face (larger vesicles typically are at the trans face). In addition, the rims of the cisternae of the Golgi apparatus are slightly dilated relative to the middle regions. RER may happen to have some of these features, but it is less likely to have all of them. So, taken collectively, these features can assist in correctly identifying the Golgi apparatus.

When considering the appearance of the Golgi apparatus on light micrographs, it is useful to re-examine cells with cytoplasmic basophilia. Recall that cytoplasmic basophilia is a feature of cells

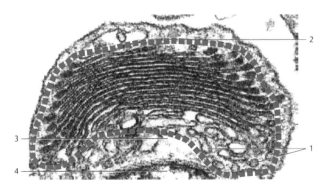

Fig. 3.18   **Electron micrograph showing prominent Golgi apparatus. Transport vesicle (1), cis-face (2), trans-face (3), nucleus (4).**

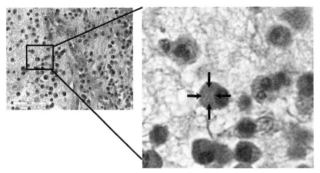

Fig. 3.19 **Plasma cell in inflammation. Golgi apparatus appears as a paler spot against the basophilic cytoplasm (Golgi ghost; outlined by the tips of the arrows).**

that have abundant RER. Since the RER and Golgi apparatus work together to synthesize and process proteins, it makes sense that a cell that has abundant RER would also have a prominent Golgi. This is indeed the case; however, the presence of the Golgi is not obvious in every cell, and even when visible, it is subtle at best.

Fig. 3.19 shows an artificially magnified region of an image of inflamed tissue. In the magnified region, the cell in the center demonstrates cytoplasmic basophilia because it is actively producing immune proteins. The nucleus of this cell is located in the right portion of the cell. In the center of the cell is the location of the Golgi apparatus (outlined by the tips of the arrows). Because the Golgi lacks ribosomes, this region demonstrates less cytoplasmic basophilia than the rest of the cytoplasm, and it appears slightly pale (relative to the rest of the cytoplasm). Many histologists refer to this phenomenon as the **Golgi ghost**.

Helpful Hint

Recognizing the Golgi ghost in light micrographs is subtle, more art than science and is typically not a crucial component of recognizing a protein-synthesizing cell, since the cytoplasmic basophilia is more reliable.

3.3.6 Smooth Endoplasmic Reticulum

Smooth endoplasmic reticulum (SER) is a network of membrane-bound organelles that are elongated, tube-shaped, and not studded with ribosomes. In **Fig. 3.20**, SER occupies most of the cell (only a portion of the cell is shown here). SER has several

functions, mostly related to lipid biosynthesis (e.g., steroid production) or glycogen metabolism. In addition, it has a major role in detoxification.

Helpful Hint

Because the SER is tube-shaped (think of a tree or ginger root), sections through the SER will generate round or short tube-shaped sections, as opposed to the longer, flattened stacks of membrane typically seen with RER or Golgi. Also, the lack of ribosomes is helpful in identifying SER.

Smooth and rough ER are continuous. In fact, they can be converted one to another, largely by the addition or removal of ribosomes. This is common in cells such as hepatocytes of the liver, which play a major role in both protein synthesis and detoxification.

In **Fig. 3.21**, which shows the same field shown in **Fig. 3.12**, recall that the RER is indicated by 1. SER is in the outlined region (2), but it is also seen to the upper left of the RER. Note that the two reticula are continuous.

3.3.7 Lysosomes

Lysosomes are membrane-bound structures containing digestive enzymes, involved in intracellular breakdown of senile organelles or of exogenous cells (e.g., bacteria) and molecules ingested by the cell. Lysosomes newly formed by budding from the Golgi apparatus are often called primary lysosomes, which become secondary lysosomes when they fuse with structures to be degraded. Secondary lysosomes are larger, and because they contain breakdown products in different stages of degradation, they are relatively easy to identify in a cell because their lumen is heterogeneous. Lysosomes typically are about half the size of mitochondria, but can be larger.

In **Fig. 3.22**, two large secondary lysosomes are shown (one is outlined), and a smaller primary lysosome is marked by the black arrow at right.

3.3.8 Other Cellular Organelles

There are other organelles within the cell that are not necessary to identify on electron micrographs at this time. These include:

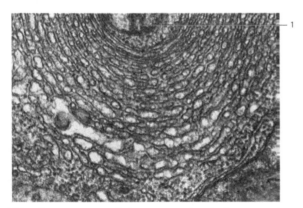

Fig. 3.20 **Electron micrograph showing smooth endoplasmic reticulum filling entire cell. Nucleus of the cell is indicated (1).**

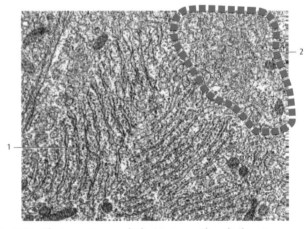

Fig. 3.21 **Electron micrograph showing smooth endoplasmic reticulum (outlined and at 2). Rough endoplasmic reticulum (1) also shown for comparison.**

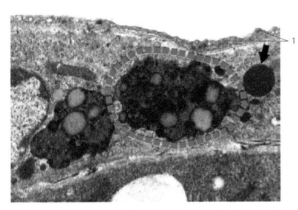

Fig. 3.22   **Electron micrograph showing lysosomes (outlined and black arrow). Capillary endothelium (1).**

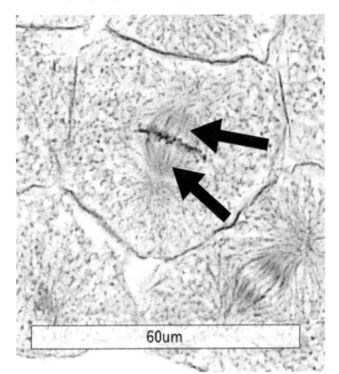

60um

Fig. 3.23   **Mitotic spindle (black arrows).**

1. **Secretory vesicles** are products of the RER and Golgi apparatus; they contain proteins or other molecular products to be secreted into the extracellular matrix.
2. **Peroxisomes** have a major role in detoxification.

3. **Lipid droplets** are for storage of fatty substances, seen prominently in adipose tissue.
4. **Glycogen** is a form of stored carbohydrate; glycogen particles are similar in appearance to ribosomes, but cluster together, often associated with SER.
5. The **cytoskeleton** is a filamentous network within the cell that is responsible for cell structure, cell movement, and movement of cellular organelles or chromosomes. There are three components to the cytoskeleton: **actin microfilaments**, **intermediate filaments**, and **microtubules**. The mitotic spindle (involved in chromosome movement during mitosis) is composed of microtubules (**Fig. 3.23**, arrows), while cytokinesis (division of the cytoplasm) is a process driven by actin filaments.

We'll come back to some of these organelles as they arise in subsequent chapters.

Helpful Hint

Staining of the cytoskeleton generates some of the most impressive images in cell biology—do a Google image search.

3.4   Chapter Review

The outer boundary of the cell is a lipid bilayer called the plasma (cell) membrane. The part of the cell excluding the nucleus is the cytoplasm, which is composed of the cytosol and organelles. Many organelles are bounded by a lipid bilayer similar to the plasma membrane, including rough and smooth endoplasmic reticulum, the Golgi apparatus, lysosomes, peroxisomes, and secretory vesicles. Mitochondria and the nucleus are unique because they are bounded by two membranes. Other structures in the cell are not membrane bound, including free ribosomes, glycogen, lipid droplets, and components of the cytoskeleton. Each structure in the cell plays a role in the functions of the cell. For example, the rough ER and Golgi apparatus are involved in protein synthesis and processing.

Questions and Answers

An online-only section of questions and answers accompanying this chapter is hosted on Thieme's MedOne Education site: https://medone-education.thieme.com. Use the code on the media page at the front of this book to gain access. An institutional license to the site is required to access these questions in an interactive format, and individual users are required to register for an individual account to track results.

4   Epithelial Classification

After completing this chapter, you should be able to:
— Identify, at the light microscope level, each of the following:
- Simple epithelia
  - Simple squamous
  - Simple cuboidal
  - Simple columnar
  - Pseudostratified
- Stratified epithelia
  - Stratified squamous (keratinized and nonkeratinized)
  - Stratified cuboidal/stratified columnar
  - Transitional
— Outline the function of each of these epithelial types
— Predict the type of epithelium present in a specific organ given the function of that organ

4.1   Overview of Tissue Types

The introductory chapters focused on cells and cell function and briefly described the extracellular matrix. This sequence of chapters 4–15 focuses on tissues.

Tissues are formed when cells and extracellular matrix combine together to achieve one or more common functions. For example, closely packed cells that form the inner lining of the esophagus (**Fig. 4.1**, green bracket) form a barrier between the **lumen** through which food passes and the underlying tissues of the body. These cells work together as one tissue type (an epithelium), while the more loosely organized cells below the bracket form another tissue type (connective tissue).

There are four main types of tissues in the body:
1. **Epithelial tissue**: closely packed sheets of cells that form linings of body spaces
2. **Connective tissue**: loosely packed cells that form a wide variety of tissues, ranging from liquid (blood) to solid (bone)
3. **Muscle tissue**: Contains cells that use energy to contract, providing movement
4. **Neural tissue**: Contains cells that use electrical potentials for cell-cell signaling

Note that most of these main tissue types have subtypes. For example, there are eight types of epithelia (or nine, depending on how they are organized); the structure and function of these will be discussed in this chapter.

This chapter will also introduce the functions of each tissue type. During this discussion, examples of where these tissues are found will be provided. It is not important at this time to memorize the complete list of where each tissue type is found in the body. However, it is a useful exercise to be able to propose tissue types that can be found in certain organs based on the function of those organs. This will enhance learning the structure of organs in later chapters.

In all anatomic disciplines, *form follows function*. In other words, a cell, tissue, or organ appears a certain way because that form best accomplishes the function of that cell, tissue, or organ. Therefore, understanding why a tissue looks the way it does will help recall what the tissue is doing, which will help in cell, tissue, and organ recognition. For example, a cell synthesizing large amounts of proteins contains abundant rough ER and therefore demonstrates cytoplasmic basophilia on H and E-stained tissues.

4.2   Overview of Epithelia

The first three chapters in this series on tissues investigate epithelia. In this chapter, an overview of epithelia is described, followed by the classification of the different types of epithelia, focusing on recognition of the types of epithelia and their functions. The following chapter focuses on specializations of epithelia and is followed by a chapter describing glands.

Epithelia form sheets of closely packed cells with very little extracellular matrix between the cells. In this way they form a barrier, separating the spaces or tissues that lie on either side. For example, in **Fig. 4.2**, there is a space above the epithelium and

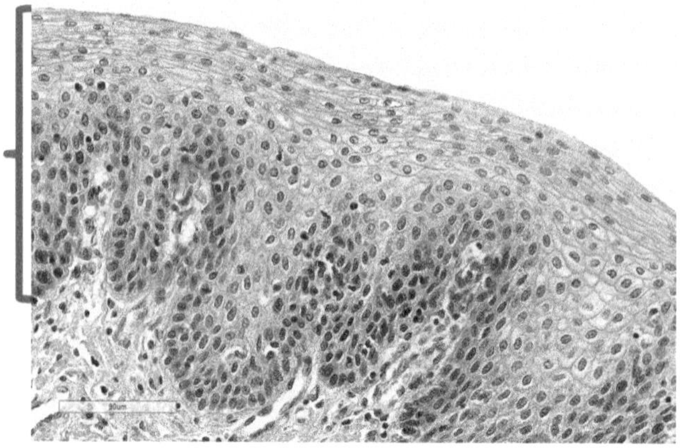

Fig. 4.1   Light micrograph of the stratified squamous epithelium (green bracket) and underlying connective tissue from the esophagus.

Typical epithelium

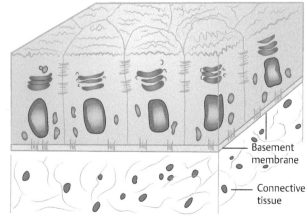

Basement membrane

Connective tissue

Fig. 4.2   **Drawing of a typical epithelium.**

connective tissue below. Not only does the epithelium form the barrier between the space and the connective tissue, but it regulates molecular movement from one side to the other (from the space to the connective tissue and vice versa). Different types of epithelia have different functions, largely related to the amount of material that passes through them.

Epithelial tissue typically is exposed to external forces (physical, chemical) more than other tissues. Therefore, epithelia contain **stem cells** that proliferate to regenerate damaged cells; often this is a continual process of cell renewal and sloughing of older cells.

Connective tissue is almost always on one side of an epithelium, separated from the epithelium by a sheet of extracellular protein called the **basement membrane**. The basement membrane is secreted by both the epithelial cells and cells of the connective tissue, and it serves as a "platform" on which the epithelial cells rest.

The "space" on the other side of the epithelia varies. In many cases, the space is the outside world (e.g., for the epithelium of the skin) or its equivalent (for example, the inner lining of the gut or respiratory system lines the lumen of these organs, which communicates with the outside world). In this way, the epithelium provides a barrier between the outside world and tissues in the body. In still other cases, the space contains body fluids. For example, the inner lining of blood vessels is an epithelium, separating blood from the connective tissue in the vessel wall.

In this regard, it is useful to note that epithelial cells, and the epithelium itself, are polarized. The side of the epithelium that is nearer the basement membrane and connective tissue is called the **basal** aspect, while the side that is nearer the space is the **apical** side. Note that this apical/basal polarization applies both to the individual cells of the epithelium and to the epithelium as a whole. Therefore, for a single cell, the terms *basal* and *apical* refer to the corresponding sides of the cell; for example, the **basal plasma membrane** and **apical plasma membrane** are the regions of the plasma membrane of that cell closer to the basement membrane and to the space, respectively. With regard to an epithelium that has many layers of cells (stratified epithelia, discussed subsequently in this chapter), the cells closer to the basement membrane can be referred to as **basal cells**, while those closer to the space are called **apical cells**.

To apply all this to a practical example, the esophagus is lined by an epithelium that separates the lumen of the esophagus from the underlying connective tissue. In **Fig. 4.3**, the location of the basement membrane is indicated by the dotted line. Above this

line is the epithelium that forms the inner lining of the esophagus (faces the lumen). Below this line is connective tissue. The nuclei just above the dotted line belong to basal cells, while those nuclei closest to the lumen belong to apical cells.

Note that the epithelium is more cellular than the underlying connective tissue. As described in previous chapters, the lines between the nuclei represent two adjacent plasma membranes, underscoring the fact that there is little extracellular space between the cells in an epithelium.

4.3 Classification of Epithelia

Before classifying epithelia, it is important to note that an epithelium is a flat sheet of cells, and a section of tissue may be cut through an epithelium at different angles. Think of the epithelium as a sheet of plywood (or any other flat object with some thickness). If viewed from the side, it will appear like the object labeled "side view" in **Fig. 4.4**. However, if viewed from above, the epithelium will look like the object labeled "top view."

> **Helpful Hint**
>
> This whole concept may seem silly to even mention, but it can get quite confusing when looking at tissue sections, which cut epithelia in a variety of angles. In addition, because some epithelia are wavy, they can transition from one view to another.
>
> Keep this in mind: An epithelium is classified based on its appearance in the *side view*; that is, when the section is cut at right angles to plane of the epithelium. Because of this, when looking at slides, ignore any other angle of an epithelium and focus on regions where the epithelium is cut nearest this angle. Never try to classify an epithelium from the top view or from an oblique angle.

As shown in **Fig. 4.5**, epithelia are classified based on two features:

1. The number of cell layers: **simple epithelia** are one cell thick, while **stratified epithelia** are composed of two or more layers of cells.
2. The shape of the cells: **squamous** (flat), **cuboidal**, or **columnar**. Here, it is important to note that it is the shape of the *surface* cells that defines the classification of the epithelium. For example, note that stratified squamous epithelium has cuboidal cells near the basement membrane, but the cells are squamous apically.

> **Helpful Hint**
>
> Remember that **Fig. 4.5** shows all side views. Think about it: When viewed from the top down, all epithelia would look pretty much the same, right?

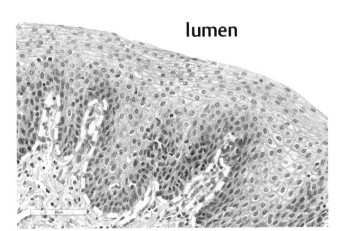

lumen

Fig. 4.3   **Epithelium of the esophagus (above dotted line).**

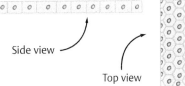
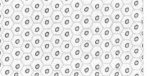

Side view

Top view

Fig. 4.4   **Epithelial orientation.**

Type of epithelium

Simple epithelium

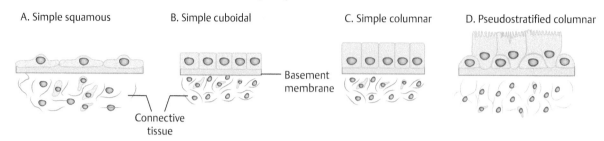

A. Simple squamous   B. Simple cuboidal   C. Simple columnar   D. Pseudostratified columnar

Basement membrane

Connective tissue

Stratified epithelium

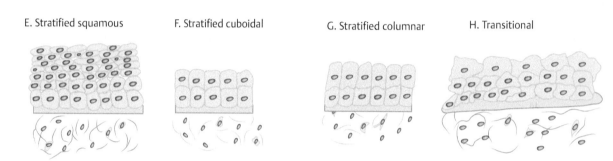

E. Stratified squamous   F. Stratified cuboidal   G. Stratified columnar   H. Transitional

Fig. 4.5   Epithelial classification.

If an epithelium is defined as either simple or stratified, *and also* as either squamous, cuboidal, or columnar, then you might expect that there would be six total epithelial types (simple squamous, simple cuboidal, simple columnar, stratified squamous, stratified cuboidal, stratified columnar). There are two other epithelial types (pseudostratified columnar and transitional) that fall into their own categories because they have features similar to both simple and stratified epithelia.

Recall that epithelia form a barrier and that the permeabilities of different epithelia vary. Simple epithelia are thinner than stratified epithelia, so, as a general rule, they allow more movement of molecules from one side of the epithelium to the other (e.g., from the apical side to the basal side). However, this increase in **permeability** comes at a cost, as simple epithelia are typically less resilient and are more likely breached by infectious agents. The stratified epithelia are less permeable but provide more protection, both physical and against pathogens.

So simple epithelia are found in such places as the intestines, where absorption of nutrients is most important, whereas stratified epithelium can be found in the skin, where protection is imperative.

4.3.1   Simple Squamous Epithelia

A **simple squamous epithelium** (A in **Fig. 4.5**) consists of a single layer of flattened cells. When viewed from the side, the cells appear flattened; in a top-down view they appear round, similar to a fried egg. Since nuclei conform to the shape of the cell, they are flattened as well, though the cell is thicker in the vicinity of the nucleus. The rest of the cell is attenuated (thin).

Recall that simple epithelia are most favorable to movement of molecules from one side of the epithelia to the other. Simple

squamous epithelial cells are thin, which minimizes the distance between the apical and basal sides of the cell and thus maximizes diffusion efficiency, both through and between the cells. Therefore, simple squamous epithelia are found in tissues and organs that utilize diffusion for molecular movement. Capillaries are an excellent example because their function is to enable molecules to move from the blood into the tissues and vice versa.

Squamous epithelia also provide a smooth surface, which makes it easier for blood or other fluid to flow over them. Therefore, all blood vessels and the heart, not just capillaries, are lined on the inside by a simple squamous epithelium.

Fig. 4.6 is a section of the inner lining of the heart. In this image, blood would be located in the space to the upper right (lumen). This tissue was processed with a special connective tissue stain, so nuclei here are red and the extracellular matrix is green. The flattened nuclei of the simple squamous epithelial cells are indicated by the arrows. The attenuated cytoplasm of most cells is barely visible. To estimate the shape of these flattened cells, it helps to draw cell borders mentally halfway between nuclei.

The pale tissue just below the epithelium is connective tissue; note the paucity of nuclei. If this were a stratified epithelium, there would be more nuclei in that region.

Video 4.1   Simple squamous epithelium

Be able to identify:
— Simple squamous epithelium
https://www.thieme.de/de/q.htm?p=opn/tp/308390101/978-1-62623-414-7_c004_v001&t=video

4.3.2 Simple Cuboidal and Simple Columnar Epithelia

Simple cuboidal and **simple columnar epithelia** are introduced together because, functionally, they are quite similar. As shown in B and C in **Fig. 4.5**, they are histologically distinct based on the shape of the cells. The nuclei conform to the shape of the cells, so cuboidal cells typically have spherical nuclei, while columnar cells have elongated nuclei.

Both simple cuboidal and simple columnar are simple epithelia, so they play a role in the movement of molecules across the epithelium. However, unlike simple squamous cells, which are flattened to maximize passive diffusion, cells in simple cuboidal or simple columnar epithelia contain more cytoplasm (and more plasma membrane due to surface modifications, discussed further in the next chapter). Cells in these epithelia are involved in more active transport of molecules from one side of the epithelium to the other using **pump** and **channel** molecules synthesized by the cells and placed in the plasma membrane. Movement of these molecules requires ATP, so these cells typically have large numbers of mitochondria as well. Simple cuboidal epithelia are found in the kidneys, and a simple columnar epithelium forms the inner lining of the intestines.

Simple Cuboidal Epithelia

The image in **Fig. 4.7** was taken from a section through the ovary. The outer surface of the ovary is lined by an epithelium that is mostly simple cuboidal (yellow brackets). Note that the borders between the cells are not visible, so they need to be mentally drawn in.

Video 4.2 Simple cuboidal epithelium

Be able to identify:
Simple cuboidal epithelium
https://www.thieme.de/de/q.htm?p=opn/
tp/308390101/978-1-62623-414-7_c004_v002&t=video

Simple Columnar Epithelia

The tissue in **Fig. 4.8** was taken from the intestines. Here, determining orientation is a little challenging because there are two epithelial sheets facing the same lumen. The lumen represents the apical side of the epithelium in both cases, while the connective tissue side is the basal side. Therefore, these epithelial sheets (black brackets) are mirror images of each other. They consist of a single layer of tall cells, with elongated nuclei in the basal half of the cells. Some cell borders are visible. Some nuclei appear to be on top of others; this is due to the thickness of the section, not because it is a stratified epithelium. The space between the epithelium and connective tissue is an artifact caused by tissue shrinkage.

Video 4.3 Simple columnar epithelium

Be able to identify:
— Simple columnar epithelium
https://www.thieme.de/de/q.htm?p=opn/
tp/308390101/978-1-62623-414-7_c004_
v003&t=video

Helpful Hint

Simple epithelia will appear stratified when cut at an angle. However, looking around the slide to find a location where the epithelium is sectioned at a right angle will reveal the tissue's true type. Note that, on the other hand, stratified epithelium can *never* appear simple, no matter at what angle it is sectioned.

4.3.3 Pseudostratified Columnar Epithelia

Pseudostratified columnar epithelium (D in **Fig. 4.5**) appears to consist of two rows of cells: small cuboidal cells with round nuclei and tall columnar cells with elongated nuclei. The nuclei of these two types of cells form two distinct rows, giving the

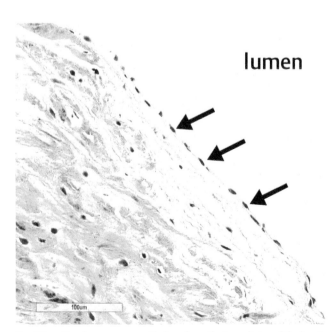

Fig. 4.6   **Simple squamous epithelium from the inner lining of the heart (black arrows).**

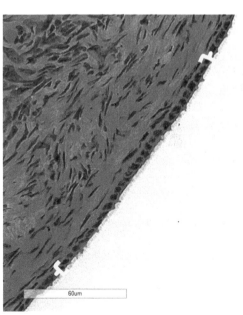

Fig. 4.7   **Simple cuboidal epithelium from the ovary (between yellow brackets).**

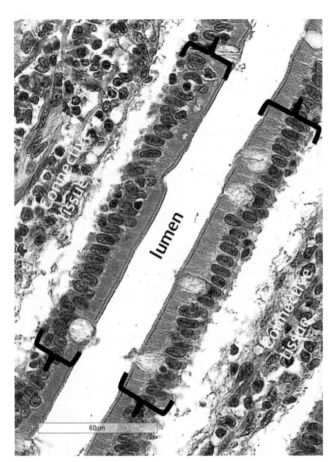

Fig. 4.8   **Simple columnar epithelium from the intestines (between black brackets).**

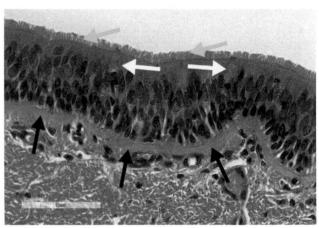

Fig. 4.9   **Pseudostratified columnar epithelium from the trachea. Basement membrane (black arrows), goblet cells (yellow arrows) and cilia (green arrows) are shown.**

Helpful Hint

This section in Fig. 4.9 is cut a little thick, so it appears that there are several rows of nuclei (note that some nuclei are faint or out of focus). However, one feature of pseudostratified epithelium is that the basal cells closer to the basement membrane are rounder, and the cells toward the apical side have larger, more elongated nuclei. In addition, the nuclei are staggered (we'll come back to this a little later in this chapter). Also note the fact that the very apical aspect of this tissue is fairly devoid of nuclei. Pseudostratified epithelium typically has surface modifications (cilia, stereocilia), but other tissue types have these modifications, so this point is less reliable.

Video 4.4   Pseudostratified columnar epithelium in the trachea

Be able to identify:
— Pseudostratified columnar epithelium
https://www.thieme.de/de/q.htm?p=opn/
tp/308390101/978-1-62623-414-7_c004_v004&t=video

appearance of a stratified epithelium. However, as shown in the figure, all of the cells rest on the basement membrane, so this epithelium is truly a simple epithelium. Thus the name *pseudostratified* (false stratified).

Pseudostratified epithelium is taller than other simple epithelia, so transport of molecules across the epithelium is not necessarily its main function (though it does occur). Instead, these cells typically have surface specializations such as cilia that aid in movement of mucus or absorption of other material. For example, mucus produced by the bronchi and bronchioles is moved by the cilia lining those structures, a feature known as the mucociliary escalator. This will be discussed in the chapters describing the respiratory system.

The tissue shown in **Fig. 4.9** was taken from the trachea. The basement membrane in the trachea is unusually thick (black arrows), which makes it easier to recognize, and easy to distinguish the epithelium from the underlying connective tissue. In this epithelium, several rows of nuclei give the immediate impression that the epithelium is stratified. However, all the cells make contact with the basement membrane (though not all reach the surface). There are surface projections (cilia, green arrows) on the apical surface of this epithelium; these will be addressed further in **Chapter 5**. This image also shows one or two goblet cells (very subtle, yellow arrows); these will be addressed in **Chapter 6**.

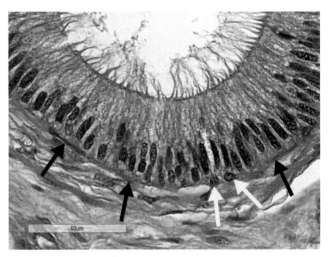

Fig. 4.10   **Pseudostratified columnar epithelium from the epididymis. Basement membrane (black arrows) and basal cells (yellow arrows).**

The tissue shown in **Fig. 4.10** was taken from the epididymis, part of the male reproductive tract that also has pseudostratified columnar epithelium. The basement membrane here is a little thinner than in the trachea (black arrows). In this image, there are fewer basal cells (yellow arrows) than in the trachea. However, the basal cells are cuboidal, with more nearly round nuclei, while the remainder of the cells are tall columnar, with much more elongated nuclei. The surface modifications here are very long and are called **stereocilia**.

Helpful Hint

As mentioned, here there are fewer basal nuclei than seen in the trachea, so this tissue might look similar to simple columnar epithelium. Therefore, pay special attention to the fact that the round nuclei are on the epithelial side of the basement membrane and not the connective tissue side. In addition, make sure to look around the slide as much as possible before making a final decision on the tissue type (this is true for any tissue).

Video 4.5 Pseudostratified columnar epithelium in the epididymis

Be able to identify:
— Pseudostratified columnar epithelium

https://www.thieme.de/de/q.htm?p=opn/tp/308390101/978-1-62623-414-7_c004_v005&t=video

4.3.4   Stratified Squamous Epithelia

In stratified epithelia, the tissue forms more than one layer of cells. **Stratified squamous epithelia** (E in **Fig. 4.5**) consists of multiple (up to 40!) layers of cells. Although the basal cells are often cuboidal, the apical cells are squamous. There are two types of stratified squamous epithelium:

1. **Stratified squamous nonkeratinized epithelium**: Here the apical cells retain their nuclei and other organelles. This epithelium lines some internal organs of the body, such as the esophagus, and remains moist.
2. **Stratified squamous keratinized epithelium**: As the apical cells mature, they lose their nuclei and other organelles. The intracellular proteins (keratins) that remain form a protective barrier. This epithelium is normally found in the skin in humans but can occur elsewhere in certain pathological conditions.

The many layers of a stratified squamous epithelium provide an excellent protective barrier to physical trauma and infectious agents. Although all epithelia have cell renewal, it is a main feature of stratified squamous epithelia. Cell proliferation in the basal region is robust, and as cells mature, they progress toward the surface, where they are sloughed off.

Stratified Squamous Nonkeratinized Epithelia

Fig. 4.11 is an image from the esophagus. The epithelium here is stratified squamous nonkeratinized. Although the basal cells are cuboidal, close examination reveals that the surface cells are squamous and retain their nuclei (arrows).

Helpful Hint

When seeing this epithelium, think moist, and exposed to mechanical forces such as friction. Stratified squamous epithelium is ideal for the esophagus, which transmits swallowed food to the stomach.

Video 4.6 Video of stratified squamous epithelium nonkeratinized

Be able to identify:
— Stratified squamous nonkeratinized epithelium

https://www.thieme.de/de/q.htm?p=opn/tp/308390101/978-1-62623-414-7_c004_v006&t=video

Stratified Squamous Keratinized Epithelia

Fig. 4.12 is an image from the ear. The basement membrane here is not visible; its location is indicated by the series of black arrows. The basal cells in this epithelium are cuboidal. As the cells move toward the apical surface, they become squamous, and the nucleus condenses (green arrows). Eventually the nucleus and other organelles are broken down, leaving the remaining intracellular proteins, which forms the keratinized layer at the surface (yellow brackets).

Helpful Hint

Skin cells called melanocytes produce the brown pigmentation seen here. More on this will be presented in **Chapter 27**.

Video 4.7 Stratified squamous epithelium keratinized in thin skin

Be able to identify:
— Stratified squamous keratinized epithelium

https://www.thieme.de/de/q.htm?p=opn/tp/308390101/978-1-62623-414-7_c004_v007&t=video

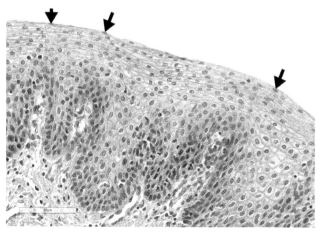

Fig. 4.11 **Stratified squamous nonkeratinized epithelium from the esophagus. Arrows indicate nuclei in apical cells.**

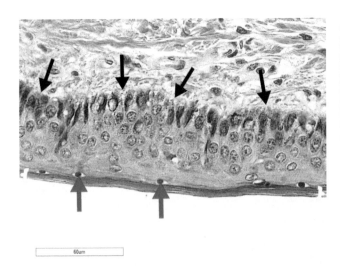

Fig. 4.12   **Stratified squamous keratinized epithelium from the ear. The keratinized layer (between yellow brackets), squamous cells (green arrows) and basement membrane (black arrows) are indicated.**

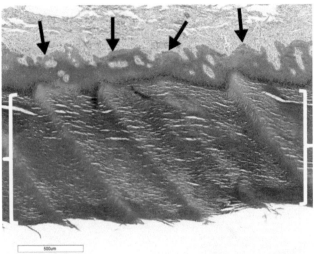

Fig. 4.13   **Stratified squamous keratinized epithelium from the sole of the foot. The keratinized layer (between yellow brackets) and basement membrane (black arrows) are indicated.**

The ear is not exposed to excessive mechanical forces, so the stratified squamous epithelium is lightly keratinized. **Fig. 4.13** shows a specimen from the sole of the foot, which, not surprisingly, has a much thicker keratinized layer to provide more protection. Note that the image was taken at low magnification in order to capture the entire thickness of the keratinized layer (yellow brackets). The basement membrane is indicated by the series of arrows. The living epithelial cells are between the black arrows and yellow brackets.

Skin (integument) will be discussed in detail in other chapters, especially **Chapter 27**. The only thing to appreciate for now is that the degree of keratinization varies in different regions of the body.

Video 4.8   Stratified squamous epithelium keratinized in thick skin

Be able to identify:
— Stratified squamous keratinized epithelium
https://www.thieme.de/de/q.htm?p=opn/
tp/308390101/978-1-62623-414-7_c004_v008&t=video

4.3.5   Stratified Cuboidal and Stratified Columnar Epithelia

Like simple cuboidal and simple columnar epithelia, which were discussed together because they have similar functions, **stratified cuboidal** and **stratified columnar epithelia** (F and G in **Fig. 4.5**) can be grouped together as well. In both cases, there are two layers of cells that form relatively uniform rows. The only difference between the two is that the apical cells are either cuboidal or columnar, respectively.

These epithelial types provide protection, albeit not as robust as stratified squamous epithelia, but without the

cellular cost from sloughing. Therefore, stratified cuboidal and stratified columnar epithelia are located in places such as the ducts of salivary glands, which require some resistance to physical trauma and friction, but not nearly as much as the skin or esophagus.

Fig. 4.14 is an image of a salivary gland duct that includes a stratified columnar epithelium. Two yellow lines have been drawn through the nuclei of each of the two rows of cells.

Correctly identifying stratified columnar epithelia is a little challenging because the thickness of the tissue gives the appearance of more than two rows of nuclei in some places. However, appreciate that most of the nuclei fall into one or the other of the rows indicated by the yellow dotted lines, and that in many places nuclei from the apical row are directly above nuclei of the basal row (rather than staggered as in pseudostratified columnar epithelium).

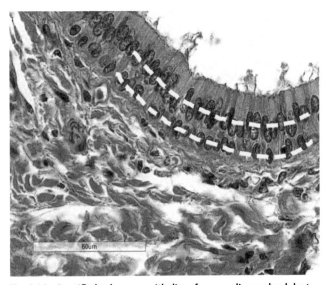

Fig. 4.14   **Stratified columnar epithelium from a salivary gland duct. The two dotted lines indicate the two rows of cells.**

Fig. 4.15 shows ducts from salivary glands that have regions lined by stratified cuboidal epithelia (rectangles). Here, cells in the apical layer are shorter, closer to cuboidal, than those in the apical layer seen in **Fig. 4.14**. Note that other regions of these ducts look more stratified; this is because these portions of the ducts are cut at an oblique angle.

Helpful Hint

The effort to distinguish stratified cuboidal epithelium from stratified columnar epithelium is *not* high yield. These two epithelia are part of a continuum anyway, and their function is the same.

Video 4.9   Stratified columnar epithelia

Video 4.10 Stratified cuboidal and stratified columnar epithelia

Be able to identify:
— Stratified cuboidal/columnar epithelia
https://www.thieme.de/de/q.htm?p=opn/
tp/308390101/978-1-62623-414-7_c004_
v009&t=video
https://www.thieme.de/de/q.htm?p=opn/
tp/308390101/978-1-62623-414-7_c004_v010&t=video

Helpful Hint

One of the look-alikes in histology is stratified columnar vs. pseudostratified epithelia. Note that the nuclei in stratified columnar epithelia tend to form nice rows, with nuclei that tend to be directly over others (**Fig. 4.14**). In pseudostratified epithelia, the nuclei usually do not form nice rows and are staggered (**Fig. 4.9**). Appreciating the difference between these two tissues is challenging and takes a little practice. When looking at tissues on slides, remember to find a region in which the plane of section is perpendicular to the epithelium.

One other distinguishing feature that can be useful is that pseudostratified epithelium typically has numerous apical surface modifications (e.g., cilia; **Fig. 4.9**, green arrows). The fluff seen in **Fig. 4.14** on the apical surface of the stratified columnar epithelium is mostly debris. This can be tricky, since the debris can appear to be surface modifications, and some surface modifications are destroyed during tissue preparation. Therefore, using surface modifications to differentiate these two tissue types is not always reliable.

4.3.6   Transitional Epithelia

Transitional epithelia (H in **Fig. 4.5**) can be found in the ureter and bladder. Because these epithelia are able to stretch (e.g., during bladder filling), the number of apparent layers of cells depends on the state of the tissue at the time of fixation. An empty bladder (less stretched epithelium) will demonstrate a clear stratified appearance, while a stretched bladder will show fewer layers. Most prepared slides are taken from empty bladders.

In addition to its ability to stretch, transitional epithelium is fairly impermeable to water and ions. Therefore, it is ideal for the bladder, which must stretch but also must retain the ion and water concentrations of the urine produced by the kidneys.

Fig. 4.16 is an image that is taken from the bladder and includes transitional epithelium. Note that this epithelium is a few cells thick. In this relaxed (bladder empty) state, the apical cells are significantly larger than the basal cells and bulge into the lumen. Binucleate cells are common (green arrow). In addition, there is band of increased eosinophilia just under the apical plasma membrane (black arrows), which represents numerous infoldings of the plasma membrane of these cells, called plaques, which unfold as the epithelium is stretched.

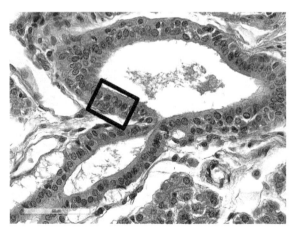
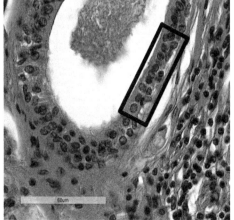

Fig. 4.15   **Stratified cuboidal epithelia from a salivary gland duct.**

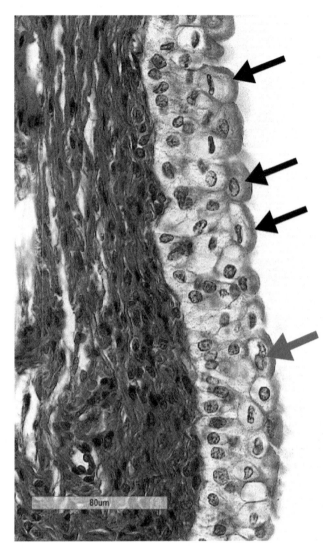

Fig. 4.16   Transitional epithelium from the bladder. Cytoplasmic plaques (black arrows) and a binucleate cell (green arrow) are indicated.

There are several features of a transitional epithelium that make it fairly easy to identify. It is easiest to look for bulging apical cells, which are a fairly reliable feature of transitional epithelium. However, note that tissue folding may cause other epithelia to have apparent bulges. In addition, some regions of transitional epithelium lack obvious bulges. If an epithelium appears transitional but has a flat surface, larger apical cells (relative to basal cells), as well as the eosinophilia just under the plasma membrane of the apical cells, are pretty reliable methods for confirming that the tissue is transitional. Binucleate cells help but are sometimes hard to find.

Video 4.11 Transitional epithelium from the bladder

Video 4.12 Transitional epithelium from the ureter

Be able to identify:
— Transitional epithelia

https://www.thieme.de/de/q.htm?p=opn/tp/308390101/978-1-62623-414-7_c004_v011&t=video

https://www.thieme.de/de/q.htm?p=opn/tp/308390101/978-1-62623-414-7_c004_v012&t=video

It is sometimes difficult to differentiate stratified squamous non-keratinized epithelium from transitional epithelium, because they both have nuclei close to the apical surface (which is usually not the case for pseudostratified or stratified columnar epithelia). When differentiating stratified squamous from transitional epithelia, it is useful to note that the surface cells in stratified squamous epithelia are smaller than the basal cells, or at least flatter, and not larger (**Fig. 4.11**). In transitional epithelium, the apical cells are almost always much larger than the basal cells (**Fig. 4.15**).

4.4   Chapter Review

There are four tissue types in the body: epithelia, connective tissue, muscle, and neural tissue. Epithelia form sheets of cells closely packed together, with little extracellular material. An epithelium forms a barrier between its apical side (usually the outside world or a fluid) and the body tissues on its basal side (usually connective tissue). Epithelia come in several types, each with a different function. In general, the permeability of an epithelium is inversely proportional to the ability of the epithelium to protect the underlying tissues. For example, simple epithelia are typically very permeable but more likely to be breached by physical trauma or infectious agents, while stratified squamous epithelia are less permeable but provide more substantial protection. Some types of epithelia, such as pseudostratified columnar and transitional epithelia, have specialized functions (ciliary motility and stretching, respectively). The ability to recognize an epithelium and to distinguish epithelial types from one another will be critical for identifying organs and describing their function.

An online-only section of questions and answers accompanying this chapter is hosted on Thieme's MedOne Education site: https://medone-education.thieme.com. Use the code on the media page at the front of this book to gain access. An institutional license to the site is required to access these questions in an interactive format, and individual users are required to register for an individual account to track results.

5 Epithelial Specializations

After completing this chapter, you should be able to:
— Identify, at the light microscope level, each of the following:
  • Cell attachments
    ◦ Cell-cell junctions
    ◦ Intercellular bridges
  • Basement membrane
  • Free surface specializations
    ◦ Cilia
    ◦ Microvilli
    ◦ Stereocilia
— Identify, at the electron microscope level, each of the following
  • Cell attachments
    ◦ Cell-cell junctions
      ▪ Tight junctions (zonula occludens)
      ▪ Belt desmosomes (zonula adherens)
      ▪ Desmosomes (macula adherens)
      ▪ Gap junctions
    ◦ Cell–basement membrane junctions
      ▪ Hemidesmosomes
  • Basement membrane / basal lamina
  • Interdigitation of basal and lateral membranes
  • Free surface specializations
    ◦ Cilia
    ◦ Microvilli
— Outline the function of each of the structures listed
— Discuss the relationship of these structures to each other and to members of the cytoskeleton (actin microfilaments, intermediate filaments, microtubules)
— Predict the surface specializations in a cell type given the function of that cell type

5.1 Plasma Membrane Specializations

Epithelial cells have specializations of their plasma membrane that perform important functions for the cell (**Fig. 5.1**). For example, the basement membrane serves as an anchor for the basal aspect of the epithelium. In addition to surface modifications of the apical surface (microvilli, cilia, stereocilia), the basal plasma membrane of epithelial cells can also have specialized folds that increase surface area. Epithelial cells also interact with each other laterally, via cell-cell junctions.

This chapter will investigate these surface specializations. Many of these surface specializations discussed here are common in epithelial cells but are found in other cells and tissues as well.

5.2 Cell-Cell Junctions

Epithelial cells interact laterally with adjacent cells through cell-cell junctions. Although these junctions can be found in any location where cells interact with adjacent cells, there is a cluster of them close to the apical surface of epithelial cells. This area, referred to as the **junctional complex,** has three components (from apical to basal):
1. Tight junctions (zonula occludens)
2. Belt desmosomes (zonula adherens)
3. Desmosomes (spot desmosomes, macula adherens)

The two zonula junctions form bands that wrap around the entire cell, interacting with several neighboring cells. Desmosomes are round structures that are found in the junctional complex but in other regions of the cell as well.

All of these junctions are composed of transmembrane proteins that have extracellular domains that interact with the extracellular domains of similar proteins in neighboring cells. The cytoplasmic domains of these transmembrane proteins interact with cytoplasmic proteins, especially the cytoskeletal elements. The junctional complex, located in the lateral plasma membrane of the cell near the apical side, divides the plasma membrane of each cell into an apical and a basolateral portion (the basolateral portion includes both the basal and most of the lateral sides of the cell).

5.2.1 Tight Junctions

Tight junctions (zonula occludens, ZO) are nearest the apical aspect of the cell (**Fig. 5.1**) and are composed of proteins such as claudins and occludins. These junctions bring the plasma membranes of adjacent cells close together, so they have been called "kissing junctions." They create a tight seal between adjacent cells, restricting movement of water and other molecules from passing between cells (i.e., from passing from the free space to the connective tissue side). The "leakiness" of these junctions can vary. For example, vessels in the brain have very restrictive tight junctions, so most molecular movement requires passage through the cells.

In addition, tight junctions also restrict movement of lipids and proteins in the plasma membrane; that is, proteins and lipids in the apical plasma membrane cannot drift into the basolateral membrane and vice versa.

The tight junction shown at ZO in **Fig. 5.2** is slightly out of the plane of section and appears a little fuzzy. However, the two plasma membranes of these cells are close together in this location (yellow arrows). In addition, note that these tight junctions are nearest the apical aspect of the cell. Finally, the other junctions (ZA and D in **Fig. 5.2**, discussed in subsequent sections) form thick densities adjacent to the plasma membrane and are more intimately associated with the cytoskeleton (fuzzy material in the cytoplasm near junctions ZA and D).

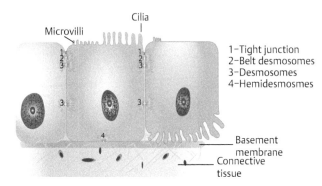

Fig. 5.1   **Specializations of the epithelial membrane.**

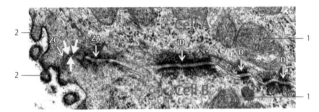

Fig. 5.2   Electron micrograph showing the junctional complex between two cells (A and B). ZO marks a zonula occludens (tight junction); ZA indicates a zonula adherens (belt desmosome); Ds indicates a desmosome; plasma membrane is indicated by the yellow arrows, and can be seen between the desmosomes.

5.2.2 Belt Desmosomes

Belt desmosomes (zonula adherens, ZA; **Fig. 5.1**) are composed of transmembrane proteins called E-cadherins. These junctions interact with actin filaments, in particular a network of actin just beneath the apical plasma membrane called the **terminal web.** Like tight junctions, belt desmosomes wrap all the way around the cell. They provide physical strength to the cell-cell interaction, whereas the tight junctions provide a seal.

In **Fig. 5.2** the belt desmosome shown at ZA appears adjacent to, and on the basal side of, the tight junction (to the right of it in this image). Note that the plasma membranes of the two cells in the region of the belt desmosome are not as close to each other as they are in the tight junction (the clear area between the membranes is the extracellular space). In addition, the proteins involved in this junction make the plasma membrane in this region thicker than in the tight junctions. The fuzzy material in the cytoplasm adjacent to the junction is mostly actin associated with the terminal web, as well as other proteins (e.g., vinculin).

5.2.3 Desmosomes

Desmosomes (macula adherens, **Fig. 5.1**) are composed of transmembrane proteins called desmocollins and desmogleins. As mentioned, these junctions are the most basal member of the junctional complex, but they can be found in numerous other locations as well. Like the belt desmosome, these junctions provide mechanical strength to the cell-cell interaction.

Desmosomes interact with the intermediate filament network of the cytoskeleton (see **Chapter 3**); together with that network, they provide considerable strength across an epithelium.

Desmosomes are easily recognized in electron micrographs (**Fig. 5.2**) because they include thick cytoplasmic plaques, seen as dense bands associated with both plasma membranes. These plaques, which interact with the cytoplasmic side of the plasma membrane, are composed of proteins such as desmoplakins and plakoglobins. The intermediate filament network in the cell loops through these dense plaques and can be seen as the fuzzy fibers adjacent to the dense plaques.

Desmosomes cannot be seen in the light microscope, but their presence can create an artifact of tissue preparation. During fixation of tissues for light microscopy, cells pull apart due to tissue shrinkage. However, cell-cell attachments through desmosomes persist. **Fig. 5.3** is a drawing of two cells joined by five desmosomes. On the left, cells are shown before tissue shrinkage, showing adjacent plasma membranes. After shrinkage (right), the cells pull apart but remain connected in the location of desmosomes. These connections between adjacent cells (outlined) can be seen in light micrographs and are referred to as **intercellular bridges**.

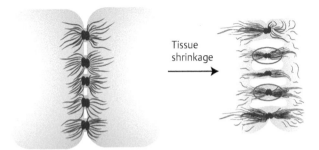

Fig. 5.3   Schematic of two cells joined by five desmosomes before (left) and after (right) tissue shrinkage; red outlines indicate intercellular bridges.

Epithelial cells in skin are joined by numerous desmosomes to provide strength to the tissue. **Fig. 5.4** is from skin, showing approximately 20 epithelial cells. Due to tissue shrinkage, the cells have pulled apart from each other, creating the light areas seen between the cells. However, note that there are thin extensions (1) or "spines" that connect adjacent cells. As mentioned, these are artifacts of tissue shrinkage. Before shrinkage, the cells were adjacent, with no clear area between the cells. The cells pulled apart during shrinkage, but remained attached by desmosomes, creating these intercellular bridges. The desmosomes cannot be seen but are located approximately in the middle of each bridge.

Video 5.1   Intercellular bridges

Be able to identify:
— Intercellular bridges
https://www.thieme.de/de/q.htm?p=opn/
tp/308390101/978-1-62623-414-7_c005_
v001&t=video

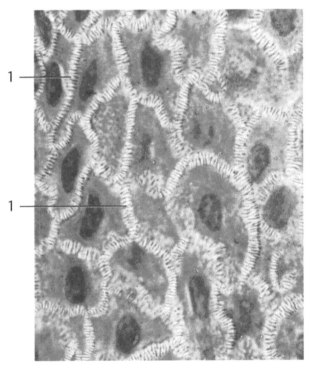

Fig. 5.4   **Epidermis of the skin, showing intercellular bridges (spines, 1).**

5.2.4 Gap Junctions

Gap junctions are located on the lateral aspect of epithelial cells. Gap junctions are composed of proteins called connexins, which assemble into pores that join with corresponding pores on neighboring cells to form channels that allow passage of water and other small molecules from the cytosol of one cell to that of another. This passage also provides electric communication between cells via small ions such as sodium (Na^+). The pores created by gap junctions can be normally in an open or a closed position but close or open in response to intracellular conditions, enabling the cells to regulate cell-cell continuity through these junctions.

5.3   Basement Membrane

The **basement membrane** is an extracellular sheet that provides support for an epithelium and separates the epithelium from the underlying connective tissue (**Fig. 5.1**). The proteins of the basement membrane (e.g., laminins and type IV collagen) are produced by both the epithelial cells and the connective tissue.

5.3.1 Basement Membrane in Light Micrographs

In light micrographs of H and E-stained slides, the basement membrane appears as an eosinophilic band (**Fig. 5.5**, arrows) and demarcates the border between the epithelium and connective tissue.

Video 5.2   Basement membrane—H and E

Be able to identify:
— Basement membrane
https://www.thieme.de/de/q.htm?p=opn/
tp/308390101/978-1-62623-414-7_c005_
v002&t=video

As shown in **Fig. 5.6**, the proteins of the basement membrane stain readily with PAS. The simple columnar epithelium that lines the lumen of the intestine is indicated by the bracket. The pale regions on this slide are connective tissue. The basement membrane (yellow arrows) appears as a thin, PAS-positive structure between the epithelium and connective tissue.

Video 5.3   Basement membrane—PAS

Be able to identify:
— Basement membrane
https://www.thieme.de/de/q.htm?p=opn/
tp/308390101/978-1-62623-414-7_c005_
v003&t=video

5.3.2 Basement Membrane in Electron Micrographs

Fig. 5.7 is an electron micrograph of the basal portion of a single epithelial cell (nucleus indicated at 1). Adjacent to the basal plasma membrane of this cell is the basement membrane (4), which appears as a thin gray line with paler regions on either side (above and below). Immediately below the basement membrane is a blood vessel, the lumen of which is indicated at 5 (the structure of blood vessels will be discussed further in a later chapter).

Figure 5.8 is an electron micrograph showing a basement membrane (4) taken from the filtration apparatus of the kidney. Note that there are two epithelial layers (3, and arrowheads) that share a basement membrane. This occurs in many locations where two epithelial layers form a thin barrier between the outside world (here the urinary space, which eventually communicates with the bladder and the outside of the body) and internal structures (here the blood vessels).

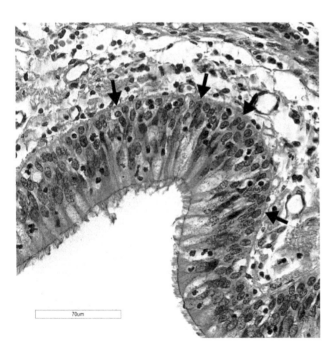

Fig. 5.5   **Light micrograph of the tracheal epithelium showing basement membrane (arrows).**

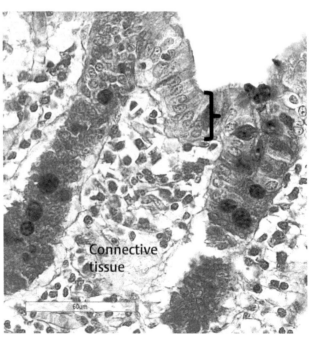

Fig. 5.6   **PAS stain of intestinal tissue showing columnar epithelium (black bracket) and basement membrane (yellow arrows).**

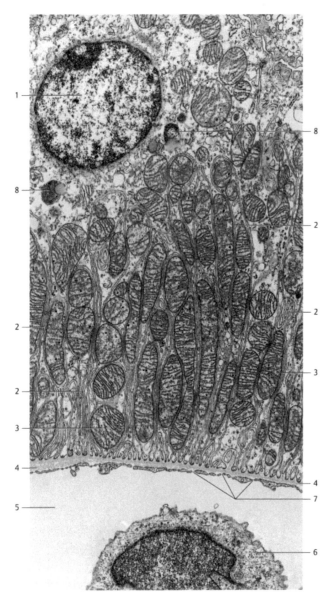

Fig. 5.7   **Electron micrograph of a single epithelial cell showing nucleus (1), basolateral infoldings (2), mitochondria (3), basement membrane (4), and lysosome (8). The connective tissue on the other (bottom) side of the basement membrane consists of a capillary with lumen of capillary (5), white blood cell (6), and capillary wall (7).**

Note that the basement membrane includes thin, lighter regions on either side of the thin gray line. These light and dark regions of the basement membrane have been named the lamina lucida and lamina densa, respectively. Some studies suggest that the lamina lucida may be an artifact. Regardless, it should be noted that many consider one lamina lucida and the lamina densa as a **basal lamina**, which is a subcomponent of the basement membrane (which would include all three layers, light-dark-light). The two terms *basal lamina* and *basement membrane* are often used interchangeably, even though there is this technical difference.

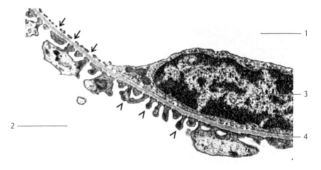

Fig. 5.8   **Electron micrograph of filtration apparatus of the kidney where two epithelial layers (3, and arrowheads) share a basement membrane (4). This filtration barrier separates the blood (1) from the urinary space (2), and will be discussed in greater detail in later chapters.**

5.3.3 Hemidesmosomes

As their name implies, **hemidesmosomes** look like half of a desmosome (**Fig. 5.1**), though they are composed of different proteins such as integrins. Located on the basal aspect of epithelial cells, hemidesmosomes attach the cell to the underlying basement membrane rather than to other cells. On the cytoplasmic side, hemidesmosomes, like desmosomes, interact with intermediate filaments.

5.4   Plasma Membrane Modifications

Along with cell-cell junctions and the basement membrane, many epithelial cells show specialized features that are either projections (microvilli, cilia, stereocilia) or infoldings (basolateral infoldings) of the plasma membrane (**Fig. 5.1**). These membrane modifications are driven and supported by the cytoskeleton, and, therefore, cytoskeletal elements often form the core of these projections.

5.4.1   Microvilli

Microvilli are relatively small, fingerlike projections on the apical aspect of the cell. They are supported by a core bundle of actin filaments that run in the same direction as the long axis of the microvillus. These actin filaments interact with the underlying terminal web. Microvilli are immotile and serve to increase the surface area of the apical surface to maximize contact with the contents of the lumen. This also increases the number of membrane proteins that can act as enzymes or transport channels. Transmembrane proteins on microvilli are heavily glycosylated on the external aspect of the cell, a feature known as the glycocalyx (see **Chapter 3**).

The size of microvilli is close to the level of resolution of the light microscope (**Fig. 5.9**). Therefore, individual microvilli are not routinely visible on light micrographs. However, *collectively*, they form a band of eosinophilia on the apical surface of the cell. **Fig. 5.9a** is an image from the small intestine stained with H and E; the epithelial cells here have numerous microvilli (black brackets) to increase surface area for enzymatic breakdown and absorption of food. This appearance of microvilli in the intestines is referred to as the striated border. (In the kidneys, a similar feature is called the brush border.)

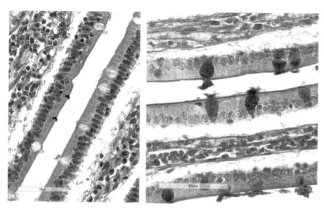

Fig. 5.9   **(a) Light micrograph showing microvilli collectively as a band of eosinophilia (brackets). (b) Microvilli stain with PAS due to their high carbohydrate content.**

Helpful Hint

When identifying surface modifications in light micrographs, it helps to compare them to the length of the elongated nuclei of the columnar cells. A good guesstimate is that microvillus height is approximately one-tenth to one-fifth the length of the nucleus. More on this will be addressed in the discussion on cilia and stereocilia.

As mentioned, the outer portion of the cell is modified with carbohydrate, forming the glycocalyx. The glycocalyx associated with microvilli is particularly robust, so microvilli stain positively with PAS, demonstrating a high carbohydrate content (**Fig. 5.9b**).

Video 5.4   Microvilli—H & E

https://www.thieme.de/de/q.htm?p=opn/
tp/308390101/978-1-62623-414-7_c005_
v004&t=video

Video 5.5   Microvilli—PAS

Be able to identify:
— Microvilli

https://www.thieme.de/de/q.htm?p=opn/
tp/308390101/978-1-62623-414-7_c005_
v005&t=video

Fig. 5.10 is an electron micrograph of the apical surface of a cell, with microvilli sectioned longitudinally, appearing as thin, fingerlike projections filled with bundled actin microfilaments. **Fig. 5.11** is an electron micrograph of microvilli cut in cross section, showing that each microvillus has an outer plasma membrane and a core of actin filaments. **Fig. 5.12** is a scanning electron micrograph of the inner lining of the uterus, showing the appearance of microvilli on the surface of these cells. In this image, the grooves represent the borders between the cells, and each cell has over one hundred microvilli visible.

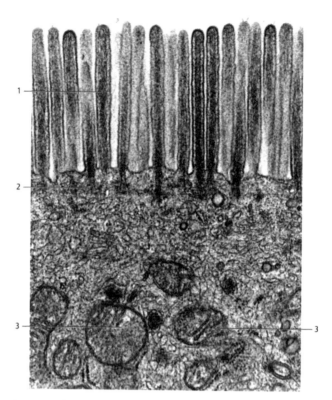

Fig. 5.10   **Electron micrograph of microvilli sectioned longitudinally (1). The terminal web (2) and mitochondria (3) are also shown.**

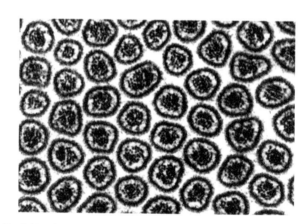

Fig. 5.11   **Electron micrograph of microvilli in cross section.**

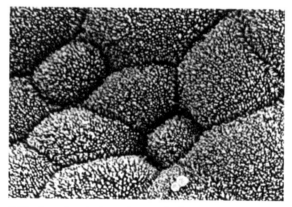

Fig. 5.12   **Scanning electron micrograph of uterine inner lining; grooves are intercellular borders and tiny projections are microvilli.**

When trying to identify surface modifications in electron micrographs, it helps to identify the core proteins. Actin microfilaments are fine structures and bundle together within the microvillus. Microvilli are relatively short (compare to mitochondria at 3 in **Fig. 5.10**).

More will be discussed on this after cilia and stereocilia are introduced.

5.4.2 Cilia

The core protein in **cilia** is microtubules (made of polymers of alpha and beta tubulin). Cilia are actively moved by the cell in an ATP-driven process. For example, cilia of the respiratory epithelium move mucus across the surface of these cells. Cilia are large enough to be seen individually in light micrographs (**Fig. 5.13**).

Video 5.6   Cilia

Be able to identify:
— Cilia

https://www.thieme.de/de/q.htm?p=opn/
tp/308390101/978-1-62623-414-7_c005_
v006&t=video

As mentioned, height is a useful tool to identify surface modifications in light micrographs. Recall that microvilli are one-tenth to one-fifth the length of the elongated nuclei. Here, cilia are closer to half the length of the nucleus.

In electron micrographs, cilia appear as elongated structures when cut longitudinally (**Fig. 5.14a**). As mentioned, the core protein in cilia is microtubules oriented longitudinally. In cross section (**Fig. 5.14b**), the microtubules are arranged such that nine microtubules form an outer ring, with two microtubules in the center (9+2 arrangement). Therefore, in longitudinal section, the microtubules are seen as three dark lines within the cilia. Compare this to microvilli (1 in **Fig. 5.14a**), which are shorter and have a finer internal structure than the dark microtubules found within cilia. Each microtubular arrangement of a cilium is anchored by a **basal body** (2).

Fig. 5.15 shows a scanning electron micrograph of the inner lining of the uterus, showing that cilia are elongated structures emanating from the apical surface of a cell. Other cells can be seen that have microvilli (appearing as short bulges) on their surface.

5.4.3 Stereocilia

Stereocilia are very long processes that are found in only a few cell types in the male reproductive system (**Fig. 5.16**) as well as the inner ear. Stereocilia were once thought to be similar to cilia, but the core protein in stereocilia is now known to be actin filaments rather than microtubules. Therefore, stereocilia are more similar to microvilli. In the male reproductive system, they serve to increase surface area for absorption.

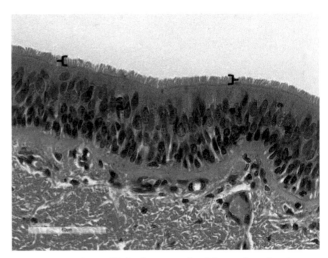

Fig. 5.13   **Pseudostratified columnar cells of the trachea showing numerus cilia (brackets).**

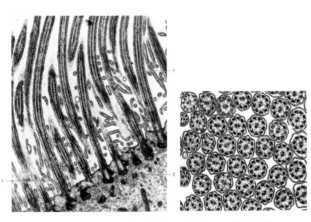

Fig. 5.14   **Electron micrographs of cilia in (a) longitudinal (cilia are marked with red Xs; microvilli [1] and basal body [2] are also visible) and (b) cross-sectional views.**

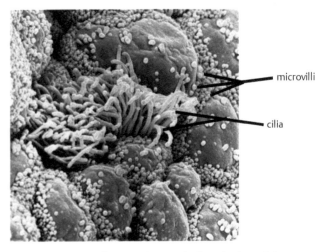

microvilli

cilia

Fig. 5.15   **Scanning electron micrograph of uterine inner lining.**

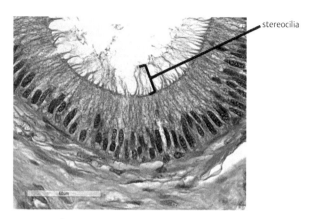

Fig. 5.16 **Light micrograph of the epididymis; note the elongated stereocilia (bracket).**

Video 5.7 Stereocilia

Be able to identify:
— Stereocilia
https://www.thieme.de/de/q.htm?p=opn/tp/308390101/978-1-62623-414-7_c005_v007&t=video

When viewing surface modifications in light micrographs, it helps to note their length. Recall that microvilli are one-tenth to one-fifth the length of the elongated nuclei, while cilia are closer to half the size of the nucleus. Stereocilia are much longer, certainly longer than the nucleus—up to half the size of the columnar cells or even longer.

5.4.4 Basolateral Infoldings

A final modification of the plasma membrane are basolateral infoldings. These are undulations of the plasma membrane on the basolateral side of the cell (**Fig. 5.17**). Note that they are quite extensive; close examination reveals that many extend close to the nucleus. Like microvilli, basolateral infoldings increase the surface area of the plasma membrane. Not surprisingly, cells involved in active transport have numerous basolateral infoldings.

5.5 Chapter Review

The plasma membrane of epithelial cells (and other cells) have specializations that provide specific functions for the cell. Epithelial cells are joined by cell-cell junctions on their lateral aspect, including tight junctions, belt desmosomes, desmosomes, and gap junctions. Tight junctions restrict movement of fluid between the epithelial cells (i.e., prevent movement between the luminal side and the connective tissue side). The two types of desmosome junctions provide strength, while gap junctions allow small molecules to pass from cell to cell. Hemidesmosomes, which are similar to desmosomes, anchor the basal plasma membrane to the underlying basement membrane. Apical surface modifications include microvilli and stereocilia, both of which

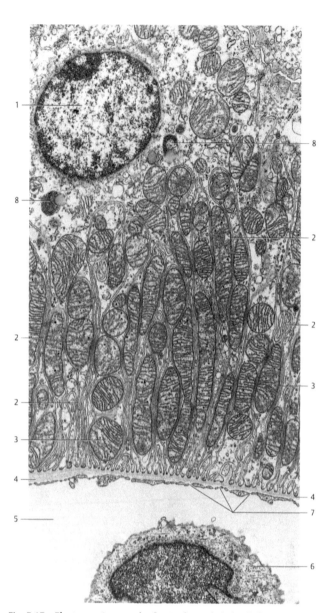

Fig. 5.17 **Electron micrograph of a single epithelial cell showing nucleus (1), basolateral infoldings (2), mitochondria (3), basement membrane (4), and lysosome (8). The connective tissue on the other bottom side of the basement membrane consists of a capillary with lumen of capillary (5), white blood cell (6), and capillary wall (7).**

contain a core of actin microfilaments and increase surface area. Cilia have a core microtubule structure and are actively moved by the cell using energy stored in ATP. On the basal aspect of the cell, basolateral infoldings can provide an increase in surface area for membrane-bound proteins.

An online-only section of questions and answers accompanying this chapter is hosted on Thieme's MedOne Education site: https://medone-education.thieme.com. Use the code on the media page at the front of this book to gain access. An institutional license to the site is required to access these questions in an interactive format, and individual users are required to register for an individual account to track results.

6   Epithelia: Glands

After completing this chapter, you should be able to:
— Identify, at the light microscope level under H and E stain, each of the following
  • Unicellular glands (goblet cells)
  • Multicellular glands
    ○ Mucous glands
    ○ Serous glands
    ○ Serous demilunes
— Outline the secretory component and function of each structure listed
— Predict the appearance of each structure on other types of stains (PAS) or in electron micrographs

6.1   Epithelial Tissues as Glands

Many epithelial cells are involved in active secretion of substances they produce. In many cases, epithelial cells become very active in secretion and are referred to as **glands**. Glands come in a variety of shapes and sizes; they can be single cells (unicellular) that remain part of the epithelial sheet or multicellular structures that grow from the epithelium to form a distinct structure. Here, the basic principles of glandular formation, structure, and secretion will be introduced. Glands are then revisited in subsequent chapters as they are encountered in discussions of structures and organs.

Glandular cells secrete their substances either **apically** into a lumen or **basally** into the connective tissue. Therefore, a feature of many of these cells is an elaborate secretory apparatus involving rough endoplasmic reticulum, Golgi apparatus, and secretory vesicles. The extent of these organelles varies, depending on the specific function of the secretory cells.

6.2   Unicellular Glands

As just stated, individual cells in an epithelium may specialize to perform a secretory function. In these cases, the cell remains continuous with the epithelial sheet but is readily distinguished because it takes on a secretory appearance. **Fig. 6.1** shows simple columnar epithelium that includes scattered **goblet cells,** which secrete mucus that protects the inner lining of the intestinal tract. These cells are easily recognized because the apical half of the cytoplasm is engorged with numerous secretory vesicles (black arrows). The mucus does not stain well with H and E, so this region of the cell is paler than neighboring cells. The nucleus is in the basal half of the cell (yellow arrows), a region that is narrower than the apical region. Therefore, these cells take on a goblet shape.

Video 6.1   Goblet cells (H & E)

Be able to identify:
— Goblet cells
https://www.thieme.de/de/q.htm?p=opn/
tp/308390101/978-1-62623-414-7_c006_v001&t=video

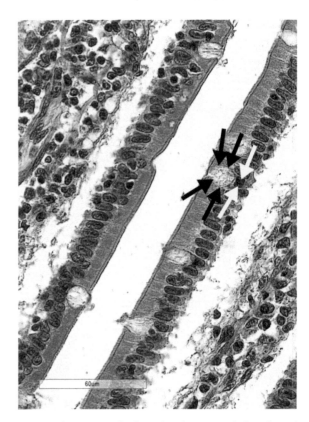

Fig. 6.1   **Light micrograph of simple columnar epithelium from the intestine. The cytoplasm (black arrows) and nucleus (yellow arrows) of a single secretory cell, called a goblet cell, is shown.**

The mucus secreted by goblet cells consists of proteins that are heavily glycosylated. Therefore, the apical region of goblet cells is intensely PAS positive (**Fig. 6.2**).

Video 6.2   Goblet cells (PAS)

Be able to identify:
— Goblet cells
https://www.thieme.de/de/q.htm?p=opn/
tp/308390101/978-1-62623-414-7_c006_v002&t=video

Helpful Hint

Sometimes it is difficult to tell which nucleus belongs to the goblet cell and which nuclei belong to neighboring cells. In most cases, making this distinction is not important.

6.3   Multicellular Glands

Multicellular glands develop from an epithelium (**Fig. 6.3**). In **Fig. 6.3a–c**, the epithelium is separated from the underlying connective tissue by a basement membrane. During development, the

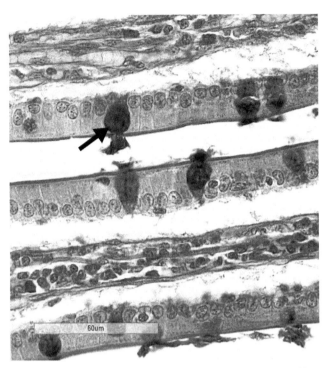

Fig. 6.2   **Light micrograph of cells from intestinal lining, stained by PAS; goblet cells are easily identified (black arrow).**

epithelial cells proliferate and grow into the underlying connective tissue. Note that the basement membrane also extends to maintain its position between the epithelium and connective tissue.

After proliferation of the epithelium, the cells can organize into one of two types of gland: endocrine or exocrine.

6.3.1 Endocrine Gland Formation

In **endocrine gland** formation (**Fig. 6.3d**), the newly formed epithelial cells separate from the original epithelium and form a cluster of cells, in most cases lacking a lumen. These cells release their products basally (blue arrows in **Fig. 6.3d**), across the basement membrane and into the connective tissue, to be picked up by the bloodstream. An example of an endocrine gland is the pituitary gland. Individual endocrine glands will be discussed in more detail later.

6.3.2 Exocrine Gland Formation

In **exocrine gland** formation (**Fig. 6.3e**), the newly formed epithelial cells remain connected to the original epithelium, and a **lumen** forms in the center. Typically, the deeper cells become the active unit, called the **gland** or **secretory unit,** and secrete their product apically (blue arrows in **Fig. 6.3e**) into the lumen. Secreted products flow toward the surface of the epithelium through a **duct,** which is lined by inactive (or less active) cells. Examples of exocrine glands include sweat glands in the skin. Exocrine glands are discussed here and then revisited as they are encountered in later chapters.

Helpful Hint

The branching pattern in exocrine glands is quite variable. The ducts can be simple (unbranched) or complex (branched). The secretory pieces can be acinar (round) or tubular (elongated) and can also branch. There is a nomenclature schema to name the types of exocrine glands based on these criteria that some may find useful. In a single section or image, it is usually not possible to classify glands in this way. However, terms referring to this morphology, such as **acinus** (plural **acini**) for a round secretory end piece, are still useful.

Gland formation

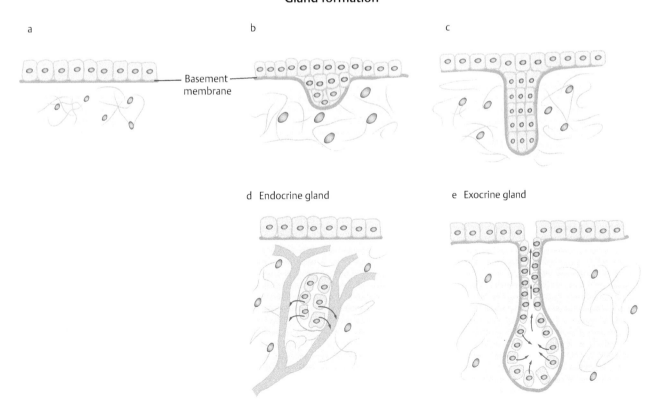

Fig. 6.3   **Development of multicellular glands. (a)–(c) Growth of epithelial cells into the connective tissue and extension of basement membrane. (d) Endocrine gland formation. (e) Exocrine gland formation.**

6.4   Exocrine Glands

Salivary glands (e.g., the parotid gland) are excellent examples of exocrine glands (**Fig. 6.4**). During development, the glandular tissue proliferates extensively to form large glands, with the secretory units packed closely together.

Fig. 6.4 shows four secretory end pieces (acini) connected to a single duct (black bracket) of a salivary gland. Closer to the secretory portion, the duct is lined by a simple cuboidal epithelium, but it transitions to a simple columnar and then stratified cuboidal/columnar as the duct enlarges.

The secretory end pieces are lined by different cell types:
1. **Serous glands** (serous-secreting cells, **Fig. 6.4**, green arrows): These cells produce a protein-based secretion. Therefore, they exhibit cytoplasmic basophilia in their basal aspect. The nucleus is round and located in the basal aspect of the cell. The apical region of these cells is eosinophilic.
2. **Mucous glands** (mucus-secreting cells, **Fig. 6.4**, blue arrows): These cells produce mucus, which does not stain well with H and E. Therefore, the cells have a pale (or washed-out) appearance. The nuclei in these cells are flattened and basally located to accommodate the abundant mucus-containing secretory vesicles.
3. **Serous demilunes** (**Fig. 6.4**, red arrow): These cells are serous-secreting cells, similar to the serous glands, but are associated with mucous glands and secrete their product into the lumen of the mucous glands.

The submandibular salivary gland contains both mucus- and serous-secreting acini, as well as serous demilunes (**Fig. 6.5**), so it provides an excellent tissue to compare these structures. In this image, two secretory units are outlined. The lumen of the secretory unit outlined in black is indicated by the X. The lumen of the secretory unit outlined in yellow is collapsed due to tissue fixation; this is typically the case for most acini. Each secretory end piece (acinus) is round, usually with 6 to 12 cells visible. Not all acini appear perfectly round, either because they are more elongated or because of sectioning.

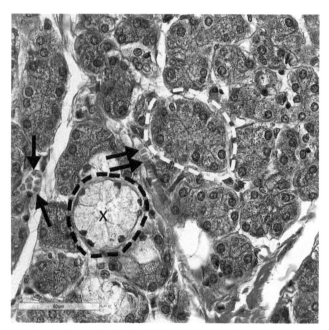

Fig. 6.5   **Submandibular gland showing mucous- (black outline) and serous- (yellow outline) secreting acini. The lumen of the mucous acinus (X) and blood vessels containing red blood cells (black arrows) are indicated.**

Fig. 6.5 highlights the histologic differences between serous and mucous acini:
1. Serous glands (serous-secreting cells, yellow outline): These cells produce a watery, protein-based secretion. Note the eosinophilic cytoplasm, with cytoplasmic basophilia in the basal aspect of the cells. The nucleus is round and located in the basal aspect of the cell.
2. Mucous glands (mucus-secreting cells, black outline): The mucus in these cells does not stain well with H & E. The nuclei in these cells are flattened against the basal side of the cell.

The black arrows in the image indicate blood vessels.

Fig. 6.6 shows more serous (yellow outline) and mucous acini (black outline), as well as a serous demilune (yellow arrow). The cells of a serous demilune are serous-secreting, so they are eosinophilic with cytoplasmic basophilia, but are associated with mucous glands. The product is secreted into the lumen of the mucous glands with which they are associated.

Organs that secrete are referred to as glands (e.g. submandibular gland). They are composed of hundreds/thousands of units called acini, which are clusters of individual secretory cells. Because each acinus or individual cell secretes product, many histologists refer to acini or even individual cells as glands. Therefore, as seen above, glands and acini are used interchangeably.

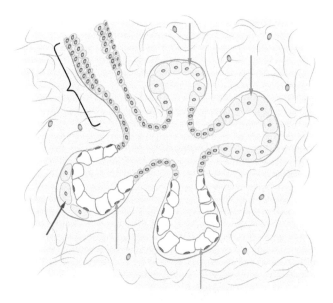

Fig. 6.4   **Schematic of a salivary gland showing serous glands (green arrows), mucous glands (blue arrows), a serous demilune (red arrow) and a duct (black bracket).**

Video 6.3   Mucous and serous glands

Be able to identify:
— Mucous glands
— Serous glands
— Serous demilunes

https://www.thieme.de/de/q.htm?p=opn/tp/308390101/978-1-62623-414-7_c006_v003&t=video

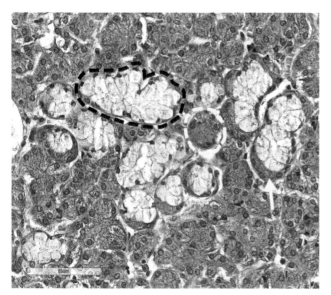

Fig. 6.6   **Submandibular gland showing serous demilune (yellow arrow), serous acinus (yellow outline), and mucous acinus (black outline).**

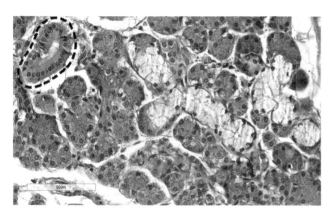

Fig. 6.7   **Submandibular gland showing duct (black outline).**

Finally, ducts of multicellular glands (**Fig. 6.7**, black outline) transmit secretory product to the surface. These ducts consist of an epithelium that is either simple cuboidal, simple columnar, or stratified cuboidal/columnar, surrounded by connective tissue. The epithelial cells of ducts are pale and eosinophilic. Ducts will be discussed in greater detail in the chapter on the oral cavity.

6.5   Chapter Review

In addition to forming sheets of cells that form a barrier, cells of an epithelium may become specialized for secretion. Epithelial cells that secrete products basally into the connective tissue are called endocrine glands (discussed in later chapters), while cells that secrete product apically are called exocrine glands (discussed in this chapter). In some cases of exocrine glands, individual cells within an epithelium become secretory. The most notable examples of this are goblet cells found in the intestine and respiratory system. In contrast to these unicellular glands, multicellular glands are formed through a proliferation of epithelial cells that extends into the underlying connective tissue. The resulting cluster of epithelial cells secretes products that flow to the surface epithelium via ducts. The clusters of cells (acini) can be either serous- or mucous-secreting.

Questions and Answers

An online-only section of questions and answers accompanying this chapter is hosted on Thieme's MedOne Education site: https://medone-education.thieme.com. Use the code on the media page at the front of this book to gain access. An institutional license to the site is required to access these questions in an interactive format, and individual users are required to register for an individual account to track results.

7   Connective Tissue Overview

After completing this chapter, you should be able to:
— Identify, at the light microscope level, each of the following components of connective tissue:
  • Collagen fibers
  • Elastic fibers (may need special stains)
  • Reticular fibers (seen with special stains only)
  • Fibroblasts
  • Mast cells (distinguished only with special stains: metachromasia)
  • Ground substance
— Identify, at the electron microscope level, each of the following components of connective tissue:
  • Collagen fibers
  • Elastic fibers
  • Fibroblast
— Outline the function of each of these structures or cells
— Predict the extracellular fibers that would be prominent in a tissue or organ given the function of that tissue or organ

7.1   Overview of Connective Tissue

Connective tissues are a diverse class, ranging from fluid (blood) to solid (bone). Although connective tissues are diverse in their overall structure and function, the unifying theme that is consistent among almost all connective tissues is that they are composed of relatively fewer cells and more extracellular matrix (ECM) than is found in epithelia. Connective tissues are all formed from a common precursor: embryonic mesenchyme.

This chapter will describe the cells and ECM of connective tissue, which will provide the foundation for discussion of specific connective tissue types. Subsequent chapters in this sequence will address these specific connective tissue types: generic connective tissues, adipose tissue, cartilage, and bone. Blood is addressed in the cardiovascular sequence beginning with **Chapter 16**.

7.2   Recognizing Connective Tissue

Before analyzing connective tissue in detail, it helps to recognize first that a tissue is indeed some form of connective tissue. Unlike epithelia, which are composed of many cells with little ECM, connective tissues typically are composed of relatively few cells, with much more ECM (**Fig. 7.1** and **Fig. 7.2**). On an H and E slide, this is readily apparent by comparing the number of nuclei in epithelia and connective tissue. The basement membrane separates the epithelium from the connective tissue (green dotted lines in **Figs. 7.1** and **7.2**).

> **Helpful Hint**
>
> It helps to remember that epithelia line a lumen, or space. Also note that epithelial cells tend to have more cytoplasm, which stains eosinophilic, while connective tissue cytoplasm is pale or sparse.

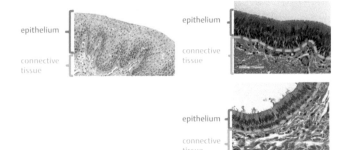

Fig. 7.1   In these three examples, connective and epithelial tissue can be seen. Note fewer nuclei and increased cellular matrix of connective tissue. In each image, the green dashed line indicates the border between epithelial and connective tissues; that is, the location of the basement membrane.

7.3   Components of Connective Tissue

The cells of connective tissue come in two types (**Fig. 7.3**):
1. "Native" cells, known as **fibroblasts**, are cells that originally developed within the connective tissue and secrete the components of the ECM. They typically have a tapered appearance, often called spindle-shaped (**Fig. 7.3**, blue arrows).
2. "Invading" cells are mostly immune cells (white blood cells) that develop in bone marrow and migrate into the connective tissue to serve an immune function. On the right side of **Fig. 7.3**, there is a row of cells that are more cuboidal and have more eosinophilic cytoplasm than fibroblasts have; these are most likely white blood cells.

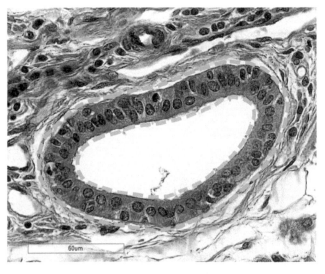

Fig. 7.2   In this specimen of a duct, the epithelial tissue is between the dashed lines and the connective tissue is everything else (except the space). The basement membrane is in the approximate location of the green dashed line.

fibroblast cytoplasm and nucleus

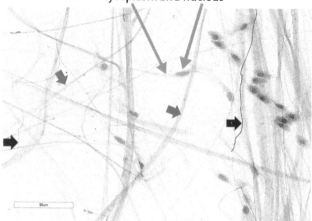

Fig. 7.3 **Light micrograph of connective tissue (H and E stain). Purple arrows indicate collagen fibers; black arrows indicate elastic fibers.**

The extracellular material in connective tissue can be broken down into two categories:

1. Fibers are elongated structures composed of proteins secreted by fibroblasts. These include **collagen fibers** (**Fig. 7.3**, purple arrows), **elastic fibers** (**Fig. 7.3**, black arrows), and **reticular fibers** (not visible in routine staining, but will be seen later with special stains).
2. **Matrix**, or **ground substance**, is the fluid component of extracellular material that fills in the space between the fibers. Ground substance (discussed later in Section 7.7) is composed of water, ions, and organic molecules such as glycosaminoglycans.

The fibers of connective tissue are addressed first, followed by a brief description of the development of connective tissue, and then a discussion of the cells of connective tissue.

7.4 Connective Tissue Fibers

Collagen fibers in H & E and electron micrographs.

7.4.1 Collagen

Collagen is the most abundant protein in the human body. Collagen provides strength to tissues, preventing stretching; this is referred to as tensile strength.

Synthesized in the rough endoplasmic reticulum (RER) and further processed in the Golgi complex, these proteins are secreted into the ECM, where they assemble into large fibers or sheets. There are different types of collagens, synthesized from combinations of different collagen polypeptides. However, for most histologic purposes, understanding four types of collagen suffices:

— Collagen Type I, found in generic connective tissues and bone, forms thick, ropelike structures.
— Collagen Type II, found in cartilage only, forms thin, threadlike structures.
— Collagen Type III, found in generic connective tissues, forms thin, threadlike structures.
— Collagen Type IV, found in basement membranes, forms sheets.

The basement membrane has already been discussed in the epithelium chapters. This chapter will focus on type I and type III collagen, as these are found in generic connective tissues. Type II collagen will be addressed in **Chapter 10** on cartilage.

Fig. 7.4a, b are two images of generic connective tissues. In routine H and E stains, type I collagen fibers appear as eosinophilic threads or bands. The thickness and abundance of collagen fibers varies; many of the fibers are much larger than the cells that secrete them. Black arrows show collagen fibers sectioned longitudinally; the purple arrows indicate collagen fibers cut in cross section. **Fig. 7.4c** shows an electron micrograph of connective tissue; note the collagen fibers in longitudinal section (red circle) and in cross section (green circle). Collagen fibers in longitudinal section demonstrate a characteristic banding pattern; in cross section they are round.

It is important to note that one collagen fiber on the electron micrograph does *not* correspond to a collagen fiber seen in **Fig. 7.4a, b**. This may be intuitive, as these are at significantly different magnifications. In fact, it is more likely that a bundle of collagen fibers (e.g., all the fibers outlined in red or green in the electron micrograph in **Fig. 7.4c**) represents one of the thinner collagen fibers in the light micrograph (**Fig. 7.4a, b**).

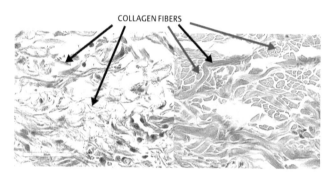

COLLAGEN FIBERS

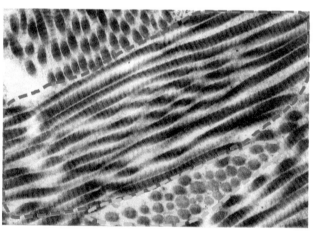

Fig. 7.4 **In H & E stained sections, collagen fibers are seen as eosinophilic extracellular structures, either as thin threads (a) or thick bundles (b). The black arrows indicate fibers oriented longitudinally; purple arrows show fibers in cross section. An electron micrograph of collagen fibers is shown in (c), showing collagen fibers in longitudinal (red outline) and cross section (green outline). For perspective, the bundle outlined in red would be similar to one of the thinner threads in a.**

Video 7.1 Collagen fibers—1

https://www.thieme.de/de/q.htm?p=opn/tp/308390101/978-1-62623-414-7_c007_v001&t=video

CHAPTER 7

Video 7.2   Collagen fibers—2

Be able to identify:
— Collagen fibers
https://www.thieme.de/de/q.htm?p=opn/
tp/308390101/978-1-62623-414-7_c007_v002&t=video

elastin core, with a somewhat darker border. Contrast this to the dark stippled appearance of the collagen fibers (labeled 1 in the figure).

Video 7.4   Elastic fibers—H and E

https://www.thieme.de/de/q.htm?p=opn/tp/308390101/978-1-62623-414-7_c007_v004&t=video

7.4.1 Reticular Fibers

The proteins making up reticular fibers (type III collagen fibers) are homologous to those that make up collagen fibers. Indeed, individual reticular fibers seen on electron micrographs are indistinguishable from those that make up collagen fibers (see **Fig. 7.4**). However, reticular fibers do not bundle as extensively as collagen fibers, so they are too thin to be seen in routine H and E-stained images (**Fig. 7.5a**). To visualize reticular fibers in light micrographs, special stains, such as silver stains, are used. **Fig. 7.5b** is a specimen from the spleen prepared using a silver stain, visualizing the reticular fibers (yellow arrows).

Video 7.5   Elastic fibers—resorcin

https://www.thieme.de/de/q.htm?p=opn/
tp/308390101/978-1-62623-414-7_c007_v005&t=video

Video 7.6   Collagen and elastic fibers

Be able to identify:
— Elastic fibers
— Collagen fibers
https://www.thieme.de/de/q.htm?p=opn/tp/308390101/978-1-62623-414-7_c007_v006&t=video

Video 7.3   Reticular fibers

Be able to identify:
— Reticular fibers
https://www.thieme.de/de/q.htm?p=opn/
tp/308390101/978-1-62623-414-7_c007_v003&t=video

7.4.2 Elastic Fibers

Elastic fibers are an entirely different type of extracellular structure from collagen or reticular fibers. Whereas collagen and reticular fibers provide resistance to stretching, elastic fibers can be stretched and are able to return to their original shape after the stretching forces are removed.

Like reticular fibers, elastic fibers are often thin and do not stain well on routine H & E sections. However, in tissues such as large elastic arteries, they form prominent eosinophilic sheets that are readily apparent on H & E (**Fig. 7.6a**, blue arrows) or with special stains (**Fig. 7.6b**, resorcin stain, yellow arrows). Also note that, because elastic fibers recoil during tissue fixation, they tend to have a wavy appearance.

As mentioned, elastic fibers are quite different from collagen fibers in terms of their protein composition and function. **Fig. 7.7** is an electron micrograph showing elastic fibrils (one is outlined in red), which demonstrate several dark microfibrils within a paler

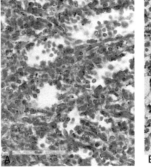

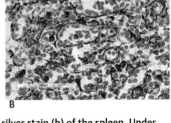

Fig. 7.5   H and E stain (a) and silver stain (b) of the spleen. Under the silver stain, reticular fibers can be seen (yellow arrows). Many of the nuclei are white blood cells; red blood cells are also visible. The spaces are the lumina of blood vessels.

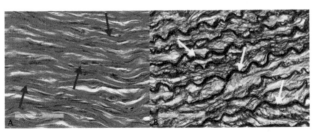

Fig, 7.6   H and E (a) and resorcin (b) stains of elastic fibers (arrows) from an elastic artery.

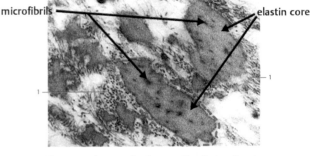

Fig. 7.7   Electron micrograph of connective tissue showing an elastic fiber (red outline) and collagen fibers (1). Elastic fibers are composed of thin microfibrils embedded in an elastin core.

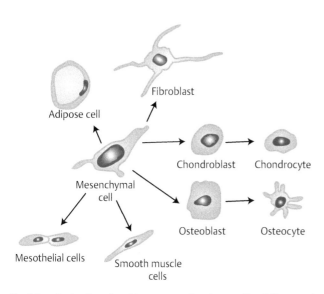

Fig. 7.8 **Derivation of resident connective tissue cells. Cell types of connective tissue, including fibroblasts, adipose cells, epithelial cells (mesothelial cells), muscle cells, cartilage cells (chondroblasts and chondrocytes) and bone cells (osteoblasts and osteocytes), are all derived from a common precursor called a mesenchymal cell.**

7.5 Development of Connective Tissue

Almost all connective tissues, and some other tissues such as muscle, are derived from an embryonic precursor tissue called mesenchyme (**Fig. 7.8**). This tissue is composed of mesenchymal cells surrounded by a matrix with very few fibers. The cells of mesenchyme will mature into a variety of cell types and secrete products consistent with the tissue type they form.

Fig. 7.9 shows a specimen from an umbilical cord and demonstrates the histologic appearance of mesenchyme. In this slide, some cells have nuclei that are paler than the cytoplasm on H & E (black arrows), while others show darker nuclei. Because mesenchyme contains little collagen or elastic fibers, most of the background is clear. Many of the thin structures in the matrix (green arrows) are cell processes; the nuclei of these cells lie outside the plane of section.

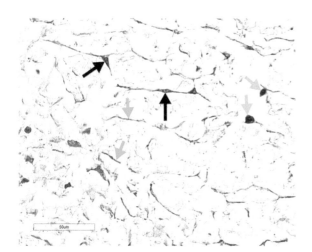

Fig. 7.9 **Light micrograph (H and E) of mesenchyme from umbilical cord specimen. Nuclei may be paler (black arrows) or darker (blue arrows) than the cytoplasm. Many cell processes (green arrows) are also visible.**

Mesenchyme is characterized by the near absence of connective tissue fibers, while loose connective tissue (discussed in Chapter 8) has some collagen and elastic fibers.

Video 7.7   Mesenchyme

Be able to identify:
— Mesenchyme
— Mesenchymal cells
https://www.thieme.de/de/q.htm?p=opn/
tp/308390101/978-1-62623-414-7_c007_v007&t=video

7.6 Connective Tissue Cells

7.6.1 Fibroblasts

Fibroblasts, derived from mesenchymal cells, are the "resident" cells of generic connective tissue that produce most, if not all, of the fibers and matrix. In **Fig. 7.3**, the cytoplasm and nucleus of a fibroblast are indicated, showing that these cells are elongated, with several cell processes.

Video 7.8   Fibroblasts in a connective tissue spread

Be able to identify:
— Fibroblasts
https://www.thieme.de/de/q.htm?p=opn/
tp/308390101/978-1-62623-414-7_c007_v008&t=video

The cytoplasm and nucleus of fibroblasts in a connective tissue spread can be distinguished because the tissue is thin. In most routine tissue sections, fibroblasts can be identified because they usually have elongated nuclei (**Fig. 7.10**, yellow arrows). In most cases, the cytoplasm of fibroblasts cannot be distinguished from surrounding collagen fibers. Cells with round nuclei (black arrows) are most likely white blood cells.

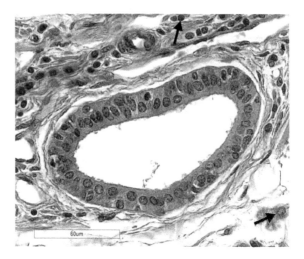

Fig. 7.10 **Fibroblasts can be identified within connective tissue by their elongated nuclei (yellow arrows). Cells with round nuclei (black arrows) are most likely white blood cells.**

Video 7.9   Fibroblasts in routine tissue sections

Be able to identify:
— Fibroblasts
https://www.thieme.de/de/q.htm?p=opn/
tp/308390101/978-1-62623-414-7_c007_v009&t=video

In electron micrographs (**Fig. 7.11**), fibroblasts are elongated or spindle-shaped cells. Active fibroblasts will have abundant RER and Golgi apparatus necessary for synthesis of the extracellular fibers, while quiescent fibroblasts will have less RER and Golgi.

Helpful Hint

Features consistent with fibroblasts include an elongated cell and secretory organelles (RER, Golgi), surrounded by connective tissue fibers. Although other cell types have not been discussed in detail, it should be noted that fibroblasts are often identified by exclusion. In other words, they are fairly generic cells, with few definitive identifying features that can be found in other cell types.

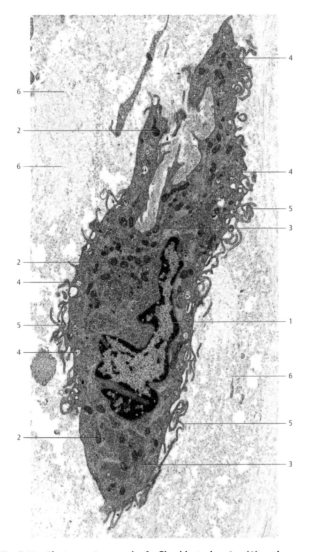

Fig. 7.11   Electron micrograph of a fibroblast, showing (1) nucleus, (2) mitochondria, (3) rough endoplasmic reticulum (RER), (4) secretory vesicles, (5) cell processes (microvilli), (6) extracellular material including collagen fibers.

7.6.2 Immune Cells

Most of the other cells in connective tissues are not permanent residents but immune cells (white blood cells) that are "visiting." These cells arise from the hematopoietic compartment (bone marrow; **Fig. 7.12**, red arrows indicate white blood cells), enter the bloodstream, and migrate into the connective tissues.

Many connective tissues contain a few of these white blood cells. However, when connective tissues are invaded by pathogens, or when some other condition stimulates an immune response (e.g., an autoimmune reaction), large numbers of white blood cells migrate from the bloodstream into the connective tissue. This is referred to as **inflammation**. **Fig. 7.13a** shows connective tissue before an inflammatory response; most of the cells are fibroblasts (green arrows). **Fig. 7.13b** shows a similar type of connective tissue in which the inflammatory response has been initiated. Note that this tissue includes large numbers of cells with round nuclei and abundant cytoplasm. Most of these are white blood cells, notably plasma cells (red arrows) and neutrophils (yellow arrow) that have infiltrated into the connective tissue in response to an infection. For comparison, a fibroblast (green arrow) can be recognized by its elongated nucleus and tapered cytoplasm.

Video 7.10 Inflammation

Be able to identify:
— Inflammation
https://www.thieme.de/de/q.htm?p=opn/
tp/308390101/978-1-62623-414-7_c007_v010&t=video

Clinical Correlate

Inflammation occurs in a wide number of conditions and is usually beneficial because it is the process by which the body destroys pathogens and repairs damaged tissue. However, the inflammatory response can be destructive, as seen in autoimmune conditions such as rheumatoid arthritis.

There are many types of white blood cells in connective tissue. Most of these will be discussed in detail in later chapters on the immune system. To provide some sense of the types of immune cells in connective tissue, two of these cell types will be briefly described here.

Macrophages

Macrophages are derived from monocytes and are found in many tissues throughout the body. The name macrophage ("big eater") aptly describes their characteristic phagocytic capacity. In addition, macrophages play roles in inflammation and in immune responses. **Fig. 7.14** shows a single macrophage surrounded by collagen fibrils.

Mast Cells

Mast cells are immune cells that play a role in inflammation. In electron micrographs (**Fig. 7.15**), they demonstrate numerous large secretory granules (arrows), which contain **histamine** and **heparin**. In inflammation, these substances are released;

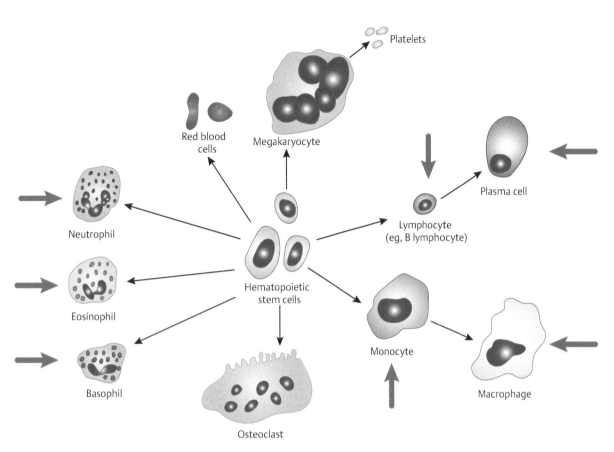

Fig. 7.12   Derivation of immune cells (red arrows) from a common precursors called hematopoietic stem cells. Red arrows indicate white blood cells.

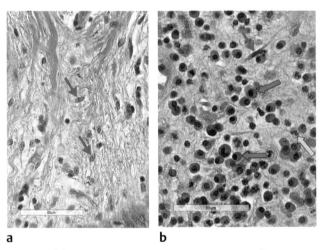

a   **b**

Fig. 7.13   (a) Generic connective tissue; green arrows indicate fibroblasts. (b) Inflammation, in which the connective tissue has been "invaded" by white blood cells (red arrows mark plasma cells, yellow arrow indicates a neutrophil).

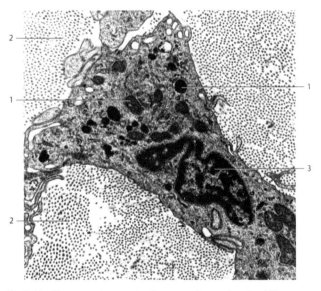

Fig. 7.14   Electron micrograph of a macrophage, showing (1) lysosomes, (2) collagen fibers, (3) nucleus.

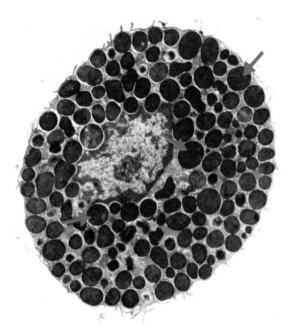

Fig. 7.15 Electron micrograph of a mast cell with secretory granules (red arrows).

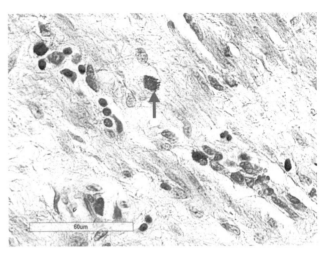

Fig. 7.16 Connective tissue specimen stained with toluidine blue, which stains collagen fibers and nuclei blue but stains secretory granules of mast cells purple (red arrow).

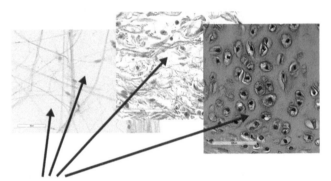

Fig. 7.17 Ground substance of connective tissue (arrows) is the extracellular substance not including the collagen and elastic fibers, and ranges from fluid (left, middle) to solid (right).

histamine increases the permeability of vessels to white blood cells, and heparin is an anticoagulant.

The components of the secretory granules in mast cells demonstrate a specific type of staining quality called **metachromasia**, in which the components of a cell or tissue changes the original color of a dye. **Fig. 7.16** shows an image from connective tissue stained with the dye toluidine blue. Here, many structures are stained blue, including collagen fibers and nuclei. The contents of the mast cell granules turn the dye a purple color (red arrow). Many of the nuclei with pale cytoplasm belong to fibroblasts, although some belong to other white blood cells.

Video 7.11 Mast cells

Be able to identify:
— Mast cells
https://www.thieme.de/de/q.htm?p=opn/
tp/308390101/978-1-62623-414-7_c007_v011&t=video

7.7 Connective Tissue Ground Substance

The ground substance of connective tissue is the ECM component that fills in the spaces between the fibers and cells (**Fig. 7.17**). It contains water, ions, glycosaminoglycans, and other molecules. The proportions of the specific components vary considerably and account for the fact that the consistency of ground substance (and connective tissues) ranges from fluid, as seen in the left and middle images in **Fig. 7.17**, which are from generic connective tissues, to solid (right image in **Fig. 7.17**, taken from cartilage).

7.8 Chapter Review

Connective tissues are a diverse class, ranging from liquid (blood) to solid (bone). Connective tissue, as well as muscle, is derived from

embryonic mesenchyme. The main feature that is consistent among most connective tissue types is the fact that they consist of few cells and large amounts of ECM. The components of connective tissue include the matrix fibers, cells, and ground substance. The matrix fibers include collagens (both type I and type III fibers), which provide tensile strength, as well as elastic fibers, which allow the tissue to stretch and then return to its original shape. The fluid portion of the extracellular matrix, known as ground substance, consists of water, ions, buffers, and other molecules. Fibroblasts are the native cells of connective tissue and produce most of the extracellular fibers and components. Most other cells found in connective tissue are white blood cells, which are produced by the bone marrow and migrate into the connective tissue to perform immune functions.

Questions and Answers

An online-only section of questions and answers accompanying this chapter is hosted on Thieme's MedOne Education site: https://medone-education.thieme.com. Use the code on the media page at the front of this book to gain access. An institutional license to the site is required to access these questions in an interactive format, and individual users are required to register for an individual account to track results.

8 Generic Connective Tissues

After completing this chapter, you should be able to:
— Identify, at the light microscope level, each of the following types of connective tissue:
  • Loose (areolar)
    ○ Reticular tissue
    ○ Elastic tissue
  • Dense irregular
  • Dense regular (e.g., tendon)
— Outline the function of the generic connective tissues listed
— Predict the type of generic connective tissue in an organ or structure given its function

8.1 Classification of Connective Tissue

Chapter 7 provided an overview of connective tissue and discussed the components of connective tissue (cells, fibers, ground substance). The types of connective tissues are presented in this and subsequent chapters. As mentioned, these range from liquid (blood) to solid (bone) and have a wide range of characteristics (e.g., strength, flexibility). The wide variety of tissues that compose the connective tissue class is created largely by the substances secreted by the connective tissue cells (e.g., fibroblasts) into the extracellular matrix (ECM). In general, all types of connective tissues have some of each basic component (collagen, elastic fibers, ground substance). However, what defines a specific type of connective tissue is the relative amount of each. For example, tissues that require resistance to stretching (e.g., tendons) are composed mostly of type I collagen fibers, while tissues that expand (e.g., the aorta) have large amounts of elastic fibers. Some tissues, such as the dermis of the skin, have a relatively balanced mixture of collagen and elastic fibers, providing both strength and flexibility.

As with epithelium, the structure and function of connective tissue will be discussed, providing examples of tissues or organs in which these are found. It is not important to memorize the list of these tissue locations at this time. It is much more important to be able to predict where a specific tissue type might be found, and why.

In a broad sense, connective tissue can be classified into generic and specialized:
  • Generic connective tissues
    ○ Loose (or areolar; includes reticular and elastic tissues and perhaps mesenchyme)
    ○ Dense irregular
    ○ Dense regular
These are addressed in this chapter.
  • Specialized connective tissues
    ○ Adipose
    ○ Cartilage (hyaline, elastic, fibrous)
    ○ Bone
    ○ Blood
These are covered in upcoming chapters.

8.2 Generic Connective Tissues

Generic connective tissues are so named because they are found in most tissues of the body. The dermis of the skin is largely composed of generic connective tissue. In addition, generic connective tissues are supporting elements that hold other tissues and organs together. For example, generic connective tissue is interspersed among cardiac muscle cells of the heart, providing support and structure.

The foregoing classification of generic connective tissues into three categories is based on two variables:
  • The density and thickness of the extracellular fibers (loose vs. dense)
  • The orientation of the extracellular fibers (irregular vs. regular)

> **Helpful Hint**
>
> Of course, two variables with two possibilities each should result in a total of four generic connective tissue types; the fourth generic connective tissue type would be "loose regular." As will become clearer after further exploration of this class of tissue, loose regular is not a useful tissue type from a functional standpoint.
>
> Loose connective tissue is irregular, even though "irregular" is not part of the name because loose regular does not exist.

8.2.1 Loose (Areolar) Connective Tissue

Loose connective tissue has the following features:
  • Appearance: Thin collagen and reticular fibers; more space, so it is *loose*; fibers oriented in all directions
  • Function: Not very strong, but is usually well vascularized

Loose connective tissue is found in many locations throughout the body, often serving the role of "filler." Because it is well vascularized, it is the connective tissue immediately adjacent to epithelia, which lack blood vessels.

Although loose connective tissue may have a slightly different appearance based on tissue preparation and staining, it always has few extracellular fibers and relatively more clear space. For example, **Fig. 8.1** is a connective tissue spread (a special type of preparation previously discussed) from the mesentery of the intestines. **Fig. 8.2** shows loose connective tissue in typical H & E-stained slices, demonstrating the appearance of loose connective tissue that will be encountered on most slides. Fibroblasts and extracellular fibers are indicated for review. **Fig. 8.3** shows the inner wall of the heart specially stained for collagen.

All connective tissues vary to some extent in the amount and relative proportion of collagen fibers, reticular fibers, and elastic fibers. The loose connective tissues include different types or subclasses, based on the fibers that predominate in that tissue. These tissues have predictably different functional features.

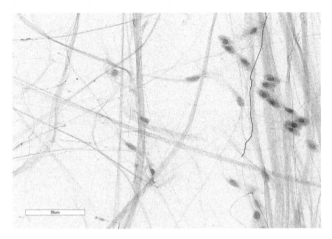

Fig. 8.1   Connective tissue spread.

Reticular Tissue

Fig. 8.4a shows a section of spleen stained with silver, which highlights reticular fibers (yellow arrows), not normally seen on routine H & E preparations. (Cells are red.)

Elastic Tissue

Fig. 8.4b shows a specimen from the lower esophagus, consisting of connective tissue with abundant elastic fibers, which appear as bright eosinophilic bands. Elastic fibers are "shinier" than collagen fibers (they are said to be refractile).

Mesenchyme

Fig. 8.5 shows a specimen from the umbilical cord, containing embryonic mesenchyme. This tissue consists of mesenchymal cells, precursors to connective tissue and muscle cells. Very few extracellular fibers are present (thin threads are cell processes).

8.2.2 Dense Irregular Connective Tissue

Dense irregular connective tissue has the following features:
- Appearance: Thick collagen (type I) fibers, packed close together, so it is *dense*; collagen fibers oriented in all directions, so it is *irregular*
- Function: Strong in multiple directions, but usually not as well vascularized as loose connective tissue

Fig. 8.6 shows dense regular connective tissue from the dermis of the skin. Note the very large collagen fibers, many of which are much thicker than the fibroblasts that made them. The collagen fibers in this tissue are in different orientations, so the fibers are cut at different angles.

Video 8.1   Loose and dense irregular connective tissue—1

https://www.thieme.de/de/q.htm?p=opn/tp/308390101/978-1-62623-414-7_c008_v001&t=video

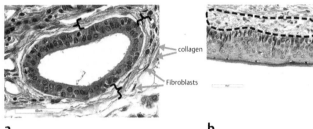

a   b

Fig. 8.2   Loose connective tissue in routine specimens. (a) Loose connective tissue surrounding the epithelium of a duct (black brackets). Fibroblasts and extracellular fibers (collagen) are indicated. (b) Loose connective tissue adjacent to the stratified squamous keratinized epithelium of the skin.

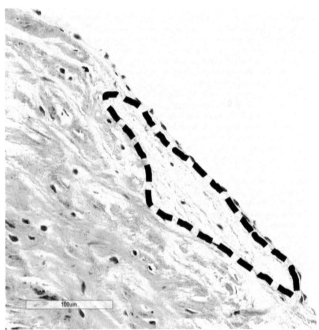

Fig. 8.3   Loose connective tissue (outlined) from the inner lining of the heart stained with Gomori trichrome stain, which highlights collagen (green). Nuclei in this image are red.

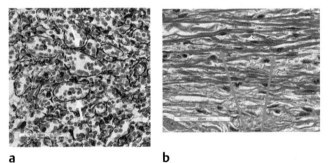

a   b

Fig. 8.4   Reticular and elastic connective tissue. (a) Spleen stained with silver to show reticular fibers (yellow arrows); (b) Lower esophagus stained with H & E, showing refractile elastic fibers.

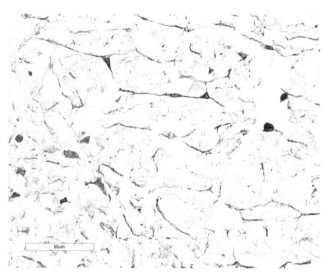

Fig. 8.5 **Embryonic mesenchyme from the umbilical cord.**

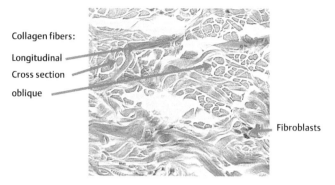

Collagen fibers:

Longitudinal

Cross section

oblique

Fibroblasts

Fig. 8.6 **Dense irregular connective tissue from the dermis of the skin, showing collagen fibers cut in different orientations, as well as a cluster of fibroblasts. Most of the clear spaces between the fibers are artifact.**

Video 8.2 Loose and dense irregular connective tissue—2

Be able to identify:
— Loose connective tissue
— Dense irregular connective tissue
https://www.thieme.de/de/q.htm?p=opn/tp/308390101/978-1-62623-414-7_c008_v002&t=video

The orientation of fibroblast nuclei in dense regular connective tissue indicates the orientation of the collagen fibers. Also note that these fibroblasts are very narrow to accommodate the collagen fibers, so their nuclei are very elongated. Nuclei in other generic connective tissues are round or oval.

Because dense regular connective tissue has a sparse blood supply, these tissues (e.g., ligaments, tendons) take a long time to heal.

In many cases, the density of extracellular fibers in a connective tissue is somewhere between the idealized examples of loose and dense irregular connective tissues just shown. Sometimes, histologists use terms such as "loosely dense" or "densely loose" to describe these.

Video 8.3 Dense regular connective tissue

Be able to identify:
— Dense regular connective tissue
https://www.thieme.de/de/q.htm?p=opn/tp/308390101/978-1-62623-414-7_c008_v003&t=video

8.2.3 Dense Regular Connective Tissue

Dense regular connective tissue has the following features:
- Appearance: Many thick (type I) collagen fibers packed so tightly that individual fibers may be difficult to distinguish, so it is *dense*; collagen fibers oriented in one direction, so it is *regular*
- Function: Strong in one direction (e.g., tendon, ligament), but usually very poorly vascularized

Fig. 8.7 shows dense regular connective tissue from a tendon. In this image, the collagen fibers are oriented from 10 o'clock to 4 o'clock, but this is difficult to appreciate because the individual collagen fibers are hard to see. Fibroblast nuclei are oriented and narrow to accommodate the large, parallel array of collagen fibers between them.

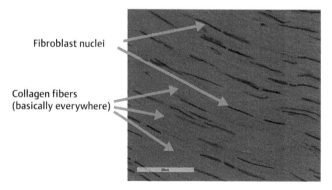

Fibroblast nuclei

Collagen fibers (basically everywhere)

Fig. 8.7 **Dense regular connective tissue from a tendon.**

8.3   Chapter Review

Connective tissues can be broadly divided into generic and specialized connective tissues. Generic connective tissues are found throughout the body, either as large portions of organs (e.g., dermis of the skin) or interspersed among other tissues (e.g., among heart muscle). In this regard, generic connective tissues provide structure and support to the tissues or organs with which they associate. There are three main types of generic connective tissues: loose, dense irregular, and dense regular. These connective tissues differ based on the density and orientation of the extracellular fibers. These differences underscore the function of these tissues. Loose connective tissue is well vascularized, while the dense connective tissues provide more strength.

Questions and Answers

An online-only section of questions and answers accompanying this chapter is hosted on Thieme's MedOne Education site: https://medone-education.thieme.com. Use the code on the media page at the front of this book to gain access. An institutional license to the site is required to access these questions in an interactive format, and individual users are required to register for an individual account to track results.

9   Adipose Tissue

After completing this chapter, you should be able to:
— Identify, at the light microscope level, each of the following
  • Adipose tissue
    ◦ Unilocular
    ◦ Multilocular
— Outline the function of the types of adipose tissue

9.1   Overview of Adipose Tissue

Adipose tissue is a connective tissue specialized to store energy in the form of lipids. In addition, adipose tissue in the skin serves as a thermal insulator to maintain body temperature. Furthermore, adipose tissue surrounds organs such as the kidneys and provides a protective function.

These functions describe the more abundant type of adipose in humans, namely **white fat**. There is a second type of adipose tissue, termed **brown fat**, which generates heat. Brown fat is abundant in hibernating animals and is found in the neck and axilla of human infants.

Fig. 9.1 depicts the development of white and brown fat. As mentioned in the connective tissue overview (**Chapter 7**), connective tissues are derived from mesenchyme. In developing adipose tissue, mesenchymal cells accumulate lipid, becoming **adipocytes (adipose cells)**. The lipid coalesces as small lipid droplets within the cytoplasm of these cells. Adipose tissue in which the cells have numerous small lipid droplets is termed **multilocular adipose tissue**. Brown fat remains multilocular. In white fat, the small lipid droplets converge into a single, large lipid droplet that occupies most of the cell, and the remaining cytoplasmic components and nucleus are thin and in the periphery of the cell; this tissue is called **unilocular adipose tissue**.

9.2   Unilocular Adipose Tissue

As mentioned, cells of unilocular adipose accumulate one large lipid droplet in the cytoplasm. This droplet occupies most of the cell, with the remaining cytoplasm and nucleus relegated to the periphery. **Fig. 9.2** shows a low-magnification image of adipose tissue; two adipocytes are outlined in black. Recall that lipid washes away during routine H & E tissue preparation, so the majority of the adipocyte appears empty. However, note that there is a thin rim of cytoplasm peripherally, and occasional nuclei (arrows) can be seen.

Sparse connective tissue fills in the space between adipocytes (a larger region of connective tissue is outlined in green in **Fig. 9.2**). Because the cytoplasm of the adipocytes and the collagen of the connective tissue between the adipocytes are both eosinophilic, it is difficult to distinguish the border between the adipocytes and the surrounding connective tissue. In addition, fibroblasts and adipocyte nuclei are difficult to distinguish definitively.

Fig. 9.3 shows unilocular adipose taken at higher magnification. Red blood cells (arrows) indicate the location of blood vessels in the connective tissue of adipose. Adipose is well vascularized, which enables rapid storage of lipids from the bloodstream after a meal and rapid mobilization of lipids from adipose into the blood during periods of need.

Adipocytes in a given tissue are roughly the same size, although, occasionally, "larger adipocytes" such as that marked by the X in **Fig. 9.3** can be seen. These are artifacts created when the thin cytoplasm and connective tissue between two or more cells breaks apart during tissue preparation.

Video 9.1   Video of unilocular adipose tissue

Be able to identify:
— Unilocular adipose tissue
https://www.thieme.de/de/q.htm?p=opn/
tp/308390101/978-1-62623-414-7_c009_
v001&t=video

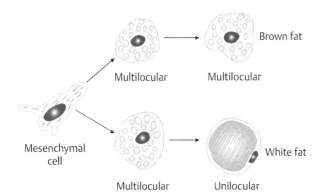

Fig. 9.1   **Development of adipose tissue.**

Development of adipose

Mesenchymal cell

Multilocular → Multilocular → Brown fat

Multilocular → Unilocular → White fat

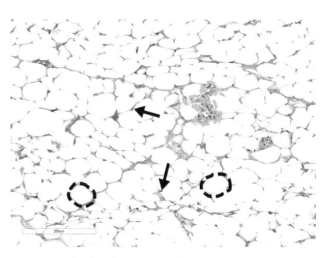

Fig. 9.2   **Unilocular adipose tissue at low magnification. Two adipocytes are outlined in black. The cytoplasm and nucleus of these cells are forced to the periphery of the cell; two nuclei are indicated by the black arrows. The green outline represents connective tissue.**

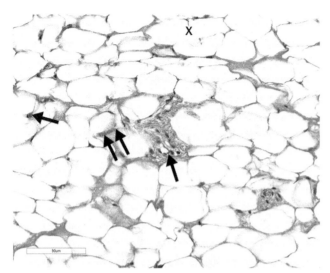

Fig. 9.3   Unilocular adipose tissue at high magnification. Blood vessels are indicated by the arrows. The X indicates a location where the border between two cells was destroyed during tissue preparation, creating the appearance of a larger cell.

Fig. 9.4 shows two scanning electron micrographs of unilocular adipose tissue. Each adipose cell appears as a rounded structure. The connective tissue between the cells has been enzymatically removed, so it appears as (dark) spaces between the cells.

9.3   Multilocular Adipose Tissue

In multilocular adipose tissue, the smaller droplets in the adipocytes do not coalesce into a single large droplet. **Fig. 9.5** is an image of multilocular adipose tissue. One multilocular adipose cell is outlined, which is approximately the same size as the unilocular cells (seen at the top of **Fig. 9.5**). Note the numerous lipid droplets within the multilocular cells, which wash away with tissue preparation; the eosinophilia within the cytoplasm represents the remaining cytoplasm that did not wash away. In contrast to unilocular adipose, the nuclei in multilocular adipose are not flattened against the plasma membrane but remain round and are either near the center of the cell or slightly off center (eccentric). The peripheral nuclei in **Fig. 9.5** likely belong to connective tissue cells (fibroblasts).

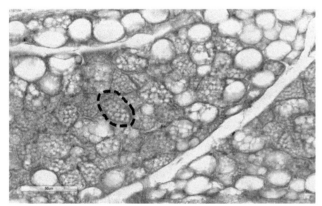

Fig. 9.5   Multilocular adipose tissue. One adipocyte filled with numerous lipid droplets is outlined. Some unilocular adipocytes are also present.

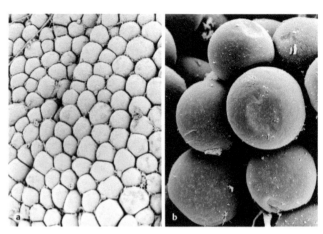

Fig. 9.4   Scanning electron micrographs of unilocular adipose tissue at (a) low and (b) high magnification.

Video 9.2   Video of multilocular adipose tissue

Be able to identify:
— Multilocular adipose tissue
https://www.thieme.de/de/q.htm?p=opn/tp/308390101/978-1-62623-414-7_c009_v002&t=video

Helpful Tip

Because multilocular adipose cells and a mucous acinus both have a washed-out appearance on H & E stain, they are often challenging to distinguish. However, note that the lipid droplets in multilocular adipose are quite large (**Fig, 9.6a**), while mucus secretory vesicles are too small to be seen individually in light micrographs (**Fig. 9.6b**). Therefore, multilocular adipose cells demonstrate many clear structures, while a mucous acinus is relatively uniformly pale. In addition, note the numerous flattened nuclei in the periphery of the mucous acinus. Even though the nucleus in the multilocular adipocyte is obscured, this cell definitely lacks the numerous flattened, peripherally located nuclei seen in the mucous acinus.

One final note (reminder). Adipose tissue is derived from mesenchyme and forms when the mesenchymal cells begin to store lipid droplets (see **Fig. 9.1**). In both brown and white fat, the cells initially store the lipid as small droplets. Therefore, both brown fat and developing white fat appear multilocular. Ultimately, the lipid droplets in white fat consolidate into one larger droplet and appear unilocular. Brown fat maintains a multilocular appearance. Therefore, unilocular adipose is always white fat. However, multilocular adipose may be developing white fat or brown fat.

Special stains can be used to distinguish brown fat from developing white fat. Brown fat has a mitochondrial protein called **uncoupling protein**, which is involved in the main function of brown fat, namely, to generate heat. Special stains for this protein can be used to identify brown fat definitively.

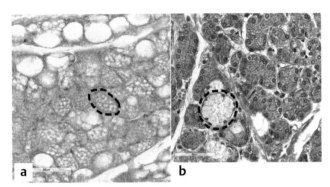

Fig. 9.6 **Comparison of multilocular adipose tissue (a) and a mucous acinus (b).** Note that in a, the outlined structure is a single, large cell, while the mucous acinus outlined in b is 6-10 cells of the acinus.

9.4 Chapter Review

Most adipose tissue in humans is white fat, which functions as a reservoir for energy storage and for insulation and protection of vital organs. Human infants have some brown fat, which functions to generate heat. All adipose tissue develops when mesenchymal cells begin to accumulate lipid droplets, becoming adipocytes. Initially, the lipid in adipocytes is in the form of numerous small lipid droplets, and the tissue is called multilocular adipose tissue. Brown fat and developing white fat have a multilocular appearance, whereas in mature white fat, the lipid droplets coalesce into a single large droplet, and the tissue is called unilocular adipose tissue.

10   Cartilage

After completing this chapter, you should be able to:
— Identify, at the light microscope level, each of the following:
  • Basic features of cartilage
    ◦ Chondrocytes
      ▪ Lacunae
      ▪ Isogenous groups
    ◦ Matrix
    ◦ Perichondrium
  • Types of cartilage
    ◦ Hyaline
    ◦ Elastic
    ◦ Fibrocartilage
— Outline the function of the cells, structures, and types of cartilage listed
— Predict the type of cartilage present in a specific organ given the function of that organ

10.1   Overview of Cartilage

Cartilage is a specialized semisolid connective tissue that provides a structural and protective function. It is located in numerous places throughout the body, most notably on the ends of bones, in the ear and nose, and in the upper respiratory tract. There are three types of cartilage: **hyaline cartilage**, **elastic cartilage**, and **fibrocartilage**. As will be described in this chapter, elastic cartilage and fibrocartilage can be considered as modifications of hyaline cartilage. Therefore, this chapter will begin by describing the basic features of cartilage, using hyaline cartilage as a model. This will be followed by a discussion of elastic cartilage and fibrocartilage, highlighting how they differ from hyaline cartilage.

10.2   Development and Basic Components of Cartilage

As mentioned in the connective tissue overview (**Chapter 7**), almost all connective tissues and muscle are derived from embryonic precursor tissue called **mesenchyme** (**Fig. 10.1**). This tissue is composed of spindle-shaped **mesenchymal cells** within a matrix that is relatively clear because it contains very few fibers and abundant ground substance (**Fig. 10.1b**). Like other connective tissues, cartilage will develop from mesenchyme.

To form cartilage, mesenchymal cells differentiate into **chondroblasts**, cuboidal cells that lack extensive cell processes characteristic of mesenchymal cells and fibroblasts (**Fig. 10.1a**). Like fibroblasts, chondroblasts develop elaborate rough endoplasmic reticulum (RER) and a Golgi apparatus. However, the matrix secreted by chondroblasts is rich in **type II collagen** and proteoglycans, forming a semisolid matrix. When this matrix surrounding the chondroblast solidifies, the cell becomes "trapped" in a space within its own matrix called a **lacuna**.

Once surrounded by semisolid matrix, chondroblasts are referred to as **chondrocytes**. Because the matrix is semisolid and not rigid, chondrocytes within lacunae can grow and divide, "pushing out" against the flexible matrix.

Fig. 10.2 is a scanning electron micrograph of a section of cartilage, showing several chondrocytes embedded within the matrix. The outer edge (plasma membrane) of one chondrocyte is indicated by the series of red arrows. The nucleus of another chondrocyte (1) is visible. These chondrocytes have large lipid droplets (2), which are not necessarily characteristic of all chondrocytes.

Connective tissue cell origin

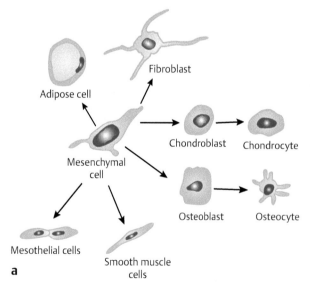

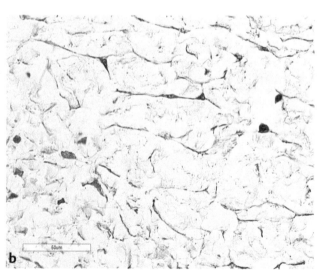

Fig. 10.1   Origin of cartilage. (a) Most cells of connective tissue and muscle are derived from a common precursor, the mesenchymal cell. (b) Mesenchyme.

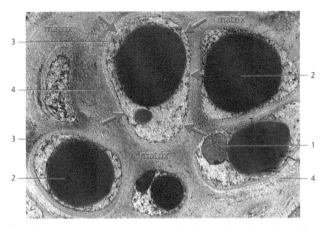

Fig. 10.2 **Scanning electron micrograph of a section of cartilage. The plasma membrane of a chondrocyte is indicated by the tips of the arrows. The matrix surrounding the chondrocytes is indicated. (1) Nucleus; (2) lipid droplet; (3) capsular matrix; (4) territorial matrix.**

Surrounding the chondrocytes is the **matrix** secreted by these cells. This matrix can be divided into the **capsular matrix** (3), which immediately surrounds the chondrocytes, and matrix that is farther away from the chondrocytes, the **territorial matrix** (4).

Fig. 10.3 is an H & E preparation of hyaline cartilage. The outer border of a single chondrocyte is indicated by the yellow arrows; its nucleus is the dark structure in the lower right of the cell. The matrix is brightly stained, in this image a pink/purple. Note that the chondrocyte indicated by the arrows has not shrunk as a result of tissue fixation, so its outer edge (plasma membrane) remains in contact with the matrix. However, many chondrocytes have shrunk, creating space between the chondrocytes and matrix (black arrows). In many cases, the chondrocyte was lost altogether, creating a space or hole (marked with an X). The "hole" is an artifact, but it represents the space in which the chondrocytes existed, and it is referred to as a lacuna.

This phenomenon happens because fixation shrinks the tissue, and the matrix, being fairly rigid, shrinks less than the cells within the matrix. The cells "pull away" from the matrix during fixation. Tissue prepared for electron microscopy shrinks less than tissue prepared for light microscopy and, therefore, shows fewer shrunken cells or empty lacunae than in light micrographs.

Although lacunae do not exist in living tissue, the presence of lacunae in prepared slides is a powerful criteria for narrowing down a tissue as either cartilage or bone.

The components of the matrix provide the unique functional properties of cartilage (**Fig. 10.4**). **Proteoglycans** are composed of a core protein to which a number of **glycosaminoglycan molecules** are attached, creating a structure similar to a bottle brush. These structures are linked to type II collagen fibers, as well as larger glycosaminoglycan molecules. The glycosaminoglycans in proteoglycans are highly negatively charged, so they repel each other. This creates space between the glycosaminoglycans, which is filled with ground substance. This structure provides rigidity as well as a porosity that enhances diffusion. Cartilage contains no blood vessels, so the living chondrocytes depend on diffusion from adjacent tissues to provide nutrients and remove waste.

10.3 Hyaline Cartilage

Hyaline cartilage is found at the ends of long bones, as part of the growth plate (see **Chapter 12**), and in the supporting structures of the respiratory system (nose, larynx, trachea). In a sense, hyaline cartilage is a "generic" cartilage, so it is a good place to begin a discussion of the features of cartilage. **Fig. 10.5** is a low-magnification image of a piece of hyaline cartilage (black bracket) surrounded by connective tissues, mucus glands (outlined), and an epithelium (arrows). Surrounding the cartilage is a specialized connective tissue called the **perichondrium** (yellow brackets, discussed subsequently).

Type I collagen fibers (e.g., dense irregular connective tissue) appear as large, eosinophilic bundles in H & E-stained slides. However, the type II collagen fibers found in cartilage are small and not visible within the matrix.

The following features of a prepared tissue specimen are consistent with cartilage:

1. There are numerous spaces (lacunae); however, note that bone also has lacunae (discussed in **Chapter 11**).
2. The matrix of cartilage is semisolid, and when sectioned appears smooth or "glassy."
3. The matrix in the central region of a piece of cartilage is more darkly stained than the matrix in the peripheral region.

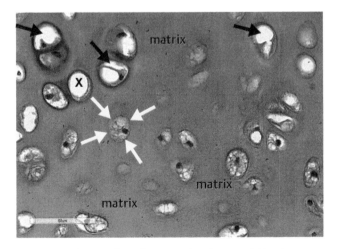

Fig. 10.3 **Hyaline cartilage showing a chondrocyte within a lacuna (yellow arrows), lacunae (black arrows and X), and the matrix.**

Cartilage matrix

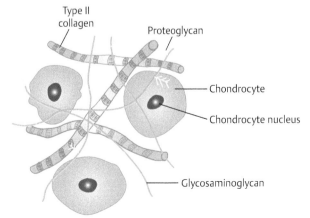

Fig. 10.4 **Components of cartilage matrix.**

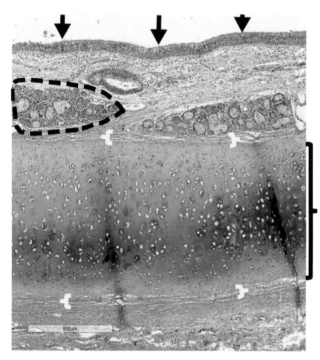

Fig. 10.5   Hyaline cartilage (black bracket) under low magnification. The perichondrium (yellow brackets), mucus glands (outline), and epithelium (arrows) are indicated.

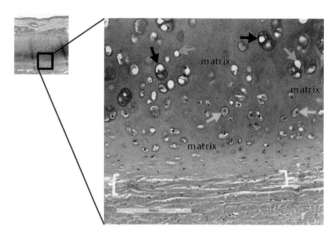

Fig. 10.6   Hyaline cartilage under high magnification. The cartilage matrix is indicated. Chondrocytes in lacunae (green arrows) as well as empty lacunae (blue arrows), from which the chondrocytes have been lost during tissue preparation, are indicated. Black arrows indicate capsular matrix. Yellow brackets delimit the perichondrium.

Fig. 10.6 is a higher-magnification image of hyaline cartilage and reveals lacunae with chondrocytes (green arrows) as well as empty lacunae (blue arrows). The matrix is smooth and glassy and shows areas of eosinophilia and basophilia; the basophilia is more intense toward the center of the piece of cartilage. The capsular matrix immediately surrounding the chondrocytes is rich in proteoglycans, and in many cases it stains more darkly (black arrows) than the territorial matrix. The perichondrium is indicated by the yellow brackets.

Fig. 10.7 provides a closer look at the perichondrium (yellow brackets), which is a specialized connective tissue that consists of two layers. The outer, fibrous portion (green bracket) has the appearance of dense irregular connective tissue. The inner, cellular portion (black bracket) shows flattened cells that are differentiating into chondroblasts. These cells secrete cartilage matrix and will become trapped within lacunae. In this way, new

cartilage is added to the outer surface of an existing cartilage piece, a process called **appositional growth of cartilage**.

Cells within cartilage continue to secrete matrix and divide. The newly formed matrix and the production of new cells result in growth of the cartilage from the inside, a process referred to as **interstitial growth of cartilage**. Because cartilage matrix is semisolid, when cells divide, the daughter cells cannot move apart from each other as readily as cells in other tissues do. This creates clusters of cells called **isogenous groups** (**isogenous nests**). **Fig. 10.8** shows two isogenous groups, each with two cells, outlined in yellow; isogenous groups of up to four cells are routinely seen. Isogenous groups are more apparent in the center of a piece of cartilage than in the periphery because the matrix in the center is older and more rigid.

Although cartilage is avascular, the perichondrium is rich in blood vessels. In order to provide nutrients to the still-living chondrocytes in lacunae, the matrix is enriched with glycosaminoglycans. As mentioned, the structure of glycosaminoglycans creates "space" that allows robust diffusion of nutrients and waste products between the perichondrium and the chondrocytes.

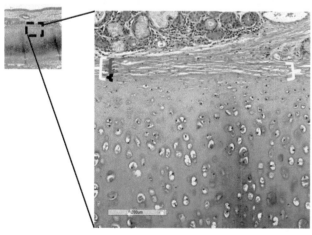

Fig. 10.7   Perichondrium of hyaline cartilage (yellow brackets), showing the fibrous perichondrium (green bracket) and cellular perichondrium (black bracket).

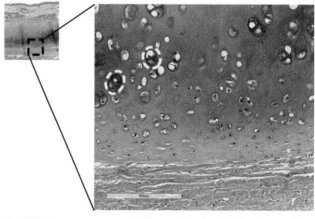

Fig. 10.8   Isogenous groups (yellow outlines) within hyaline cartilage.

CHAPTER 10

Video 10.1 Hyaline cartilage

Be able to identify:
— Hyaline cartilage
— Lacunae
— Chondrocytes
— Matrix
— Perichondrium
— Isogenous groups (nests)
https://www.thieme.de/de/q.htm?p=opn/tp/308390101/978-1-62623-414-7_c010_v001&t=video

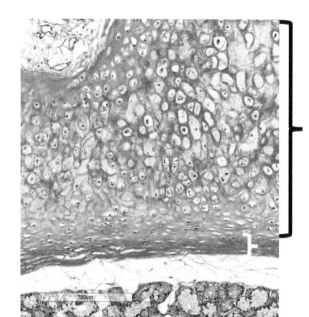

Fig. 10.10 **Elastic cartilage under low magnification, showing the cartilage (black bracket) and perichondrium (yellow bracket).**

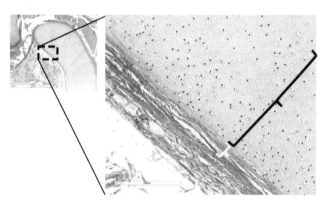

Fig. 10.9   **Developing cartilage. The cartilage (black bracket) shows chondrocytes within lacunae. The perichondrium is indicated by the yellow bracket.**

10.4   Developing Cartilage

Developing cartilage has features similar to mature cartilage, such as cells within lacunae. However, because newly formed cartilage has yet to produce significant quantities of extracellular matrix components (e.g., less glycosaminoglycans), developing cartilage has less intense basophilia and fewer isogenous cell nests than mature cartilage, as seen in **Fig. 10.9**. Developing cartilage has features similar to hyaline cartilage. As the name implies, developing cartilage is the precursor for hyaline, elastic, or fibrocartilage.

Video 10.2 Developing cartilage

Be able to identify:
— Developing cartilage having a similar appearance to hyaline cartilage
https://www.thieme.de/de/q.htm?p=opn/tp/308390101/978-1-62623-414-7_c010_v002&t=video

10.5   Elastic Cartilage

Elastic cartilage contains elastic fibers in the matrix in addition to the components described for hyaline cartilage. This provides more flexibility. Elastic cartilage is the cartilage in structures such as the ear.

Fig. 10.10 is a low-magnification image of elastic cartilage (black bracket). The elastic fibers are the brightly eosinophilic structures within the matrix. Elastic cartilage typically has a

similar number of cells as hyaline cartilage, and it has a perichondrium (yellow bracket).

Helpful Hint

Elastic cartilage is simply hyaline cartilage plus elastic fibers. Therefore, like all cartilage, the matrix of elastic cartilage has type II collagen and proteoglycans, in addition to elastic fibers.

Fig. 10.11 shows elastic cartilage at higher magnification. Thin elastic fibers are visible (e.g., numerous fine threads in the region outlined in black) as well as larger elastic bundles (black arrows), which are particularly abundant in the capsular matrix.

Helpful Hint

Remember, type II collagen fibers, characteristic of all cartilage including elastic cartilage, are too thin to visualize in routine H & E-prepared slides. Type II fibers are present, but the visible fibers in elastic cartilage are elastic fibers. The elastic fibers in elastic cartilage are refractile, so they appear shinier. This feature is best appreciated with the condenser on a microscope lowered.

Video 10.3 Elastic cartilage—H & E

Be able to identify:
— Elastic cartilage
— Lacunae
— Chondrocytes
— Matrix
— Elastic fibers
— Perichondrium
— Isogenous groups
https://www.thieme.de/de/q.htm?p=opn/tp/308390101/978-1-62623-414-7_c010_v003&t=video

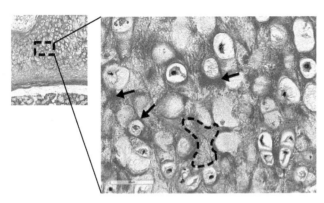

Fig. 10.11 **Elastic cartilage under high magnification, showing thin elastic fibers (within outlined region) as well as regions of thicker bundles (arrows).**

Special stains can be used to highlight the elastic fibers in elastic cartilage. The specimen shown in **Fig. 10.12** was prepared using resorcin, which stains elastic fibers. Thin fibers and thicker bundles of elastic fibers can be seen (purple), similar to those seen on H & E slides. The cells (brownish-yellow) are poorly preserved within their lacunae. The perichondrium is in the upper right of the image.

Video 10.4 Elastic cartilage—resorcin

Be able to identify:
— Elastic cartilage
— Elastic fibers
https://www.thieme.de/de/q.htm?p=opn/
tp/308390101/978-1-62623-414-7_c010_v004&t=video

10.6 Fibrocartilage

Fibrocartilage (fibrous cartilage) contains type I collagen fibers in the matrix in addition to the components described for hyaline

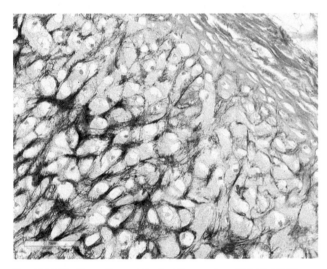

Fig. 10.12 **Elastic cartilage stained with resorcin, which highlights elastic fibers (purple). Chondrocytes are brownish-yellow, and the perichondrium is to the upper right.**

cartilage. The type I collagen fibers provide additional tensile strength; fibrocartilage is found in intervertebral disks, the pubic symphysis, articular disks, and the menisci of the knee.

Fig. 10.13 is an image of the edge of a piece of fibrocartilage. Fibrocartilage typically has fewer chondrocytes than hyaline or elastic cartilage, with fewer isogenous nests. Due to the presence of type I collagen, the matrix is highly eosinophilic and is broken up into large bundles similar to collagen seen in dense irregular connective tissue. In addition, fibrocartilage lacks a perichondrium.

Helpful Hint

Fibrocartilage is simply hyaline cartilage plus type I collagen fibers. Therefore, like all cartilage, the matrix of fibrocartilage has type II collagen and proteoglycans in addition to type I collagen fibers.

Fig. 10.14 is an image of fibrocartilage taken at higher magnification. Cells within lacunae (blue arrows) are evident. The matrix has bundles of collagen fibers in multiple orientations, which, unfortunately, gives fibrocartilage an appearance similar to dense irregular connective tissue (see the hints).

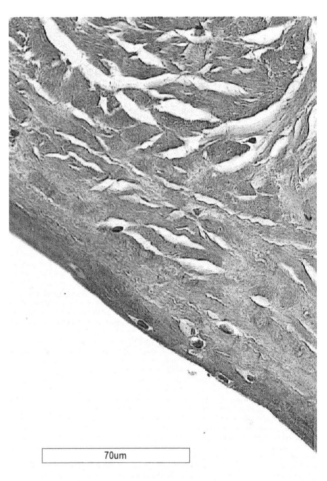

70um

Fig. 10.13 **Fibrocartilage under medium magnification. Note the strongly stained matrix and absence of perichondrium.**

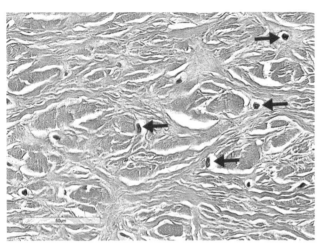

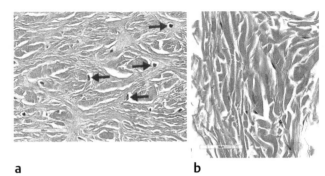

a   **b**

Fig. 10.15 **Comparison of (a) fibrocartilage (note the cells within lacunae, marked with arrows) and (b) dense regular connective tissue.**

Fig. 10.14 **Fibrocartilage under high magnification, showing chondrocytes in lacunae (arrows).**

10.7   Chapter Review

Cartilage is a semisolid tissue found in places such as the trachea, ear, and joints, and provides support and protection, with some flexibility. The cells of cartilage (chondrocytes) secrete a matrix that is rich in type II collagen fibers, as well as other components such as glycosaminoglycans that provide rigidity and enhance diffusion. The space in which the chondrocytes are located are called lacunae, which are evident when the cells are lost or shrink on tissue preparation. There are three types of cartilage: hyaline, elastic, and fibrous. Hyaline cartilage is recognized by the glassy appearance of the matrix. It is found in organs that require support and protection (such as the trachea) and at the ends of long bones. Elastic cartilage contains elastic fibers in the matrix and provides greater elasticity and flexibility in locations such as the ear. Fibrous cartilage contains abundant type I collagen in the matrix, which provides tensile strength useful for cartilage of the intervertebral disks, pubic symphysis, and menisci.

> **Helpful Hint**
>
> Remember, type II collagen fibers, which are characteristic of all cartilage, are too thin to visualize in routine H & E slides. Type II fibers are still present, but the visible fibers in fibrocartilage are type I collagen fibers.

Video 10.5 Fibrocartilage

Be able to identify:
— Fibrocartilage
— Lacunae
— Chondrocytes
— Matrix

https://www.thieme.de/de/q.htm?p=opn/tp/308390101/978-1-62623-414-7_c010_v005&t=video

> **Questions and Answers**
>
> An online-only section of questions and answers accompanying this chapter is hosted on Thieme's MedOne Education site: https://medone-education.thieme.com. Use the code on the media page at the front of this book to gain access. An institutional license to the site is required to access these questions in an interactive format, and individual users are required to register for an individual account to track results.

> **Helpful Hint**
>
> It is usually fairly easy to distinguish fibrocartilage from other types of cartilage because fibrocartilage has fewer cells and has thick type I collagen bundles. Surprisingly, it is often challenging to distinguish fibrocartilage (**Fig. 10.15a**) from dense irregular connective tissue (**Fig. 10.15b**). The best way to make this distinction is to note the cells within lacunae (arrows) in fibrocartilage, which are not present in dense irregular connective tissue. However, not all nuclei in fibrocartilage are obviously in a lacuna, and some nuclei in dense irregular connective tissue lie in an artefactual space that appears to be a lacuna. The trick is to note that most true lacunae are round or oval. It is also important to consider several nuclei in a tissue to get a best assessment of whether or not most nuclei are in lacunae (or not) before making a final decision.

11   Bone Histology

After completing this chapter, you should be able to:
— Identify in a gross anatomical bone, each of the following
  • Diaphysis
  • Epiphysis
  • Endosteum
  • Periosteum
  • Spongy bone
  • Compact bone
  • Marrow cavity
— Identify, at the light microscope level, each of the following
  • Cells of bone
    ○ Osteoblasts
    ○ Osteocytes
    ○ Osteoclasts
  • Cancellous (spongy) bone
    ○ Osteocytes
    ○ Lacuna
    ○ Canaliculi
  • Compact bone
    ○ Osteon (Haversian system)
      ▪ Central (Haversian) canal
      ▪ Osteocytes
      ▪ Lacunae
      ▪ Canaliculi
      ▪ Lamellae
        – Concentric
        – Interstitial
— Identify, at the electron microscope level, each of the following
  • Osteoblasts
  • Osteoclasts
  • Bone
— Outline the function of these bone cells and structures
— Predict the effect of pathologic conditions on the activity of bone cells

11.1   Histologic Bone (Bone Tissue) versus Anatomic Bone

It is useful to begin a discussion of bone histology by first clarifying the difference between bone, as a histologic term (i.e., osseous tissue), and an anatomic bone (e.g., the humerus).

The histologic terms **bone** and **osseous tissue** both describe a tissue, ultimately derived from mesenchyme and consisting of bone cells (osteoblasts, osteocytes) within a calcified extracellular matrix secreted by those cells. In this regard, bone or osseous tissue is similar to dense irregular connective tissue or cartilage.

An anatomic bone (such as the humerus or scapula) is a gross structure that is composed of osseous tissue but, in a living human, also includes connective tissues, blood vessels, and adipose or marrow, which are all integral parts of the anatomic bone.

11.2   Features of Anatomical Bones

Fig. 11.1 shows a dried bone, which consists of only the extracellular matrix of the osseous tissue of the bone. The bone cells, as

well as the other connective tissues, blood vessels, adipose, and marrow, were removed in preparing this specimen.

Long bones such as the humerus shown in **Fig. 11.1** consist of a **diaphysis** (shaft) and an **epiphysis** (head) at each end. A space in the center of the diaphysis called the **marrow (medullary) cavity** houses red or yellow bone marrow. The outer portion of the entire bone is solid osseous tissue, referred to as **compact bone**. In the center of the epiphyses, and adjacent to the marrow cavity, is **spongy (cancellous) bone**, which consists of spicules of osseous tissue. In the living, the spaces between the spicules are filled by red or yellow marrow.

Like cartilage (**Chapter 10**), the outer portion of a living bone is lined by a dense irregular connective tissue; this layer over bone is called a **periosteum**. The marrow cavity is lined by a similar layer of connective tissue, referred to as an **endosteum**. Because **Fig. 11.1** represents a specimen of dried bone, these layers are not present in the figure.

Fig. 11.2 is a drawing comparing a long bone (A) with a flat bone such as many found in the skull (B). The organization of flat bones is similar to that of long bones, including an outer compact bone and a central region consisting of spongy bone (called the diploë). There is no medullary cavity in a flat bone, but marrow still occupies the spaces between the spicules of spongy bone in the diploë.

11.3   Cells of Osseous Tissue

Fig. 11.3 is a drawing showing the cells of osseous tissue, which can be divided into two groups, based on lineage and function:
— The *bone makers* are derived from mesenchyme and mature in the following sequence:
  1. **Mesenchymal cells** are precursors for connective tissue cells and were presented in **Chapter 7.**
  2. **Osteoprogenitor cells** (not shown) are cells that differentiate from mesenchymal cells and are committed to the bone lineage but have yet to secrete bone matrix.
  3. **Osteoblasts** are cells that have begun to secrete the characteristic matrix of bone. Bone matrix is composed of type I collagen, onto which is precipitated inorganic calcium (Ca^{2+}) and phosphate (PO_4^{3-}) in large crystals called **hydroxyapatite**.
  4. **Osteocytes** are cells trapped within the matrix that they secreted.
— The *bone breakers*, or **osteoclasts**, are derived from bone marrow and break down bone matrix and osseous tissue.

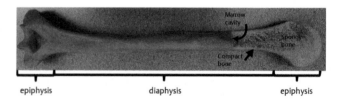

Fig. 11.1   **Anatomy of a long bone.**

a   Long bones

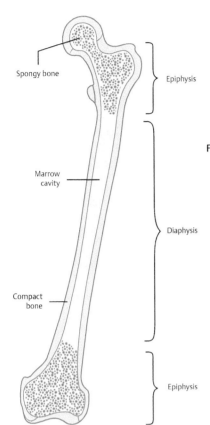

b   Flat bone

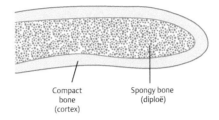

Fig. 11.2   **Drawing of (a) a long and (b) a flat bone.**

Bone makers

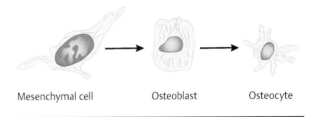

Bone breakers

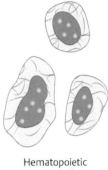

Hematopoietic
stem cells

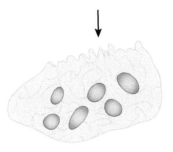

Osteoclast

Fig. 11.3   **Cells of osseous tissue.**

Helpful Hint

Note the parallel between the bone maker cell lineage (mesenchymal cell → osteoprogenitor cell → osteoblast → osteocyte) and cartilage-forming cells (mesenchymal cell → chondroblast → chondrocyte).

11.3.1   Progenitor Cells (Mesenchymal and Osteoprogenitor Cells)

Mesenchymal cells and osteoprogenitor cells are relatively undifferentiated cells. On routine H & E-stained tissues, these cells have a histologic appearance similar to fibroblasts (see **Chapters 7** and **8**). Mesenchymal cells are in embryonic mesenchyme, while osteoprogenitor cells are typically located within the periosteum and endosteum.

Helpful Hint

Because fibroblasts, mesenchymal cells, and osteoprogenitor cells have similar histologic features (round or oval nucleus, tapered cell with cell processes), it is usually not possible to distinguish these cell types on routine H & E-stained tissues.

11.3.2 Osteoblasts

Osteoblasts are derived from osteoprogenitor cells that have begun to secrete bone matrix. Because osteoblasts are actively secreting components of bone matrix, they have histologic features consistent with protein-synthesizing cells, including abundant RER and a prominent Golgi apparatus for collagen production. **Fig. 11.4** is an electron micrograph of an osteoblast secreting bone matrix; note the abundant rough ER within the cell. Type I collagen surrounds the osteoblast; the dark, electron-dense regions are locations where the collagen is calcified.

> **Helpful Hint**
>
> There are many cells with abundant RER and Golgi (e.g., plasma cells, chondroblasts), but the presence of these organelles in a cell adjacent to electron-dense bone matrix helps identify this as an osteoblast.

In light micrographs (**Fig. 11.5**), osteoblasts have an intense cytoplasmic basophilia due to the abundant RER. The osteoblasts are adjacent to bone, to which they are adding matrix components. Most of the cells not adjacent to bone and not demonstrating cytoplasmic basophilia are mesenchymal cells/fibroblasts/osteoprogenitor cells.

Note that, in H & E-stained tissues, the color of calcified bone varies, ranging from pink to purple. Regardless of the color, calcified bone is typically dark or intense. This contrasts with cartilage, which typically has a less intensely stained matrix.

The pink region along the periphery of each piece of bone (i.e., between the dark calcified bone and osteoblasts), consists of type I collagen secreted by the osteoblasts that has yet to be calcified. This matrix is called **osteoid**, which will be discussed in greater detail in **Chapter 12**.

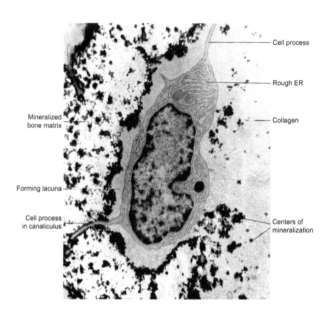

Fig. 11.4 **Electron micrograph of osteoblast surrounded by bone matrix. Image courtesy of Michael Hortsch, University of Michigan, © 2005 The Regents of the University of Michigan.**

11.3.3 Osteocytes

As shown in **Fig. 11.4**, osteoblasts have several cell processes. These processes extend toward, and make contact with, processes of adjacent osteoblasts before the cells begin secreting matrix. As osteoblasts secrete bone matrix, they become trapped in **lacunae**, becoming osteocytes (**Fig. 11.6**, arrows). However, the cell-cell connections made by these cells are maintained and are housed in tunnels called **canaliculi**, which connect adjacent lacunae. Canaliculi are too small to be seen in routine H & E-stained slides, but they will be examined later in this chapter. The connections between adjacent bone cells via these canaliculi are crucial because they provide a mechanism for transport of nutrients and waste products between adjacent bone cells.

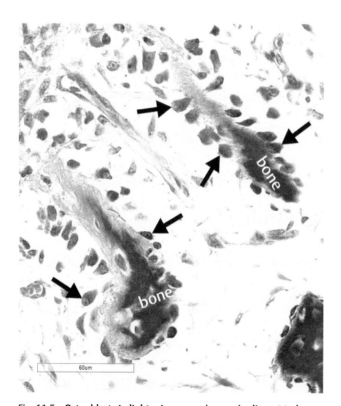

Fig. 11.5 **Osteoblasts in light microscopy (arrows) adjacent to bone spicules. Fetal pig snout.**

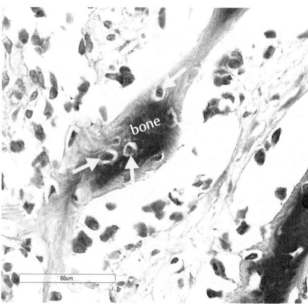

Fig. 11.6 **Osteocytes in lacunae (arrows) in fetal pig snout.**

Chondrocytes trapped in lacunae do not need cell-cell processes because diffusion is efficient in cartilage matrix. However, calcification of bone matrix prevents diffusion (as well as cell movement). Therefore, these cell-cell contacts that enable nutrient exchange must be made before the matrix surrounding these cells calcifies.

Though it may not be obvious in **Fig. 11.6**, osteocytes have less extensive RER and Golgi than when they were osteoblasts. In fact, since the matrix is solidified, these cells are unable to secrete much additional matrix. Although osteocytes are active, they are much less so than osteoblasts.

The images in **Fig. 11.5** and **Fig. 11.6** were from a fetal pig snout, showing developing bone. **Fig. 11.7** is an image from a section of the shaft of a long bone, demonstrating mature bone, showing osteocytes in lacunae (yellow arrows) as well as osteoblasts (black arrows). Note the cytoplasmic basophilia of the osteoblasts. At the top and bottom of the image, the osteoblasts have separated from the osseous tissue during tissue preparation.

Video 11.1 Osteoblasts, osteocytes, and bone—fetal pig snout

Be able to identify:
— Osteoblasts
— Osteocytes
— Bone
https://www.thieme.de/de/q.htm?p=opn/tp/308390101/978-1-62623-414-7_c011_v001&t=video

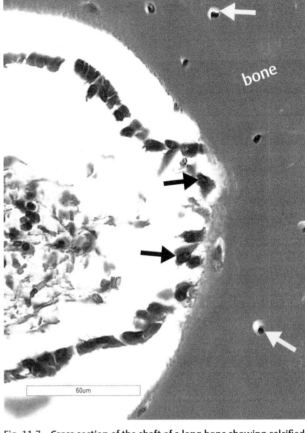

Fig. 11.7   **Cross section of the shaft of a long bone showing calcified bone, osteoblasts (black arrows), and osteocytes (yellow arrows).**

Video 11.2 Osteoblasts, osteocytes, and bone—shaft of long bone

Video 11.3 Osteocytes and bone—flat bone

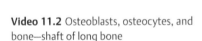

Be able to identify:
— Osteoblasts
— Osteocytes
— Bone

https://www.thieme.de/de/q.htm?p=opn/tp/308390101/978-1-62623-414-7_c011_v002&t=video
https://www.thieme.de/de/q.htm?p=opn/tp/308390101/978-1-62623-414-7_c011_v003&t=video

11.3.4   Osteoclasts

Osteoclasts are derived from hematopoietic stem cells in bone marrow (**Fig. 11.3**) and are closely related to the monocyte/macrophage lineage. Osteoclasts arise from fusion of multiple cells and, therefore, are large, multinuclear cells (**Fig. 11.8**).

To degrade bone, osteoclasts produce lysosomes, which are released into the extracellular space onto the surface of the bone

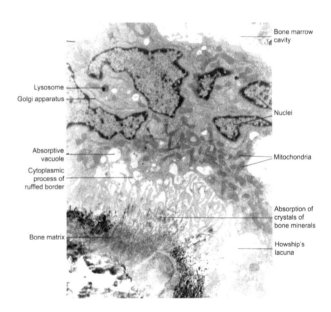

Fig. 11.8   **Electron micrograph showing osteoclast with adjacent bone matrix. Image courtesy of Michael Hortsch, University of Michigan, © 2005 The Regents of the University of Michigan.**

matrix. The plasma membrane adjacent to the bone is extremely undulated, which increases the surface area for proton pumps and release of the secretory lysosomes. This undulated region is referred to as a **ruffled border**. Degraded bone material is taken up by the osteoclast in **absorptive vacuoles**. The space between the osteoclast and the bone matrix is referred to as a **Howship's lacuna**.

In H & E sections, osteoclasts (**Fig. 11.9**, outlined) are recognized as large cells with multiple nuclei and eosinophilic cytoplasm (due to numerous secretory vesicles). As they degrade the bone, the depression created is a Howship lacuna (black arrows), which may not be readily visible in this image, but note its location. Osteoblasts are indicated with green arrows for comparison.

Video 11.4 Osteoclasts—fetal pig snout

Be able to identify:
— Osteoclasts
https://www.thieme.de/de/q.htm?p=opn/
tp/308390101/978-1-62623-414-7_c011_v004&t=video

The previous image of osteoclasts was taken from fetal pig snout and shows developing bone. **Fig. 11.10** is an image from the shaft of a mature long bone, showing an osteoclast (green arrow). Again, note that it is a large cell with multiple nuclei and intense cytoplasmic eosinophilia.

Video 11.5 Osteoclasts—shaft of long bone

Be able to identify:
— Osteoclasts
https://www.thieme.de/de/q.htm?p=opn/
tp/308390101/978-1-62623-414-7_c011_v005&t=video

11.4   Organization of Bone

Recall that the periphery of an anatomic bone is compact bone, which consists entirely of osseous tissue (**Fig. 11.2**). The

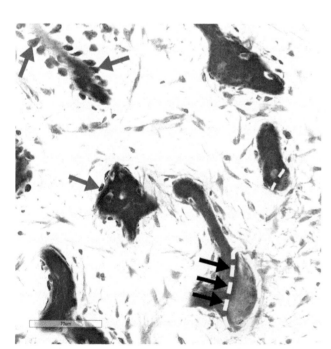

Fig. 11.9   **Osteoclasts in light microscopy (yellow outline) adjacent to bone spicules in fetal pig snout. The space between the lower osteoclast and the bone spicule it is degrading is a Howship lacuna (black arrows). Osteoblasts (green arrows) are indicated for comparison.**

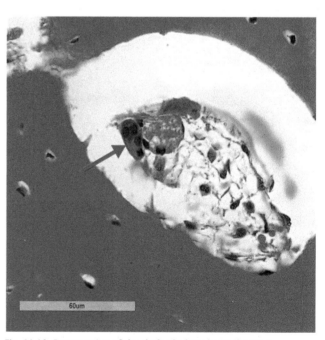

Fig. 11.10 **Cross section of the shaft of a long bone showing osteoclast (green arrow).**

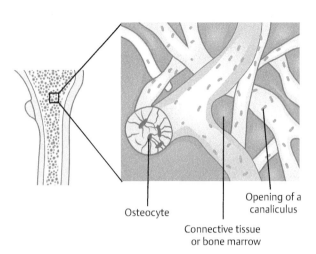

Fig. 11.11 **Organization of spongy bone.**

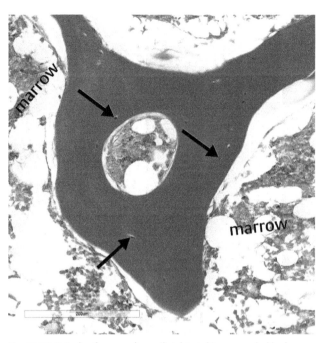

Fig. 11.12 **Spicule of spongy bone (bright pink) surrounded by bone marrow. Osteocytes are indicated (arrows).**

inside lining of the marrow cavity, the inside of the epiphysis, and the middle portion of a flat bone are all composed of spongy bone. The osseous pieces in spongy bone are referred to as **spicules** or **trabeculae** (trabeculae are larger, but the terms are often used interchangeably). The space between the spicules in spongy bone, empty in a dried specimen, is occupied by mesenchyme, marrow, adipose, or connective tissue in living tissue.

Since diffusion cannot occur through calcified bone matrix, osteocytes in lacunae obtain nutrients and eliminate waste by maintaining contact with tissues that contain blood vessels or with other osteocytes. This is achieved via cellular processes (see **Fig. 11.4**), which extend into narrow tunnels within the matrix called canaliculi and connect lacunae containing the osteocytes. As previously mentioned, note that the osteoblasts must establish these connections with neighboring cells or tissues before the matrix surrounding them calcifies.

Helpful Hint

Like lacunae, canaliculi are "spaces" in the bone matrix. They are long, narrow tunnels and contain osteocyte cell processes. Lacunae are round and contain the part of the osteocyte that includes the nucleus. Keep in mind that in living tissue, when cells and cell processes are present, there is no empty space at all.

11.4.1   Organization of Spongy Bone

In spongy bone, the spicules/trabeculae are not thick (**Fig. 11.11**). Therefore, the osteocytes within are usually near enough to the edge of the osseous spicule that their cell processes can extend to the surface to access nutrients from the tissue (e.g., marrow) between the spicules. Alternatively, a short chain of a few osteocytes can pass nutrients to an osteocyte in the middle of a spicule.

Fig. 11.12 shows a light micrograph of a bone spicule; osteocytes within lacunae are indicated (black arrows). Each osteocyte maintains contact to the adjacent marrow through canaliculi, which are not visible in this slide.

Video 11.6 Spongy bone

Be able to identify:
— Spongy bone
— Osteocyte
— Lacunae

https://www.thieme.de/de/q.htm?p=opn/tp/308390101/978-1-62623-414-7_c011_v006&t=video

11.4.2   Organization of Compact Bone

Compact bone is thicker than spicules of spongy bone and, therefore, requires more organization to deliver nutrients to osteocytes effectively. Compact bone consists of **osteons** (or Haversian systems), which are cylinders of osseous tissue that run lengthwise along the long axis of a bone (**Fig. 11.13**). Each osteon is composed of several **concentric lamellae** (rings). In the center of each osteon is a **central (Haversian) canal**, which contains connective tissue, including blood vessels that feed the osteocytes within the osteon. Lamellae between osteons are incomplete and referred to as **interstitial lamellae**. In the outer and inner portions of a wedge of bone, large inner and outer **circumferential lamellae** are present (inner circumferential lamella not shown in **Fig. 11.13**), which go all the way around the circumference of the bone.

Fig. 11.14 is a drawing of a single osteon in which all but five osteocytes have been removed. Tan is bone matrix. The osteocytes (light blue arrows) within their lacunae (black arrows) are situated in the borders between the lamellae. Osteocyte processes (green arrows) extend into tunnels in the matrix called canaliculi (red arrows), which connect adjacent lacunae but also connect the inner lacunae to the central canal. Nutrients from the vessels in the central canal are passed to osteocytes in the inner layer,

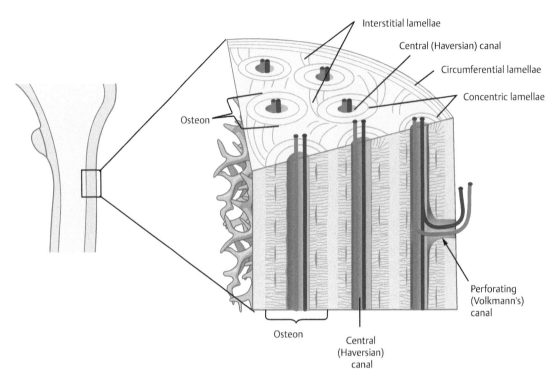

Fig. 11.13 Organization of compact bone.

which then pass nutrients to osteocytes in the outer layers. In this manner, all osteocytes in an osteon receive nutrients from the vessels within the central canal.

As shown in the bottom right of **Fig. 11.14**, each osteocyte process extends halfway through a canaliculus, so that the tips of two processes from adjacent osteocytes meet in the middle. Nutrient and waste movement occurs via diffusion in the small space between the cell processes and calcified matrix, as well as via gap junctions made by the adjacent osteocytes.

Figs. 11.15a, b are images from a thick section of a dried piece of compact bone. The osteocytes and other living cells were removed during the drying process, leaving only calcified bone matrix. The tissue was then ground, creating dust that filled in all the spaces where cells and connective tissue once existed. **Fig. 11.15a** is a low-magnification image; the osteon outlined in red is shown at higher magnification in **Fig. 11.15b**. The central (Haversian) canal, lacunae (blue arrows), and canaliculi (red arrows) of this osteon are indicated in **Fig. 11.15b**. Lamellae within a complete osteon are called concentric lamellae; those that are not part of a complete osteon are termed interstitial lamellae (e.g., **Fig. 11.15a**, blue outline).

Video 11.7 Ground compact bone

Be able to identify:
— Osteon
  • Central (Haversian) canal
  • Concentric lamella
  • Lacuna
  • Canaliculi
— Interstitial lamella
https://www.thieme.de/de/q.htm?p=opn/tp/308390101/978-1-62623-414-7_c011_v007&t=video

Fig. 11.16 shows images from a sample of the shaft of a long bone cut in cross section and stained with H & E. This tissue was not dried, so marrow, osteocytes, and other connective tissues are present. However, the details of the osteon are more obscure than in **Fig. 11.15**, so individual osteons need to be visualized mentally (one osteon is outlined) based on the location of central canals (Xs) and surrounding lacunae (blue arrows). Connective tissue can be seen in the central canals, and osteocytes are visible in most lacunae. Canaliculi and lamellae are not visible in this preparation. The larger spaces (R) are resorption canals, which will be discussed in the next chapter.

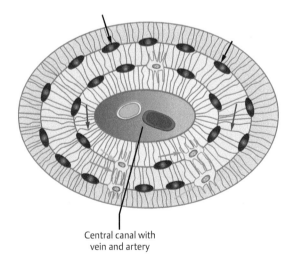

Fig. 11.14 Organization of an osteon showing osteocytes (light blue arrows) and empty lacunae (black arrows). Osteocyte cell processes (green arrows) occupy canaliculi (red arrows). Note that osteocyte processes have been drawn thicker than canaliculi. In real bone, the osteocyte processes are within canaliculi.

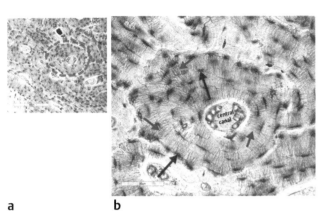

a b

Fig. 11.15 Compact bone showing the organization of osteons. A sample of bone was dried, removing living cells and tissues and leaving only calcified matrix. The tissue was sectioned, and the sections ground. Debris from the grinding process filled in spaces previously occupied by living tissue, making them appear dark. (a) Low-magnification view showing several osteons; complete osteon outlined in red; blue outline indicates interstitial lamellae. (b) Osteon outlined in red (a) at higher magnification. Blue arrows indicate lacunae; red arrows indicate canaliculi.

Video 11.8 Compact bone—1

Video 11.9 Compact bone—2

Be able to identify:
— Osteon
  • Central (haversian) canal
  • Lacuna
https://www.thieme.de/de/q.htm?p=opn/tp/308390101/978-1-62623-414-7_c011_v008&t=video
https://www.thieme.de/de/q.htm?p=opn/tp/308390101/978-1-62623-414-7_c011_v009&t=video

As mentioned, osteons, and thus haversian canals, run parallel to the long axis of the bone (**Fig. 11.13**). These, and the vessels within them, are connected to each other, and to the outside tissue and marrow cavity, by **perforating (Volkmann) canals**, which run perpendicular to the long axis of the bone. Note that perforating canals are spaces (tunnels) within the bone matrix, similar to canaliculi; the difference is that Volkmann canals are larger and contain connective tissue and vessels, while canaliculi are much smaller and contain osteocyte cell processes. **Fig. 11.17** is an image from ground bone, showing most of a Volkmann canal (red arrows) connecting two adjacent central canals (Xs).

Video 11.10 Volkmann canal

Be able to identify:
— Perforating (Volkmann) canal
https://www.thieme.de/de/q.htm?p=opn/tp/308390101/978-1-62623-414-7_c011_v010&t=video

Helpful Hint

Volkmann canals provide an important communication between osteons, allowing blood vessels to reach osteons within compact bone. However, they are not necessarily high-yield histologic structures.

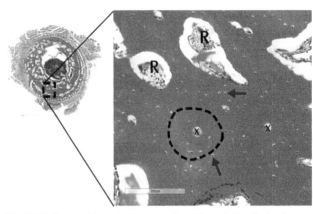

Fig. 11.16 Compact bone in tissue sections through the shaft of a long bone. One osteon is outlined; Xs mark central canals; arrows indicate lacunae. Canaliculi and lamellae are not visible. Rs mark resorption canals, discussed in the next chapter.

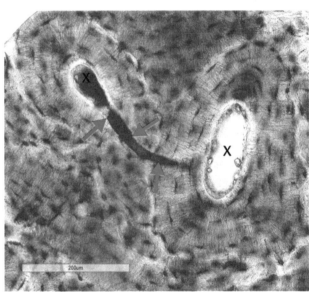

Fig. 11.17 Ground bone showing a perforating (Volkmann) canal (red arrows) connecting the central canals (Xs) of two adjacent osteons.

Like cartilage, bone is surrounded by a layer of connective tissue. In bone this layer is called **periosteum**, which is well developed and serves as a point of attachment for tendons and ligaments. **Fig. 11.18** shows that periosteum consists of an inner cellular (black bracket) and outer fibrous (blue bracket) regions. A thinner endosteum (not shown) forms the inner lining of the bone, adjacent to the marrow cavity.

Video 11.11 Periosteum

Be able to identify:
— Periosteum
— Endosteum
https://www.thieme.de/de/q.htm?p=opn/tp/308390101/978-1-62623-414-7_c011_v011&t=video

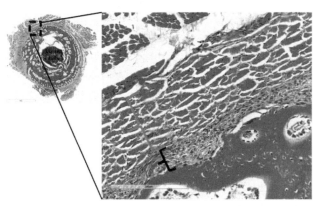

Fig. 11.18 Periosteum of bone, showing the inner cellular layer (black bracket) and outer fibrous layer (blue bracket).

11.5   Chapter Review

Anatomic bones (e.g., humerus, femur) consist of histologic bone (i.e., osseous tissue) as well as connective tissue, marrow, adipose tissue, and vessels. Osseous tissue is produced and maintained by a lineage of cells derived from mesenchymal cells, similar to the lineages that produce cartilage. Mesenchymal cells committed to the bone lineage are called osteoprogenitor cells. When osteoprogenitor cells begin to secrete bone matrix, they are referred to as osteoblasts and demonstrate intense cytoplasmic basophilia characteristic of protein-synthesizing cells. Eventually, osteoblasts become surrounded by calcified bone matrix, becoming osteocytes trapped in lacunae. Osteoclasts are cells with a

different lineage, being derived from hematopoietic cells (blood cell lineage), and serve to degenerate bone matrix, which is useful for bone remodeling (see next chapter).

Unlike cartilage, which consists of a matrix that allows diffusion of nutrients to chondrocytes trapped in lacunae, bone matrix consists of type I collagen and crystalline calcium phosphate, which restricts diffusion. Therefore, osseous tissue is organized to allow osteocytes within lacunae access to nutrients. This is achieved through canaliculi, which are tunnels in the matrix containing osteocyte cell processes that connect osteocytes to adjacent osteocytes, connective tissue, or marrow. Compact bone is thick, so it requires an organized system to ensure that all osteocytes have access to nutrients. Therefore, compact bone is organized into cylinders called osteons, which contain a central canal containing blood vessels. Osteocytes within an osteon obtain nutrients from this central canal via canaliculi. Adjacent osteons communicate through Volkmann canals. Spongy bone pieces (spicules) are not as thick as compact bone, so osteocyte processes can reach nearby vessels through canaliculi; organization into osteons is not required.

Questions and Answers

An online-only section of questions and answers accompanying this chapter is hosted on Thieme's MedOne Education site: https://medone-education.thieme.com. Use the code on the media page at the front of this book to gain access. An institutional license to the site is required to access these questions in an interactive format, and individual users are required to register for an individual account to track results.

12   Bone Development

After completing this chapter, you should be able to:
- Identify, at the light microscope level, each of the following
  - Cells of bone (review)
    - Mesenchymal cell
    - Osteoblast
    - Osteocyte
    - Osteoclast
  - Bone formation
    - Intramembranous ossification
      - Spicule or trabecula
      - Osteoid
      - Calcified bone matrix
    - Endochondral ossification
      - Hyaline cartilage
      - Calcified cartilage
      - Osteoid
      - Calcified bone matrix
      - Epiphyseal growth plate
        - Zone of resting cartilage
        - Zone of proliferation
        - Zone of hypertrophy
        - Zone of calcification
        - Zone of bone deposition
    - Bone remodeling
      - Resorption canals
- Identify, at the electron microscope level, each of the following:
  - Osteoblast
  - Osteocyte
  - Osteoclast
  - Osteoid
  - Calcified bone matrix
- Outline the function of each cell type listed

- Predict the appearance of these cells and extracellular components in light micrographs based on their appearance in electron micrographs and vice versa
- Appraise the influence of hormones on bone growth, with a focus on pathologic conditions relating to bone growth

12.1   Bone Matrix Secretion

The previous chapter presented the cell types of bone and introduced their development and role in synthesis of **bone matrix**. This chapter focuses on the formation of bone, called **ossification**, with particular emphasis on the production of the components of bone matrix.

Osteoblasts are the cells that actively secreting bone matrix, which is composed of:
- Type I collagen
- Inorganic calcium (Ca^{2+}), and phosphate (PO_4^{3-}) in large crystals called **hydroxyapatite**

It is important to note that type I collagen is secreted first and forms matrix that is called **osteoid**. Calcium and phosphate are then deposited onto osteoid to form **calcified bone matrix**.

Fig. 12.1 is a drawing showing one of the processes of bone formation, called **intramembranous** ossification (see subsequent discussions). This type of bone formation can serve as a model to describe the production of bone matrix. To form bone, **mesenchymal cells** differentiate into **osteoprogenitor cells** and then to **osteoblasts**, which cluster together to form a **center of ossification**. Each osteoblast extends several cell processes that interact with neighboring osteoblasts (A in **Fig. 12.1**). The osteoblasts first secrete osteoid, which is rich in **type I collagen** (B in **Fig. 12.1**, osteoid in pink). Osteoblasts then secrete inorganic components (calcium and phosphate), which deposit onto the collagen fibers, converting the osteoid to calcified bone matrix (C in **Fig. 12.1**,

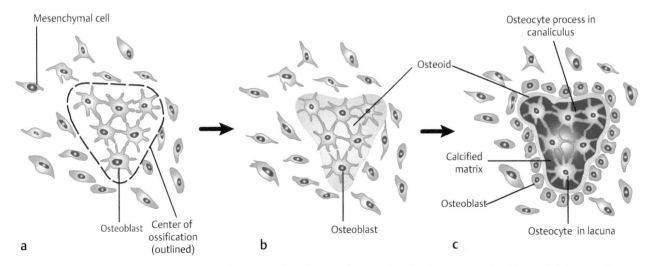

Fig. 12.1   **Intramembranous ossification starts when mesenchymal cells gather together, forming a center of ossification (a). These cells differentiate into osteoblasts, and begin secreting components of bone matrix. Secretion of type I collagen forms osteoid (b) which later becomes calcified (c).**

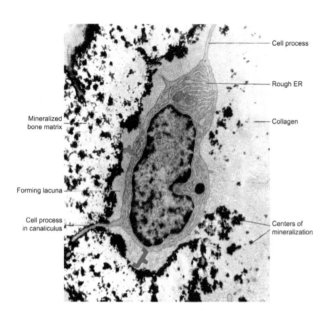

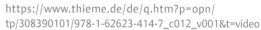

Fig, 12.2   Osteoblast secreting bone matrix. The region indicated by the red bracket is osteoid. Image courtesy of Michael Hortsch, University of Michigan, © 2005 The Regents of the University of Michigan.

magenta is calcified bone matrix). Osteoblasts trapped in the calcified matrix become less active **osteocytes**. During this entire process, the cell-cell connections made by the osteoblasts before they began secreting matrix are maintained, while bone matrix surrounds the cells and these processes. The spaces within the matrix where the osteoblasts are located are called **lacunae**, and the tunnels that contain the osteoblast cell processes are called

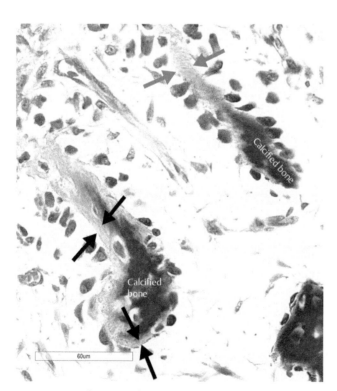

Fig. 12.3   Bone formation showing osteoid (between arrows). Calcified bone is labeled.

canaliculi. Continued bone growth involves surrounding mesenchymal cells, which differentiate into osteoblasts and begin to secrete osteoid onto the surface of the piece of bone; the osteoid will be converted to calcified bone matrix (see further discussion).

Fig. 12.2 is an electron micrograph of an osteoblast producing bone matrix. The matrix immediately adjacent to the edge of the osteoblast (brackets) is osteoid, which consists of type I collagen fibers. Further away from the osteoblasts, the mineralized (calcified) bone matrix is characteristically dark, except where it has washed away on tissue preparation.

Since collagen is protein, it is eosinophilic on H & E-stained sections. **Fig. 12.3** is an image of developing bone, which shows osteoid as pale pink (between the arrows), either on the outer surface of the bright purple calcified bone (black arrows) or as a region that has yet to calcify (blue arrows).

Video 12.1 Osteoid

Be able to identify:
— Osteoid
— Calcified bone

https://www.thieme.de/de/q.htm?p=opn/
tp/308390101/978-1-62623-414-7_c012_v001&t=video

Because bone is undergoing constant turnover throughout the lifetime of an organism (discussed later in the chapter), osteoid is present on mature bone. **Fig. 12.4** is a section of mature bone, showing osteoid (between black arrows) between the osteoblasts (blue arrows) and calcified bone (bright pink).

Video 12.2 Osteoid

Be able to identify:
— Osteoid
— Calcified bone

https://www.thieme.de/de/q.htm?p=opn/
tp/308390101/978-1-62623-414-7_c012_v002&t=video

12.2   Bone Development

Bone is formed from two distinct processes:
- **Intramembranous ossification**, in which bone develops directly from embryonic mesenchyme
- **Endochondral ossification**, in which bone develops from a model of hyaline cartilage

Because cartilage is derived from mesenchyme, all bone is ultimately derived from mesenchyme. In some places, especially in the head and neck, neural crest cells contribute to mesenchyme, so in this region, at least some parts of bone are derived from neural crest cells.

12.2.1 Intramembranous Ossification

As described in the previous section, in intramembranous ossification, mesenchymal cells cluster together and then mature first into osteoprogenitor cells and then into osteoblasts (A in **Fig. 12.1**). The region where this is occurring is often referred to as a

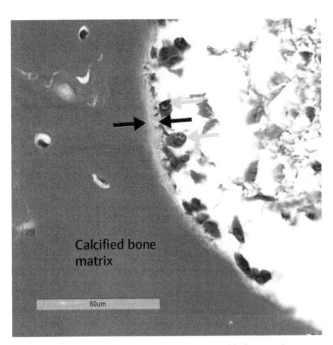

Fig. 12.4 Mature bone showing osteoid (between black arrows) secreted by osteoblasts (blue arrows). Calcified bone matrix is bright pink.

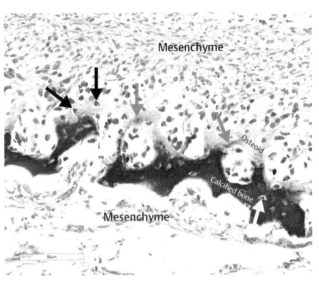

Fig. 12.5 Intramembranous ossification. Mesenchyme is labeled, as are osteoid and calcified bone. An osteocyte in a lacuna is indicated (yellow arrow). Osteoblasts surrounded by osteoid (black arrows) are shown, as well as osteoid in the initial stages of calcification (blue arrows).

center of ossification (outlined). After clustering and extending processes that make contact with their neighbors, osteoblasts secrete the characteristic molecules of bone matrix: first the organic osteoid (B in **Fig. 12.1**, pink) and then the inorganic component (C in **Fig. 12.1**, purple). Many of the osteoblasts become trapped in lacunae, becoming osteocytes, and their processes are housed in canaliculi.

Bone formed through intramembranous ossification is shown in **Fig. 12.5**. Previously, this entire region was mesenchyme, so it had histologic features similar to the top and bottom of this image. To form this piece of bone, mesenchymal cells differentiated into osteoblasts that secreted bone matrix. Cells that differentiated into osteoblasts at an early stage of this process are surrounded by calcified bone matrix as osteocytes trapped in lacunae (yellow arrow). Osteoblasts along the edge of this piece of bone continue to secrete matrix components, so that this piece of bone can grow through **appositional growth** (growth by adding to the surface of an existing piece of bone). Many of these osteoblasts are in the process of becoming trapped in osteoid (black arrows) and will soon be osteocytes after the osteoid is calcified. Osteoid that is partially calcified can also be seen (blue arrows).

Helpful Hint

Recall that, in addition to appositional growth, cartilage can enlarge by interstitial growth. This later process can occur because cartilage matrix is semisolid, so chondrocytes in the center of a piece of cartilage are able to secrete matrix and divide. Because calcified bone matrix is solid, bone tissue cannot grow by interstitial growth.

Fig. 12.6 shows a schematic of intramembranous ossification, stepping back in terms of magnification to look at the big picture. In this schematic, the tan background represents mesenchyme, and the blue regions indicate bone formed by intramembranous ossification from that mesenchyme. Early intramembranous ossification occurs in spots or regions within the mesenchyme to form bone spicules (A in **Fig. 12.6**; blue blobs represent bone

spicules in cross section). Further development includes simple enlargement of existing spicules (B in **Fig. 12.6**, blue spicules), adding additional projections onto existing spicules (light blue spicules), and the appearance of new bone spicules from mesenchyme (B in **Fig. 12.6**, dark blue spicules).

Helpful Hint

In fact, most or all of the bone spicules grow and add projections, but this figure highlights these processes separately.

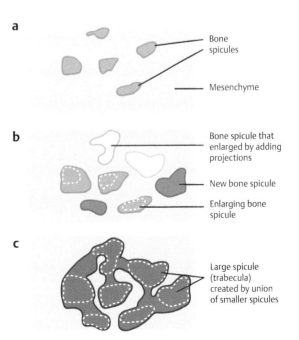

Fig. 12.6 Schematic of intramembranous ossification. Bone formation from mesenchyme results in bone spicules (a). Expansion of bone tissue occurs through growth of existing spicules (b, light blue and blue regions) or generation of new bone spicules (b, dark blue). Further growth results in fusion of existing spicules to form larger pieces (c).

Eventually, continued enlargement of existing pieces and new centers of ossification will connect the smaller pieces of bone to form larger pieces (C in **Fig. 12.6**, dark blue blob), which are sometimes called **trabeculae** (*spicule* and *trabecula* are fairly interchangeable terms).

Once formed, spicules/trabeculae can get thicker through appositional bone formation. In addition, new spicules of bone can grow in the surrounding mesenchyme and eventually connect to the larger mass. In fact, the appearance of spicules, enlargement of spicules, and fusion with adjacent spicules to form larger pieces are all happening constantly. Furthermore, osteoclasts begin degrading the newly formed bone for remodeling almost as soon as these pieces are formed, so this entire process is very dynamic.

Video 12.3 Intramembranous ossification

Be able to identify:
— Intramembranous ossification
Review the following:
— Bone cells
— Spicule or trabecula
— Osteoid
— Calcified bone matrix
https://www.thieme.de/de/q.htm?p=opn/tp/308390101/978-1-62623-414-7_c012_v003&t=video

12.2.2 Endochondral Ossification

Endochondral ossification is development of bone from a framework of hyaline cartilage; it is the process of formation of long bones such as the humerus. This is a much more complicated process than intramembranous bone formation, so it is helpful to consider the big picture first.

Fig. 12.7 is a drawing showing endochondral ossification. Endochondral ossification is the formation of bone from a hyaline cartilage model. The process begins with a piece of hyaline cartilage (1). This cartilage can grow both appositionally and interstitially, and it will continue to do so during its conversion to bone. In fact, it's actually the growth of cartilage that allows bones to grow lengthwise before maturity (as will be discussed).

The conversion of cartilage to bone begins with the formation of a bone collar around the diaphysis (2). This bone collar consists of bone tissue applied onto the surface of the cartilage model. This is followed by the appearance of a **primary ossification center** in the diaphysis (3, purple shading). In the primary ossification center, chondrocytes enlarge, and the matrix calcifies. The chondrocytes undergo apoptosis, leaving the calcified cartilage matrix. An artery invades the primary ossification center, bringing osteoprogenitor cells, which develop into osteoblasts, which in turn deposit bone onto the cartilage matrix. This initial cartilage/bone composite is subsequently converted to bone by osteoclasts and osteoblast activity (4). This process initially occurs radially from the center of the shaft, but because the bone is long, ultimately, conversion from this primary ossification center occurs lengthwise in two directions (toward each epiphysis).

In each epiphysis, **secondary ossification centers** develop (5, purple shading), and the same processes that occurred in the primary ossification center occur in these locations. The secondary ossification centers also grow radially (6), so that at birth (or in some cases after birth), each epiphysis has two regions of hyaline cartilage remaining:

1.   At the ends of the developing bone, this hyaline cartilage will remain forever as **articular** (**joint) cartilage**, which covers the ends of long bones (6 and 7).
2.   At the location where the primary and secondary ossification centers meet is an **epiphyseal growth plate** (outlined in 6). This region of the developing bone at the junction of the diaphysis and epiphysis is called the **metaphysis**, so the term **metaphyseal growth plate** is sometimes used.

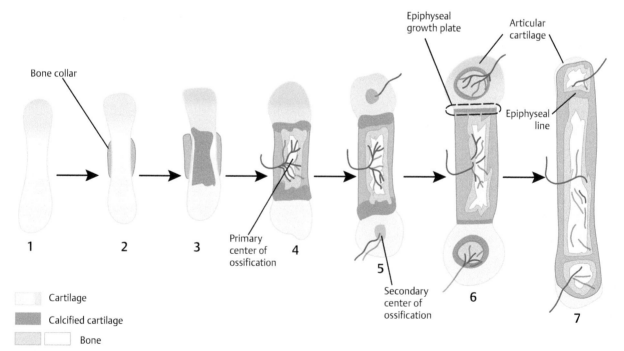

Fig. 12.7   Schematic of endochondral ossification in a long bone.

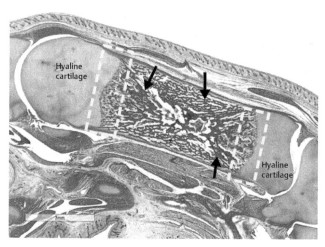

Fig. 12.8   Endochondral ossification of a long bone. Hyaline cartilage is indicated; black arrows mark bone spicules; boxed regions are the metaphyses containing the epiphyseal growth plates.

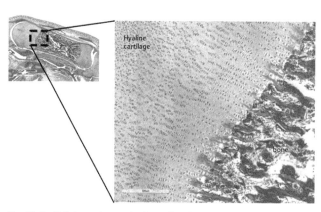

Fig. 12.9   Epiphyseal growth plate of endochondral ossification under medium magnification.

The cartilage in the epiphyseal growth plate continues to grow, and the new cartilage is converted to bone, allowing the bone itself to elongate during childhood. Sometime after puberty, bone completely replaces the cartilage in the epiphyseal plate, and lengthwise growth of the anatomic bone stops, leaving a thickened region of osseous tissue called the **epiphyseal line** (7, green arrow).

Fig. 12.8 is a low-magnification image from a developing bone that is similar to stage 4 in **Fig. 12.7**. The epiphyses consist of hyaline cartilage. The numerous dark spicules of bone (arrows) that have already formed from endochondral ossification in the primary ossification center fill the shaft where the marrow cavity will eventually form. The two yellow rectangles indicate the metaphyses, which contain the epiphyseal growth plates, where cartilage is being converted to bone; these regions are the focus of the next several figures.

Helpful Hint

The two regions in the yellow boxes in **Fig. 12.8** are mirror images of each other. The epiphyseal growth plate at left is moving toward the left as the cartilage there is growing and being replaced by bone, while the one on the right is moving to the right. In this way the bone grows lengthwise.

Fig. 12.9 is taken at slightly higher magnification, showing one end of the long bone, and focusing on the epiphyseal growth plate. The epiphysis (upper left) consists of hyaline cartilage, and the diaphysis (lower right) is composed of osseous spicules with marrow spaces. The region between these two is the metaphysis. The hyaline cartilage in the upper left is proliferating, so it is growing toward the upper left in this image. Because the cartilage is converting to bone, the epiphyseal growth plate is also progressing toward the upper left.

The conversion of cartilage to bone in the epiphyseal plate occurs in five stages:
1. Cartilage grows (similar to other cartilage).
2. Chondrocyte division becomes oriented longitudinally.
3. Chondrocytes swell.
4. The cartilage matrix becomes calcified.
5. Bone is laid down over pieces of cartilage.

In a snapshot of a growing bone, such as seen in **Fig, 12.9**, these processes manifest as regions in the epiphyseal growth plate. These regions (and their names) are described in the following paragraphs.

Zone of Reserve (Resting) Cartilage

The zone of reserve cartilage (**Fig. 12.10**, red outline) is similar to the hyaline cartilage discussed previously; it contains many chondrocytes in lacunae, clear matrix with glassy appearance, and no visible fibers.

The term "resting cartilage" for this region is unfortunate, because chondrocytes in hyaline cartilage are actively dividing and secreting matrix; this is the case here as well. In fact, it is the growth of this cartilage that is responsible for the lengthwise growth of long bones during development and childhood.

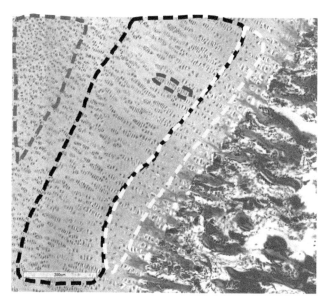

Fig. 12.10 Epiphyseal growth plate showing zone of resting cartilage (red outline); zone of proliferation (black outline) with a column of cells indicated (brown outline); zone of hypertrophy (yellow outline).

Zone of Proliferation

In the zone of proliferation (**Fig. 12.10**, black outline), division of chondrocytes is oriented so that progeny separate from each other along the long axis of the bone, creating columns of chondrocytes (one such column is outlined in brown).

> **Helpful Hint**
>
> This region is still growing cartilage, like the zone of resting cartilage. It is essentially the orientation of cell division that is the difference between these two regions.

Zone of Hypertrophy

Chondrocytes in this region (**Fig. 12.10**, yellow outline) hypertrophy (enlarge), and the cartilage matrix between the cells thins.

Zone of Calcification

The cartilage matrix becomes calcified in the last region of cartilage before bone deposition (**Fig. 12.11**, blue outline).

> **Helpful Hint**
>
> This is indeed calcified cartilage, meaning type II collagen + glycosaminoglycans + calcium. Like calcified matrix in bone, calcified cartilage matrix stains darker than its uncalcified counterpart (i.e., darker than the matrix in the zone of proliferation, see **Fig. 12.11**, arrows).

Zone of Bone Deposition

In the zone of bone deposition (**Fig. 12.11**, green outline), chondrocytes undergo apoptosis. Some cartilage matrix is removed by osteoclasts, while bone matrix is deposited on top of the remaining pieces of calcified cartilage.

    Fig. 12.12 is a medium-power image of the zone of bone deposition. Osteoclast degradation is targeted to occur in columns along the same orientation as the cell columns created by chondrocytes in the zone of proliferation (green arrows show the path of osteoclasts). This leaves spicules of calcified cartilage (black arrows) oriented along the long axis of the bone, and upon which bone matrix is added.

    Fig. 12.13 is a higher-power view of the zone of bone deposition highlighting the process of bone deposition. The core of the spicules in this region is calcified cartilage (Xs; trace the central core of these spicules up to the matrix in the zone of calcification). The darker magenta is calcified bone matrix that has been deposited by osteoblasts onto the surface of these spicules of calcified cartilage (black arrows indicate osteoblasts). In some places, paler osteoid between the osteoblasts and dark calcified bone matrix is visible (green arrow).

    Although the original spicules that form in the zone of bone deposition are composed of a core of calcified cartilage covered by calcified bone, subsequent remodeling of this tissue will eventually convert all of the tissue to bone.

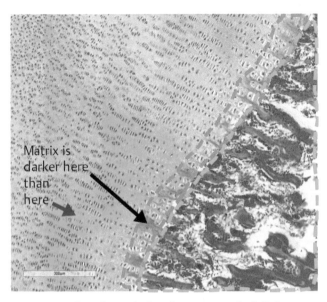

Fig. 12.11 **Epiphyseal growth plate showing zone of calcified cartilage (blue outline) and zone of bone deposition (green outline).**

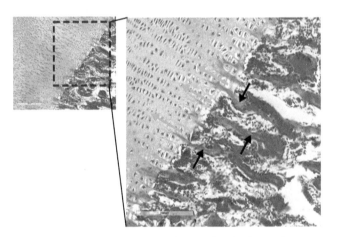

Fig. 12.12 **Epiphyseal growth plate showing details of osteoclast degradation of cartilage. Green arrows indicate the path of osteoclast degradation of calcified cartilage; black arrows show pieces of calcified cartilage that remain after osteoclast activity.**

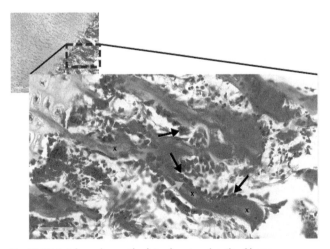

Fig. 12.13 **Epiphyseal growth plate showing details of bone deposition. Xs indicate calcified cartilage; black arrows point to osteoblasts; green arrow marks osteoid; the dark magenta bands between the osteoid and calcified cartilage are calcified bone matrix.**

Video 12.4 Endochondral ossification

Be able to identify:
— Endochondral ossification
Review bone cells
Be able to identify:
— Hyaline cartilage
— Calcified cartilage
— Osteoid
— Calcified bone matrix
— Epiphyseal growth plate
— Zone of resting cartilage
— Zone of proliferation
— Zone of hypertrophy
— Zone of calcification
— Zone of bone deposition
https://www.thieme.de/de/q.htm?p=opn/tp/308390101/978-1-62623-414-7_c012_v004&t=video

Final Notes about Growth at the Epiphyseal Growth Plate

The following are two final notes about the epiphyseal growth plate.

1. In a slide such as those presented here, five zones of the epiphyseal growth plate are defined. However, as with other biologic processes such as mitosis, there is a gradual transition from one zone to the next, so there are no absolute borders between these zones, and the borders between zones do not necessarily form straight lines.

2. In this static slide, five spatial zones are evident. However, a region, area, or cell passes through the five stages temporally. For example, the tissue in a particular region of the zone of resting cartilage will sequentially transition through the stages of proliferation, hypertrophy, cartilage calcification, and bone deposition. In fact, this is what occurs during the initial formation of the primary and secondary zones of ossification. The epiphyseal growth plate is thus a traveling wave that follows the proliferating cartilage, converting it to bone. In this way, the bone can grow lengthwise.

Growth of long bones *lengthwise* occurs via the epiphyseal growth plates as just described. An increase in the *diameter* of long bones involves appositional growth onto the outer surface by osteoblasts that differentiate from the surrounding periosteum. Bone degradation on the inner surface (the bone adjacent to the marrow cavity) balances this process, so the cross-sectional diameter of a long bone increases at the same time the bone grows lengthwise.

Basic Science Correlate: Physiology

Many hormones affect bone growth and remodeling, including growth hormone. The increase in sex hormones estrogen and testosterone at puberty stimulates proliferation of cartilage and increases the conversion of cartilage to bone in the epiphyseal growth plate. This results in the growth spurt seen during puberty. Eventually, the cartilage in the epiphyseal plate stops dividing and is completely replaced by bone, halting the lengthwise growth of bone. The location where the epiphyseal plate was located may show a thin region of slightly thicker bone called the epiphyseal line. Note that after the growth plates are lost, the only remaining cartilage is at the ends of the long bones: the articular cartilage.

Clinical Correlate

There are many abnormalities related to abnormal bone growth. By way of example, two can be presented here, both related to excess growth hormone production, which can occur with pituitary tumors (some pituitary cells secrete growth hormone). If excess growth hormone is produced while the epiphyseal growth plate is still active, then the bones will grow lengthwise to a more significant extent, but consistently with their girth and with the growth of other tissues stimulated by the excess growth hormone. This person will be proportionally tall, a condition called **gigantism**. If, however, excess growth hormone is produced after the growth plate has fused, then no lengthwise growth of the bones can occur. However, excess growth hormone will stimulate bone deposition onto the surface of the bones, resulting in thicker bones. This condition, called **acromegaly**, is most evident in thin bones of the face, hands, and feet.

Helpful Hint

A final note needs to be made regarding intramembranous and endochondral ossification in relation to spongy and compact bone. Because intramembranous ossification initially forms spongy bone, and endochondral ossification occurs in long bones, much of which is compact, it is tempting to equate intramembranous ossification with spongy bone and endochondral ossification with compact bone. This is absolutely not the case. Intramembranous and endochondral ossification are processes that produce bone, while spongy and compact describe the histologic features of bone (described in **Chapter 11**).

Both processes (intramembranous and endochondral) produce both types of bone (spongy and compact). For example, during endochondral ossification as described previously, spongy bone is formed (see **Fig. 12.8** and **Fig. 12.12**). After endochondral ossification, newly formed osseous tissue is remodeled so that some is compact, some is spongy. The same is true for intramembranous ossification; spicules and trabeculae from intramembranous ossification can thicken enough to form compact bone. For example, the flat bones of the skull (see B in **Fig. 11.2**) form via intramembranous ossification but contain both compact and spongy bone.

12.3 Bone Remodeling

Initial bone matrix formed by intramembranous and endochondral ossification is called **woven** or **primary bone**. The collagen fibers in woven bone are disorganized; therefore, woven bone is not very strong. Once bone is formed, it is remodeled, creating new matrix, called **lamellar** or **secondary bone**, in which the collagen fibers are more organized, creating bone that is stronger.

Remodeling occurs throughout the entire lifespan of the organism and includes degradation of bone by osteoclasts and deposition of bone by osteoblasts. The rate of osteoclast degradation and osteoblast deposition is well regulated so that there is no net loss or gain of bone under normal circumstances. However, certain conditions can result in a change in bone mass. For example, exercise stimulates bone deposition. Hormones also have a major effect; for example, estrogen and testosterone stimulate a net bone deposition.

osteons, so that portions of adjacent osteons and interstitial lamellae are degraded.

As osteoclasts are creating a resorption canal (A in **Fig. 12.15**), blood vessels in the center of the resorption canal bring osteoblasts in, which deposit osseous tissue along the inner edge of the canal to form the outermost concentric lamella (B in **Fig. 12.15**). Eventually, these osteoblasts become surrounded by matrix, becoming osteocytes (osteoblasts/osteocytes not shown). New matrix is laid down toward the center of the osteon, forming additional lamellae (C and D in **Fig. 12.15**), with osteoblasts becoming trapped in lacunae between lamellae. The process proceeds until all that remains is the **central canal** containing the blood vessels, which will supply the osteocytes in the newly formed osteon.

As osteoclasts create resorption canals down the length of the bone, they are immediately followed by osteoblasts, which lay down osseous tissue to fill in the canal as shown in **Fig. 12.15**. Therefore, bone resorption/deposition in this process is like a traveling wave down the shaft of compact bone. Lamella (tan) are laid down against the bone such that the outermost lamella are laid down first, followed by inner lamella (B–D).

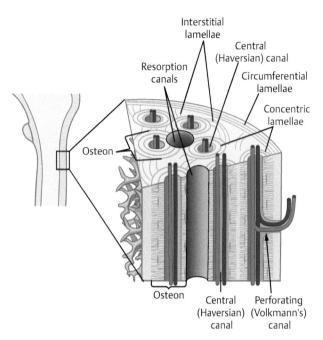

Fig. 12.14 **Organization of compact bone showing resorption canals.**

For spongy bone, remodeling is fairly straightforward because bone spicules are not thick. Osteoclasts degrade existing osseous tissue, which is replaced through osteoblast activity.

Remodeling of compact bone requires a more nuanced process because the newly produced osseous tissue must maintain an organized blood supply so that new osteocytes can obtain nutrients. This is achieved by the creation of new **osteons** as part of the remodeling process. The process begins with osteoclast activity, which creates a tunnel in existing compact bone. These tunnels, called **resorption canals** (**Fig. 12.14**), are parallel to the long axis of the bone and are approximately the size of a complete osteon. Typically, these canals are "staggered" with existing

Video 12.5 Resorption canals

Be able to identify:
— Resorption canals
https://www.thieme.de/de/q.htm?p=opn/
tp/308390101/978-1-62623-414-7_c012_
v005&t=video

12.4   Bone Fracture and Repair

When bone fractures occur, the blood supply is disrupted and local osteocytes die. In addition, torn vessels bleed into the fracture, and the blood clots, forming a blood hematoma. Immune cells (e.g., macrophages) migrate into the area to clean up the damaged tissue and clot. Progenitor cells in the periosteum and endosteum migrate into the damaged area and initially lay down fibrocartilaginous tissue, which forms a callus. This tissue is remodeled into woven bone and subsequently to lamellar bone, similar to the ossification processes described here.

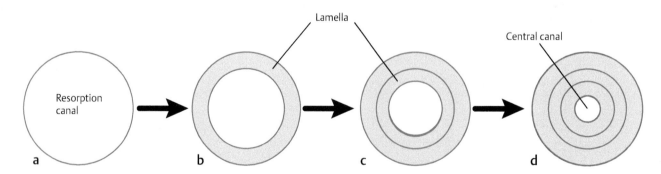

Fig. 12.15 **Remodeling of compact bone by creation of a new osteon. The clear space in the center of the circle is the resorption canal created by osteoclasts. Note that the tissue outside the circle is bone, so the circle (a) represents the inner edge of bone of the resorption canal. Lamellae (tan) are laid down against the bone such that the outermost lamellae are laid down first, followed by inner lamellae (b–d).**

12.5 Chapter Review

Chapter 11 focused on the cells of bone and the organization of mature bone. This chapter focused on bone formation, called ossification. Bone formation begins when osteoblasts secrete type I collagen, forming osteoid. Calcification of the osteoid produces calcified bone matrix. The osteoblasts that become surrounded by this matrix reside in lacunae as osteocytes. Before laying down matrix, osteoblasts extend cell processes that connect to adjacent osteoblasts; these processes lie in tunnels in the calcified matrix called canaliculi. There are two types of ossification. In intramembranous ossification, bone develops directly from mesenchyme. In endochondral ossification, a cartilage model is created first, which is subsequently converted to bone. This occurs through a series of steps that include cartilage proliferation, specialized proliferation of chondrocytes into columns, hypertrophy of chondrocytes, and calcification of the cartilage matrix. After portions of the calcified cartilage are broken down, bone is deposited onto the cartilage spicules. This process occurs during fetal development; a region called the epiphyseal growth plate persists after birth and provides a mechanism for lengthwise growth of long bones. Lengthwise growth of long bones ceases when the cartilage in the epiphyseal plate ceases to divide and is converted to bone. Bones grow in diameter by appositional growth onto the outer surface and concomitant removal of bone adjacent to the marrow cavity. Bone remodeling occurs in both spongy and compact bone. Initial bone formed is disorganized bone called woven bone, which is quickly replaced by organized, lamellar bone. Bone is continually remodeled, involving resorption of old bone by osteoclasts and deposition of new bone by osteoblasts. Remodeling in compact bone requires an organized resorption and deposition to ensure that osteocytes maintain a sufficient blood supply. Repair of fractured bone has features similar to ossification.

Questions and Answers

An online-only section of questions and answers accompanying this chapter is hosted on Thieme's MedOne Education site: https://medone-education.thieme.com. Use the code on the media page at the front of this book to gain access. An institutional license to the site is required to access these questions in an interactive format, and individual users are required to register for an individual account to track results.

CHAPTER 12

13   Skeletal Muscle

After completing this chapter, you should be able to:
— Identify, at the light microscope level, each of the following:
  • Skeletal muscle
    ○ Muscle fibers (myofibers, muscle cells)
      ▪ Myofibrils
    ○ Fascicle
    ○ Connective tissues of skeletal muscle
      ▪ Endomysium
      ▪ Perimysium
      ▪ Epimysium
    ○ Bands and lines seen in skeletal muscle
      ▪ A band
      ▪ I band
      ▪ H band
      ▪ Z line
      ▪ M line
      ▪ Zone of overlap
      ▪ Sarcomere
— Identify, at the electron microscope level, each of the following:
  • Skeletal muscle
    ○ Muscle fibers (myofibers, muscle cells)
    ○ Myofibrils
    ○ Myofilaments
      ▪ Thick filaments
      ▪ Thin filaments
    ○ Sarcolemma
    ○ Bands and lines noted for light microscopy
    ○ Sarcoplasmic reticulum
    ○ Triad
      ▪ Terminal cisternae of sarcoplasmic reticulum
      ▪ Transverse tubule (T tubule)
— Outline the function of each cell and structure listed
— Diagram skeletal muscle contraction, and compare and contrast structures of the sarcomere in the contracted and relaxed state
— Illustrate the transmission of an action potential in skeletal muscle to an increase in cytoplasmic calcium

13.1   Overview of Muscle Tissue

Muscle tissue has one common function: it shortens (contracts). This is accomplished by **muscle cells**, which are bundled together by connective tissues that also contain the blood vessels and nerves that support the muscle cells.

There are three types of muscle tissue:
• **Skeletal muscle** is involved in voluntary contraction and is associated with the body wall. As described below, it is **striated**, meaning that, when skeletal muscle cells are oriented longitudinally and examined under high magnification, alternating dark and light bands are visible. With a few exceptions, named muscles (biceps brachii, pectoralis major) are composed of skeletal muscle.
• **Cardiac muscle** is found in the heart. Cardiac muscle is also striated but is involuntary.

• **Smooth muscle** is involuntary and is found in visceral organs, such as the gastrointestinal, respiratory, urinary, and reproductive systems. It is also found in the body wall, specifically as smooth muscle of blood vessels as well as arrector pili muscles of the hair follicles. Smooth muscle is so named because it is not striated.

This chapter will focus on skeletal muscle structure and function, which serves as a model system for muscle in general. The next chapter will describe cardiac and smooth muscle, with a focus on how these muscle types differ from skeletal muscle.

13.2   Organization of Skeletal Muscles

Skeletal muscles such as the biceps brachii are composed of **skeletal muscle cells**, bundled together by connective tissue (**Fig. 13.1**). Skeletal muscle cells are commonly called **muscle fibers** (**myofibers**) because they are very long compared to their diameter, which is also large. Muscle fibers within most muscles are aligned parallel to the long axis of the muscle, so that they all shorten in the same direction.

Within a muscle, groups of muscle cells are bundled together into **fascicles** (**Fig. 13.1**).

The connective tissue component of a muscle is organized into three types:
• **Epimysium** surrounding the entire muscle
• **Perimysium** around fascicles
• **Endomysium** between individual muscle cells

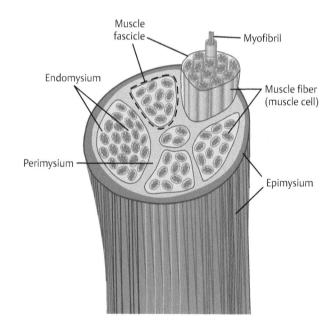

Fig. 13.1   **Diagram of a skeletal muscle (e.g., biceps brachii). Connective tissue elements lie between muscle fibers (endomysium), bundle cells into fascicles (perimysium), and surround the entire muscle (epimysium).**

Consistent with connective tissue organization in most organs, the connective tissue surrounding the entire muscle is denser than the connective tissues within the muscle. Therefore, the epimysium is dense irregular connective tissue, endomysium is loose connective tissue, and perimysium is somewhere in between ("loosy-dense" connective tissue).

Fig. 13.2 is a scanning image of a cross section of an entire muscle. A single fascicle is outlined, and the epimysium (black arrows) and perimysium (blue arrows) are indicated.

Basic Science Correlate: Gross Anatomy

The epimysium is the deep fascia that surrounds muscles, as encountered in the gross anatomy lab.

Fig. 13.3 is a high-magnification image of the edge of the cross section of skeletal muscle, showing a portion of a fascicle. A single muscle fiber (muscle cell) is outlined. The epimysium (black arrow), perimysium (blue arrows), and endomysium (green arrows) are indicated.

Apart from the difference in density, these layers appear similar because they are all connective tissue. These connective tissues are named based on their position within the muscle and among the muscle fibers.

Video 13.1 Skeletal muscle showing epimysium, perimysium, and endomysium

Be able to identify:
— Skeletal muscle
  • Fascicle
  • Endomysium
  • Perimysium
  • Endomysium

https://www.thieme.de/de/q.htm?p=opn/tp/308390101/978-1-62623-414-7_c013_v001&t=video

13.3   Skeletal Muscle Cells (Muscle Fibers)

Skeletal muscle cells develop from the fusion of **myoblasts**, resulting in large, multinuclear cells (**Fig. 13.4**). The cells then synthesize proteins involved in contraction (particularly actin and myosin), which assemble into large bundles in the cytoplasm called **myofibrils**. Each myofibril has an alternate dark-light banding pattern when viewed from the side. These myofibrils fill the cell and push the nuclei to the periphery of the cell.

Fig. 13.5 shows a longitudinal view of skeletal muscle taken at high magnification, showing five to seven muscle cells, of which two are indicated by the brackets. Typically, within a single muscle, all muscle cells are the same diameter; the apparent difference seen in the diameters of these cells is due to sectioning (i.e., the section goes through the middle of some cells and cuts closer to the edge of others).

Muscle cells are very long cells, extending far beyond the upper and lower borders of **Fig. 13.5**. They also have a wide

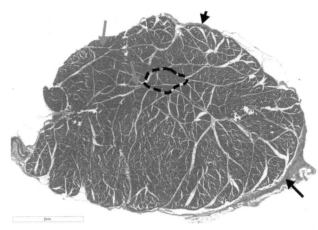

Fig. 13.2   **Skeletal muscle in cross section, scanning magnification. A fascicle is outlined; epimysium (black arrows) and perimysium (blue arrows) are indicated.**

diameter (compare to the size of the nuclei). The striated appearance of these cells (alternating dark-light pattern) is evident. Most nuclei are situated in the periphery of the cell.

Helpful Hint

Actually, some nuclei in **Fig. 13.5** belong to the muscle cells, while others are of fibroblasts of the endomysium. It is difficult to tell for sure, but nuclei in muscle cells usually are more euchromatic than fibroblast nuclei, so the nuclei indicated by the black arrows likely belong to muscle cells, whereas those indicated by the blue arrows belong to fibroblasts. Also note that the fibroblast nuclei (blue arrows) are surrounded by extracellular matrix (light pink).

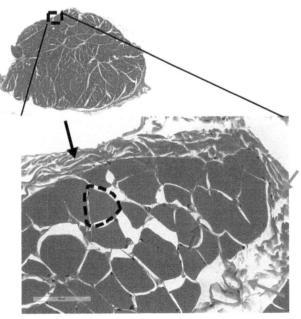

Fig. 13.3   **Skeletal muscle in cross section under high magnification, showing a muscle fiber (muscle cell, outlined), epimysium (black arrow), perimysium (blue arrows), and endomysium (green arrows).**

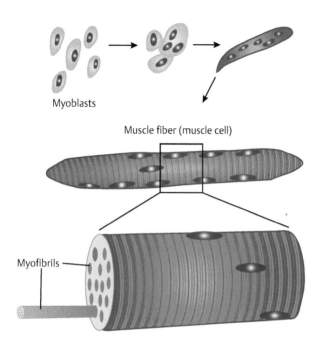

Fig. 13.4   Formation of skeletal muscle cells. During development, muscle cell precursors called myoblasts fuse together to make large, multinuclear muscle cells (muscle fibers). These cells synthesize contractile proteins, which organize into myofibrils in the cytoplasm, pushing the nuclei to the periphery of the cell.

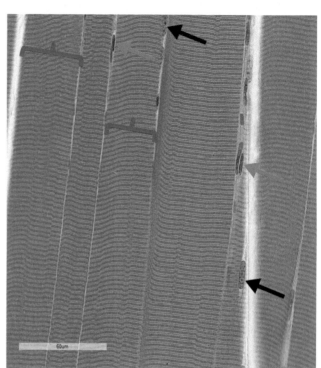

Fig. 13.5   Skeletal muscle in longitudinal section. Muscle cells are indicated by the brackets. Nuclei are indicated: muscle cell nuclei indicated by black arrows, fibroblast nuclei indicated by blue arrows.

Video 13.2 Skeletal muscle cells

Be able to identify:
— Skeletal muscle cells
https://www.thieme.de/de/q.htm?p=opn/
tp/308390101/978-1-62623-414-7_c013_
v002&t=video

As mentioned, because skeletal muscle cells are very long, they are called muscle fibers or myofibers. **Fig. 13.6** is a drawing of a small portion of a skeletal muscle fiber near the plasma membrane, showing that the cytoplasm of skeletal muscle cells is packed with contractile proteins organized into rodlike structures called myofibrils that are oriented with the longitudinal axis of the muscle fiber. Each muscle fiber contains hundreds of myofibrils.

Cellular components of muscle cells are named using the prefix *sarco-* :

• The cytoplasm of a muscle cell is referred to as **sarcoplasm**.

• The smooth endoplasmic reticulum of a muscle cell is referred to as **sarcoplasmic reticulum**.

• The plasma membrane of a muscle cell is referred to as the **sarcolemma**.

Helpful Hint

Because skeletal muscle has rods within rods within rods, it's easy to lose perspective and get lost in the terminology. The drawing in **Fig. 13.6** is only a small part of a single muscle cell (and not four separate cells). Organelles such as nuclei or mitochondria are helpful aids to orient to size.

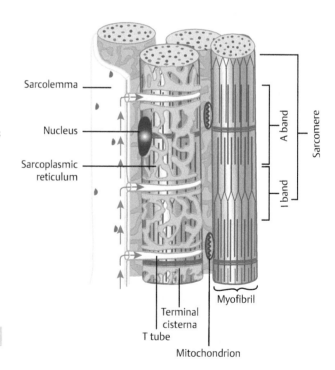

Fig. 13.6   Drawing of a portion of a skeletal muscle fiber (muscle cell), showing four myofibrils, as well as other organelles. The blue arrows represent the path of an action potential along the surface of the muscle fiber and into the T tubule system (discussed subsequently).

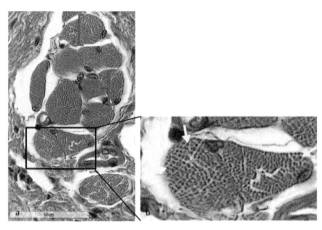

Fig. 13.7 **(a) Skeletal muscle in cross section. Two muscle fibers (cells) are indicated by the green brackets. (b) Enlargement of the single muscle fiber outlined in black in (a), showing myofibrils (yellow arrows).**

Fig. 13.7 shows skeletal muscle cut in cross section. **Fig. 13.7a** shows a fascicle with about 10 muscle fibers; two muscle fibers are indicated by the green brackets, and a single muscle fiber is within the black rectangle. When skeletal muscle cells are cut in perfect cross section, stippling in the cells can be seen owing to the myofibrils cut in cross section. The single muscle fiber (cell) within the black rectangle in **Fig. 13.7a** is artificially magnified in **Figure**

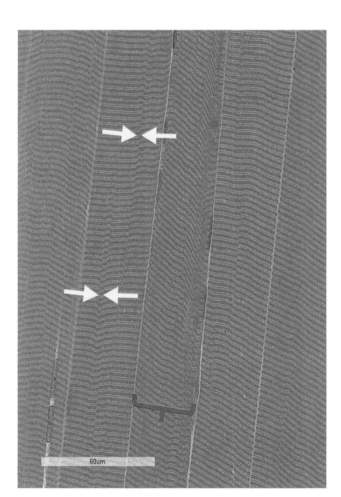

Fig. 13.8 **Skeletal muscle in longitudinal section showing myofibrils. A muscle fiber (cell) is indicated by the bracket. Yellow arrows indicate the width of one (or possibly two) myofibrils.**

13.7b, showing that each muscle fiber is filled with myofibrils (yellow arrows). Muscle cells can have hundreds of myofibrils.

> **Helpful Hint**
>
> Myofibrils are oriented longitudinally inside the muscle fiber (cell). The muscle fibers in **Fig. 13.7** are cut in cross section, so the myofibrils are also cut in cross section.

Fig. 13.8 shows another high-magnification image, this time of a longitudinal section of five to six skeletal muscle fibers (muscle cells); the green bracket indicates one cell. The alternating dark and light banding pattern (explained in detail in the next section) is caused by the alternating light and dark bands of each myofibril in the cell; and the myofibrils are arranged so that their dark bands line up side by side, as do the light bands (i.e., they are "in register").

About 30 to 50 myofibrils span the diameter of a single cell. Because the myofibrils are in register, most individual myofibrils cannot be seen. However, during fixation, some myofibrils "slide," putting them out of register with their neighbors. Between each set of yellow arrows in **Fig. 13.8** is a single myofibril (possibly two) that has slid, providing an idea of the diameter of a single myofibril relative to the entire cell.

> **Helpful Hint**
>
> As mentioned above, a skeletal muscle cell contains hundreds of myofibrils, while **Fig. 13.8** shows 30 to 50 spanning the diameter of a cell. That is because a section through the diameter of the cell will cut through only some of the myofibrils.

Video 13.3 Skeletal muscle showing myofibrils in longitudinal section

Be able to identify:
— Skeletal muscle
— Myofibers
— Myofibrils
https://www.thieme.de/de/q.htm?p=opn/tp/308390101/978-1-62623-414-7_c013_v003&t=video

13.4   Banding Pattern of Skeletal Muscle Cells

As mentioned, the banding pattern seen in light micrographs of skeletal muscle is created by the collective banding present on each myofibril. In **Fig. 13.9**, the dark bands called **A bands** (e.g., the one spanned by the yellow bracket) alternate with light bands called **I bands** (e.g., the one spanned by the black bracket) in a repetitive manner; this alternation extends over the entire length of the muscle fiber. A dark line within each I band is called the **Z line** (black arrows). Less obvious is a pale region within the A band, referred to as the **H zone** or **H band** (maroon arrows).

The functional contractile unit of skeletal muscle, the **sarcomere**, extends from one Z line to the next (blue bracket). Note that the sarcomere includes an A band plus two halves of

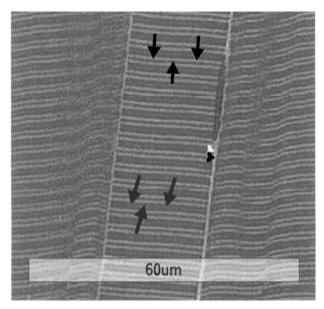

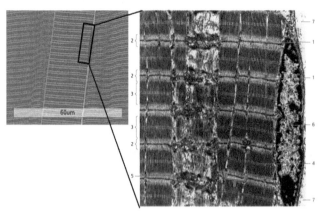

Fig. 13.10 Electron micrograph of a region similar to that outlined in black on the light micrograph. A myofibril is indicated by the red bracket. (1) Z lines; (2) I bands; (3) A bands; (4) H zone containing M line; (5) mitochondria; (6) nucleus; (7) extracellular material.

Fig. 13.9   Skeletal muscle in longitudinal section (an enlargement of part of Fig. 13.8) showing banding pattern in detail. The yellow bracket spans an A band, and the black bracket spans an I band; the blue bracket spans a sarcomere. The Z line (black arrows) and H zone (maroon arrows) are also indicated.

adjacent I bands. Adjacent sarcomeres share the Z line; for example, in this orientation, a single Z line is the "upper" end of one sarcomere and the "lower" end of another.

Video 13.4 Skeletal muscle showing banding pattern

Be able to identify:
— Skeletal muscle
— A band
— I band
— Z line
— H zone (H band)
— Sarcomere
https://www.thieme.de/de/q.htm?p=opn/tp/308390101/978-1-62623-414-7_c013_v004&t=video

Fig. 13.10 shows an electron micrograph of a portion of a muscle fiber that includes a nucleus (6) and five to seven myofibrils (one myofibril indicated by the red bracket). The banding pattern seen in the light micrographs can be visualized in greater detail in the electron micrograph, including the lighter I bands (2) and dark A bands (3). Within the A bands is a pale band, the H zone containing the **M line** (4). Dark lines in the middle of the I bands are Z lines (1).

Fig. 13.11 is a higher-magnification electron micrograph, showing the details of a sarcomere (one sarcomere is within the yellow rectangle). The orientation of **Fig. 13.11** is rotated 90° from that of **Fig. 13.10**, so the myofibrils are oriented from left to right. Note the Z lines (1), I band (2 and orange bracket) and A band (3 and green bracket). The H band within the A band is difficult to see (yellow bracket), but note the presence of a dark line within the H band (red arrows); this is the M line (M line within H band is better seen in **Fig. 13.10**, 4).

Because a sarcomere extends from Z line to Z line, an I band is shared by two adjacent sarcomeres. Also, note that one myofibril (red bracket in **Fig. 13.11**) has "slid" relative to the others during tissue preparation.

13.5   Myofilaments

Close examination of the electron micrograph in **Fig. 13.11** reveals filamentous structures oriented longitudinally along the axis of the sarcomere (horizontally). **Fig. 13.12** shows one of the sarcomeres from this same electron micrograph, along with a corresponding drawing showing these filaments and how they are assembled within a sarcomere. These filaments are called **myofilaments**, of which there are two types:

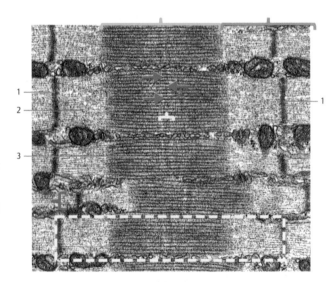

Fig. 13.11 Electron micrograph of skeletal muscle showing sarcomeres (one sarcomere outlined by the yellow bracket); note that myofibrils are not all the same diameter due to sectioning. Orange bracket: I band; green bracket: A band; yellow bracket: H zone; red arrows indicate the M line. Other features include (1) Z line; (2) part of I band; (3) part of A band. The red bracket indicates a myofibril that has "slid" relative to neighboring myofibrils.

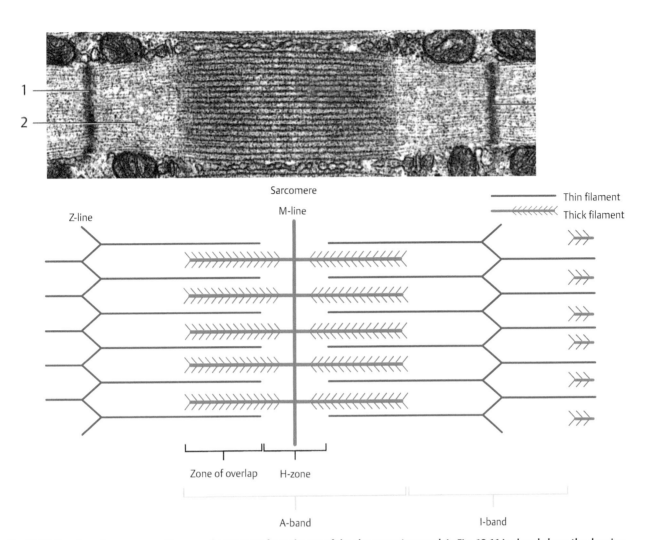

Fig. 13.12 Drawing of a sarcomere. The second sarcomere from the top of the electron micrograph in Fig. 13.11 is placed above the drawing, aligned so that the components in the micrograph line up with the structures in the drawing.

- **Thin filaments**, made up of **actin** (the same protein that makes up microfilaments in the cytoskeleton)
- **Thick filaments**, made up of proteins called **myosin**

Each type of myofilament is anchored by a collection of proteins that form specific lines:
- The Z line anchors the thin filaments.
- The M line anchors the thick filaments.

Helpful Hint

From a different perspective, each Z line has numerous thin filaments extending from it in both directions, and each M line has numerous thick filaments extending from it in both directions.

Also note that thin and thick filaments extend past each other, creating a new component of the sarcomere, the **zone of overlap**.

It should also be pointed out that the myofibrils are cylindrical structures, not flat. Therefore, although the terms "Z lines" and "M lines" are used in reference to longitudinal sections of muscle, these structures are actually disk shaped and can be better called Z disks and M disks.

The thick filaments extending from either side of the M line are in opposite orientations, as shown in the drawing in **Fig. 13.12**.

In other words, the thick filaments to the right of the M line are mirror images of the ones to the left. The same is true for the thin filaments relative to the Z line.

Fig. 13.13 shows the sarcomere from **Fig. 13.12**, with the myofilaments marked:
- Thin filaments (orange arrows), made up of actin
- Thick filaments (purple arrows), made up of myosin

The thin filaments extend into the A band (between the thick filaments) to create the zone of overlap. The H zone is the region of the A band that does not include thin filaments (see drawing in **Fig. 13.12**).

To solidify understanding of the organization of a sarcomere, it is useful to think about the proteins that are present in cross sections through each region of a sarcomere. **Fig. 13.14** is an artificially magnified sarcomere from **Fig. 13.10**, with vertical lines indicating cross sections through regions of the sarcomere listed here:
- M line (orange line): thick filaments cross-linked by M line proteins
- H zone (pink line): thick filaments only
- Zone of overlap (red line): both thick and thin filaments
- I band (purple line): thin filaments only
- Z line (blue line): thin filaments cross-linked by Z line proteins

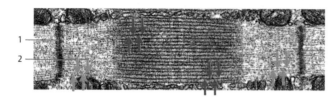

Fig. 13.13 Sarcomere from the electron micrograph in Fig. 13.12. Thick filaments (purple arrows) and thin filaments (orange arrows) are shown. Other structures marked: (1) Z line; (2) part of I band.

13.6   Contraction of Skeletal Muscle

Muscle contraction is a function of the action of myofilaments. Each thick filament is made up of hundreds of myosin proteins. Individual myosin proteins that make up the thick filaments consists of a filamentous portion and a globular (head) domain (**Fig. 13.15**). The angle of the globular domain can be in either the "cocked" (**Fig. 13.15a**) or the "flexed" (**Fig. 13.15b**) position. The filamentous portions of hundreds of myosin proteins bundle together to create a thick filament with the head domains sticking out around the periphery of the filament (**Fig. 13.15c**). These bundles of myosin proteins are the thick filaments shown in the drawing in **Fig. 13.12**; the myosin heads are the "bristles" shown on the thick filaments and are shown in the cocked position.

Remember that the thick filaments on either side of the M line are mirror images of each other. In the presence of ATP, the globular domains cycle from a cocked position (**Fig. 13.15a**) to a flexed

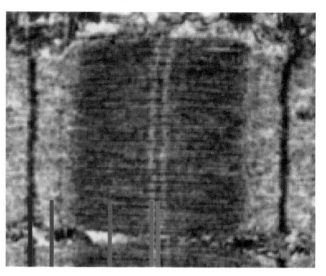

Fig. 13.14 Single sarcomere from the electron micrograph in Fig. 13.10. Lines indicate cross sections, each containing a different set of sarcomere proteins.

position (**Fig. 13.15b**). In addition, in the presence of calcium, the myosin heads can bind to and release actin thin filaments. In this way, during contraction, each head domain in the cocked position can cross bridge with an adjacent thin filament, flex, and then release. By repeating the cycle, and with all myosin heads working in the same fashion, the Z lines in a sarcomere can be pulled toward the M lines.

Fig. 13.16 shows contraction of a single sarcomere. **Fig. 13.16a** shows the sarcomere before contraction (relaxed state); **Fig. 13.16b** shows the sarcomere after contraction. During contraction, as a result of the action of the myosin heads, the thin filaments are pulled toward the M line. The thin and thick filaments slide past each other, a phenomenon known as the **sliding filament model** of muscle contraction. As a result, the Z lines are moved closer together. Note that the lengths of the thick and thin filaments do not change during contraction. In addition, the A band remains the same width. However, because the thin and thick filaments "telescope" past each other, the width of the zone of overlap increases, while the H zone and I band both decrease in width.

> **Helpful Hint**
>
> Understanding how structures and zones in a sarcomere change during contraction will solidify understanding of the structure and function of skeletal muscle. This is fairly high yield.

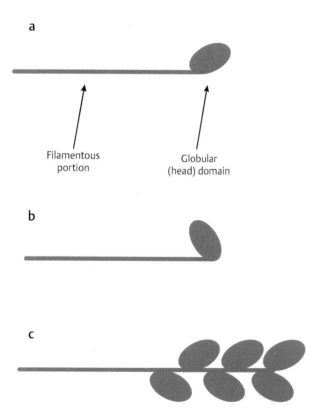

Fig. 13.15 Structure of myosin proteins that make up thick filaments, shown in the (a) "cocked" and (b) "flexed" positions, and (c) a bundle of six myosin proteins.

Taking a step back, both figuratively but also in terms of magnification, recall that each myofibril in a muscle cell (see **Fig. 13.10**, red bracket) is composed of hundreds of sarcomeres linked end to end. So, even if a single sarcomere shortens only slightly (as shown in **Fig. 13.16**), collectively they result in a significant shortening of the entire myofibril. Myofibrils are connected to the sarcolemma of the muscle fiber, so if all the myofibrils in a muscle fiber (muscle cell) shorten at the same time, this results in a significant and powerful shortening of the muscle cell. Since muscle cells are attached to the surrounding connective tissue (endomysium, perimysium, and epimysium), which is continuous with tendons or other structures, contraction of muscle cells in a muscle can generate movement.

a   **Sarcomere**

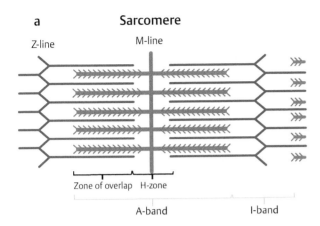

Z-line   M-line

Zone of overlap   H-zone

A-band   I-band

b   **Sarcomere contracted**

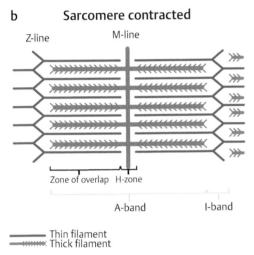

Z-line   M-line

Zone of overlap   H-zone

A-band   I-band

———— Thin filament
—❮❮❮❮❮— Thick filament

Fig. 13.16 **Sarcomere (a) in relaxed and (b) contracted state.**

The attachment of myofibrils in muscle cells to, ultimately, the surrounding connective tissue occurs through a number of intracellular, membrane-bound, and extracellular proteins that interact with each other. One such protein is **dystrophin**, which is a cytoplasmic protein that anchors actin filaments to the sarcolemma. The two most common forms of muscular dystrophy, **Duchenne muscular dystrophy** and **Becker muscular dystrophy**, are caused by mutations in dystrophin. Muscular dystrophy is characterized by weakness due to muscle fiber degeneration. The heart and cognitive abilities can also be affected.

13.7   Tubule System of Skeletal Muscle

Elevated cytoplasmic calcium is required to allow interaction of myosin heads with thin filaments and, therefore, is required for contraction. Calcium concentration in the cytoplasm of most cells, including resting muscle cells, is very low. Calcium is stored in the sarcoplasmic reticulum, and muscle contraction is stimulated by a release of this calcium from the sarcoplasmic reticulum into the cytoplasm.

The large diameter of skeletal muscle fibers requires an elaborate cellular architecture to ensure that all myofibrils receive this calcium signal at the same time. This architecture has two major components (see **Fig. 13.6**):

- Invaginations of the sarcolemma (plasma membrane) forming **transverse tubules**, or **T tubules**. Neural stimulation of a skeletal muscle fiber occurs in a specialized location on the sarcolemma called the **neuromuscular junction**, which results in action potentials that spread along the sarcolemma (**Fig. 13.6**, vertical blue arrows). These action potentials travel down the T tubule system to bring the excitation wave to the center of the cell (curved blue arrows).

- The elaborate sarcoplasmic reticulum is highlighted by dilations called **terminal cisternae**, which are adjacent to the T tubules. Upon arrival of an action potential in the T tubule, calcium channels in the membrane of the sarcoplasmic reticulum open, and calcium diffuses into the cytoplasm. Relaxation requires calcium reuptake by the sarcoplasmic reticulum.

In some tissues, the T tubules are flanked on either side by terminal cisternae. The three tubules together, a central T tubule flanked by two terminal cisternae, form a **triad**. In human skeletal muscle, the triad is located near the A–I band junction. Human cardiac muscle has only one terminal cisterna associated with each T tubule, forming **diads**. Some other organisms have diads in their skeletal muscle as well.

Star Wars fans might think of the action potential traveling along the muscle surface sarcolemma (**Fig. 13.6**, vertical blue arrows) as Luke's shot as it traveled along the surface of the Death Star. These action potentials make 90° turns to travel down the T tubule system (**Fig. 13.6**, curved blue arrows) into the depths of the cell, like Luke's shot dropping into the hole to travel down into the depths of the Death Star.

The T tubules and terminal cisternae of the sarcoplasmic reticulum can be seen in electron micrographs as small vesicle-shaped structures (**Fig. 13.17**, arrows). They are often challenging to identify clearly, and often only one or two components of the triad can be seen. Occasionally all three are visible (**Fig. 13.17**, yellow arrows). In this case, the central vesicle is the T tubule, which is usually more elongated, flanked by rounder terminal cisternae on either side. As mentioned, in human

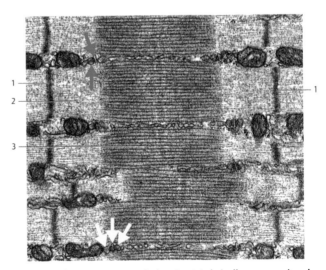

Fig. 13.17 **Electron micrograph showing triads (yellow arrows) and other tubular systems in which only two of the three components are clearly identifiable (red arrows).**

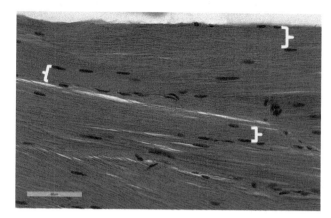

Fig. 13.18 **Skeletal muscle in tissues in (mostly) longitudinal view, high magnification. The diameter of skeletal muscle fibers (muscle cells) is indicated by the brackets.**

skeletal muscle, a triad is typically found near the A–I junction, while in cardiac muscle and muscle in some other organisms, the location and number of tubules varies.

Helpful Hint

The specific identification of these components in electron micrographs is not likely to be high yield. However, they are important physiologically, so a mental image is helpful.

13.8   Skeletal Muscle in Routinely Prepared Slides

Up to this point, most of the images in this chapter were from skeletal muscle embedded in plastic, which allows better resolution of the components of skeletal muscle fibers. In addition, the images were oriented so that most of the muscle fibers were cut longitudinally. However, routine preparations of tissues containing skeletal muscle (embedded in paraffin instead of plastic) are not as ideally positioned as these images, so it is useful to consider these because they represent the more common presentation of skeletal muscle tissue. **Fig. 13.18** shows a typical longitudinal view of skeletal muscle. The diameter of a few muscle fibers (cells) is indicated by the brackets. Note the intense cytoplasmic eosinophilia due to the tremendous amount of contractile proteins in these cells. In this longitudinal orientation, striations are still visible in some locations, but cell borders are not as obvious. However, most nuclei are toward the periphery of the cell, which helps to estimate cell borders. Skeletal muscle nuclei are elongated, but are fairly euchromatic, so they look "plump."

Fig. 13.19 shows a slightly oblique cut through skeletal muscle from a different specimen. The diameter of a single fiber (cell) is indicated by the bracket. Because the cut is slightly oblique, it is harder to see the striations. However, note that the cells are very large, with a large diameter, intense cytoplasmic eosinophilia, and peripheral nuclei (most nuclei are not clear in this preparation).

Fig. 13.20 shows a cut that is more oblique, such that no striations are visible. The wide diameter of muscle fibers can still be appreciated (yellow brackets), based on the positioning

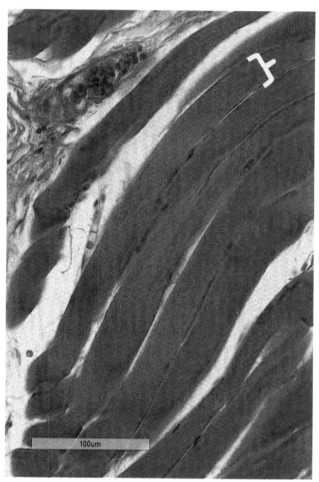

Fig. 13.19 **Skeletal muscle in tissues in slightly oblique view, medium-high magnification. The diameter of a skeletal muscle fiber (muscle cell) is indicated by the bracket.**

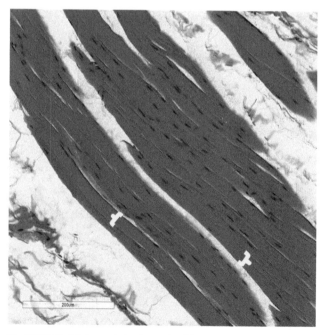

Fig. 13.20 **Skeletal muscle in tissues in oblique view, medium magnification. The diameter of skeletal muscle fibers (muscle cells) is indicated by the brackets.**

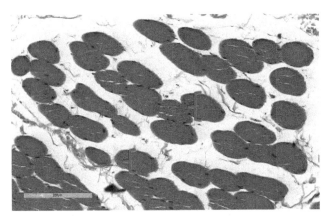

Fig. 13.21 **Skeletal muscle in tissues in cross section, medium magnification. The diameter of skeletal muscle fibers (muscle cells) is indicated by the brackets.**

of the nuclei and the loose connective tissue (endomysium) that separates the cells.

Finally, **Fig. 13.21** shows skeletal muscle cut in cross section. Note that these skeletal muscle fibers (green brackets) have a wide diameter and are, for the most part, the same size. The cytoplasm has intense eosinophilia, and most of the nuclei are peripheral.

In cross sections, it is usually easier to see the cell borders and peripheral nuclei. Close examination sometimes reveals stippling within the cytoplasm (not visible on this image, but see **Fig. 13.7**), which represents the myofibrils cut in cross section.

Video 13.5 Skeletal muscle

Be able to identify:
— Skeletal muscle
https://www.thieme.de/de/q.htm?p=opn/tp/308390101/978-1-62623-414-7_c013_v005&t=video

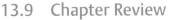

13.9 Chapter Review

Muscle tissues provide movement by contracting (shortening). There are three types of muscle tissue: skeletal, cardiac, and smooth. Skeletal muscles (e.g., biceps brachii) are composed of large cells called muscle fibers, which are bundled together by connective tissue. The muscle cells are packed with hundreds of myofibrils: cylindrical units composed of sarcomeres linked together end to end. These myofibrils are composed of many proteins, the most abundant of which are those making up the myofilaments. Myofilaments are of two types: thin filaments are composed of actin, and thick filaments are composed of myosin. Thin filaments extend from a structure called the Z line, and thick filaments are anchored at an M line. The regular arrangement of these myofilaments within a myofibril creates a regular banding pattern, called striations, within skeletal (and cardiac) muscle cells. These regions include the A band, I band, H zone, and the aforementioned Z line and M line. In addition, the location where the thick and thin filaments overlap (zone of overlap) enables the interaction between these proteins required for contraction. Each thick filament is composed of hundreds of myosin proteins, each with a globular and a filamentous domain. The globular domains can alternate between the flexed and cocked positions in an ATP-dependent manner, which drives sliding of the thin filaments relative to the thick filaments. The sliding filament theory explains how this motion brings the Z lines of a sarcomere closer together, the shortening action that results in contraction of the muscle. This process requires calcium, which is stored in the sarcoplasmic reticulum and released when an action potential travels down the T tubule system. Skeletal muscle in routine tissue preparations can be recognized because the muscle fibers are very large cells, striated on longitudinal section, with a very eosinophilic cytoplasm and numerous peripheral nuclei.

Questions and Answers

An online-only section of questions and answers accompanying this chapter is hosted on Thieme's MedOne Education site: https://medone-education.thieme.com. Use the code on the media page at the front of this book to gain access. An institutional license to the site is required to access these questions in an interactive format, and individual users are required to register for an individual account to track results.

14   Cardiac and Smooth Muscle

After completing this chapter, you should be able to:
— Identify, at the light microscope level, each of the following:
  • Muscle
    ◦ Skeletal muscle
    ◦ Cardiac muscle
      ▪ Intercalated disks
    ◦ Smooth muscle
— Identify, at the electron microscope level, each of the following:
  • Cardiac muscle
    ◦ Intercalated disks
  • Smooth muscle
    ◦ Myofilaments (mostly actin filaments)
    ◦ Dense bodies
    ◦ Pinocytotic vesicles
— Outline the function of each structure and muscle type listed
— Correlate the main function of muscle types with histological features
— Indicate the locations of types of muscle

14.1   Types of Muscle Tissue

Recall that there are three types of muscle tissue:
• **Skeletal muscle** is involved in voluntary contraction, is striated, and is associated with the body wall. This is the tissue of named muscles (biceps brachii, pectoralis major).
• **Cardiac muscle** is found in the heart, is striated, and is involuntary.
• **Smooth muscle** is found in visceral organs, such as the gastrointestinal, respiratory, urinary, and reproductive systems. It is also found in the body wall, specifically smooth muscle of blood vessels as well as arrector pili muscles of the hair follicles. It is not striated and is involuntary.

Chapter 13 described skeletal muscle in detail. This chapter will focus on cardiac and smooth muscle, followed by comparisons to each other, skeletal muscle, and connective tissue.

14.2   Cardiac Muscle

Cardiac muscle is composed of branched muscle cells, which are smaller than skeletal muscle cells and are connected to each other by **intercalated disks** (**Fig. 14.1**). These intercalated disks, which are unique to cardiac muscle tissue, include adherent junctions for cell-cell strength as well as gap junctions to allow electrical synchrony (so that the cells contract at the same time). As in skeletal muscle, the myofilaments in cardiac muscle fibers are organized into sarcomeres. These sarcomeres are assembled into myofibrils, which are in-register and give the tissue a striated appearance. Each cardiac muscle cell has a single nucleus that is centrally located.

Helpful Hint

The term "smaller cells" is sometimes used for cardiac muscle cells as a comparison to skeletal muscle cells. In fact, cardiac muscle cells are large when compared to most other cells, including smooth muscle cells. They just happen to be smaller than the very large skeletal muscle cells to which they are often compared.

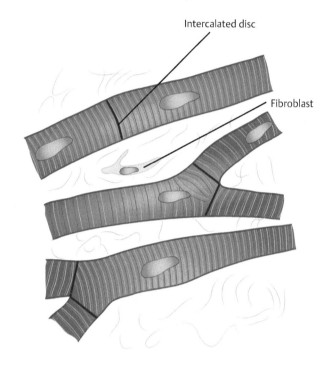

Fig. 14.1   **Cardiac muscle. Several cardiac muscle cells are shown, joined to each other by intercalated disks. The pale region surrounding the cardiac muscle cells is connective tissue.**

Fig. 14.2 is an image of cardiac muscle in which most of the muscle cells are in longitudinal section. As in skeletal muscle, striations are readily apparent in cardiac muscle viewed perpendicular to the long axis of the cells. Also as in skeletal muscle, the fibers are long, with a relatively consistent diameter throughout the length of the cell (green brackets). The diameters of the cells are similar; the slight variation observed on a slide is due to sectioning (either through the thickest part of the cell or catching the edge). However, the diameter of each cell is narrower than that of a skeletal muscle fiber.

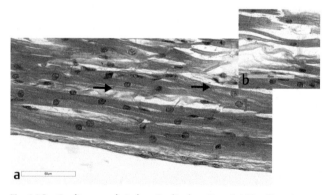

Fig. 14.2   **Cardiac muscle in longitudinal section. (a) The diameters of cardiac muscle cells are indicated by the green brackets. Intercalated disks are indicated by the arrows. (b) Branched cell.**

This image gives the impression that the diameter of each cell is comparable to the size of the nucleus. This is not the case; in fact, cardiac muscle cells have a fairly wide diameter relative to most cells (though much smaller than those of skeletal muscle). This will be better demonstrated in cross section.

Also note the single, centrally located nucleus per cell. The nuclei here appear round. Typically they are oval, but not as elongated as seen in skeletal muscle. The ends of the cells are joined by intercalated disks (black arrows), which appear as dense bands in the same orientation as the striations. The cells are branched: a nice example of a branched cell is shown in **Fig. 14.2b**.

Fig. 14.3a is a cross section through cardiac muscle tissue. Three cells are outlined, color coded to the section they represent in the cartoon in **Fig. 14.3b**. Cardiac muscle cells have centrally located nuclei, although the nucleus is only visible in cells sectioned through the nucleus (black), while in other cells the nucleus is not in the same plane as the section (green).

Like skeletal muscle cells, cardiac muscle cells have approximately the same diameter throughout their length, so, in cross section, the cells are approximately the same diameter. Cells with oval or irregular shapes (purple) are sections through branch points.

Note that there is a significant amount of cytoplasm surrounding the nuclei in cardiac muscle cells (**Fig. 14.3**, black outline). The relatively large amount of cytoplasm around the nucleus is useful when comparing to smooth muscle.

Video 14.1 Cardiac muscle

Be able to identify:
— Cardiac muscle
— Intercalated disks
https://www.thieme.de/de/q.htm?p=opn/
tp/308390101/978-1-62623-414-7_c014_v001&t=video

Fig. 14.4 is a specially stained slide (Bencosme stain) of cardiac muscle; intercalated disks are easier to see in this preparation (arrows).

Video 14.2 Cardiac muscle showing intercalated disks

Be able to identify:
— Cardiac muscle
— Intercalated disks
https://www.thieme.de/de/q.htm?p=opn/tp/308390101/978-1-62623-414-7_c014_v002&t=video

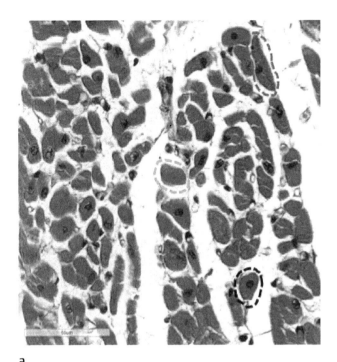

a

b

Fig. 14.3 **Cardiac muscle in cross section (a) and a drawing of cardiac muscle in longitudinal section (b). The outlined structures in a correspond to sections through cells indicated by the lines in b. Green is through the cell in a region away from the nucleus; black is through the cell in the region of the nucleus; purple is through a branch point.**

Fig. 14.5 is a transmission electron micrograph from cardiac muscle. In this image, cells are oriented longitudinally from upper left to lower right (two are indicated, A and B). The narrow extracellular space between cells is dark because of a special preparation. Myofibrils are visible within the cells, as well as

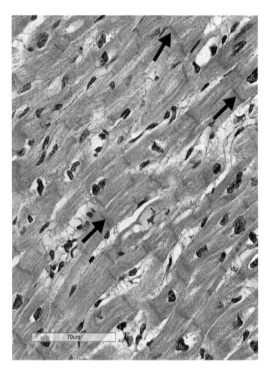

Fig. 14.4   Cardiac muscle in longitudinal section, specially stained (Bencosme, a trichrome stain) to highlight intercalated disks (arrows).

mitochondria (3), which are positioned between the myofibrils. The jagged line (1) is an intercalated disk, joining the ends of cells A and B. Capillaries (2) are also shown.

Cardiac muscles are almost completely dependent on aerobic metabolism, underscored by the abundance of mitochondria.

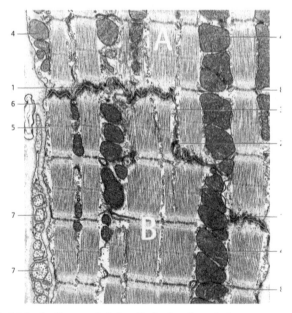

Fig. 14.6   Cardiac muscle in longitudinal section, electron micrograph. Two cells (A and B) are shown. (1) fascia adherens; (2) macula adherens; (3) gap junction; (4) mitochondria; (5) plasma membrane with pinocytotic vesicles; (6) basal lamina (external lamina); (7) axons within myelin sheath.

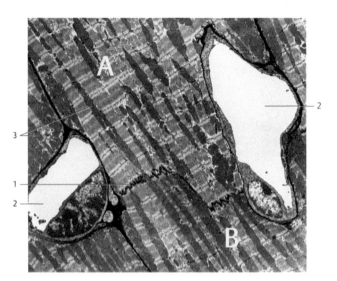

Fig. 14.5   Cardiac muscle in longitudinal section, electron micrograph. At least two cells (A and B) are shown. Other structures: (1) intercalated disk; (2) capillaries; (3) mitochondrion.

Fig. 14.6 is a higher-power transmission electron micrograph from cardiac muscle; the cells are oriented vertically (cells A and B indicated). A portion of an intercalated disk (1–3) is shown in more detail. Note that the junctions providing cell-cell adhesion, **fascia adherens** (1, equivalent to zonula adherens or belt desmosomes; see **Chapter 5**) and **macula adherens**, also known as desmosomes (2), are located in or near the "horizontal" portion of the disk, joining the ends of the cells, while the **gap junctions** (3) are located along the "vertical" portion of the intercalated disks.

The position of these junctions makes sense. The adherent junctions provide strength, and since the muscle cells are shortening, they have a tendency to pull apart from each other. The adherent junctions keep the ends of the cells together during contraction.

Gap junctions, as you recall, electrically connect adjacent cells and do not provide much resistance to external forces. Therefore, their placement in these lateral borders between cells, where stress is minimal, is ideal.

The ends of cardiac muscle cells are not flat. As shown in **Fig. 14.6**, the two cells shown each have irregular faces that fit together like a jigsaw puzzle. The intercalated disk therefore has a jagged outline, as shown in the electron micrographs in **Fig. 14.5** and **Fig. 14.6**, which reflects this interdigitation between the ends of the cardiac muscle cells. In light micrographs, this detail is lost, so the intercalated disk appears as a relatively straight line (**Fig. 14.4**).

14.3   Smooth Muscle

Smooth muscle tissue is composed of many smooth muscle cells. Although there are connective tissue elements (e.g., collagen) between the cells, smooth muscle is much more cellular than connective tissue. In addition, smooth muscle cells are smaller than cardiac and skeletal muscle cells. These features result in a tissue that has a high nuclear density (**Fig. 14.7**). Depending on the orientation of the cells, the nuclei appear slightly elongated (in longitudinally oriented cells, L) or round (in cross sections, C).

The contractile proteins within smooth muscle cells give the tissue a highly eosinophilic color, though it is usually (not always) less eosinophilic than cardiac or skeletal muscle (in **Fig. 14.7** the smooth muscle is more red than typical smooth muscle).

Individual smooth muscle cells are spindle shaped (**Fig. 14.8**). Because smooth muscle cells are smaller than cardiac or skeletal muscle cells, they have less cytoplasm than their larger counterparts. Even though smooth muscle utilizes similar contractile proteins as skeletal and cardiac muscle (i.e., actin and myosin), these proteins are not organized into sarcomeres or myofibrils. Therefore, smooth muscle is not striated (thus the name).

The ratio of actin to myosin in smooth muscle is much higher than in skeletal or cardiac muscle. Therefore, smooth muscle cells are packed with thin filaments, which are anchored to **dense bodies**. The dense bodies are either attached to the inner portion of the plasma membrane or anchored within the cytoplasm.

Whereas skeletal and cardiac muscle cells contract in a linear fashion, smooth muscle cells twist when they contract, similar to wringing out water from a towel. Smooth muscle cells also synthesize and secrete much of their surrounding extracellular matrix.

Because smooth muscle cells are embedded in extracellular matrix, which is eosinophilic like the smooth muscle cell cytoplasm, it is often difficult to see distinct cell borders of smooth muscle cells (see **Fig. 14.7**). **Fig. 14.9** is an image of smooth muscle oriented longitudinally, taken at high magnification. An approximate outline of a single smooth muscle cell is drawn in yellow. Again, note that the cells are small (actually, their size is typical as far as cells go, but small when compared to skeletal and cardiac muscle). They are tapered or cigar shaped, so they are thinner at the tips and fatter in the middle. In the middle portion of the cell, there is relatively little cytoplasm surrounding the nucleus.

Fig. 14.10a is a cross section through smooth muscle. Green and blue arrows indicate sections through cells that correspond to sections indicated in the drawing in **Fig. 14.10b**. The cells cut through the center of the cell (green) show nuclei and are largest in diameter, with a central nucleus and thin rim of cytoplasm. Sections through the periphery of the cell (blue) lack a nucleus and vary in diameter due to tapering of the cell.

Helpful Hint

Cross sections through smooth muscle in which individual cells are evident, as shown in the middle region of **Fig. 14.10a**, are the exception rather than the rule. In most cases, such as the top and bottom of **Fig. 14.10a**, cross sections of smooth muscle are cut at a slightly oblique angle, and individual cell borders are less distinct.

Video 14.3 Colon showing smooth muscle

Be able to identify:
— Smooth muscle

https://www.thieme.de/de/q.htm?p=opn/
tp/308390101/978-1-62623-414-7_c014_v003&t=video

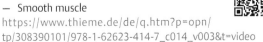

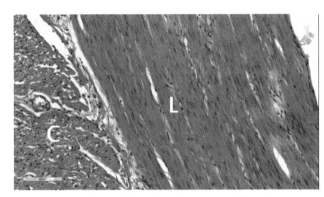

Fig. 14.7 **Smooth muscle from the colon, in cross (C) and longitudinal (L) sections.**

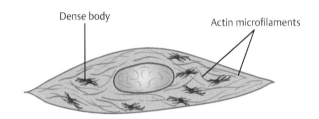

Dense body   Actin microfilaments

Fig. 14.8 **Drawing of a smooth muscle cell.**

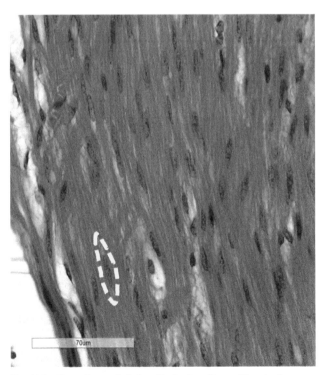

70um

Fig. 14.9 **Smooth muscle in longitudinal section, with a single smooth muscle cell outlined.**

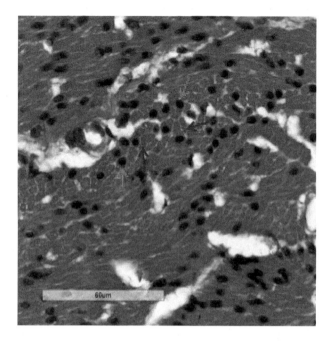

a

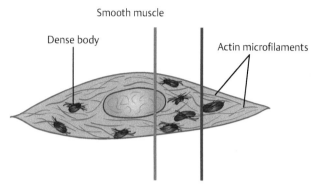

b

Fig. 14.10 **Smooth muscle in cross section (a) and a drawing of a smooth muscle cell in longitudinal orientation (b). The cells indicated by the arrows in a correspond to sections through the smooth muscle cell indicated by the lines in b. Green is through the center of the cell containing the nucleus; blue is through a tapered region of the cell outside of the nucleus.**

Fig. 14.11 is a more typical image of smooth muscle because it is difficult to see individual cells. The area between the brackets, and some tissue near the top, is dense irregular connective tissue.

Note that:

- Smooth muscle tissue has an overall appearance that is more red in color than other tissues, but typically is slightly pinker (less red) than skeletal or cardiac muscle. Note that in **Fig. 14.11** the connective tissue is unusually eosinophilic and appears red.
- In longitudinal section, smooth muscle nuclei are oval shaped (blue arrows). Also note that the nuclei are relatively evenly

dispersed throughout the tissue. Connective tissues tend to have fewer nuclei, which are more clustered or unevenly distributed.

- The contractile proteins in smooth muscle are not arranged in an ordered fashion; thus, there are no visible striations in smooth muscle.
- In cross section, smooth muscle tends to form bundles. These are not organized into fascicles as in skeletal muscle, but it often has this appearance nonetheless.
- There is no distinct border surrounding smooth muscle; it blends in with the surrounding connective tissue. This feature will help contrast it with neural tissue in the next chapter.

Because the appearance of smooth muscle is diverse, mostly related to the amount and type of interspersed connective tissue, **Fig. 14.12** is provided to show more examples. In **Fig. 14.12a**, from the uterus, the bundles of smooth muscle are intertwined a little more than in the colon or bladder, which have more organized longitudinal and cross-sectional areas. **Fig. 14.12b** shows smooth muscle bundles in the nipple (outlined) surrounded by dense irregular connective tissue. Note that there are more nuclei in smooth muscle than in the surrounding connective tissue.

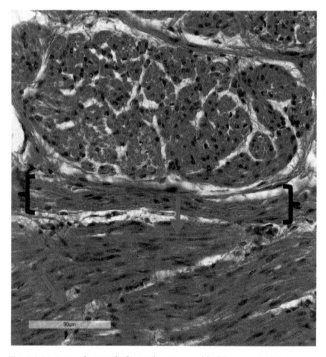

Fig. 14.11 **Smooth muscle from the urinary bladder. Most of this image is smooth muscle, but there are significant bundles of dense irregular connective tissue (black brackets). Smooth muscle nuclei are oval shaped in longitudinal sections (blue arrows).**

Video 14.4 Urinary bladder showing smooth muscle

Be able to identify:
— Smooth muscle

https://www.thieme.de/de/q.htm?p=opn/tp/308390101/978-1-62623-414-7_c014_v004&t=video

Not surprisingly, electron micrographs of smooth muscle taken at low magnification demonstrate spindle-shaped cells with central nuclei. **Fig. 14.13** shows portions of 6 to 10 smooth muscle cells, two with visible nuclei (N). Note that the cells are packed with fine microfilaments, just barely visible in the cytoplasm at this magnification. In smooth muscle, actin

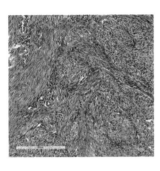
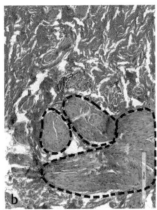

a   b

Fig. 14.12 **Smooth muscle from (a) uterus and (b, outlined) nipple.**

microfilaments are more predominant than myosin. The dark, elongated structures are mitochondria.

At higher magnification, more cellular detail of smooth muscle cells can be seen (**Fig. 14.14**). Here, portions of two or three cells are shown; part of a nucleus is visible (1). Most of the cytoplasm is filled with thin filaments. The dense structures indicated by the arrows are dense bodies, which are analogous to Z lines in skeletal and cardiac muscle because thin (actin) filaments attach to them. Tiny invaginations of the plasma membrane, termed **pinocytotic vesicles** (3), are characteristic of smooth muscle (and endothelial cells of blood vessels). In smooth muscle cells, these invaginations are thought to be analogous to the T tubule system in skeletal and cardiac muscle. Extracellular collagen fibers (4) are synthesized and secreted by the smooth muscle cells.

14.4 Comparison of Skeletal and Smooth Muscle

Now that the three types of muscle have been discussed, it is useful to make a direct comparison between skeletal muscle, smooth muscle, and connective tissue, especially since these tissues are often found in the same location. **Fig. 14.15** is an image from the esophagus, in a region of transition from skeletal (voluntary) muscle to smooth (autonomic) muscle, both of which are in longitudinal section. Note the following:
- Skeletal muscle is typically more eosinophilic (red rather than pink) and has large-diameter cells with peripheral nuclei.

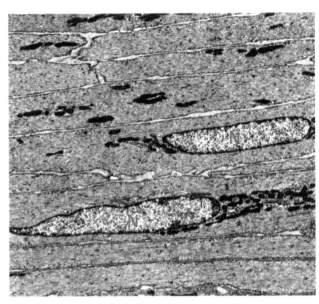

Fig. 14.13 **Smooth muscle, electron micrograph, low magnification. Two nuclei (N) are indicated. Very dark structures are mitochondria.**

- Smooth muscle cells are smaller, so there are more nuclei, and they are evenly distributed. The nuclei are more heterochromatic than those of skeletal muscle, and some even look "twisted" (arrow in **Fig. 14.15**); this may not be apparent at this magnification.
- Dense irregular connective tissue has fewer cells, so there are fewer nuclei, and there are extracellular elements such as collagen fibers.

Fig. 14.16 is another image from the esophagus with most of the muscle cut in cross section. Note the following:
- Skeletal muscle is typically more eosinophilic and has large-diameter cells with peripheral nuclei.
- Smooth muscle cells are smaller, so there are more nuclei, and they are relatively evenly distributed. The increase in the

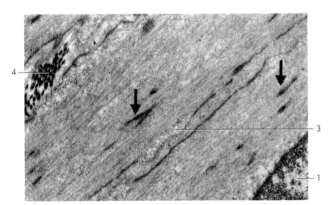

Fig. 14.14 **Smooth muscle, electron micrograph, low-medium magnification. (1) smooth muscle cell nucleus; (3) pinocytotic vesicles; (4) extracellular collagen fibers; arrows indicate dense bodies.**

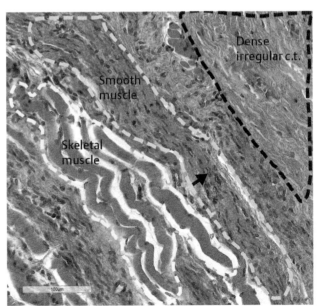

Fig. 14.15 **Comparison of skeletal muscle, smooth muscle and dense irregular connective tissue in longitudinal section. The arrow within the smooth muscle indicates a "twisted" nucleus.**

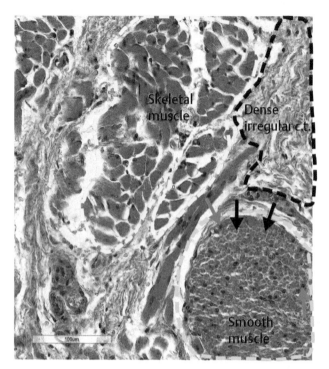

Fig. 14.16 **Comparison of skeletal muscle, smooth muscle, and dense irregular connective tissue in cross section. The blue arrows within the smooth muscle indicate nuclei, while the black arrows indicate tapered portions of cells.**

number of nuclei is not as obvious in cross section as it is in longitudinal section. However, close examination reveals individual cells, some with central nuclei and a thin rim of cytoplasm (blue arrows); others are smaller in diameter without nuclei, representing tapered ends of cells (black arrows). There are hundreds of smooth muscle cells in the outlined region.

- Dense irregular connective tissue has fewer cells, so there are fewer nuclei, and there are extracellular elements such as collagen fibers.

Video 14.5 Skeletal and smooth muscle

Be able to identify:
- Skeletal muscle
- Smooth muscle
- Dense irregular connective tissue

https://www.thieme.de/de/q.htm?p=opn/tp/308390101/978-1-62623-414-7_c014_v005&t=video

14.5   Chapter Review

Fig. 14.17 and **Fig. 14.18** show side-by-side comparisons of skeletal, smooth, and cardiac muscle in longitudinal and cross sections, respectively.

The following reviews the characteristics of each type of muscle.

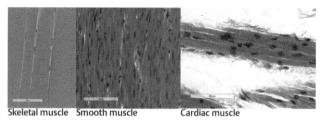

Skeletal muscle   Smooth muscle   Cardiac muscle

Fig. 14.17 **Comparison of skeletal muscle, smooth muscle, and cardiac muscle in longitudinal sections.**

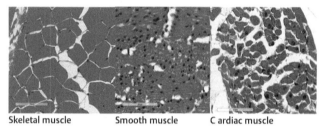

Skeletal muscle   Smooth muscle   C ardiac muscle

Fig. 14.18 **Comparison of skeletal muscle, smooth muscle and cardiac muscle in cross sections.**

14.5.1 Characteristics of Skeletal Muscle Cells

- Long cells
- Wide fibers (cells) of constant diameter
- Multiple nuclei, located in periphery of the cell
- Striated
- Voluntary
- Found in named muscles (e.g., biceps brachii)

14.5.2 Characteristics of Cardiac Muscle Cells

- Longer than typical cells, though much shorter than skeletal muscle cells
- Fibers (cells) of constant diameter, intermediate diameter
- Central nucleus
- Striated
- Involuntary
- Found in heart
- Branched cells
- Intercalated disks

14.5.3 Characteristics of Smooth Muscle Cells

- Spindle-shaped cells (cigar-shaped)
- Central nucleus
- Not striated
- Involuntary
- Found in visceral organs, blood vessels

14.5.4 Common Characteristics of Two of Three Muscle Types

The following is a list of features common to two types of muscle, but not all three:

- Striations are evident in skeletal and cardiac muscle, but not smooth muscle.
- Nuclei are located in the center of cardiac and smooth muscle cells but are located near the plasma membrane in skeletal muscle.
- Skeletal muscle cells are large and multinuclear, while cardiac and smooth muscle cells are smaller, with only a single nucleus each.
- The diameter of skeletal muscle is very consistent between cells. Cardiac muscle cells are somewhat consistent in diameter (but vary in shape), while the smooth muscle cell diameter varies depending on whether the cell is sectioned through the middle (with nucleus) or near the periphery of the cell (without nucleus).

14.5.5 Other Distinguishing Characteristics

Following are some other features that can be helpful in distinguishing muscle cell types:

- Skeletal muscle cells have the largest diameter, cardiac muscle cells are smaller, and smooth muscle cells have the smallest diameter.
- Because smooth muscle cells are smaller than either cardiac or skeletal muscle cells, smooth muscle typically has a higher nuclear density than the other two tissues.
- Cardiac muscle is the only tissue that has intercalated disks.
- In cuts through the nucleus of a cell, there is significant cytoplasm in skeletal and, to a lesser extent, cardiac muscle, while smooth muscle has a thin rim of cytoplasm around the nucleus.

Questions and Answers

An online-only section of questions and answers accompanying this chapter is hosted on Thieme's MedOne Education site: https://medone-education.thieme.com. Use the code on the media page at the front of this book to gain access. An institutional license to the site is required to access these questions in an interactive format, and individual users are required to register for an individual account to track results.

15   Neural Tissue

After completing this chapter, you should be able to:
— Identify, at the light microscope level, each of the following:
  • Spinal cord
    ◦ Gray matter
      ▪ Neuronal cell body
        – Nucleus
        – Nucleolus
        – Nissl substance (RER)
      ▪ Axons and dendrites (indistinguishable)
    ◦ White matter
      ▪ Axons and dendrites (indistinguishable)
  • Prepared nerve specimen
    ◦ Myelinated axon
    ◦ Node of Ranvier
  • Peripheral nerve
    ◦ Connective tissue of peripheral nerve
      ▪ Epineurium
      ▪ Perineurium
      ▪ Endoneurium
    ◦ Fascicle
    ◦ Axon
    ◦ Myelin
    ◦ Schwann cell nuclei
  • Ganglia
    ◦ Neuronal cell bodies
    ◦ Satellite cells
    ◦ Bundles of axons and dendrites
— Identify, at the electron microscope level, each of the following:
  • Peripheral nerve
  • Schwann cell
    ◦ Myelin
  • Axon
    ◦ Myelinated
    ◦ Ensheathed (unmyelinated)
— Outline the function of each cell and structure listed
— Correlate the appearance of each cell type or structure with its function
— Describe the organization of the nervous system

15.1   Overview of the Nervous System

The nervous system consists of the **central nervous system** (brain and spinal cord) and **peripheral nervous system** (peripheral nerves and ganglia). The organization and anatomic detail of the nervous system is vastly complicated. However, at its core, the main function of the nervous system is cell-cell communication. This chapter will focus on cells of the nervous system, the spinal cord, and peripheral nerves and ganglia. Sensory nerve endings will be considered in **Chapter 27**.

15.1.1   Cells of the Nervous System

Although there are several cell types in neural tissue, the main player involved in cell-cell communication is the **neuron. Fig. 15.1** shows several illustrations of some neurons. The main

portion of a neuron is the **cell body** (**soma**, **perikaryon**), where the nucleus and most organelles reside. Neurons extend numerous processes called **dendrites** and **axons**. Dendrites receive input from other cells and transmit that signal to the cell body of the neuron. In general, axons carry signals away from the cell body. Neurons come in all shapes and sizes, but for the purposes of this chapter, the focus will be on the **multipolar neuron** and, to a lesser extent, the **unipolar neuron** (or **pseudounipolar neuron**).

A neuron is an excitable cell that sends an electrical signal (action potential) down its axon to reach a distant target cell. When the action potential reaches the terminal end of the axon, **neurotransmitters** are released, which bind to receptors on target cells (e.g., skeletal muscle, other neurons). This site at which cell-cell communication takes place via neurotransmitter release is called the **synapse**.

For each neuron, the decision to send an action potential or not at any given moment is based on synaptic input from other cells. In most cases, this comes in the form of axons from other cells, which synapse on either the dendrites or the cell body of the neuron.

Other cells in the nervous system that support the function of neurons are called **glial cells**. There are several types of glial cells, including microglia, ependymal cells, and astrocytes. The glial cells that will be the focus of this chapter are **Schwann cells** (in the peripheral nervous system) and **oligodendrocytes** (in the central nervous system). These cells wrap around axons and some dendrites to provide protection and support (**Fig. 15.2**). In some cases, the Schwann cell simply envelops the axon, a process referred to as **ensheathment** (**Fig. 15.2a**). In other cases, the Schwann cell or oligodendrocyte wraps around the axon multiple times, a process known as **myelination** (**Fig. 15.2b, c**).

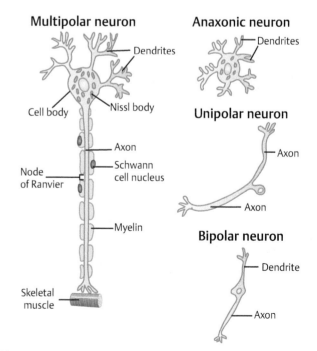

Fig. 15.1   **Neurons.**

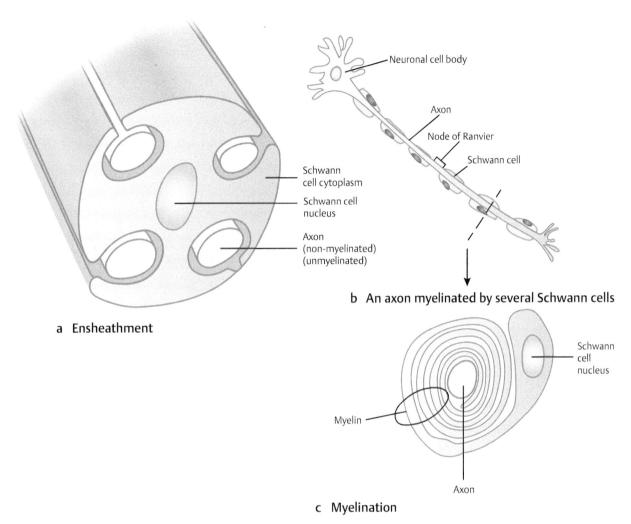

Fig. 15.2 **Interaction of glial cells with neuronal axons. (a) Ensheathment, a process in which a glial cell envelops axons. (b, c) Myelination. (b) shows a longitudinal drawing of a neuron that is myelinated by several glial cells (Schwann cells). (c) shows a cross section through the axon, showing the Schwann cell wrapping around the axon multiple times.**

Because the plasma membrane and its membrane proteins are hydrophobic, this stack of membranes of the Schwann cell or oligodendrocyte, called **myelin**, provides a significant insulator that increases action potential velocity up to 100-fold. In these cases, the axon (or neuron) is referred to as **myelinated**. Axons that are surrounded by Schwann cells but are not myelinated (**Fig, 15.2a**) are called **ensheathed** or **unmyelinated** axons.

Helpful Hint

Myelin does not preserve well on routine H & E-stained tissues, so it imparts a washed-out appearance similar to mucus. Special fixation techniques can be used to stain for myelin. However, in most routinely stained slides, myelin is recognized by the lack of stain.

15.1.2 Organization of the Nervous System

As mentioned, the organization of neurons in the nervous system is quite complex. **Fig. 15.3** is a drawing of a cross section of the spinal cord and peripheral nerves. In this image, colored dots represent cell bodies of neurons, while lines extending from these

represent axons. Orange arrows indicate the direction of a putative signal (action potential). The diagram shows a simple example of a reflex arc. A stimulus from the skin activates an afferent or sensory neuron (blue), which is a pseudounipolar neuron with one axon extending to the skin and the other to the spinal cord. The stimulus travels along the peripheral axon (in the form of an action potential), bypasses the cell body in the dorsal root ganglion, to travel down the central axon into the spinal cord. (The peripheral axon of this type of neuron is an exception to the general rule that axons carry action potentials away from the cell body.) In the spinal cord, the sensory neuron synapses with an interneuron (green), which passes the stimulus to an efferent or motor neuron (red). The motor neuron relays the signal to a target tissue, either muscle or glands.

Helpful Hint

One can learn a great detail about the nervous system in a neuroscience text or course, such as details of action potential transmission, synaptic function, and organization of structures in the spinal cord and brain. The focus of this chapter is the histology of the spinal cord and peripheral nervous system; this simplified overview is designed to provide just enough background to interpret images.

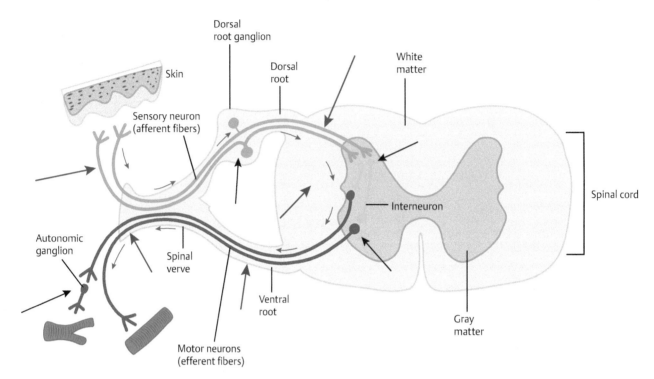

Fig. 15.3 General organization of the nervous system at the level of the spinal cord. Cell bodies are represented by colored dots; axons are represented by lines extending from these cell bodies. Locations in which numerous cell bodies are clustered are indicated by the black arrows; purple arrows indicate bundles of axons. Orange arrows show the direction of flow of action potentials.

For the most part, neuronal cell bodies gather together in specific locations (**Fig. 15.3**, black arrows), while axons are bundled together in others (purple arrows). Terminology used for these structures is based on whether the structure is a collection of cell bodies or of axons, and whether the structure is in the central nervous system (brain or spinal cord) or peripheral nervous system:

- A **nucleus** is a collection of cell bodies in the central nervous system; here it will be called gray matter.
- A **tract** is a collection of axons in the central nervous system; here it will be called white matter.
- A **ganglion** is a collection of cell bodies in the peripheral nervous system.
- A **nerve** is a collection of axons in the peripheral nervous system.

Fig. 15.3 shows only a few cells, but in real tissue there are hundreds or thousands of cells or cell processes in each region. Also note that in regions where cell bodies are gathered, there are also axons and dendrites that are coming from and going to the cell bodies, so expect to see both cell bodies and axons/dendrites in those locations.

15.2 Spinal Cord

This discussion will begin with a look at the spinal cord. **Fig. 15.3** includes the spinal cord in cross section. Histologically, the spinal cord has two major regions:

- **Gray matter** contains neuronal cell bodies (grouped into nuclei) and forms a butterfly-shaped region in the center of the spinal cord.
- **White matter** consists of axons (grouped into tracts), many of which are myelinated, located in the periphery of the spinal cord. Most of these axons extend to higher or lower levels of the brain or spinal cord. Therefore, in a cross section of the spinal cord, these processes are cut in cross section.

The myelin that surrounds axons is fatty and, in fresh tissue, appears white or light yellow, which is why tissue containing mostly axons is called white matter. Cell bodies are not myelinated, so tissue containing mostly cell bodies appears gray in fresh specimens.

15.2.1 Spinal Cord Gray Matter

Many neurons in the spinal cord are large, multipolar neurons, which have an axon and several dendrites. Motor neurons are excellent examples of multipolar neurons; their cell bodies are located in the gray matter of the spinal cord.

Fig. 15.4a is a scanning image of a cross section through the spinal cord stained with Nissl stain; the approximate outer border of the gray matter is indicated with a dotted line. Nissl stain highlights rough endoplasmic reticulum (RER); these motor neuron cell bodies have abundant RER and can be seen even at low magnification (**Figure 15.4b**, arrows).

Fig. 15.5 is a medium- to high-power view of the gray matter showing several motor neurons. The location of the plasma membrane (green arrows) and nuclear envelope (black arrows) of motor neurons are indicated. The nuclei of the motor neurons are large and round, with a prominent nucleolus (yellow arrow) and abundant euchromatin (pale area surrounding nucleolus). The extensive cytoplasm of these cells is filled with RER, which stains purple with Nissl stain (thus the name **Nissl substance** or **Nissl bodies** for RER in these cells). Cell processes (orange arrows) extending from the cell bodies are probably dendrites, but may be axons (it can be challenging to identify axons versus dendrites positively). The smaller, round nuclei (red arrows) belong to glial cells; the cytoplasm of these cells is sparse and so is not visible or barely so.

Helpful Hint

It is often useful at this point to take a moment and appreciate the difference in size between motor neurons and glial cells (**Fig. 15.5**). Like most neurons, the motor neuron is a huge cell; the Nissl substance occupies the cytoplasm and extends to the outer boundary of these cells (green arrows). The pale central structure is the nucleus, which is very large and euchromatic, with a prominent nucleolus (yellow arrow). On the other hand, glial cells (**Fig. 15.5**, red arrow) are extremely small in comparison; they appear as a small dot, which is the entire condensed nucleus. Note that the nuclei of glial cells are about the same size as nucleoli of motor neurons. The cytoplasm of glial cells is sparse and barely seen in most glial cells here. The entire glial cell can fit easily inside the nucleus of a motor neuron.

Nissl stain is useful for highlighting rough endoplasmic reticulum and nucleoli, but it does not stain axons and dendrites very well. **Fig. 15.6** shows an area of gray matter similar to that shown in **Fig. 15.4** and **Fig. 15.5**, but stained with a silver stain that highlights proteins. A neuronal cell body with a process extending to the right is indicated (red arrow). Neuronal cell processes contain abundant proteins, mostly cytoskeletal elements such as microtubules and intermediate filaments. Most of the threadlike structures throughout this slide are dendrites and axons from this or neighboring cells, which were not readily visible in the Nissl-stained images.

15.2.2 Spinal Cord White Matter

White matter of the spinal cord contains axons that extend up and down the spinal cord (see **Fig. 15.3**). Because the fibers are oriented in a cranial-caudal fashion, they are seen in cross section in sections of the spinal cord cut in cross section. Because

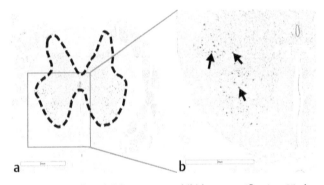

Fig. 15.4 **Spinal cord, (a) scanning and (b) low magnification, Nissl stain. The dotted outline in a indicates the border between gray matter (inside) and white matter (outside). Arrows in b indicate motor neuron cell bodies.**

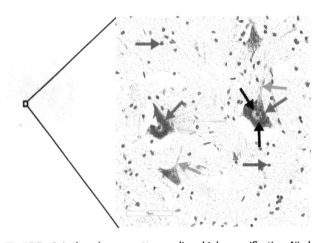

Fig. 15.5 **Spinal cord, gray matter, medium-high magnification, Nissl stain. Motor neurons are the large cells; arrows indicate locations of the plasma membrane (green arrows), the nuclear envelope (black arrows), the nucleolus (yellow arrow), and cell processes (orange arrows). Red arrows indicate glial cell nuclei.**

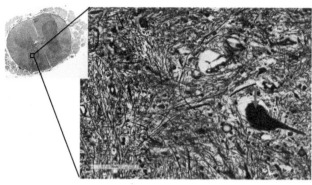

Fig. 15.6   **Spinal cord, gray matter, medium magnification, silver stain. The numerous threadlike structures are axons and dendrites. A motor neuron cell body is indicated (arrow).**

axons have little to no endoplasmic reticulum, they stain very poorly with Nissl stain.

> **Video 15.4**   Spinal cord showing white matter with Nissl stain
>
> Be able to identify:
> — Cell processes (dendrites and axons)
> https://www.thieme.de/de/q.htm?p=opn/
> tp/308390101/978-1-62623-414-7_c015_
> v004&t=video

Although white matter does not stain well with Nissl, special stains can be used to visualize the components of white matter. **Fig. 15.7** is an image of white matter stained with silver, which highlights the cytoskeletal elements abundant in axons (yellow arrow). The axons are surrounded by pale regions representing myelin, which was dissolved away during tissue preparation.

> **Video 15.5**   Spinal cord showing white matter with silver stain
>
> Be able to identify:
> — Axons
> — Myelin
> https://www.thieme.de/de/q.htm?p=opn/tp/308390101/978-1-
> 62623-414-7_c015_v005&t=video

Specific tissue preparation methods and special stains can be used to visualize myelin. **Fig. 15.8** is an image from a spinal cord carefully prepared to preserve and stain myelin (between arrows). Recall that myelin is composed of glial cell membranes wrapped many times around neuronal axons. The axons do not stain well with this preparation, so they are represented by the pale centers in the middle of the dark myelin rings.

> **Video 15.6**   Spinal cord showing white matter with myelin stain
>
> Be able to identify:
> — Axons
> — Myelin
> https://www.thieme.de/de/q.htm?p=opn/tp/308390101/978-1-
> 62623-414-7_c015_v006&t=video

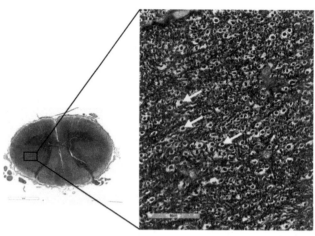

Fig. 15.7   **Spinal cord, white matter, medium magnification, silver stain. Axons (yellow arrows) stain darkly with silver, surrounded by pale regions representing myelin.**

There are several types of disorders that affect myelinating cells. For example, **multiple sclerosis** is thought to be caused by immune destruction of myelin. The resulting decreased speed of action potentials causes sensory and motor dysfunction. Brain and spinal cord tissues from these patients at autopsy show decreased myelin staining.

15.3   Peripheral Nerves

Peripheral nerves are bundles of axons (see **Fig. 15.3**, purple arrows), supported by connective tissues. Nuclei seen in peripheral nerves belong to glial cells.

As shown in **Fig. 15.3**, anatomically, there are many types of peripheral nerves, referred to as roots, spinal nerves, and so on. From a histologic standpoint, all these structures are bundles of axons with supporting glial cells and connective tissue, so they are indistinguishable.

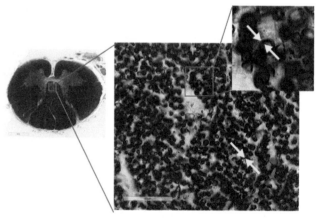

Fig. 15.8   **Spinal cord, white matter, high magnification, myelin stain. Myelin (between yellow arrows) stains darkly, while the axons surrounded by myelin are pale. The image to the upper right is pseudo-magnified.**

In the peripheral nervous system, individual axons are surrounded by **Schwann cells** rather than oligodendrocytes (see **Fig. 15.2**). During embryogenesis, a Schwann cell initially surrounds several axons with portions of its cytoplasm and plasma membrane. This arrangement is termed **ensheathment** (**Fig. 15.2a**).

Smaller-caliber axons remain ensheathed. When large axons are present, the Schwann cell selects a single axon to support and wraps its cytoplasm and plasma membrane around that axon numerous times (**Fig. 15.2b, c**). After the cytoplasm of the Schwann cell is squeezed out, the remaining layers of cell membrane are called **myelin**. A single axon is myelinated by many Schwann cells. Regularly spaced regions of bare axon not surrounded by myelin, called **nodes of Ranvier**, are important for propagation of the action potential.

15.3.1 Ultrastructure of Peripheral Nerves

Fig. 15.9 is an electron micrograph of a peripheral nerve, showing about 40 axons cut in cross section, ensheathed by several Schwann cells. An axon is indicated at (1); the diameter of another is indicated by the double red arrow. Stippling within the axons is due to cytoskeletal elements that run longitudinally within the axon.

In this micrograph, the cytoplasm of Schwann cells is darker than the axons they surround. The nucleus of a Schwann cell is indicated (2); note that this Schwann cell is ensheathing over two dozen axons. Other axons are ensheathed by Schwann cells whose nuclei are out of the plane of section. The extracellular dots at (3) and (4) are collagen fibers.

Fig. 15.10 is an electron micrograph of 20 to 30 myelinated axons in cross section. The axons are pale (1); the diameter of one is indicated by the double red arrow. Note that many are irregular in shape in this preparation. Stippling in the axon cytoplasm (barely visible at this magnification) represents cytoskeletal elements. The myelin surrounding the axons is electron dense (between purple arrows) and, as mentioned, consists of multiple layers of Schwann cell plasma membrane. The main portion of Schwann cells can be seen in some locations (3), while others lie outside the plane of section. Other axons in this image are ensheathed (unmyelinated, 2).

15.3.2 Peripheral Nerve in a Teased Preparation

Now that axons in electron micrographs have been presented, a discussion of their appearance in light micrographs follows. First, recall that myelinated axons have regular intervals of bare axon (i.e., no myelin) called nodes of Ranvier (see **Fig. 15.2b**).

Helpful Hint

Imagine an extremely long hot dog covered with many buns, one after the other, with a small gap between one bun and the next. The hot dog represents the axon, and the buns represent Schwann cell myelin. Then the nodes of Ranvier correspond to the gaps between the buns along the hot dog.

Fig, 15.11 is a light micrograph of a longitudinal view of a nerve bundle that has been teased apart to separate individual axons and then stained with osmium tetroxide, which labels myelin (similar to **Fig. 15.8**). The bare portion of one axon, a node of Ranvier, is indicated by the arrow.

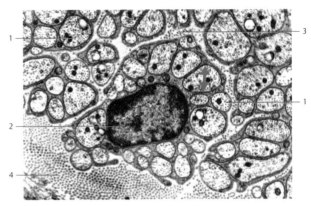

Fig. 15.9 **Peripheral nerve, cross section, electron micrograph, showing (1, and double red arrow) ensheathed axons; (2) Schwann cell nucleus; and (3, 4) collagen.**

Video 15.7 Teased nerve stained for myelin

Be able to identify:
— Axons
— Myelin
— Node of Ranvier
https://www.thieme.de/de/q.htm?p=opn/tp/308390101/978-1-62623-414-7_c015_v007&t=video

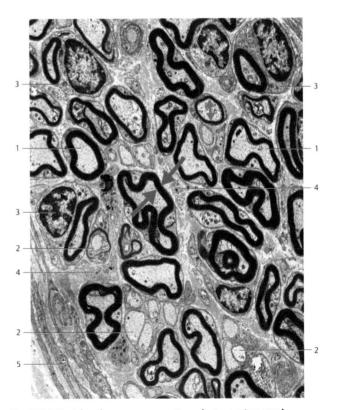

Fig. 15.10 **Peripheral nerve, cross section, electron micrograph showing myelin (between purple arrows); myelinated axons (1, and double arrow); ensheathed (unmyelinated) axon (2); Schwann cell (3); collagen (4); and a cell of the perineurium (5).**

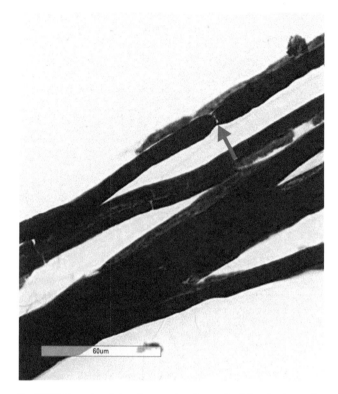

Fig. 15.11 **Teased peripheral nerve showing node of Ranvier (arrow).**

15.3.3 Peripheral Nerves Stained with H & E

A peripheral nerve is a bundle of axons with supporting glial cells and connective tissues. **Fig. 15.12** shows light micrographs of a large peripheral nerve (from the axilla) stained with H & E. In **Fig. 15.12a**, the top portion of the image shows the axons in longitudinal section, while the bottom shows them in cross section. In H & E-stained tissues, the axons are eosinophilic (green arrows) due to abundant proteins, though they often appear a little purple. Much of the myelin washes out in tissue preparation, so the area around the axon is pale pink (edge of the myelin indicated by the blue arrows). In some fortuitous images (**Fig. 15.12b**), nodes of Ranvier can be seen. Note that the myelin tapers on either side of the node, but the axon is continuous through the node.

Video 15.8   Axilla showing peripheral nerves

Be able to identify:
— Axons
— Myelin
— Node of Ranvier
https://www.thieme.de/de/q.htm?p=opn/tp/308390101/978-1-62623-414-7_c015_v008&t=video

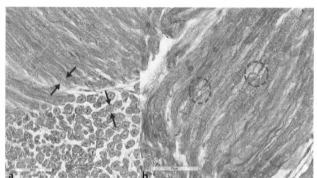

Fig. 15.12 **Large peripheral nerve (from axilla), medium-high magnification. (a) Longitudinal and transverse sections showing axons (green arrows) and the outer edge of the myelin sheath (blue arrows). (b) Longitudinal section showing nodes of Ranvier (outlined).**

Smaller peripheral nerves (**Fig. 15.13a**, **b**, outlined) can be found throughout the body. In these smaller nerves, the details of individual axons and their myelin sheaths are not visible. Several features distinguish a peripheral nerve from the surrounding connective tissue:
— Pale eosinophilia: Due to washed-out myelin, the nerve is more of a salmon color than red.
— Wavy appearance: Nerves are elastic and recoil on tissue preparation, so the tissue appears wavy.
— **Perineurium**: Note the distinct outer boundary (**Fig. 15.13a**, **b**, arrows). Perineurium will be discussed in detail in the following section.
— Numerous nuclei: Most of these belong to Schwann cells that myelinate the axons.

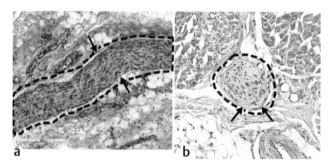

Fig. 15.13 **Small peripheral nerves (outlined), medium magnification. The perineurium is indicated by the arrows. (a) Longitudinal section of the nerve. (b) Oblique or cross section.**

Video 15.9 Esophagus showing peripheral nerves

https://www.thieme.de/de/q.htm?p=opn/tp/308390101/978-1-62623-414-7_c015_v009&t=video

Video 15.10 Esophagus showing peripheral nerves

https://www.thieme.de/de/q.htm?p=opn/tp/308390101/978-1-62623-414-7_c015_v010&t=video

Video 15.11 Lung hilus showing peripheral nerves

https://www.thieme.de/de/q.htm?p=opn/tp/308390101/978-1-62623-414-7_c015_v011&t=video

Video 15.12 Spermatic cord showing peripheral nerves
Be able to identify:
— Peripheral nerve

https://www.thieme.de/de/q.htm?p=opn/tp/308390101/978-1-62623-414-7_c015_v012&t=video

In addition to demyelination of axons in the central nervous system, demyelination of peripheral nerves can also occur. For example, **Guillain-Barré syndrome** is caused by an autoimmune reaction that occurs subsequent to bacterial infection due to molecular mimicry (antibodies against the bacteria cross-react with myelin). Patients with Guillain-Barré syndrome have sensory and motor dysfunction, mostly affecting the peripheral portion of the limbs (nerves supplying these regions are longest), but it can also have more central effects.

15.3.4 Connective Tissues of Peripheral Nerves

Fig. 15.14 is a light micrograph taken at low magnification from the same specimen of the axilla/brachial plexus shown in **Fig. 15.12**. The organization of connective tissues surrounding and bundling axons is similar to that present in skeletal muscle (with some differences). In peripheral nerves, axons are bundled together to form fascicles (in **Fig. 15.14**, a **fascicle** is outlined.)

There are three levels of connective tissue that bundle axons in peripheral nerves together:

• **Epineurium** (green bracket in **Fig. 15.14**): Dense irregular connective tissue that is the outer border of an entire nerve and encloses one or more bundled nerve fascicles

• **Perineurium** (black arrows in **Fig. 15.14**): Cellular layer that bounds one fascicle, eosinophilic, but with a little purple tinge

• **Endoneurium**: Loose connective tissue between myelinated and ensheathed axons

Fig. 15.15 is a medium-magnification image of the edge of the same fascicle, highlighting the connective tissue layers of peripheral nerves. Note that epineurium is dense irregular connective tissue, while endoneurium is loose connective tissue between the myelinated axons (green arrows). The perineurium (between black arrows) is very cellular; the cells of this layer form tight

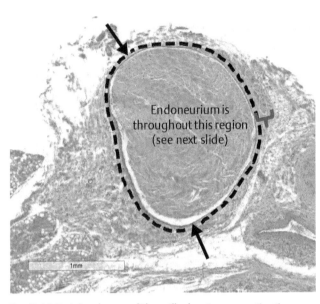

Fig. 15.14 Peripheral nerve of the axilla showing connective tissues, low magnification. A fascicle is outlined, its perineurium is marked with black arrows, and the thickness of the epineurium is marked with a green bracket.

junctions that provide a protective environment for the axons and glial cells within the nerve.

Video 15.13 Connective tissue of peripheral nerves

Be able to identify:
— Endoneurium
— Perineurium
— Fascicle
— Epineurium

https://www.thieme.de/de/q.htm?p=opn/tp/308390101/978-1-62623-414-7_c015_v013&t=video

As larger nerves (i.e., bundles of fascicles), branch and enter the organs or structures they serve, they become smaller

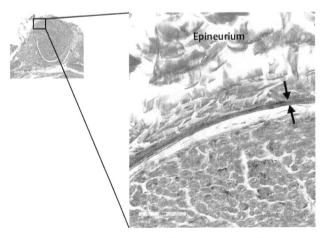

Fig. 15.15 Peripheral nerve of the axilla showing connective tissues, medium-high magnification. Epineurium is indicated; black arrows mark perineurium; green arrows mark endoneurium.

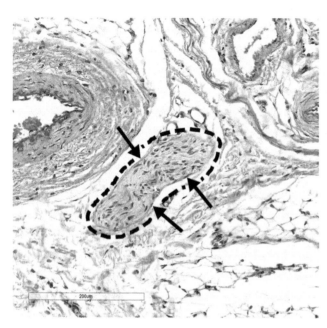

Fig. 15.16 **Small peripheral nerve (outlined), medium magnification showing connective tissue layers. The perineurium is indicated by the arrows.**

peripheral nerves (**Fig. 15.16**, outlined), which are each essentially a single fascicle. Therefore, these small peripheral nerves contain only endoneurium and perineurium (black arrows); there is no epineurium. These fascicles are surrounded by connective tissues of the organ or structure in which they are located. The perineurium delineates the peripheral nerve from the surrounding connective tissue and is useful in distinguishing peripheral nerves from connective and other tissues (e.g., smooth muscle).

Video 15.14 Connective tissue of peripheral nerves

Be able to identify:
— Perineurium
https://www.thieme.de/de/q.htm?p=opn/
tp/308390101/978-1-62623-414-7_c015_v014&t=video

15.4   Ganglia

Ganglia are clusters of neuronal cell bodies in the peripheral nervous system, together with supporting cells, contained within a connective tissue capsule (see **Fig. 15.3**; e.g., dorsal root ganglion, autonomic ganglion). Note that axons project from the neuronal cell bodies, so a ganglion will have many features of a peripheral nerve (myelinated axons, endoneurium, etc.)

Helpful Hint

Several different ganglia will be used as examples, and their specific names indicated for completeness. However, it is usually not necessary to name specific ganglia based on a histologic specimen.

Fig. 15.17 is a scanning image of a dorsal root ganglion, which contains sensory neuronal cell bodies, visible even at this low

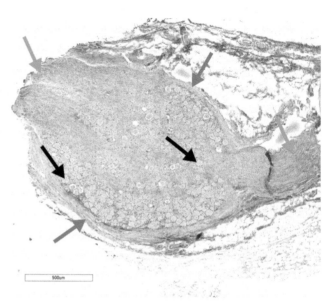

Fig. 15.17 **Dorsal root ganglion, scanning magnification. Black arrows indicate neuronal cell bodies; green arrows point to peripheral nerves; blue arrows point to the connective tissue.**

magnification (black arrows). Among the cell bodies are central and peripheral axons. The ganglion is surrounded by a connective tissue capsule (blue arrows). Peripheral nerves enter and exit the ganglion (green arrows).

Fig. 15.18 is a higher-magnification image of this same ganglion, showing large neuronal cell bodies with euchromatic nuclei (black arrows mark the edge of one nucleus) and prominent nucleoli (blue arrow). The smaller nuclei surrounding the neuronal cell bodies belong to glial cells called **satellite cells** (green arrows). The tissue between the neurons is mostly axons, with a small amount of loose connective tissue.

Helpful Hint

The neurons in ganglia are very similar to motor neurons in the spinal cord: very large cells with abundant basophilic cytoplasm (although the basophilia is not prominent in **Fig. 15.17** and **Fig. 15.18**) and a very large, euchromatic nucleus with a prominent nucleolus.

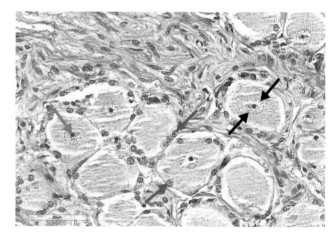

Fig. 15.18 **Dorsal root ganglion, medium-high magnification. The nucleus of a neuronal cell body is framed by black arrows; a nucleolus is indicated by a blue arrow; green arrows point to satellite cells. The horizontal "tears" through the neurons are artifact.**

Video 15.15 Dorsal root ganglion

Be able to identify:
— Ganglion
— Neuronal cell bodies
— Satellite cells
— Axons and dendrites
https://www.thieme.de/de/q.htm?p=opn/tp/308390101/978-1-62623-414-7_c015_v015&t=video

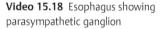

Smaller ganglia are located within peripheral tissues such as the intestinal tract (**Fig. 15.19a**, **b**, outlined). Although there are fewer neuronal cell bodies in these ganglia than in the larger, named ganglia, the characteristic features are the same: frothy eosinophilia due to washed-out myelin, with large neuronal cell bodies with cytoplasmic basophilia (green arrows). Some, but not all, neurons have their large, euchromatic nuclei in the plane of section (e.g., the middle neuron in **Fig. 15.19a**). Most of the other nuclei in these ganglia belong to Schwann cells.

Video 15.16 Trigeminal ganglion

https://www.thieme.de/de/q.htm?p=opn/tp/308390101/978-1-62623-414-7_c015_v016&t=video

Video 15.17 Sympathetic ganglion SL051_x264.mp4
Be able to identify:
— Ganglion
— Neuronal cell bodies
— Satellite cells
— Axons and dendrites
https://www.thieme.de/de/q.htm?p=opn/tp/308390101/978-1-62623-414-7_c015_v017&t=video

Fig. 15.20 shows images of two other ganglia. **Fig. 15.20a** is an image of the trigeminal ganglion, a structure belonging to the fifth cranial nerve that is analogous to a dorsal root ganglion in that it contains cell bodies and central and peripheral axons. **Fig. 15.20b** is a sympathetic ganglion, where preganglionic axons synapse on postganglionic neurons. In both images, black arrows indicate nuclear membranes, blue arrows mark nucleoli, and green arrows indicate satellite cells. Note the same features as seen in **Fig. 15.18**; the cytoplasmic basophilia in these neurons is more pronounced.

Video 15.18 Esophagus showing parasympathetic ganglion

https://www.thieme.de/de/q.htm?p=opn/tp/308390101/978-1-62623-414-7_c015_v018&t=video

Video 15.19 Colon showing parasympathetic ganglion
Be able to identify:
— Ganglion
— Neuronal cell bodies
— Axons and dendrites
https://www.thieme.de/de/q.htm?p=opn/tp/308390101/978-1-62623-414-7_c015_v020&t=video

Video 15.20 Jejunum showing parasympathetic ganglion

https://www.thieme.de/de/q.htm?p=opn/tp/308390101/978-1-62623-414-7_c015_v019&t=video

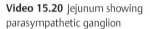

Helpful Hint

The neuronal cell bodies in parasympathetic ganglia are smaller than their counterparts in the larger ganglia. However, they are still very large cells (compare to the Schwann cell nuclei in **Fig. 15.20**).

15.5 Chapter Review

The nervous system is perhaps the most complicated of all the organ systems. However, at its core histologically, neural tissues are composed of neuronal cell bodies and processes, supported by glial cells and bundled together by connective tissue. The principal cells of the nervous system—neurons—are very large cells with large, euchromatic nuclei and prominent nucleoli. Neurons are heavily involved in protein synthesis, so they have abundant RER in their cell bodies, which stains readily with Nissl stain and therefore is called Nissl substance. Neuronal processes are axons and dendrites. Supporting cells are called glial cells, and

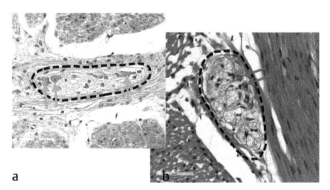

Fig. 15.19 (a,b) Ganglia in tissues (outlined), high magnification. Green arrows indicate neuronal cell bodies.

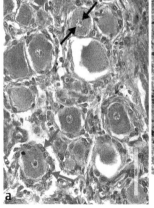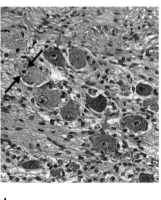

Fig. 15.20 (a) Trigeminal ganglion, high magnification. **(b)** Sympathetic ganglion, medium-high magnification. Nuclei of neuronal cell bodies are framed by black arrows; nucleoli are indicated by blue arrows; green arrows point to satellite cells.

the most prominent of them are oligodendrocytes in the central nervous system (brain and spinal cord) and Schwann cells in the peripheral nervous system. Both of these types of cells either wrap loosely around axons (ensheathment) or wind very tightly around one axon a large number of times (myelination).

The nervous system is organized such that cell bodies are clustered together and axons are bundled together. Clusters of cell bodies are called nuclei in the central nervous system and ganglia in the peripheral nervous system. Bundles of axons are called tracts in the central nervous system and nerves in the peripheral nervous system. In the spinal cord, most cell bodies are in a butterfly-shaped central region called the gray matter. Axons, many of them myelinated, are in the white matter, located in the outer portions of the spinal cord. Special stains can be used to visualize axons (silver stain) or myelin in the spinal cord.

Peripheral nerves can be teased apart to show individual axons with their myelin wrapping and nodes of Ranvier, which are locations on axons that are not myelinated. Peripheral nerves in routinely stained tissue can be recognized because the myelin washes away on tissue preparation, so peripheral nerves appear a pale salmon color, with numerous nuclei belonging to Schwann cells. Peripheral nerves are also elastic, so they appear wavy, and

are bounded by a perineurium, so they form bundles distinct from the surrounding connective tissues. Bundles of axons are called fascicles. Loose connective tissue between axons within a fascicle is called endoneurium. The outer boundary of a fascicle is perineurium, which is a very cellular layer; the cells have tight junctions and provide a protected environment for nerves. Fascicles can be bundled with other fascicles into larger nerves by a dense irregular connective tissue called epineurium. Ganglia are collections of neuronal cell bodies outside the nervous system. Large ganglia have numerous neuronal cell bodies, while smaller ganglia are scattered throughout tissues (e.g., intestines).

Questions and Answers

An online-only section of questions and answers accompanying this chapter is hosted on Thieme's MedOne Education site: https://medone-education.thieme.com. Use the code on the media page at the front of this book to gain access. An institutional license to the site is required to access these questions in an interactive format, and individual users are required to register for an individual account to track results.

16   Cardiovascular Overview

After completing this chapter, you should be able to:
— Identify, at the light microscope level, each of the following:
  • Layers of vessel walls
    ◦ Tunica intima
      ▪ Endothelium
    ◦ Tunica media
    ◦ Tunica externa (adventitia)
    ◦ Internal and external elastic lamina
  • Arteries
  • Veins
  • Capillaries
  • Lymphatic channels
— Outline the function of each organ or structure and cell type listed
— Describe the overall organization and function of the cardiovascular and lymphatic systems

16.1   Overview of the Cardiovascular and Lymphatic Systems

Vessels in the body transport fluids (blood and lymphatic fluid), enabling distribution of nutrients, waste products, hormones, and other substances as well as certain types of cells. There are two components of the vascular system:
• The **cardiovascular system** (**Fig. 16.1a**) transports blood; it includes the heart, arteries, capillaries, and veins.
• The **lymphatic system** (**Fig. 16.1b**) returns tissue fluid (lymph) from the tissues back to the cardiovascular system.

This series of chapters (from this chapter through **Chapter 26**) discusses the histology of the different components of these systems and includes chapters focusing on blood, blood cell development, blood vessels, the heart, lymphoid tissues, and lymphoid organs. This chapter provides a brief introduction to the vascular systems by overviewing the structure of vessels.

16.2   General Structure of Vessels

Fig. 16.2 is a drawing showing a typical vessel. The walls of vessels have three basic components (from inside to outside):
1. The **tunica intima** consists of a simple squamous epithelium (called the **endothelium**), a basement membrane, and underlying loose connective tissue.
2. The **tunica media** is a thicker layer composed mostly of smooth muscle and elastic fibers.
3. The **tunica externa** (or **adventitia**) consists of dense connective tissue that blends with surrounding tissues.
Some vessels have elastic sheets, called **internal** and **external elastic laminae**, situated between these layers. The internal elastic lamina is between the tunica intima and tunica media, and the external elastic lamina lies between the tunica media and the adventitia.

Fig. 16.3 is a cross section of a blood vessel (an artery); the blood in the lumen is indicated. The double arrow indicates the extent of the tunica media, which consists mostly of smooth muscle in this vessel. The smooth muscle cells in the tunica media are circularly arranged; in other words, the cells lie perpendicular to the long axis of the vessel.

Basic Science Correlate: Physiology

The circularly arranged smooth muscle in the tunica media can constrict, like a sphincter, reducing the diameter of the lumen. This is called vasoconstriction. Relaxation of this muscle results in vasodilation, which increases the diameter of the lumen. These changes in diameter regulate flow through the vessel.

Fig. 16.4 is a higher-magnification image focusing on the wall of the same vessel. At this magnification, it is easier to see the tunica intima (green double arrow), tunica media (black double arrow), and adventitia (blue double arrow). Brown arrows indicate nuclei of endothelial cells, which form the inner lining of vessels. The internal elastic lamina (marked by a yellow dotted line) separates the intima from the media. The external elastic lamina is not visible, which is not unusual for most vessels.

Video 16.1   Vessel layers

Be able to identify:
— Blood vessel
  • Tunica intima
    ◦ Endothelium
  • Tunica media
  • Tunica externa (adventitia)
https://www.thieme.de/de/q.htm?p=opn/tp/308390101/978-1-62623-414-7_c016_v001&t=video

Fig. 16.5 is an image of a smaller artery. The simple squamous endothelial cells that form the inner lining of blood vessels have nuclei along the inner aspect of the vessel wall (black arrows). In many cases, these nuclei are flattened (see **Fig. 16.4**), but here they are small and round lumen. Smooth muscle cells in the tunical media exhibit larger nuclei (yellow arrow) than the endothelial cells.

16.3   Comparison of Major Types of Vessels

There are four major categories of vessels: **arteries**, **veins**, **capillaries**, and **lymphatic vessels**. These vessels are variations on the general vessel structure described in the preceding section. There are subcategories of most of these categories, which will be described in a subsequent chapter. For example, small arteries are called arterioles, and small veins are venules. For now, it is useful to note ways that these vessels differ from each other (**Fig. 16.6**):
• The major histological difference between arteries and veins lies in the thickness and muscularity of the tunica media; arteries have a thicker, more muscular tunica media.
• Capillaries are composed simply of endothelial cells, without a tunica media or adventitia.
• Lymphatic vessels (not shown in **Fig. 16.6**) have a thinner tunica media than veins, and the smallest lymphatic vessels have valves.

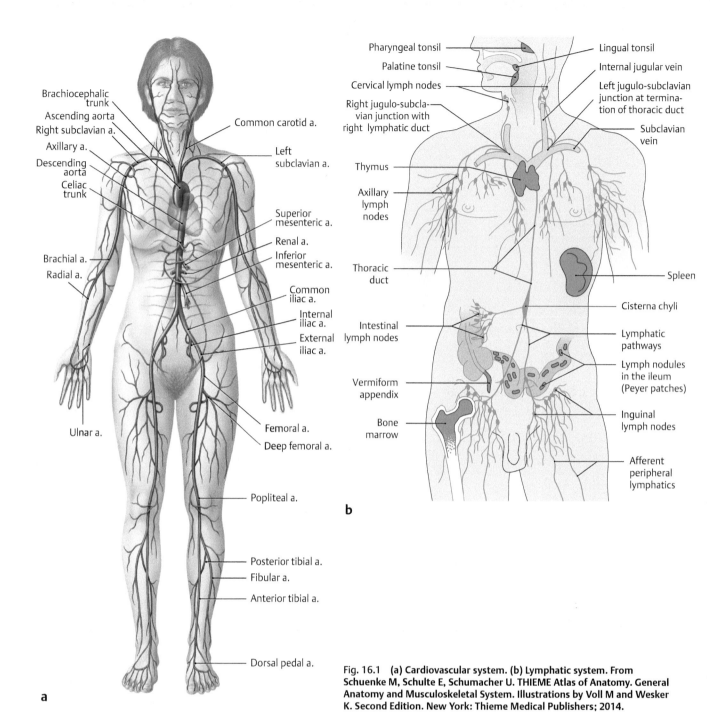

a

Brachiocephalic trunk
Ascending aorta
Right subclavian a.
Axillary a.
Descending aorta
Celiac trunk
Brachial a.
Radial a.
Ulnar a.

Common carotid a.
Left subclavian a.
Superior mesenteric a.
Renal a.
Inferior mesenteric a.
Common iliac a.
Internal iliac a.
External iliac a.
Femoral a.
Deep femoral a.
Popliteal a.
Posterior tibial a.
Fibular a.
Anterior tibial a.
Dorsal pedal a.

b

Pharyngeal tonsil
Palatine tonsil
Cervical lymph nodes
Right jugulo-subclavian junction with right lymphatic duct
Thymus
Axillary lymph nodes
Thoracic duct
Intestinal lymph nodes
Vermiform appendix
Bone marrow

Lingual tonsil
Internal jugular vein
Left jugulo-subclavian junction at termination of thoracic duct
Subclavian vein
Spleen
Cisterna chyli
Lymphatic pathways
Lymph nodules in the ileum (Peyer patches)
Inguinal lymph nodes
Afferent peripheral lymphatics

Fig. 16.1 (a) Cardiovascular system. (b) Lymphatic system. From Schuenke M, Schulte E, Schumacher U. THIEME Atlas of Anatomy. General Anatomy and Musculoskeletal System. Illustrations by Voll M and Wesker K. Second Edition. New York: Thieme Medical Publishers; 2014.

Fig. 16.7 is a tissue section that highlights the difference between arteries and veins. Histologically, differentiating between arteries/arterioles (black outline) and veins/venules (yellow outline) is best done by comparing vessels of approximately the same size. Note that veins are typically larger but have thinner walls, so they tend to collapse (flatten). Arteries have more smooth muscle in the tunica media than veins, and, therefore, the arterial wall is relatively thicker compared to the size of the vessel itself, with a narrower lumen. In addition, arteries tend to be rounder because of the muscle and elastic fibers in the tunica media. Both may contain blood cells in the lumen, as shown here, but cells may be difficult to see clearly, or the lumen may be empty.

Fig. 16.8 is a section including a capillary (arrow). Capillaries are very thin-walled, round, small vessels. The capillary wall is composed of a single layer of endothelial cells (nucleus of one

appears at approximately the 4 o'clock position in this figure). This thin simple squamous endothelial lining allows efficient diffusion of molecules from the blood into the surrounding tissue and vice versa. The diameter of the capillary lumen is typically 8 µm, the diameter of a red blood cell.

Video 16.2 Artery, vein, and capillary

Be able to identify:
— Artery/arteriole
— Vein/venule
— Capillary

https://www.thieme.de/de/q.htm?p=opn/tp/308390101/978-1-62623-414-7_c016_v002&t=video

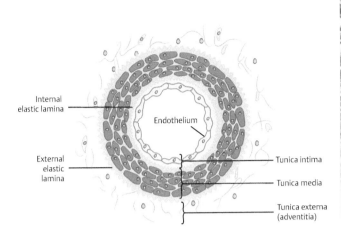

Fig. 16.2 **General structure of vessels.**

Internal elastic lamina

Endothelium

External elastic lamina

Tunica intima

Tunica media

Tunica externa (adventitia)

Fig. 16.9 shows examples of lymphatic vessels. Lymphatic vessels typically have thinner walls than veins; this is evident in the vessel in **Fig. 16.9a**. The lymphatic vessel in **Fig. 16.9b** has a slightly thicker wall than is usually seen in lymphatic vessels, but it shows the flap of a valve (black arrows), which are commonly seen in small lymphatic vessels in tissues. Lymphatic vessels are typically devoid of red blood cells and are filled with either numerous white blood cells (nuclei in the lumen), a "colloid" from precipitated lymph fluid, or both.

Video 16.3 Lymphatic vessels

Be able to identify:
— Lymphatic vessels

https://www.thieme.de/de/q.htm?p=opn/tp/308390101/978-1-62623-414-7_c016_v003&t=video

Fig. 16.3 **Medium-sized artery at low/medium magnification. Blood occupies the lumen; the double arrow indicates the extent of the tunica media.**

Helpful Hint

Valves in vessels and in the heart prevent backflow of fluid. Veins have valves also, but only in veins of medium and large size, not in small vessels found within tissues.

Functional Correlate

The lymphatic system returns tissue fluid (lymph) back to the blood vascular system. Along the way, lymph passes through lymph nodes, which, as discussed in a later chapter, are the site for initiating the immune response. Because they are involved in immunity, lymphatic vessels and lymph nodes contain numerous white blood cells.

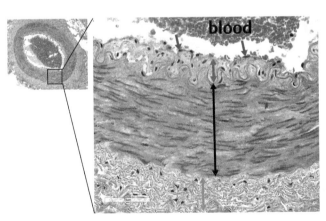

Fig. 16.4 **Wall of a medium-sized artery at higher magnification. Blood in the lumen is indicated. The double arrows indicate the extent of the layers: green, tunica intima; black, tunica media; blue, tunica externa. The brown arrows indicate nuclei of endothelial cells. The wavy dotted line is over the internal elastic lamina.**

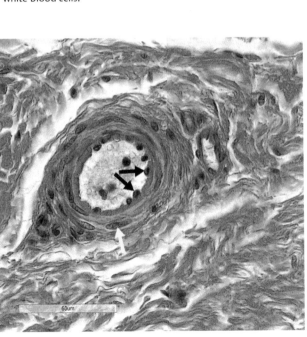

Fig. 16.5 **Small artery, showing endothelial cell (black arrows) and smooth muscle nuclei (yellow arrow).**

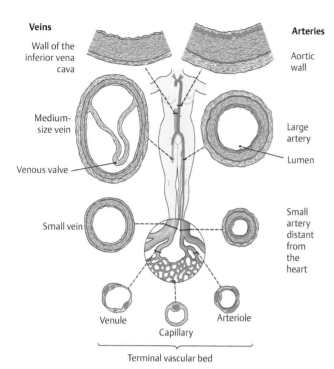

Veins

Wall of the inferior vena cava

Medium-size vein

Venous valve

Small vein

Venule

Capillary

Arteriole

Arteries

Aortic wall

Large artery

Lumen

Small artery distant from the heart

Terminal vascular bed

Fig. 16.6   Comparison of arteries, capillaries, and veins. From Schuenke M, Schulte E, Schumacher U. THIEME Atlas of Anatomy. General Anatomy and Musculoskeletal System. Illustrations by Voll M and Wesker K. Second Edition. New York: Thieme Medical Publishers; 2014.

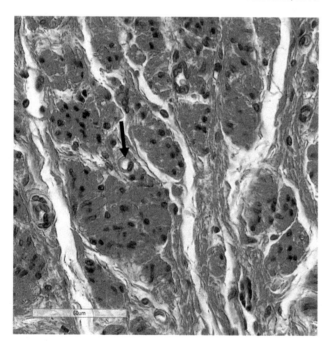

Fig. 16.8   Capillary (black arrow).

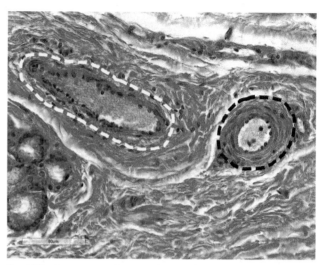

Fig. 16.7   Comparison of a typical artery (black outline) and vein (yellow outline).

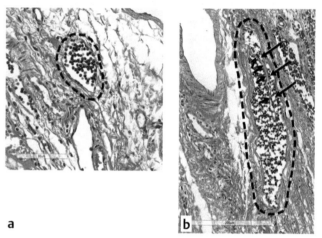

a   **b**

Fig. 16.9   (a, b) Lymphatic vessels (outlined). A valve is indicated (black arrows).

of which typically are composed of three layers. The tunica intima consists of a simple squamous endothelium, basement membrane, and underlying connective tissue; the tunica media consists mostly of smooth muscle and elastic fibers; and the tunica externa consists of dense irregular connective tissue. Some vessels have elastic laminae between these layers. Different types of vessels have variations on this three-layered structure. Arteries typically have a thicker tunica media than veins, owing to more abundant smooth muscle and elastic fibers. Capillaries are the smallest vessels and are composed of endothelial cells and associated basement membrane. Lymphatic vessels have walls thinner than those of veins.

Questions and Answers

An online-only section of questions and answers accompanying this chapter is hosted on Thieme's MedOne Education site: https://medone-education.thieme.com. Use the code on the media page at the front of this book to gain access. An institutional license to the site is required to access these questions in an interactive format, and individual users are required to register for an individual account to track results.

16.4   Chapter Review

Organisms larger than a few cells must have a mechanism to transport nutrients, wastes, and other molecules such as hormones. In humans, two systems accomplish this task. The cardiovascular system circulates blood, and the lymphatic system returns tissue fluid to the bloodstream. These systems consist of vessels, the walls

17   Blood

After completing this chapter, you should be able to:
— Identify, at the light microscope level, each of the following:
  • In a normal blood smear:
    ○ Red blood cells
    ○ Platelets
    ○ White blood cells
      ▪ Neutrophils
      ▪ Eosinophils
      ▪ Basophils
      ▪ Monocytes
      ▪ Lymphocytes
  • In peripheral tissues (inflammation):
    ○ Erythrocytes
    ○ Neutrophils
    ○ Lymphocytes
    ○ Plasma cells
    ○ Macrophages
    ○ Eosinophils
— Identify, at the electron microscope level, each of the following:
  • Red blood cells
  • Platelets
  • White blood cells
    ○ Eosinophils
    ○ Basophils
    ○ Macrophages
— Outline the function of each cell type listed
— Predict the appearance of the cells listed in light micrographs based on their appearance in electron micrographs, and vice versa
— Begin to make predictions about a patient's condition using a differential blood count, and predict a patient's differential blood count based on clinical presentation

17.1   Components of Blood

Blood is composed of **plasma** and **formed elements** (cells or cell fragments). These components can be separated by centrifugation (**Fig. 17.1**). Plasma is a clear-yellow fluid composed of water, ions, buffers, and proteins such as albumin and clotting factors. Because plasma is a clear fluid, it is not routinely seen in micrographs. Therefore, from a histologic standpoint, the main focus when analyzing blood smeared on a slide are the formed elements. These formed elements are:
• **Red blood cells** (**erythrocytes**), involved in oxygen transport
• **Platelets** (**thrombocytes**), involved in clotting
• **White blood cells** (**leukocytes**), involved in immunity
There are five types of white blood cells distinguishable in light and electron micrographs (described below)..

17.2   Preparation of Blood Smears

Slides of peripheral blood (and bone marrow) are prepared by placing a drop of blood onto one end of the slide (**Fig. 17.2**, red dot in image). Using another slide, the drop of blood is then smeared across the slide (in the direction of the arrows). This creates a gradient of cell density, such that there is a high density of cells on one end of the slide (the left side in this image) and a lower density at the other (right) end. Within this gradient, an optimal area of the slide is somewhere in the middle, where the density of cells is high enough to assess cell numbers but not so high that the cells are piled on top of one another or distorted (**Fig. 17.3**).

Helpful Hint

This point may seem trivial, but many first-time users waste time searching areas of the slide that are not optimal. Digital scanners are typically set to scan only the central region of optimal cell density.

After the blood is smeared on the slide, special stains (e.g., Wright stain, Giemsa stain) are then used, which are similar to H & E in that the nucleus appears blue and cytoplasm appears pink, but have additional dyes that visualize **azurophilic** (dark blue to purple) **granules** in white blood cells.

Helpful Hint

The strict definition of azure is a shade of blue. However, as will be seen, azurophilic granules seen in white blood cells are closer to purple in color.

17.3   Red Blood Cells

The most common formed elements in blood are red blood cells (or erythrocytes), approximately 5 million per microliter of blood. These elements are biconcave disks, so they exhibit a pale central region (**Fig. 17.4**). The diameter of red blood cells (shown by double arrows in **Fig. 17.4**) is 7–8 μm, which is useful to keep in mind when estimating the size of neighboring structures. Red blood cells circulate for about 120 days before they are destroyed and their components recycled.

Fig. 17.5 is a scanning electron micrograph demonstrating the biconcave shape of red blood cells. Red blood cells are able to achieve this shape because they lack a nucleus; in fact, they lack most organelles. This shape is advantageous because it increases the surface area of the plasma membrane to maximize diffusion of soluble gases. In addition, the biconcave shape provides flexibility to red blood cells, allowing them to pass through capillaries more easily. In addition, several red blood cells can stack as they pass through a capillary in single file.

Red blood cells are full of **hemoglobin**, an iron-containing protein that carries oxygen. Therefore, in transmission electron micrographs, they appear as disks with homogeneous, electron-dense cytoplasm. **Fig. 17.6** is an electron micrograph of an arteriole with about a dozen red blood cells within the lumen.

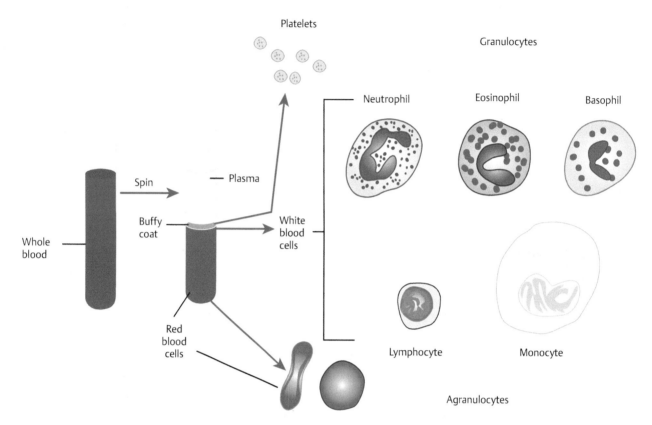

Fig. 17.1   **Components of blood. Blood is withdrawn from an artery or vein into a tube containing anticoagulant. Centrifugation separates the cells from the plasma. Red blood cells, being the heaviest due to iron, are in the bottom half of the spun sample. White blood cells and platelets form a thin layer in the middle referred to as the buffy coat.**

17.4   Platelets

Platelets (**Fig. 17.7**, arrows) are cell fragments that vary in size but are smaller than red blood cells. Normal blood contains 150,000–450,000 platelets per microliter. Platelets are involved in clotting and have a lifespan of about 10 days. Close examination reveals that platelets contain dense structures within a pale blue cytoplasm. These dense structures are **alpha granules**, which contain secretory components important for blood clotting.

Fig. 17.8 is an electron micrograph showing several platelets. In peripheral blood, platelets are elongated disks. They have no nucleus, but other cytoplasmic organelles can be seen. These include alpha granules (2), which are visible in light micrographs and contain proteins, and **delta (dense) granules** (3), which are too small to be seen in light micrographs and contain small molecules such as serotonin and calcium. Platelets release the contents of these granules to stimulate clotting, inflammation, and wound repair. The periphery of the platelet cytoplasm contains a bundle of **microtubules** (1) and other cytoskeletal elements, which maintain the shape of platelets while allowing them to change shape during activation.

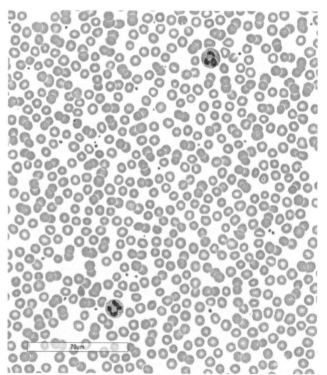

Fig. 17.3   **Peripheral blood smear.**

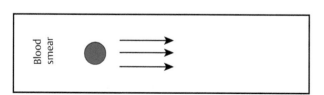

Fig. 17.2   **Preparation of a blood smear. A drop of blood is placed on a slide (red dot), and the edge of another slide is used to spread the drop of blood in the direction of the arrows.**

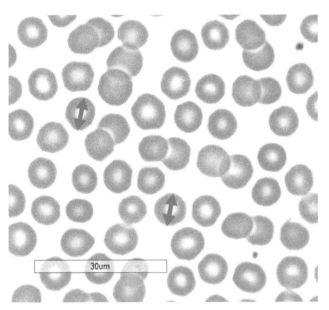

Fig. 17.4 **Red blood cells (the blue double arrows indicate the diameter of two of them).**

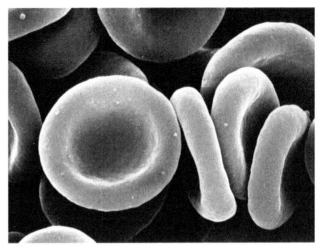

Fig. 17.5 **Red blood cells in scanning electron micrograph.**

Video 17.1 Red blood cells and platelets

Be able to identify:
— Red blood cells
— Platelets
https://www.thieme.de/de/q.htm?p=opn/
tp/308390101/978-1-62623-414-7_c017_v001&t=video

Fig. 17.9 is an electron micrograph of a larger platelet. Platelets contain elaborate **canaliculi** (2), which are continuous with the plasma membrane; alpha granules (1) release their contents into the extracellular space via the system of these canaliculi. When a platelet is activated, it extends numerous **pseudopodia** (6), cell processes that enable the platelet to adhere to neighboring platelets and other cells. In addition, this increases plasma membrane surface area, which is a platform for clot formation.

17.5 White Blood Cells

White blood cells play a role in immunity. There are 5,000–10,000 white blood cells per microliter of blood. Though white blood cells vary in size and appearance, all are larger than red blood cells. There are five types of white blood cells distinguishable on routine blood smears, and they can be grouped into two categories:

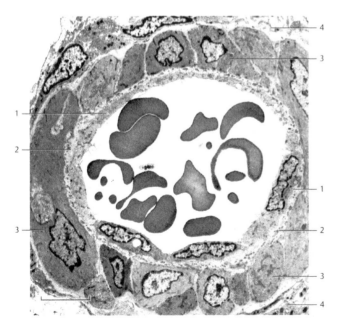

Fig. 17.6 **Electron micrograph showing red blood cells in a blood vessel. (1) endothelial cell of tunica intima; (2) connective tissue of tunica intima; (3) smooth muscle cells of tunica media; (4) tunica adventitia.**

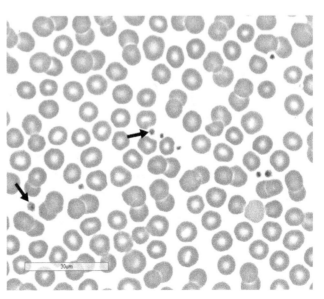

Fig. 17.7 **Platelets (arrows).**

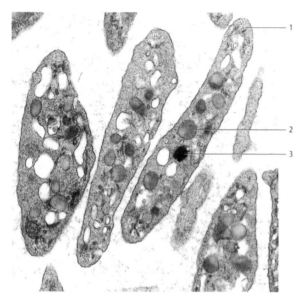

Fig. 17.8   **Electron micrograph showing platelets in peripheral blood. (1) microtubules; (2) alpha granules; (3) delta (dense) granules.**

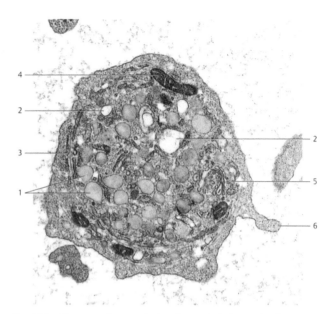

Fig. 17.9   **Electron micrograph showing a single large platelet in peripheral blood. (1) alpha granules; (2) canaliculi; (3) microtubules; (4) mitochondrion; (5) Golgi apparatus; (6) pseudopodia.**

- **Granulocytes**, which contain abundant granules in their cytoplasm (top row of white blood cells in **Fig. 17.1**)
- **Agranulocytes**, which have fewer cytoplasmic granules (bottom row of white cells in **Fig. 17.1**)

17.5.1 Neutrophils

Neutrophils are 10–12 μm in diameter and contain numerous small granules (**Fig. 17.10**). **Azurophilic granules**, also called nonspecific granules, are similar to lysosomes and are just large enough to see in the light microscope (purple granules indicated by the arrows). Smaller granules, called **neutrophilic granules**, cannot be seen individually in the light microscope but collectively give the cytoplasm an overall pale eosinophilic (salmon) color. Since mature neutrophils in the blood have already produced the proteins they will need during their short lifespan, they lack significant rough endoplasmic reticulum (RER) and Golgi apparatus, so they show little to no cytoplasmic basophilia. The contents of the granules in neutrophils are used to destroy bacteria that they have phagocytosed.

The nucleus is typically segmented, or polymorphonuclear; these cells are often called "polys" or "segs" by physicians. The segmented nucleus may produce more than one nuclear profile in thin sections on electron micrographs. The DNA in the nucleus is "clumpy."

17.5.2 Eosinophils

Like neutrophils, **eosinophils** are also 10–12 μm in diameter, but they contain numerous large **eosinophilic granules** that have an intense, refractory eosinophilia in the light microscope (blue

arrow, showing eosinophilic granule with pale center, in **Fig. 17.11**). Eosinophils are involved in inflammation and destruction of large parasites. The nucleus is characteristically bilobed. As in neutrophils, the DNA in the nucleus is "clumpy."

Fig. 17.12 is an electron micrograph of an eosinophil. The large **eosinophilic granules** contain a characteristic central crystalloid region (dark band indicated by the arrow) rich in a protein called **major basic protein**. The contents of these eosinophilic granules are toxic to large organisms such as parasitic worms. Eosinophils also have a few azurophilic granules (not shown), also involved in destruction of parasites and in allergies.

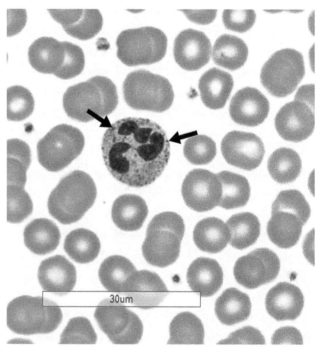

Fig. 17.10 **Neutrophil showing azurophilic granules (arrows).**

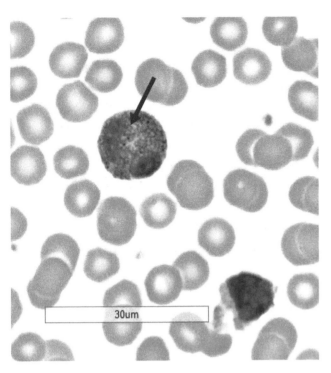

Fig. 17.11 **Eosinophil showing eosinophilic granule (arrow).**

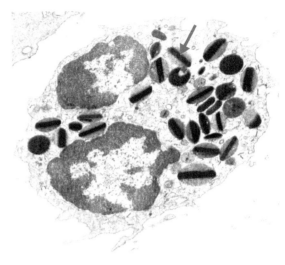

Fig. 17.12 **Eosinophil in electron micrograph. The arrow indicates the crystalloid region within an eosinophilic granule.**

Helpful Hint

Because eosinophilic granules have such a unique appearance in electron microscopes, they are a useful resource for question writers; recognizing them is often "high yield."

17.5.3 Basophils

Basophils are related to mast cells found in tissues (see **Chapter 7**). They are 10–12 μm in diameter, like other granulocytes, and contain numerous large, dark granules within their cytoplasm (**Fig. 17.13**). The large **basophilic granules** contain highly sulfated glycosaminoglycans, notably **heparin** and heparin sulfate, which are intensely basophilic (arrows). The heparin and **histamine** in these granules play a role in inflammation.

The nucleus is characteristically bilobed, though the presence of the large basophilic granules often obscures the nucleus, as seen in **Fig. 17.13**. The DNA in the nucleus is "clumpy."

Helpful Hint

The contents of basophilic granules tend to wash out during glass slide blood smear preparation. In **Fig. 17.13**, areas where the granules have washed away can be seen in the top portion of the cell. In some cases, basophils may appear devoid of granules, making them difficult to identify.

In electron micrographs, basophils appear similar to mast cells found in tissues. The large granules visible in blood smears, and in mast cells in tissues, appear as large, dark structures on electron micrographs. **Fig. 17.14** is of a mast cell (from **Chapter 7**). Basophilic granules have a similar appearance but are typically larger.

Video 17.2   Neutrophil

https://www.thieme.de/de/q.htm?p=opn/tp/308390101/978-1-62623-414-7_c017_v002&t=video

Video 17.3   Eosinophil

https://www.thieme.de/de/q.htm?p=opn/tp/308390101/978-1-62623-414-7_c017_v003&t=video

Video 17.4   Basophil

Be able to identify:
— Neutrophils
— Eosinophils
— Basophils

https://www.thieme.de/de/q.htm?p=opn/tp/308390101/978-1-62623-414-7_c017_v004&t=video

17.5.4 Monocytes

Although **monocytes** are agranulocytes, they have a few granules. **Fig. 17.15** shows a monocyte; several azurophilic granules are visible in the cytoplasm just to the left of the nucleus. Monocytes have the potential to produce proteins, so the cytoplasm of these cells typically demonstrates a basophilic background, though the one in **Fig. 17.15** has eosinophilic regions as well. Monocytes are the largest white blood cells (~18 μm). The nucleus is typically indented or horseshoe-shaped, with a finer chromatin pattern (rather than clumpy).

Fig. 17.16 is an electron micrograph of a small blood vessel. A small monocyte is the nucleated cell adjacent to the red blood cell (1), recognized by its indented nucleus. Monocytes are relatively inactive in blood, so they have sparse RER and a less developed Golgi apparatus. However, when they leave the bloodstream and enter the tissues, they mature into **macrophages**, which are active in phagocytosis and antigen presentation and exhibit more robust cytoplasmic organelles.

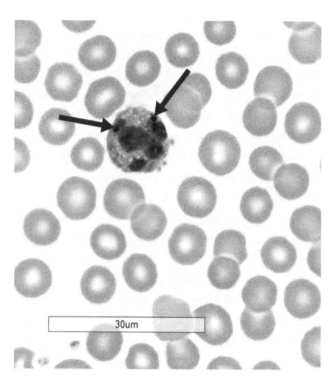

Fig. 17.13 **Basophil showing basophilic granules (arrows).**

17.5.5 Lymphocytes

Most **lymphocytes** in blood have very little cytoplasm; therefore, most are slightly larger than a red blood cell (**Fig. 17.17**). Lymphocytes often have no visible granules. Like monocytes, lymphocytes have the potential for future protein synthesis, so they contain a small amount of RER and Golgi, which gives the thin rim of cytoplasm a basophilic color. The nucleus is round, with a condensed chromatin pattern. Lymphocytes are involved in specific immunity.

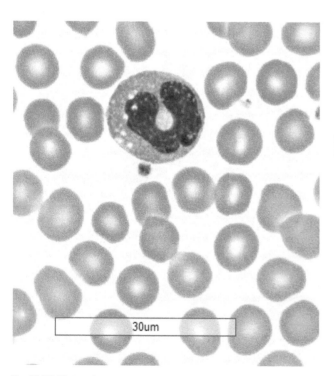

Fig. 17.15 **Monocyte.**

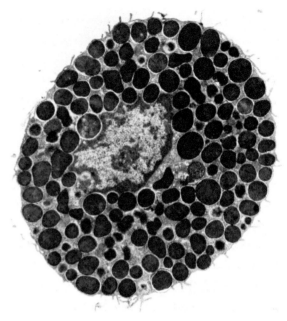

Fig. 17.14 **Electron micrograph of mast cell. Basophils have a similar appearance as this mast cell.**

Fig. 17.18 is an electron micrograph of a small lymphatic vessel. Most of the cells in the lumen of this vessel are lymphocytes. Note the small nuclei and thin rim of cytoplasm with few organelles.

Video 17.5   Monocyte

https://www.thieme.de/de/q.htm?p=opn/
tp/308390101/978-1-62623-414-7_c017_
v005&t=video

Video 17.6   Lymphocyte

Be able to identify:
— Monocytes
— Lymphocytes
https://www.thieme.de/de/q.htm?p=opn/
tp/308390101/978-1-62623-414-7_c017_v006&t=video

Clinical Correlate

A patient's blood sample is a routine test used to assist in diagnosing a number of conditions. In a **complete blood count**, the number of red blood cells, platelets, and white blood cells is determined, along with other parameters (e.g., hemoglobin). An increase or decrease in the number of blood cells from reference values can provide clues to numerous pathologic conditions. In addition, a **differential blood cell count** calculates the percentage of each type of white blood cell relative to the total number of white blood cells. Normal values are: neutrophils, 40–60%; lymphocytes, 20–40%; monocytes, 4–8%; eosinophils, 1–3%; basophils, 0–1%. Note that different sources have slightly different reference values. Comparison of a patient's test results to these reference values can provide clues to pathologic conditions, especially when considering the function of these cells. For example, an elevated eosinophil count is seen in parasitic infections or allergies.

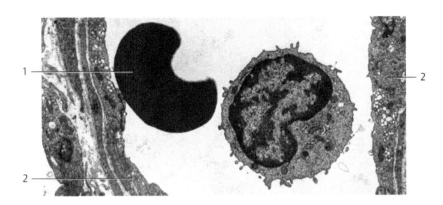

Fig. 17.16 **Electron micrograph of a monocyte. (1) red blood cell; (2) endothelial cell.**

17.6   White Blood Cells in Tissues

Although white blood cells are found in blood, they mostly function in peripheral tissues. **Inflammation** is a complex series of reactions that is the body's response to tissue damage, often caused by infectious agents or other pathologic conditions. Histologically, inflammation is seen as an increase in white blood cells in tissues.

As described in **Chapter 7**, connective tissue (**Fig. 17.19a**) consists of fibroblasts (green arrows) and extracellular matrix (collagen, elastic fibers, tissue fluid). When inflammation occurs, white blood cells migrate into the affected tissue. This continually happens in small numbers throughout the body, particularly in tissues exposed to the external environment. However, when white blood cells migrate into a tissue in large numbers, the result is quite striking (**Fig. 17.19b**).

The appearance of white blood cells in normal H & E-stained tissues (**Fig. 17.19b**) is slightly different from, but parallel to, the appearance of these cells in Wright-stained blood smears. Although the resolution of these cells in tissues is not as good as

that seen in blood smears, it is important to recognize these cells in tissues in order to ascertain specific pathologies.

Clinical Correlate

Neutrophils play a major role in bacterial infections. Therefore, inflammation caused by bacteria, as well as acute inflammation, is characterized by the presence of high numbers of neutrophils. Macrophages and lymphocytes are prominent cell types in chronic inflammation and are more likely to be predominant in viral or autoinflammatory conditions.

17.6.1 Neutrophils in Tissues

Recall that neutrophils have a segmented nucleus and a pale eosinophilic cytoplasm. **Fig. 17.20** shows a neutrophil in inflammation (blue arrow) that displays these two characteristics.

17.6.2 Lymphocytes in Tissues

Fig. 17.20 shows two lymphocytes (black arrows) in inflammation. The cytoplasm of these cells is more eosinophilic than the basophilic cytoplasm seen in lymphocytes in blood. This feature is not unusual for lymphocytes in tissues. More important is that these cells have a small, round nucleus and sparse cytoplasm, which identifies them as lymphocytes.

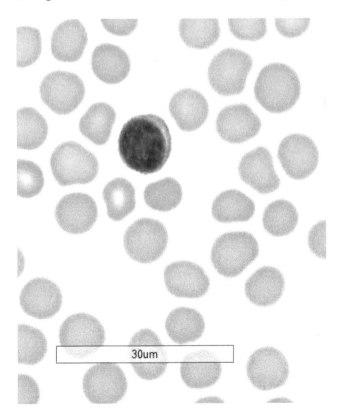

Fig. 17.17 **Lymphocyte.**

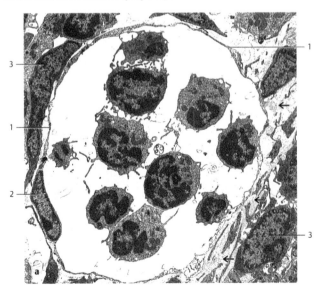

Fig. 17.18 **Electron micrograph of small lymphatic vessel, containing several lymphocytes. (1) endothelial cell process; (2) endothelial cell nucleus; (3) fibroblast. Collagen in tunica intima (black arrows).**

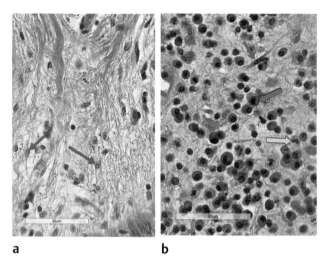

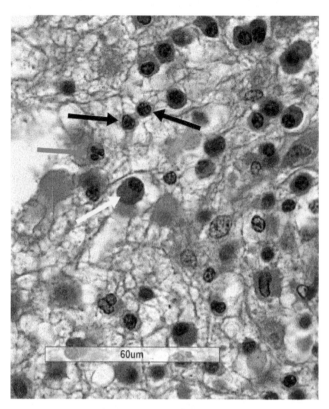

a   b

Fig. 17.19 **(a) Dense irregular connective tissue in a healthy condition, showing fibroblasts (green arrows). (b) Similar tissue with inflammation, showing fibroblasts (green arrow), plasma cells (red arrow), and neutrophils (orange arrow).**

17.6.3 Plasma Cells in Tissues

Some lymphocytes (B cells) can mature into antibody-secreting **plasma cells** (**Fig. 17.21**). Because these cells are very active in protein synthesis, their cytoplasm is loaded with RER, with several Golgi profiles (red outline). However, this cell is synthesizing large numbers of copies of only a few proteins. Therefore, the nucleus is expressing only a few genes, so it has a large amount of heterochromatin for an active cell.

In H & E-stained sections, plasma cells (**Fig. 17.20**, yellow arrow) have intense cytoplasmic basophilia (compare to nearby neutrophil, blue arrow). Careful observation reveals a paler perinuclear region (in the center of the cell), indicating the location of the Golgi apparatus. This region is paler than the surrounding cytoplasm because the Golgi is a relatively ribosome-free zone. Also note the relatively small, heterochromatic nucleus.

17.6.4 Macrophages in Tissues

As mentioned, monocytes migrate into tissues and become macrophages. **Fig. 17.22** and **Fig. 17.23** are electron micrographs of an isolated macrophage and one in tissue, respectively. Macrophages are very large cells with a mostly euchromatic nucleus, a prominent Golgi apparatus, and numerous secretory granules. Macrophages are very active in **phagocytosis**; they envelop foreign organisms and digest them in their lysosomal compartment.

In H & E-stained tissue sections, macrophages can be challenging to identify. **Fig. 17.24** shows a good example of a macrophage. Macrophages are large cells; the black arrows indicate the approximate location of the plasma membrane of this macrophage. Macrophages have a large, euchromatic nucleus; in many cases, the nucleolus is prominent and has a pink color. The cytoplasm is extensive, staining a very pale eosinophilia, but is typically ill defined and frothy, blending in with the surrounding connective tissue matrix.

60um

Fig. 17.20 **White blood cells in inflammation, showing neutrophil (blue arrow), lymphocytes (black arrows), and plasma cell (yellow arrow).**

Clinical Correlate

Because both macrophages and neutrophils are involved in phagocytosis, physicians typically refer to macrophages as **mononuclear** phagocytes and to granulocytes, in particular neutrophils, as **polymorphonuclear cells**, or **polys**. This is based on the nuclear profile; monocytes have an indented nucleus that often appears as a single structure, while neutrophil nuclei have multiple lobes that often appear to be multiple nuclei.

Video 17.7   Overview of inflammation

https://www.thieme.de/de/q.htm?p=opn/tp/308390101/978-1-62623-414-7_c017_v007&t=video

Video 17.8   Inflammation showing cells of inflammation
Be able to identify:
— Lymphocytes
— Neutrophils
— Plasma cells
— Macrophages
— Fibroblasts

https://www.thieme.de/de/q.htm?p=opn/tp/308390101/978-1-62623-414-7_c017_v008&t=video

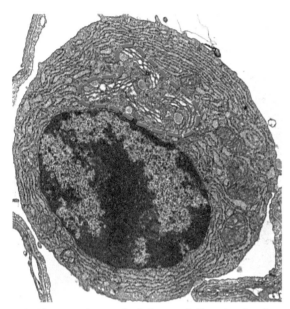

Fig. 17.21 **Electron micrograph of plasma cell.** Note the abundant rough endoplasmic reticulum and profiles of Golgi apparatus (Golgi outlined, rough endoplasmic reticulum occupies most of the rest of the cytoplasm).

17.6.5 Eosinophils in Tissues

In blood smears, eosinophils are recognized by their large, intensely eosinophilic granules and bilobed nucleus. This translates into H & E-stained tissues nicely. **Fig. 17.25** is an image of the stratified squamous epithelium of the esophagus, showing eosinophils that have infiltrated into the epithelium (black arrows). The eosinophilia is intense, nearly red when compared to the pink eosinophilia in the cytoplasm of the surrounding epithelial cells. Note that the two cells identified clearly have bilobed nuclei, but in many eosinophils, one of the lobes may be out of the plane of section, giving the appearance of a round nucleus that is not lobed.

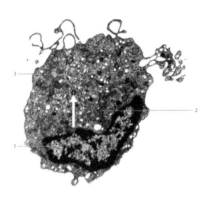

Fig. 17.22 **Electron micrograph of macrophage. (1) nucleus; (2) mitochondrion; (3) Golgi apparatus. White arrow marks a centriole.**

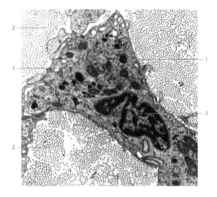

Fig. 17.23 **Electron micrograph of macrophage in tissue. (1) granules; (2) extracellular collagen; (3) nucleus.**

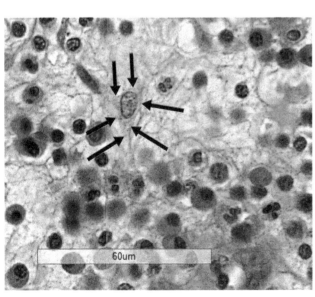

Fig. 17.24 **Macrophage in connective tissue.** The black arrows indicate the approximate location of the macrophage plasma membrane.

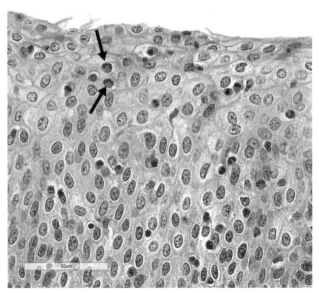

Fig. 17.25 **Eosinophils in stratified squamous epithelium.**

Video 17.9   Eosinophils in the esophagus

Be able to identify:
— Eosinophils

https://www.thieme.de/de/q.htm?p=opn/
tp/308390101/978-1-62623-414-7_c017_
v009&t=video

17.7   Chapter Review

Blood is composed of plasma and formed elements. The formed elements of blood include red blood cells, platelets, and white blood cells. Red blood cells are biconcave disks that contain few or no organelles and are filled with hemoglobin for oxygen transport. Platelets are small cell fragments that contain numerous granules and cytoskeletal elements and are involved in clotting. There are five types of white blood cells, divided into granulocytes and agranulocytes. Of the granulocytes, neutrophils display a pale eosinophilic cytoplasm and multilobed nucleus and are involved in bacterial infections. Eosinophils have large, eosinophilic granules and a bilobed nucleus and are involved in parasitic infections and allergies. Basophils also have a bilobed nucleus, but this is often obscured by the large basophilic granules in the cytoplasm, which contain mediators of inflammation such as histamine and heparin. Agranulocytes include monocytes and lymphocytes. Monocytes are large, with a pale basophilic cytoplasm and indented or horseshoe-shaped nucleus. In tissues, monocytes become macrophages, which are large cells with very pale cytoplasm that are active in phagocytosis. Lymphocytes are involved in specific immunity and are small cells with a round nucleus and a very thin rim of basophilic cytoplasm. Some lymphocytes become antibody-secreting plasma cells, large cells with intense cytoplasmic basophilia due to abundant RER. Many of the cells in blood can be identified in tissue sections. A blood test can ascertain the number or percentage of these cell types in a patient's blood and, by comparing to reference values, provide clues about a patient's condition.

Questions and Answers

An online-only section of questions and answers accompanying this chapter is hosted on Thieme's MedOne Education site: https://medone-education.thieme.com. Use the code on the media page at the front of this book to gain access. An institutional license to the site is required to access these questions in an interactive format, and individual users are required to register for an individual account to track results.

18 Hematopoiesis Overview

After completing this chapter, you should be able to:
— Identify, at the light microscope level, each of the following:
  • Cytoplasmic granules
    ◦ Azurophilic (nonspecific) granules
    ◦ Eosinophilic granules
    ◦ Basophilic granules
    ◦ Neutrophilic granules
  • Nucleoli
  • Nuclear shape
    ◦ Round
    ◦ Indented
    ◦ Kidney bean–shaped
    ◦ Band
    ◦ Segmented
  • Chromatin pattern
    ◦ Fine
    ◦ Clumped
  • Cytoplasmic staining
    ◦ Cytoplasmic basophilia
    ◦ Cytoplasmic eosinophilia
— Assign significance to each of the structures listed for developing and mature blood cells

18.1 Overview of Hematopiesis

As described in the last chapter, blood cells (or blood cell fragments such as platelets) have a relatively short lifespan. These cells need to be continually renewed throughout the lifetime of the individual. This process of production of blood cells is called **hematopoiesis**, or **hemopoiesis**, which occurs in bone marrow after birth. Hematopoiesis occurs in other locations in developing fetuses, such as the yolk sac, liver, and spleen, and certain pathologic conditions can stimulate hematopoiesis in these organs after birth. A number of diseases cause either underdevelopment of sufficient mature blood cells (e.g., **anemia**) or overproduction of some types of them (e.g., **leukemia**).

All blood cells are derived from a common precursor, the **hematopoietic stem cell** (HSC, **Fig. 18.1**). This precursor cell is histologically indistinguishable from circulating lymphocytes; it has a small round nucleus with a thin rim of cytoplasm.

Clinical Correlate

In fact, a small number of hematopoietic stem cells can be found in the circulation and may be used as a form of bone marrow transplant.

The hematopoietic stem cell gives rise to a number of more differentiated stem cells, specific for each cell lineage: red blood cells (RBCs), platelets (fragments of megakaryocytes), and white blood cells. Most of these progenitor cells are also histologically similar to the common progenitor cell, though they can be differentiated from each other and mature lymphocytes with molecular techniques (e.g., antibodies to cell surface markers).

However, in most applications, specific identification of these early precursor cells is not necessary and will not be discussed here.

Ultimately, the early progenitor cells give rise to more differentiated progeny with specific histologic features that can be recognized on light and electron microscopy (**Fig. 18.2**). It is the identification of these later stages that will be the focus of upcoming chapters and is useful for clinical practice.

Hematopoiesis is a considerably challenging topic partially because it is complicated, but also because many of the cellular features that are the hallmarks of this process are subtle. For example, different stages of granulocyte development require recognition of cytoplasmic granules, probably the smallest structures visible in light microscopy. In addition, other structures such as nucleoli are challenging to recognize due to subtle differences in chromatin density.

This chapter will focus on the major cellular features that allow differentiation of specific cell types, without any attempt at identifying the cell types in **Fig. 18.2**. Once identification of these key cellular features is mastered, subsequent chapters will utilize these features to describe the histologically distinct stages of developing of blood cells.

18.2 Cellular Features Used to Differentiate Hematopoietic Cells

Five cytologic features are used to differentiate among developing blood cell types. They are:
• Cytoplasmic granules
• Presence or absence of nucleoli
• Shape of the nucleus
• Extent of nuclear chromatin clumping
• Degree of cytoplasmic basophilia

Helpful Hint

Recall that blood cells are stained routinely with specific hematologic dyes, not H & E, and this results in a slightly wider range of coloration than seen with H & E. A new color is recognized: azure, a bluish purple. To view these critical cytologic features of blood cells, images are magnified to a much greater degree than seen in previous chapters. RBCs (7.5 μm in diameter) in the field of view are useful to gauge the size of cells.

18.3 Cytoplasmic Granules

Four types of cytoplasmic granules can be visible in developing blood cells: azurophilic (primary, nonspecific), eosinophilic, basophilic, and neutrophilic. Although these have all been described in the previous chapter, it is useful to review them here in the context of developing blood cells.

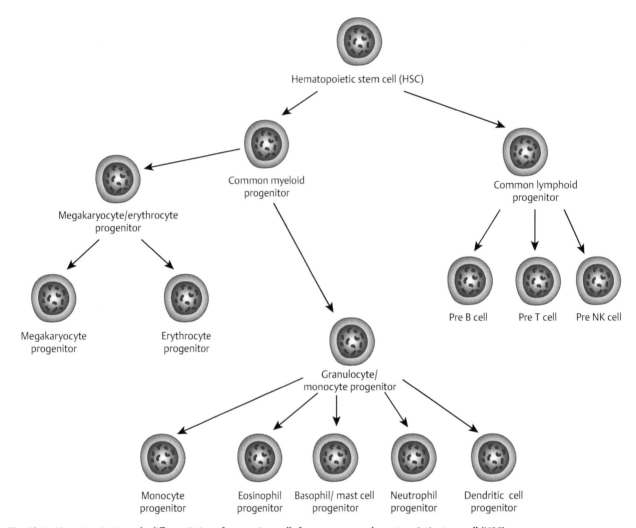

Fig. 18.1   **Hematopoiesis: early differentiation of progenitor cells from a common hematopoietic stem cell (HSC).**

18.3.1   Azurophilic (Primary, Nonspecific) Granules

Azurophilic (**primary**, or **nonspecific**) **granules** are purple and readily recognized because of their small size. The larger cell in **Fig. 18.3** has many azurophilic granules; two are indicated at the arrows. The smaller nucleated cell has fewer of these granules.

As will be discussed in an upcoming chapter, the azurophilic granules are described as nonspecific because their appearance during granulocyte maturation is no help in distinguishing among precursors of the neutrophil, eosinophil, and basophil lineages. The other three granules (eosinophilic, basophilic, neutrophilic) are called specific because their appearance allows one to place the cell definitively in a specific granulocyte lineage. Azurophilic granules are also called primary granules because they appear earlier in development than the specific granules.

18.3.2   Eosinophilic Granules

Eosinophilic granules are very large, red-pink, and have a glassy appearance. The large cell to the right in **Fig. 18.4** is chock-full of these granules (arrows). For comparison, the large cell to the left is loaded with azurophilic granules, which are smaller and purple.

18.3.3   Basophilic Granules

Basophilic granules are large and blue, almost black. The large cell in the center of **Fig. 18.5** is full of these granules (arrows). Compare to the nucleated cell near the top, which is filled with smaller azurophilic granules.

18.3.4   Neutrophilic Granules

Neutrophilic granules are too small (0.1–0.2 μm) to be seen as individual structures with the light microscope. Their presence in neutrophilic granulocytes is signified by a salmon-colored appearance of the cytoplasm. As Cell A in **Fig. 18.6**, a granulocyte precursor with a basophilic cytoplasm and many azurophilic granules, matures to stage B, then C, then D, synthesis of neutrophilic granules renders the cytoplasm pink.

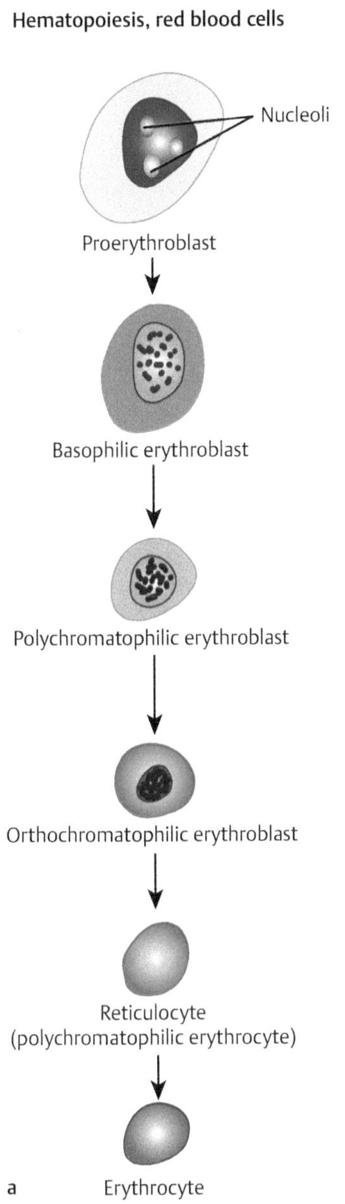

Hematopoiesis, red blood cells

Nucleoli

Proerythroblast

Basophilic erythroblast

Polychromatophilic erythroblast

Orthochromatophilic erythroblast

Reticulocyte
(polychromatophilic erythrocyte)

a   Erythrocyte

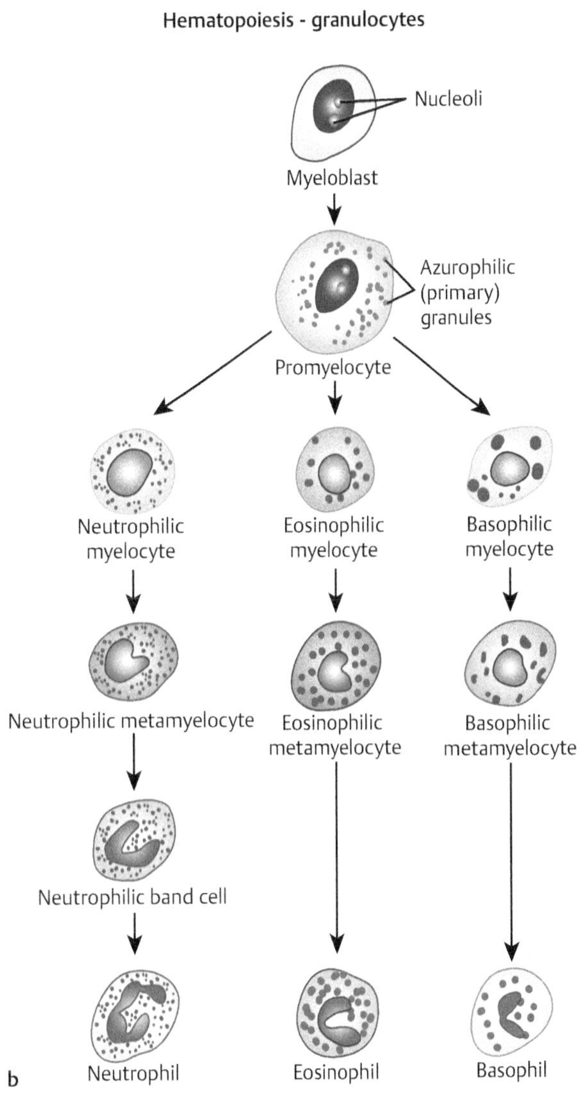

Hematopoiesis - granulocytes

Nucleoli

Myeloblast

Azurophilic
(primary)
granules

Promyelocyte

Neutrophilic
myelocyte

Eosinophilic
myelocyte

Basophilic
myelocyte

Neutrophilic metamyelocyte

Eosinophilic
metamyelocyte

Basophilic
metamyelocyte

Neutrophilic band cell

b   Neutrophil

Eosinophil

Basophil

Fig. 18.2 Hematopoiesis: differentiation of identifiable stages of blood cell development of (a) red blood cells and (b) granulocytes.

Video 18.1 Azurophilic (nonspecific) granules

https://www.thieme.de/de/q.htm?p=opn/
tp/308390101/978-1-62623-414-7_c018_
v001&t=video

Video 18.2 Eosinphilic granules

https://www.thieme.de/de/q.htm?p=opn/
tp/308390101/978-1-62623-414-7_c018_
v002&t=video

Video 18.3 Basophilic granules

https://www.thieme.de/de/q.htm?p=opn/
tp/308390101/978-1-62623-414-7_c018_
v003&t=video

Video 18.4 Neutrophilic granules
Be able to identify:
— Azurophilic (nonspecific, primary) granules
— Specific granules
  • Eosinophilic granules
  • Basophilic granules
  • Neutrophilic granules (recognize the presence of these)

https://www.thieme.de/de/q.htm?p=opn/tp/308390101/978-1-
62623-414-7_c018_v004&t=video

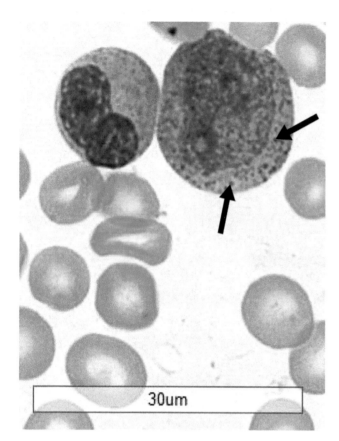

Fig. 18.3   Azurophilic granules (arrows).

18.4   Nucleoli

Cells in the earliest recognizable stages of blood cell development have **nucleoli**. With hematologic stains, these nucleoli appear as pale spots against a darker nuclear background; one to three nucleoli per nucleus may be apparent.

> **Helpful Hint**
>
> Note that with routine H & E stains, nucleoli were seen as dark densities within a pale, euchromatic nucleus. The opposite is true with hematologic stains.

   Nucleoli are very subtle structures to identify, so it is useful to begin with an obvious example. The cell in **Fig. 18.7** has no cytoplasm; only the large nucleus remains. Three nucleoli are readily seen (between pairs of red arrows). Note that these nucleoli are oval, pale (but not white), and often accented by condensed chromatin immediately surrounding them.

   Fig. 18.8 shows four more cells, each with at least one nucleolus (between red arrows); some of these are more subtle than those in **Fig. 18.7**.

Video 18.5   Nucleoli

Be able to identify:
— Nucleoli

https://www.thieme.de/de/q.htm?p=opn/
tp/308390101/978-1-62623-414-7_c018_v005&t=video

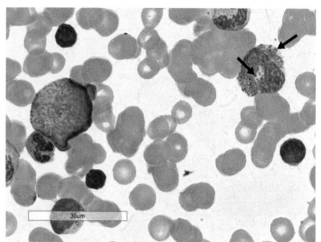

Fig. 18.4   Eosinophilic granules (arrows).

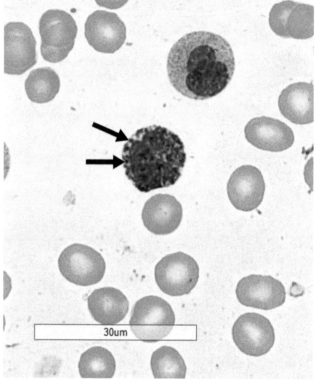

Fig. 18.5   Basophilic granules (arrows).

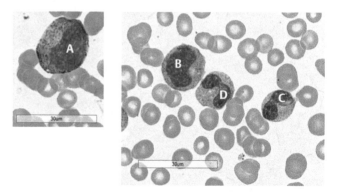

Fig. 18.6   Neutrophilic granules, recognized by a change in the cytoplasmic color to pink as the cell matures from A to B to C to D.

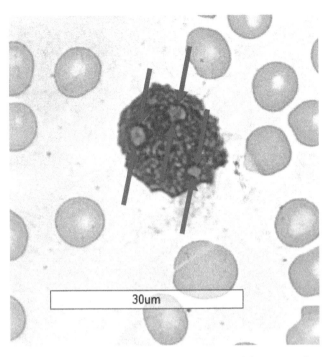

Fig. 18.7 **Nucleus (without cytoplasm) with nucleoli between red arrows.**

18.5 Nuclear Shape

In the early stages of all lineages of developing blood cells that can be identified, nuclei tend to be large and round. **Fig. 18.9** shows two early stages of developing blood cells; the nuclear envelope is indicated by the tips of the red arrows.

> **Helpful Hint**
>
> Some irregularities may be observed in nuclear shape, caused by impinging adjacent cells or tissue preparation.

All recognizable cells in the RBC lineage maintain a round-shaped nucleus during maturation, though the nuclei become significantly smaller. For example, in **Fig. 18.10**, the cell marked A is the earliest RBC precursor, and the cell marked C is the latest nucleated RBC precursor. B shows two intermediates adjacent to each other.

As shown in **Fig. 18.11**, cells of the granulocyte lineages are quite different. During maturation, the early, nearly round nucleus (A) undergoes shape changes that include indentations, forming a kidney bean shape (B), and then segmentation to a band (horseshoe-shaped) form (C), ultimately leading to a fully segmented mature nucleus (D). This is easiest to see in neutrophils because nuclei are readily visible.

In eosinophils and basophils, nuclei are less prominently segmented. In addition, the cytoplasmic granules often make it difficult to distinguish the exact shape of the nucleus. Nevertheless, these maturing forms do demonstrate nuclear indentation, as in the eosinophil in **Fig. 18.12** (black arrow), and nearly complete segmentation, as demonstrated by the basophil (green arrow). Compare to the fully segmented nucleus in the neutrophil (blue arrow).

Video 18.6 Nuclear shape

Be able to identify:
— Changes in nuclear shape
  • Round
  • Indented
  • Kidney bean
  • Band

https://www.thieme.de/de/q.htm?p=opn/tp/308390101/978-1-62623-414-7_c018_v006&t=video

18.6 Chromatin

The chromatin content of the nucleus is described as either fine (threadlike) or clumped. In the early stages of blood cell development shown in **Fig. 18.13** (when nucleoli are visible), the chromatin in the remainder of the nucleus is fine (cells at arrows).

> **Helpful Hint**
>
> In the marked cell in **Fig. 18.13b**, a few azurophilic granules overlie the nucleus, which gives a more clumped appearance than the cell on the left. These must be mentally subtracted in assessing the chromatin pattern.

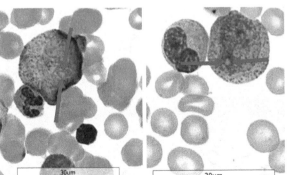
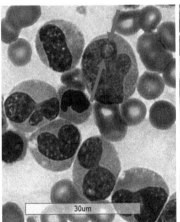
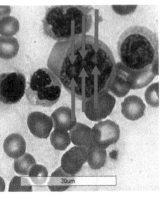
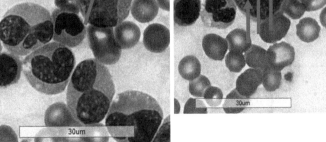

Fig. 18.8 **Nucleoli (between red arrows) in these cells are more subtle to find than those in Fig. 18.7. Note that not all possible nucleoli are indicated.**

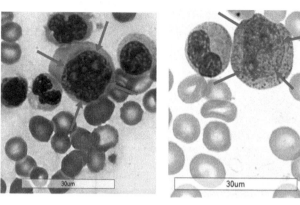

Fig. 18.9   Nuclei in early identifiable blood cell precursors (red arrows indicate the outer edge of the nuclei).

As blood cells mature, chromatin often becomes clumped. A good example of this is shown in the two basophilic erythroblasts marked by the red arrow in **Fig. 18.14**. The clumping of the chromatin in these nuclei results in a distinctive dark, ropy pattern (solid black arrows) that leaves some areas white (dashed black arrows). An earlier stage of erythroblast is shown in **Fig. 18.13a** for comparison. A similar dark and ropy staining pattern due to condensation of chromatin is visible in the nuclei of developing granulocytes (**Fig. 18.14**, blue arrows). An extreme kind of condensation called **pyknosis** is seen in late-stage erythroblasts (**Fig. 18.14**, green arrow), in which the chromatin condenses completely and the nucleus is reduced in size.

Video 18.7   Chromatin

Be able to identify:
— Fibrillar (fine) chromatin
— Clumpy chromatin

https://www.thieme.de/de/q.htm?p=opn/tp/308390101/978-1-62623-414-7_c018_v007&t=video

Helpful Hint

It is often useful to compare spaces in clumpy chromatin patterns with nucleoli. The spaces in clumpy chromatin patterns are almost white and are small and irregular in shape (**Fig. 18.14**). Contrast this with nucleoli (**Fig. 18.8**), which are larger, pale but not white, and oval.

18.7   Degree of Cytoplasmic Basophilia

Generally speaking, immature cells have a basophilic cytoplasm due to large amounts of ribosomal RNA (rRNA). In the case of erythroblasts preparing to make hemoglobin, this is in the form of free ribosomes. In granulocytes, the basophilia is due to rough ER necessary to synthesize granules. The early-stage cells in **Fig. 18.15** (black arrows) demonstrate intense cytoplasmic basophilia.

In general, as cells mature, there is a gradual decrease in the rRNA content and a concomitant increase of protein or organelles that render the cytoplasm less basophilic and more eosinophilic.

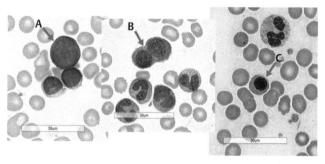

Fig. 18.10   Nuclei in maturing red blood cells.

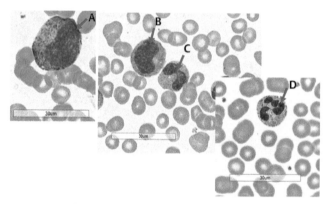

Fig. 18.11   Nuclei in maturing granulocytes (neutrophils).

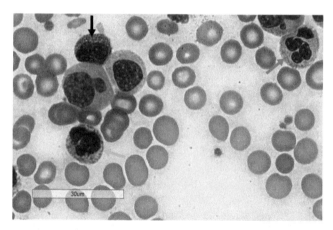

Fig. 18.12   Nuclei in maturing granulocytes: eosinophil (black arrow); basophil (green arrow); neutrophil (blue arrow).

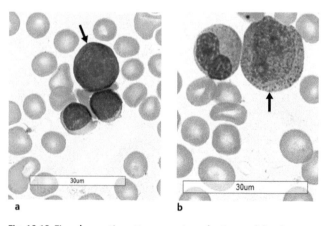

Fig. 18.13   Fine chromatin pattern seen in early stages of development of (a) RBCs and (b) white blood cells.

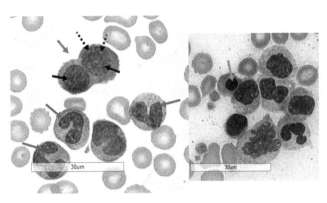

Fig. 18.14 Chromatin pattern as developing blood cells mature. The two cells indicated by the red arrow demonstrate good examples of clumps (black arrows) and white areas (dashed black arrows). Granulocytes also display this clumpy chromatin pattern (blue arrows). Extreme chromatin condensation, called pyknosis, is seen in late-stage erythroblasts (green arrow).

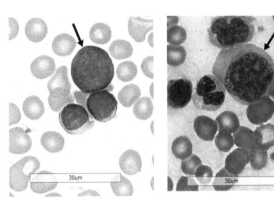

Fig. 18.15 Cytoplasmic basophilia seen in early stages of blood cell development.

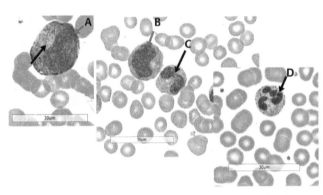

Fig. 18.16 Cytoplasmic changes in maturing granulocytes A to D (neutrophils). Black arrow in cell A indicates early cytoplasmic change in the Golgi region.

In neutrophil development (**Fig. 18.16**), the cytoplasm gets pinker due to accumulation of neutrophil granules. Cell A is an early stage of development and has a roughly evenly blue cytoplasm. However, this cell has begun to synthesize granules, which initially accumulate in the region of the Golgi, resulting in a prominent patch of pink (black arrow) in the formerly exclusively blue cytoplasm. Gradually, the cytoplasm changes from blue to pink (cells B through D) as the cell matures.

In the developing RBC lineage, the rRNA and hemoglobin are cytosolic. Therefore, as shown in **Fig. 18.17**, the mix of pink/blue color possibilities is greater than in developing neutrophils. The erythrocyte precursor cytoplasm is pure blue (red arrow) at early stages; as the cells mature (green arrow), eosinophilic hemoglobin is added, resulting in a dull purple or gray color. As the rRNA is lost in more mature cells, the cytoplasm becomes progressively pinker (blue arrows).

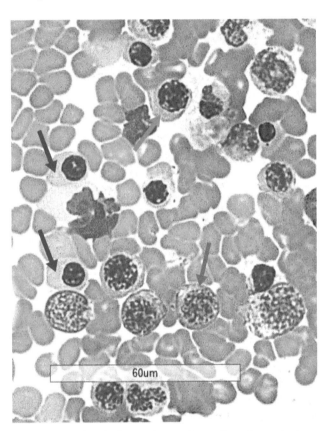

Fig. 18.17 Cytoplasmic changes in maturing erythrocytes: early stage (red arrow), middle stage (green arrow), late stage (blue arrows).

Video 18.8   Cytoplasm color change in neutrophil series

https://www.thieme.de/de/q.htm?p=opn/tp/308390101/978-1-62623-414-7_c018_v008&t=video

Video 18.9   Cytoplasm color change in erythrocyte series—part 1

https://www.thieme.de/de/q.htm?p=opn/tp/308390101/978-1-62623-414-7_c018_v009&t=video

Video 18.10 Cytoplasm color change in erythrocyte series—part 2
Be able to identify:
— Maturity of cell based on cytoplasmic basophilia/eosinophilia

https://www.thieme.de/de/q.htm?p=opn/tp/308390101/978-1-62623-414-7_c018_v010&t=video

18.8   Chapter Review

Because blood cells have a short lifespan, the bone marrow must continually generate new blood cells. This process, termed hematopoiesis or hemopoiesis, is driven by a self-replicating hematopoietic stem cell that is a common precursor for all blood cells. This cell, and its early progeny, have the histologic appearance of lymphocytes, so they are not identified routinely. Later stages take on specific characteristics that place these cells in identifiable stages. These characteristics include cytoplasmic granules (azurophilic, eosinophilic, basophilic, neutrophilic), the presence or absence of nucleoli, nuclear shape, chromatin pattern (fine or clumped), and cytoplasmic staining (basophilic or eosinophilic). Recognition of these cellular features makes it possible to identify specific developmental stages in blood cell maturation, which will be discussed in upcoming chapters.

Questions and Answers

An online-only section of questions and answers accompanying this chapter is hosted on Thieme's MedOne Education site: https://medone-education.thieme.com. Use the code on the media page at the front of this book to gain access. An institutional license to the site is required to access these questions in an interactive format, and individual users are required to register for an individual account to track results.

19 Hematopoiesis: White Blood Cells and Platelets

After completing this chapter, you should be able to:
— Identify, at the light microscope level, each of the following:
- Stages of granulocyte development
  ○ Myeloblast
  ○ Promyelocyte
  ○ Myelocyte
    ▪ Neutrophilic myelocyte
    ▪ Eosinophilic myelocyte
    ▪ Basophilic myelocyte
  ○ Metamyelocyte
    ▪ Neutrophilic metamyelocyte
    ▪ Eosinophilic metamyelocyte
    ▪ Basophilic metamyelocyte
  ○ Band
    ▪ Neutrophilic band cell
  ○ Mature cells (neutrophil, eosinophil, basophil)
- Megakaryocyte
— Evaluate the significance of the appearance of white blood cell precursors in peripheral blood

19.1 Overview of White Blood Cell Development

As mentioned in the previous chapter, all blood cells are derived from a common **hematopoietic stem cell** (**Fig. 19.1**). This cell differentiates into precursors for each of the mature cell types. All of these early precursors are similar histologically. However, during the later stages of hematopoiesis, these cells transition through histologically identifiable stages. This is especially true for the **granulocytes**, which will be the main focus of this chapter. **Megakaryocytes**, the precursors that generate **platelets**, will also be presented. The next chapter will focus on the stages of red blood cell development.

Monocytes, lymphocytes, and dendritic cells also go through developmental stages as they mature. These stages do not have clear histologically identifiable features, so they will be mentioned only briefly in the chapters discussing lymphatic tissues and organs.

> **Helpful Hint**
>
> A full understanding of the cells discussed in the next two chapters requires the ability to recognize the cellular features discussed in the previous chapter: cytoplasmic granules, nucleoli, nuclear shape, chromatin pattern, and cytoplasmic basophilia. If some uncertainty exists in recognizing these features, it is best to review them before proceeding.

19.2 Hematopoiesis of Granulocytes

The identifiable stages of granulocyte development are shown in **Fig. 19.2**. The granulocyte series consists of maturation of cells from a common granulocyte precursor, similar in appearance to a lymphocyte, to one with features of a cell actively synthesizing proteins and producing secretory granules. These features, which are evident in the early stages of **Fig. 19.2** (myeloblast, promyelocyte) include a large cell, a large round nucleus with nucleoli and fine chromatin, and a basophilic cytoplasm due to abundant rough endoplasmic reticulum (RER).

The products of granulocyte maturation are mature cells that have granules and other products that are used in the immune response. Therefore, as these cells mature, they transition from cells that are actively synthesizing these products to cells that have accumulated these products but are synthetically less active. These changes can be evident in both the nucleus and the cytoplasm. The nucleus takes on the appearance of a less active cell; it loses its nucleoli, the chromatin becomes clumped, and the nucleus becomes smaller and segmented. In the cytoplasm, as granules accumulate, the cytoplasm becomes less basophilic due to the loss of RER because mature cells no longer need to produce granules.

> **Helpful Hint**
>
> Understanding this principle will help mentally organize the stages of granulocyte production, which will aid in learning. If this concept is unclear, it may help to reread it before proceeding.

19.2.1 Myeloblast and Promyelocyte

In the granulocyte series, the first two recognizable stages, the **myeloblast** and **promyelocyte**, are large cells with a basophilic cytoplasm and a large, round nucleus with a fine chromatin pattern and nucleoli (see **Fig. 19.2**). They can be distinguished from each other because the promyelocyte has **nonspecific (azurophilic, primary) granules**, while the myeloblast does not.

At these early stages, it cannot be determined in routine smears whether the myeloblast or promyelocyte is committed to the neutrophilic, eosinophilic, or basophilic cell lineage. (This can be determined with cell type–specific markers, but that is beyond the scope of this textbook.)

> **Helpful Hint**
>
> Because routine hematologic staining of hematopoietic cells does not distinguish a myeloblast or promyelocyte as a neutrophil or eosinophil or basophil, it is not advisable to identify a cell as a "basophilic myeloblast" or a "neutrophilic promyelocyte." "Myeloblast" and "promyelocyte" are sufficient terms at this stage.

Fig. 19.3 shows a myeloblast (arrow). Features of a myeloblast include:
- Large cell
- Large round nucleus

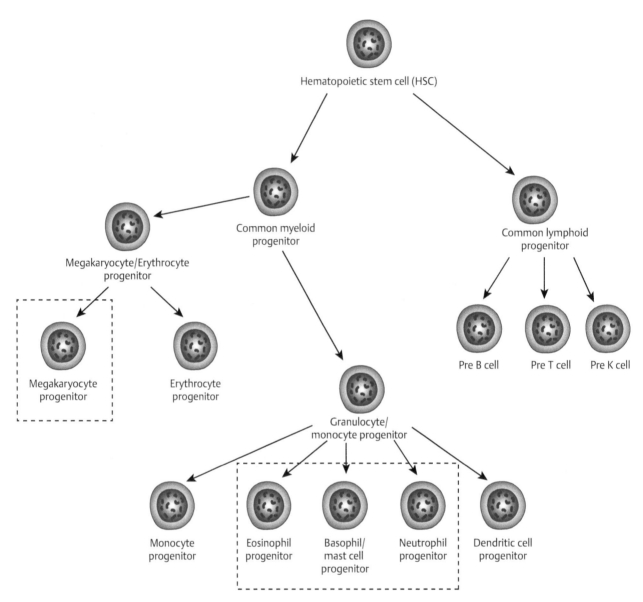

Fig. 19.1 **Hematopoiesis: early differentiation of progenitor cells from a common hematopoietic stem cell (HSC). Boxed cells are progenitors of granulocytes and platelets, cell types covered in this chapter.**

- Nucleoli (at least one; this cell has at least three)
- Fine chromatin pattern
- Basophilic cytoplasm
- Absence of granules

Fig. 19.4 shows a promyelocyte (arrow). Features of a promyelocyte include:
- Large cell
- Large round nucleus
- Nucleoli (at least one, this cell has two to three)
- Fine chromatin pattern

- Basophilic cytoplasm
- *Azurophilic granules*
- *More often than not, larger than a myeloblast*

In the description of the promyelocyte, the features that have changed from the previous stage (myeloblast) are in italics. This will be done for the remaining stages.

Note that the promyelocyte in **Fig. 19.4** has many azurophilic granules in the cytoplasm "over" the nucleus; this obscures the fine chromatin pattern characteristic of a cell at this early stage.

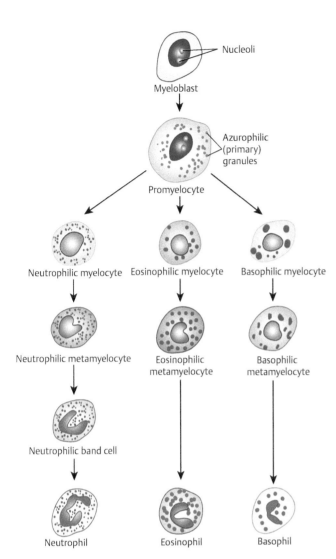

Fig. 19.2 **Hematopoiesis: differentiation of identifiable stages of granulocyte development.**

Video 19.1 Myeloblasts and promyelocytes

Be able to identify:
— Myeloblast
— Promyelocyte
https://www.thieme.de/de/q.htm?p=opn/
tp/308390101/978-1-62623-414-7_c019_v001&t=video

Helpful Hint

Remember that developing cells belong to a continuum. Therefore, many cells have features consistent with two stages, and some cells do not appear to belong to any stage at all. This is not unusual, particularly in slides prepared of peripheral blood from patients with leukemia.

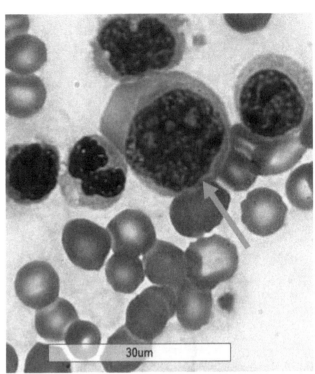

Fig. 19.3 **Myeloblast.**

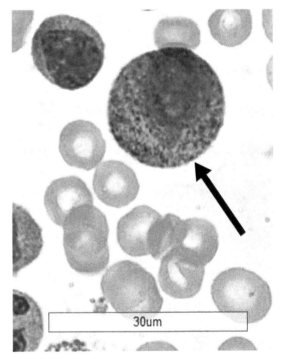

Fig. 19.4 **Promyelocyte.**

Leukemia is a cancer of white blood cells that causes increased numbers of abnormal developing white blood cells in the bone marrow and bloodstream. Note that the presence of increased white blood cells in the bone marrow may compromise production of red blood cells and platelets, so patients with leukemia often have associated **anemia** or bleeding disorders. There are many types of leukemia. One type, called **acute promyelocytic leukemia**, results in an increase in the number of promyelocytes. These cells have abnormal azurophilic granules, often in the form of elongated structures called **Auer rods**, which enable fairly rapid diagnosis.

19.2.2 Myelocyte

The next cells in the granulocyte series, the **myelocytes**, lose their nucleoli and accumulate specific granules (see **Fig. 19.2**). **Fig. 19.5** shows an **eosinophilic myelocyte** (EM) and a **neutrophilic myelocyte** (NM). Features of myelocytes include:

- *Medium-sized cell*
- *Medium-sized round nucleus*
- *No nucleoli*
- *Clumped chromatin pattern*
- *(Mostly) basophilic cytoplasm*
- *Azurophilic granules*
- *Specific granules*

Note that there are many changes at this stage.

The neutrophilic myelocyte in **Fig. 19.5** is not a perfect example, since the cytoplasm is more basophilic than pink, suggesting that production of specific (neutrophilic) granules has just begun. However, the nucleus is smaller with clumpy chromatin and no nucleoli, so it is definitely a myelocyte. **Fig. 19.6** shows another neutrophilic myelocyte (NM) in which the cytoplasm is more convincingly pink, but the nucleus is less round.

   Basophilic myelocytes are very challenging to find. **Figure 19.7** shows a basophilic myelocyte (BM) with a nucleus that is roundish, though quite lumpy because it is beginning to become segmented.

Video 19.2   Myelocytes

Be able to identify:
- Myelocyte
  - Neutrophilic myelocyte
  - Eosinophilic myelocyte
  - Basophilic myelocyte

https://www.thieme.de/de/q.htm?p=opn/tp/308390101/978-1-62623-414-7_c019_v002&t=video

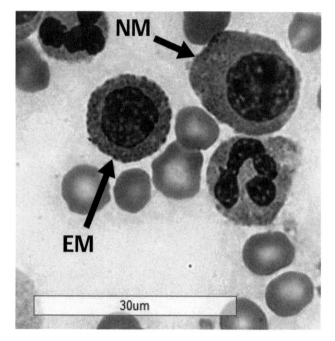

Fig. 19.5   Eosinophilic myelocyte (EM) and neutrophilic myelocyte (NM).

As mentioned, the myeloblast and promyelocyte cannot be placed into a specific granulocyte lineage with routine hematologic stains. Myelocytes (and later stages), on the other hand, contain specific granules, so proper identification includes the type of granulocyte (e.g., *basophilic* myelocyte).

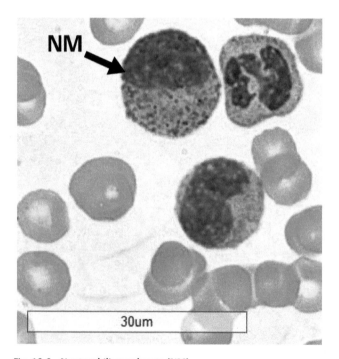

Fig. 19.6   Neutrophilic myelocyte (NM).

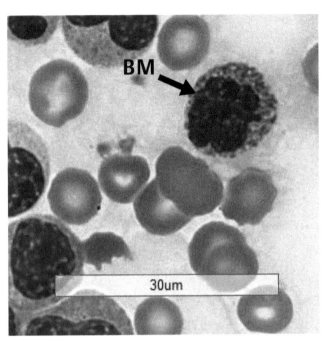

Fig. 19.7   **Basophilic myelocyte (BM).**

19.2.3   Metamyelocytes, Band Cells, Mature Cells

In the final sequence of granulocyte development, the nucleus changes shape. The myelocyte (see **Fig. 19.5**, **Fig. 19.6**, and **Fig. 19.7**) has a round nucleus, which becomes indented to form the **metamyelocyte** (**Fig. 19.8**, black arrow). At the **band cell** (or **stab cell**) stage, the nucleus is horseshoe-shaped (**Fig. 19.8**, green arrow). Finally, the nucleus becomes segmented to form the mature neutrophil (**Fig. 19.8**, blue arrow).

Nuclear shape changes are accompanied by other "minor" changes, such as a general decrease in the overall size of the

cell and nucleus, an even clumpier chromatin pattern, and an increase in specific granules. The most recognizable feature that differentiates these stages, however, is nuclear shape.

The eosinophil and basophil series of cells also undergo similar maturation of their nuclei. These cells are not as common, however, and their large granules usually obstruct the nucleus. Therefore, the neutrophil series provides a much better model of these stages.

Video 19.3   Later neutrophil stages

Be able to identify:
— For neutrophils:
   • Myelocyte
   • Metamyelocyte
   • Band
   • Mature

https://www.thieme.de/de/q.htm?p=opn/tp/308390101/978-1-62623-414-7_c019_v003&t=video

Video 19.4   Later eosinophil stages

Be able to identify:
— For eosinophils and basophils:
   • Myelocyte
   • Metamyelocyte
   • Mature

https://www.thieme.de/de/q.htm?p=opn/tp/308390101/978-1-62623-414-7_c019_v004&t=video

As a final note, it should be emphasized one more time that all cell development is a continuum, and the stages described here are a way to organize the content, similar to stages of mitosis. Many cells will be between stages. For example, in **Fig. 19.9**, the large cell is best identified as a promyelocyte with large cell, large round nucleus, fine chromatin, at least one very clear

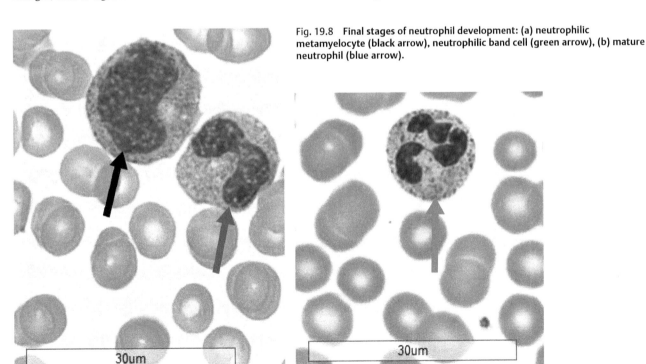
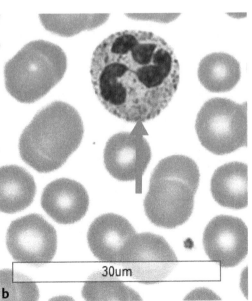

Fig. 19.8   **Final stages of neutrophil development: (a) neutrophilic metamyelocyte (black arrow), neutrophilic band cell (green arrow), (b) mature neutrophil (blue arrow).**

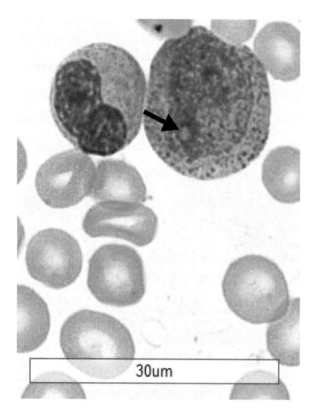

Fig. 19.9 **Promyelocyte that has some features consistent with the myelocyte stage. Arrow indicates a nucleolus.**

nucleolus (black arrow), and azurophilic granules. If you look closely, however, you will see cytoplasmic eosinophilia, particularly near the bottom of the cell. This is due to the production of neutrophilic specific granules, which is a feature of the myelocyte stage and not the promyelocyte. This occurrence is referred to as "nuclear-cytoplasmic mismatch"—a feature often seen in leukemias.

19.3   Megakaryocytes

Cells that produce platelets progress through developmental stages that include a **megakaryocyte progenitor cell** (see **Fig. 19.1**), which gives rise to the **megakaryoblast** and **megakaryocyte** (not shown in **Fig. 19.1**). During maturation,

megakaryoblasts duplicate their genome several times (i.e., $2N \rightarrow 4N \rightarrow 8N \rightarrow 16N \rightarrow 32N \rightarrow 64N \rightarrow \cdots$) without nuclear division. This process produces a large, often multilobed nucleus. In addition, the cell expands its basophilic cytoplasm, which will be "shed" to produce platelets. The resulting megakaryocytes are large cells, with extensive eosinophilic cytoplasm, often foamy, with granules and a multilobed nucleus.

Fig. 19.10 is an image from a bone marrow smear that shows a single, really large megakaryocyte (outlined, compare to neighboring red blood cells and developing white blood cells), with clear lobulation of the nucleus. The cytoplasm shows some remaining basophilia, but eosinophilic regions are visible as well. (The eosinophilic disk that appears to be in the center of the cell is actually a red blood cell lying either on top of or below the megakaryocyte.)

Fig. 19.11 is an image taken from a red bone marrow section, so the cells are more closely packed than they are in a bone marrow smear. The numerous nuclei observed throughout the slide represent different stages of blood cell development, but staging is not routinely accomplished in such material because the magnification is insufficient and because the features of each cell are obscured by both the superimposition of cells in the thickness of a routine section and the proximity of cells to one another. Despite this, in this figure three megakaryocytes are easily identified (outlined): really large cells with multilobed nuclei and eosinophilic cytoplasm.

Once the megakaryocyte is formed, it resides in the marrow next to the **sinuses** (capillaries in the marrow), where it "sheds" portions of its cytoplasm and plasma membrane into the bloodstream. These released cell fragments of the megakaryocyte

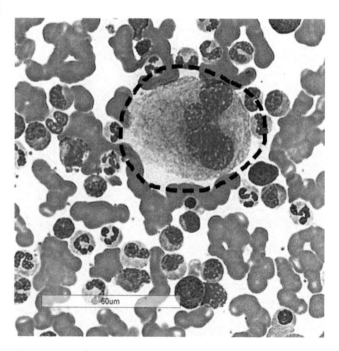

Fig. 19.10 **Megakaryocyte in a bone marrow smear (outlined).**

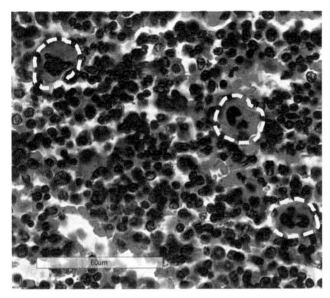

Fig. 19.11 **Megakaryocytes in tissue section of bone marrow (outlined).**

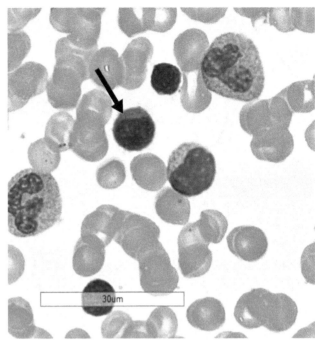

Fig. 19.12 **Lymphocyte in bone marrow smear (arrow).**

are the mature platelets. A single megakaryocyte will produce thousands of platelets. The remaining nucleus is then recycled.

Video 19.5 Megakaryocyte in bone marrow smear

https://www.thieme.de/de/q.htm?p=opn/ tp/308390101/978-1-62623-414-7_c019_ v005&t=video

Video 19.6 Megakaryocyte in bone marrow tissue

Be able to identify:
— Megakaryocyte

https://www.thieme.de/de/q.htm?p=opn/ tp/308390101/978-1-62623-414-7_c019_v006&t=video

19.4 Lymphocytes and Plasma Cells

Occasionally, lymphocytes (**Fig. 19.12**, arrow), plasma cells, and mature granulocytes are seen in bone marrow. These cells have the same features previously described in the chapter on blood.

19.5 Chapter Review

Hematopoiesis consists of the process of development of mature blood cells (and cell fragments) from a common hematopoietic stem cell. Later stages of granulocyte maturation include cells with characteristics that can be visualized by routine hematologic staining (Wright stain). The first identifiable stage, the myeloblast, is a large cell with multiple nucleoli, fine chromatin, and basophilic cytoplasm that lacks granules. This cell enlarges and begins to generate azurophilic (nonspecific) granules, becoming a promyelocyte. From here, the cell begins to produce specific granules (neutrophilic, eosinophilic, basophilic). The production of specific granules occurs at the same time that nucleoli cease to be visible and the chromatin appears clumpy. The loss of nucleoli and appearance of specific granules mark the progression of the cell into the myelocyte stage. Continued maturation of these cells largely features changes in nuclear shape, from round (myelocyte) to indented (metamyelocyte) to horseshoe (band or stab) and, finally, to segmented (mature cell). Megakaryocytes generate platelets and are recognized in bone marrow as very large cells with a large, multilobed nucleus and abundant cytoplasm.

Questions and Answers

An online-only section of questions and answers accompanying this chapter is hosted on Thieme's MedOne Education site: https://medone-education.thieme.com. Use the code on the media page at the front of this book to gain access. An institutional license to the site is required to access these questions in an interactive format, and individual users are required to register for an individual account to track results.

20 Hematopoiesis: Red Blood Cells

After completing this chapter, you should be able to:
— Identify, at the light microscope level, each of the following stages in erythroid development:
  • Proerythroblast
  • Basophilic erythroblast
  • Polychromatophilic erythroblast
  • Orthochromatophilic erythroblast
  • Reticulocyte
  • Mature red blood cell
— Outline the rationale for the appearance of each of the red blood cell precursors listed
— Predict the effects of high altitude on reticulocyte and red blood cell counts in peripheral blood

20.1   Erythrocyte versus Granulocyte Development

The previous chapter focused on granulocyte and platelet development. This chapter will focus on the development of **red blood cells** (**RBCs**), also known as **erythrocytes** (**Fig. 20.1a–f**).

A key difference between development of RBCs and that of granulocytes is that RBCs lack cytoplasmic granules. However, the main concept that early precursors are "producers" that develop into a final product that contains functional proteins is consistent with granulocytes. The final cell, the erythrocyte, is filled with hemoglobin, a soluble cytosolic protein. In order to produce a cell filled with hemoglobin, early RBC precursors contain numerous free ribosomes and, therefore, will have intense cytoplasmic basophilia. As the cells mature, hemoglobin is produced, with a concomitant reduction in the number of ribosomes; therefore, maturing red blood cells will gradually become less basophilic and more eosinophilic.

Mature RBCs (erythrocytes) lack a nucleus. During the final stages of RBC development, the nucleus gradually condenses until it is fully compact. The nucleus is then ejected from the nearly mature cell. The resulting cell, which contains hemoglobin and a few ribosomes, is the reticulocyte that is released into the bloodstream. This eventually loses its ribosomes to become the mature erythrocyte.

20.2   Proerythroblasts

The first recognizable cell in the red blood cell series, the **proerythroblast** (**Fig. 20.2**, arrow; see also **Fig. 20.1a**), has all the features of a cell synthesizing large amounts of proteins, including an active nucleus and intense cytoplasmic basophilia due to numerous free (cytosolic) ribosomes.

Characteristics of a proerythroblast include:
• Large cell
• Large round nucleus
• Nucleoli (at least one)
• Fine chromatin pattern
• Basophilic cytoplasm
• Absence of granules

The proerythroblast (**Fig. 20.2**) and the myeloblast from the granulocyte series (Chapter 19; **Fig. 20.3**) have very similar features. The difference is very subtle; the typical proerythroblast has more intense cytoplasmic basophilia than a myeloblast does. However, in many cases it is difficult to distinguish the two with certainty on routine staining.

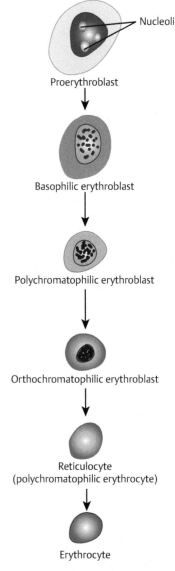

Fig. 20.1   **Erythrocyte hematopoiesis.**

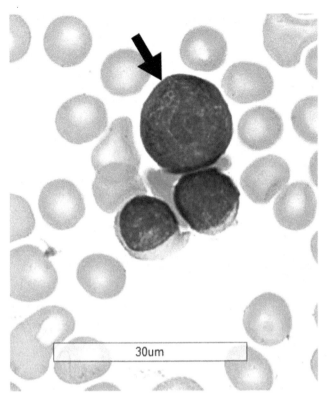

Fig. 20.2 **Proerythroblast.**

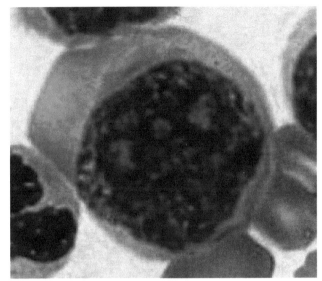

Fig. 20.3 **Myeloblast.**

20.3 Basophilic Erythroblasts

Basophilic erythroblasts (**Fig. 20.4**) are similar to proerythroblasts, except that the nucleus has changed to a clumpy pattern of chromatin without nucleoli. This signifies that the cell has shut down ribosome production (which happens in the nucleoli) but still has plenty of ribosomes in the cytoplasm to maintain cytoplasmic basophilia.

Characteristics of a basophilic erythroblast include (changes from the preceding cell type are shown in italic type):

- Large cell
- Large round nucleus
- *Absence of nucleoli*
- *Clumpy chromatin pattern*
- Basophilic cytoplasm
- Absence of granules

Helpful Hint

The pattern of dark and light regions of the nucleus are sometimes referred to by histologists as a "checkerboard" appearance.

Video 20.1 Proerythroblasts and basophilic erythroblasts

Be able to identify:
— Proerythroblast
— Basophilic erythroblast

https://www.thieme.de/de/q.htm?p=opn/tp/308390101/978-1-62623-414-7_c020_v001&t=video

20.4 Polychromatophilic and Orthochromatophilic Erythroblasts

The basophilic erythroblast has abundant ribosomes but has yet to synthesize hemoglobin. In the next sequence of events, the cell begins to synthesize hemoglobin, with a concomitant loss of ribosomes (**Fig. 20.1b–d**). The mixture of hemoglobin (eosinophilia) and ribosomes (basophilia) in the cytoplasm produces a purple/gray color, which gives way to increasing eosinophilia as hemoglobin concentration increases and ribosomes are degraded. In addition, the nucleus becomes less active and continues to condense.

Characteristics of a **polychromatophilic erythroblast** (**Fig. 20.5**) include:

- *Smaller cell*
- *Smaller nucleus*
- Absence of nucleoli

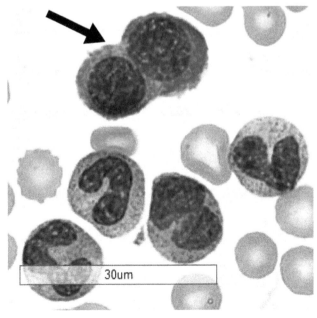

Fig. 20.4 **Basophilic erythroblasts.**

- *More clumpy chromatin pattern*
- *Basophilic and eosinophilic cytoplasm*
- Absence of granules

Characteristics of an **orthochromatophilic erythroblast** include (**Fig. 20.6**):
- *Small cell*
- *Small nucleus*
- Absence of nucleoli
- *Mostly clumpy chromatin pattern*
- *Mostly eosinophilic cytoplasm*
- Absence of granules

Helpful Hint

Again, note the general trends here as the cell matures from the basophilic erythroblast to the orthochromatophilic erythroblast: cell gets smaller, nucleus gets smaller, chromatin condenses with more clumps and less spaces, cytoplasm turns from blue to pink.

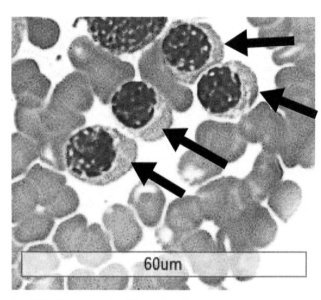

Fig. 20.5   **Polychromatophilic erythroblasts.**

Video 20.2   Basophilic erythroblast → polychromatophilic erythroblast → orthochromatophilic erythroblast

Be able to identify:
— Basophilic erythroblast
— Orthochromatophilic erythroblast
— Polychromatophilic erythroblast
https://www.thieme.de/de/q.htm?p=opn/tp/308390101/978-1-62623-414-7_c020_v002&t=video

Helpful Hint

Another look-alike to distinguish is between maturing red blood cells (**Figs. 20.4**, **Fig. 20.5**, and **Fig. 20.6**, black arrows) and lymphocytes (**Fig. 20.7**, green arrow). Recall that a lymphocyte has a small condensed nucleus, with a thin rim of blue cytoplasm. The cell in the RBC series that has a blue cytoplasm similar to the lymphocyte is the basophilic erythroblast (**Fig. 20.4**). These cells can be distinguished because the basophilic erythroblast is larger, with a larger nucleus and a chromatin pattern that is clumpy but has clear areas within the nucleus. As an RBC matures, the nucleus condenses to appear more like that in the lymphocyte. However, by the time the nucleus of the RBC condenses enough to look like the nucleus of the lymphocyte, the cell has already begun to synthesize hemoglobin, so its cytoplasm has enough eosinophilia to distinguish it from the basophilic cytoplasm of the lymphocyte.

20.5   Reticulocyte

After the maturing RBC loses its nucleus, it is called a **polychromatophilic erythrocyte**, or **reticulocyte**, and is released into the

circulation (**Fig. 20.1e**, **Fig. 20.8**, arrows). The reticulocyte still has a small number of ribosomes, so although it is fairly eosinophilic, it is tinged with a little basophilia.

Helpful Hint

RBCs last about 120 days in the bloodstream. This means that the body has to turn over 0.8–1% of these cells every day. Therefore, one would expect that around 1% of red blood cells are reticulocytes.

Clinical Correlate

In cases where blood is lost and RBCs need to be replaced, the **reticulocyte count** will increase until normal RBC values are restored. In anemias caused by pathology involving the bone marrow, the patient will have fewer RBCs (i.e., a low **hematocrit**) but will not have an expected increase in reticulocytes because the bone marrow is not able to produce sufficient reticulocytes to boost the RBC population.

Video 20.3   Reticulocytes in peripheral blood smears

Be able to identify:
— Reticulocyte
https://www.thieme.de/de/q.htm?p=opn/tp/308390101/978-1-62623-414-7_c020_v003&t=video

Reticulocytes actually got this name because supravital dyes stain the remaining ribosomes in these cells. The result of staining reticulocytes this way appears as a reticulum, or mesh, as seen in **Fig. 20.9**.

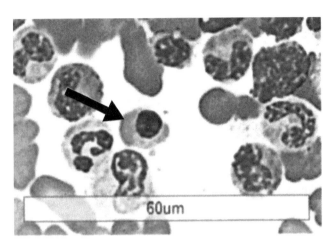

Fig. 20.6   **Orthochromatophilic erythroblast.**

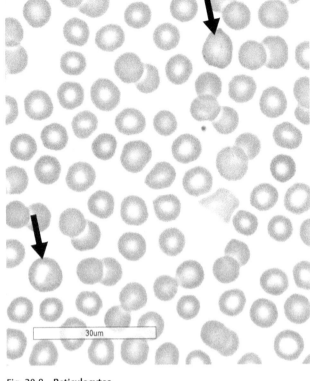

Fig. 20.8   **Reticulocytes.**

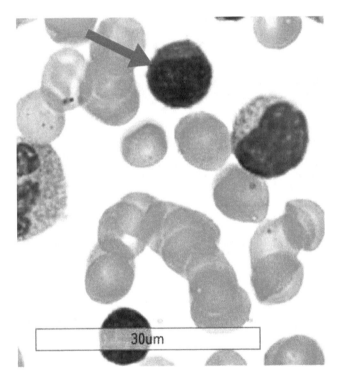

Fig. 20.7   **Lymphocyte.**

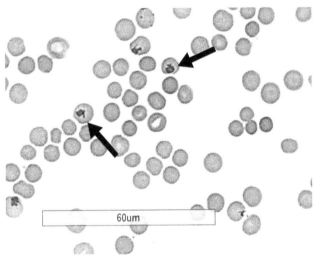

Fig. 20.9   **Reticulocytes stained with new methylene blue.**

Video 20.4   Reticulocyte with supravital staining

Be able to identify:
— Reticulocyte (stained with supravital dye)
https://www.thieme.de/de/q.htm?p=opn/
tp/308390101/978-1-62623-414-7_c020_v004&t=video

Table 20.1 Features of developing red blood cells

Fig. 20.2	Fig. 20.4	Fig. 20.5	Fig. 20.6
Proerythroblast	Basophilic erythroblast	Polychromatophilic erythroblast	Orthochromatophilic erythroblast
— Large cell — Large round nucleus — Nucleoli (at least one) — Fine chromatin pattern — Basophilic cytoplasm — Absence of granules	— Large cell — Large round nucleus — Absence of nucleoli — Clumpy chromatin pattern with spaces — Basophilic cytoplasm — Absence of granules	— Smaller cell — Smaller nucleus — Absence of nucleoli — More clumpy chromatin pattern with fewer spaces — Basophilic and eosinophilic cytoplasm — Absence of granules	— Small cell — Small nucleus — Absence of nucleoli — Mostly clumpy chromatin pattern with occasional or absent spaces — Mostly eosinophilic cytoplasm — Absence of granules

20.6   Chapter Review

The first recognizable stage of red blood cell development is the proerythroblast, a large cell with prominent nucleoli and pronounced cytoplasmic basophilia due to abundant ribosomes. As the cell matures, nucleoli disappear and the nuclear chromatin gradually condenses. Synthesis of hemoglobin introduces eosinophilia to the cytoplasm; this and the loss of ribosomes cause the cytoplasm to transition from a basophilic to eosinophilic color as the cell matures. The cell loses its nucleus and is subsequently released into the bloodstream. These changes are summarized in **Table 20.1.**

Questions and Answers

An online-only section of questions and answers accompanying this chapter is hosted on Thieme's MedOne Education site: https://medone-education.thieme.com. Use the code on the media page at the front of this book to gain access. An institutional license to the site is required to access these questions in an interactive format, and individual users are required to register for an individual account to track results.

21 Blood Cell Production: Bone Marrow and Thymus

After completing this chapter, you should be able to:
— Identify, at the light microscope level, each of the following:
  • Bone marrow
  • Thymus
    ◦ Capsule
    ◦ Trabeculae
    ◦ Cortex
    ◦ Medulla
    ◦ Lobules
    ◦ Hassall corpuscles
    ◦ Epithelial reticular cells
    ◦ Lymphocytes
— Explain the lifetime changes that occur in the organs listed above
— Outline the function of the organs listed above

21.1 Development of Blood Cells

As mentioned in previous chapters, blood cells develop in **bone marrow** from a common precursor. Once mature, these cells leave the bone marrow and enter the bloodstream. Red blood cells function within the bloodstream, while white blood cells are largely active after they leave the blood and enter peripheral tissues and organs. Platelets are activated with vessel wall damage. Therefore, most cells that leave the bone marrow are functional, or nearly so. However, specific lymphocytes called **T lymphocytes (T cells)** complete their maturation in the **thymus** before they are released as active cells.

Bone marrow and thymus are the producers of blood cells and are the focus of this chapter. Subsequent chapters will examine tissues and organs of the lymphatic system and locations where white blood cells are active in fighting infections.

21.2 Bone Marrow

Bone marrow is the site of synthesis of all formed elements of the blood. Because these elements have a limited lifespan, bone marrow is a very mitotically active tissue. **Fig. 21.1a** is a cross section through the shaft of a growing long bone, while **Fig. 21.1b** is from the sternum, a flat bone. The bright pink tissue is bone (osseous tissue), including compact (black arrows) and spongy bone (blue arrows). Bone marrow (green arrows) occupies the marrow cavity of the shaft of long bones as well as the spaces between the spicules of spongy bone.

There are two types of bone marrow:
• **Red bone marrow** contains developing and mature blood cells and adipose tissue.
• **Yellow bone marrow** is mostly (or exclusively) adipose tissue.

Fig. 21.2 shows more detail of the bone marrow from the shaft of a growing long bone. Note that the marrow contains little, if any, adipose tissue. Therefore, this is red marrow, which is highly cellular; most of these cells are developing red and white blood cells. Megakaryocytes can be seen (yellow arrows). What appear to be spaces (X) are specialized capillaries of the bone marrow, called **sinusoids** (sinuses). The endothelial cells of these

capillaries are specialized in that they allow newly formed blood cells to pass through them to enter the circulation (from the marrow compartment into the bloodstream).

Fig. 21.3 is a section of the sternum taken at higher magnification and shows a bone spicule (X) and marrow. Adipocytes (A) can be seen in the marrow. Although this tissue, by volume, is approximately half hematopoietic cells and half adipose, it is still considered red marrow due to its hematopoietic activity.

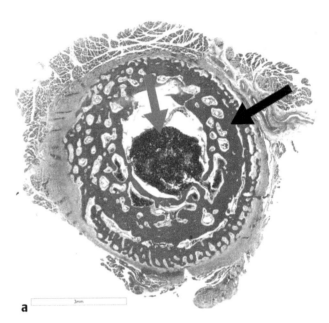

a ___3mm___

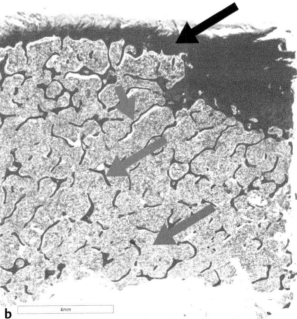

b ___4mm___

Fig. 21.1 **Scanning images of bone marrow. (a) Cross section through the shaft of a long bone. (b) Flat bone. Bone marrow (green arrows), compact bone (black arrows), and spicules of spongy bone (blue arrows) are indicated.**

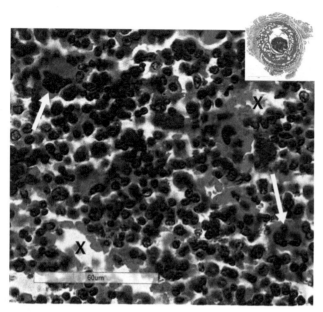

Fig. 21.2   **Bone marrow from the medullary cavity of a long bone.** Xs indicated capillaries (sinusoids) of the bone marrow; yellow arrows indicate megakaryocytes.

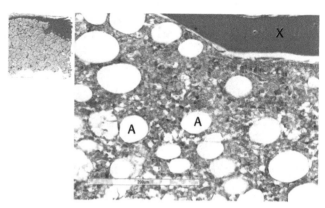

Fig. 21.3   **Bone marrow in a flat bone. X indicates osseous tissue; the As represent adipose cells.**

Because both **Fig. 21.2** and **21.3** are tissue specimens and not a bone marrow smear, cellular detail of hematopoietic cells is not optimal, though the highly cellular nature of this tissue is readily seen.

Yellow marrow is essentially adipose tissue and is identified as yellow marrow only by its location in a marrow compartment. Therefore, no image of yellow marrow need be shown here.

Nearly all bone marrow in the newborn is red marrow. As a person reaches adulthood, the marrow in the shafts of long bones loses hematopoietic activity and becomes yellow marrow. Blood cell production is maintained by the remaining red marrow in the epiphyseal regions of long bones and in flat bones. Under certain conditions, regions containing yellow marrow may become active red marrow again by growth of existing red marrow or seeding from circulating stem cells.

Clinical Correlate

In certain pathologic conditions (e.g. anemias), bone marrow becomes hypercellular in response to an increase in erythropoietin. In this setting, yellow marrow is converted to red marrow.

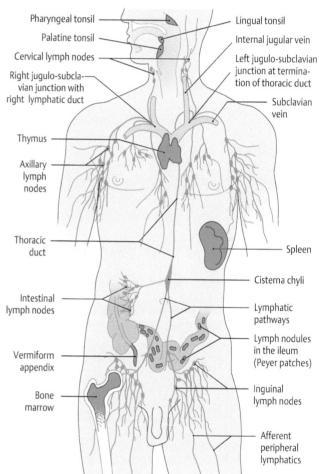

Fig. 21.4   **The lymphatic system.**

Video 21.1   Red bone marrow in situ 1

https://www.thieme.de/de/q.htm?p=opn/tp/308390101/978-1-62623-414-7_c021_v001&t=video

Video 21.2   Red bone marrow in situ 2

Be able to identify:
— Red bone marrow
— Hematopoietic cells
— Adipose
— Yellow bone marrow (essentially adipose in the marrow cavity)
https://www.thieme.de/de/q.htm?p=opn/tp/308390101/978-1-62623-414-7_c021_v002&t=video

21.3 Thymus

As mentioned, most blood cells are mature when they are released into the blood from the bone marrow. The notable exception to this is cells of the **T lymphocyte (T cell)** lineage, which undergo further maturation in the thymus (**Fig. 21.4**). This is a complicated and not well understood selection process, part of which includes removal of T cells that would bind to self-antigen if released into the general circulation.

The thymus develops from the oral cavity, namely the pharyngeal pouches. These pouches are spaces of oral cavity lined by epithelial cells that separate the oral cavity from the underlying connective tissue. In **Fig. 21.5**, the pharyngeal pouches are numbered (1–4), and the tissue that lines each pouch is color coded, matched to the organ derived from each pouch. The thymus develops from the right and left third pharyngeal pouches (light blue). Tissue from these pouches separate from the oral cavity, migrate into the neck, and come to lie anterior to the trachea, where they fuse into a single organ.

The epithelial cells from the third pharyngeal pouches that migrate to form the thymus are called **epithelial reticular cells**. Like other epithelial cells, epithelial reticular cells form a network (cords) in which the cells are joined to their neighbors by cell-cell junctions (e.g., desmosomes, tight junctions). T cells from the bone marrow occupy the spaces within this network (the space in the network is similar to a lumen of a gland). Epithelial reticular cells not only provide the blood-thymus barrier (a protected environment necessary for T cell maturation) but are involved in the antigen presentation necessary for T cell selection. The epithelial cords are surrounded by connective tissue.

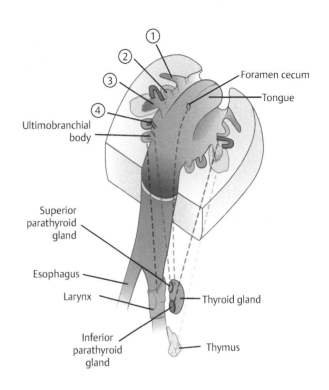

Fig. 21.5 **Derivatives of the pharyngeal pouches.**

> **Helpful Hint**
>
> The migration of pharyngeal arch derivatives is challenging to visualize. Try this: The inside lining of the pharynx (throat) is an epithelium, with connective tissue deep to that epithelium. Imagine epithelial cells lining the pharynx burrowing deeper into the connective tissue, creating pits. The epithelial cells eventually burrow deep enough to separate from the pharynx and migrate down into the neck, under the skin, muscles, and fascia, to reach a location just in front of the trachea near the top of the sternum. This burrowing and migration may seem kind of creepy, but, like food references, sometimes these descriptions help.

21.3.1 Structure of the Thymus

The thymus is surrounded by a connective tissue **capsule** (**Fig. 21.6**, blue arrows), the thickness of which varies due to tissue removal. Extensions of the capsule, called **trabeculae** (yellow arrows), partition the thymus into **lobules** (yellow outline) that vary in size, though some of this variation is due to sectioning. Each lobule has a darker outer portion, the **cortex**, containing mostly immature T cells, and a lighter **medulla**, where more mature T cells are located. The trabeculae do not penetrate through the entire organ, so the lobules are not completely separate structures. The medulla is a single, convoluted structure, the extensions of which are covered by cortical tissue.

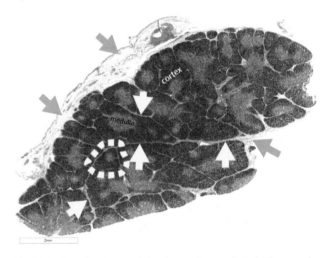

Fig. 21.6 **Scanning image of the thymus from an infant. The capsule (blue arrows) and trabeculae (yellow arrows) are indicated. One lobule is outlined in yellow.**

Video 21.3   Overview of the thymus

Be able to identify:
— Thymus
— Capsule
— Trabecula
— Cortex
— Medulla
— Lobules

https://www.thieme.de/de/q.htm?p=opn/tp/308390101/978-1-62623-414-7_c021_v003&t=video

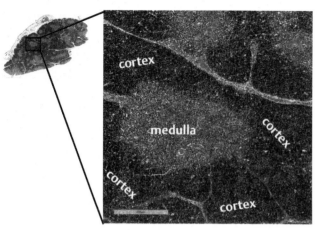

Fig. 21.7   **Thymus of an infant at medium magnification showing medulla and cortex.**

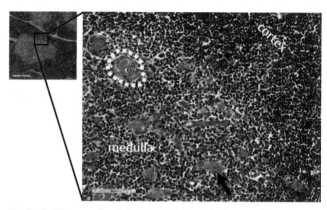

Fig. 21.8   **Thymus of an infant at medium to high magnification showing an epithelial reticular cell (arrow) and Hassal's corpuscle (outlined).**

Fig. 21.7 shows a view of a lobule, with the cortex and medulla indicated. The thymus contains numerous T lymphocytes, which are small cells with little cytoplasm. Because these lymphocytes are closely packed together, the tissue is very basophilic due to high numbers of nuclei. The basophilia is more prominent in the cortex because there are more lymphocytes than in the medulla.

Fig. 21.8 is a more detailed image of a portion of one lobule of the thymus; the cortex and medulla are indicated. The numerous small nuclei are T lymphocytes, which are more numerous in the cortex. Epithelial reticular cells (black arrow) are seen more easily in the medulla, characterized by a large, euchromatic nucleus and abundant, eosinophilic cytoplasm. As mentioned, epithelial reticular cells create tight junctions with each other to provide a protective environment for the developing T cells and are thought to play a role in T cell maturation and selection.

Over time, epithelial reticular cells come together and condense to form a concentric arrangement in structures called **Hassall's corpuscles** (yellow outline). Ultimately, these corpuscles undergo keratinization, so larger corpuscles have little cellularity. Hassall's corpuscles are a characteristic feature of the thymus, though the function of these structures is unclear.

Helpful Hint

The keratinization in Hassall's corpuscles is similar to what occurs in stratified squamous keratinized epithelia, which makes sense because they consist of epithelial reticular cells, which are epitelial in origin.

Although Hassall's corpuscles are a useful way to definitively identify the thymus, they are not always present, especially in a thymus from a young person (see next section).

Video 21.4   Details of the thymus

Be able to identify:
— Thymus
— Lymphocytes
— Epithelial reticular cells
— Hassall corpuscles
https://www.thieme.de/de/q.htm?p=opn/tp/308390101/978-1-62623-414-7_c021_v004&t=video

21.3.2   Aging of the Thymus

As the thymus ages, it undergoes histologic changes. In a newborn, the thymus largely consists of epithelial reticular cells and T lymphocytes, and Hassall's corpuscles are absent (**Fig. 21.9**). As a person ages, Hassall's corpuscles (black arrows) form and increase in size throughout early childhood and adolescence. During adult life, the thymus undergoes involution, being replaced by adipose tissue, so it no longer resembles the thymus at all. Presumably, by that time, enough T cells have been produced to last a lifetime, although pathologic conditions can restimulate T cell production in the thymus.

Video 21.5   Thymus maturation and aging

Be able to:
— Identify the thymus
— Describe the changes in the thymus during aging
https://www.thieme.de/de/q.htm?p=opn/tp/308390101/978-1-62623-414-7_c021_v005&t=video

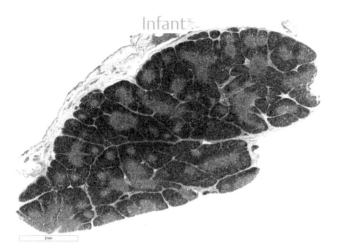

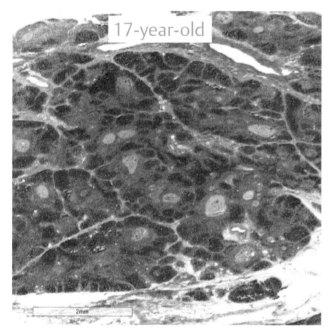

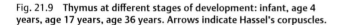

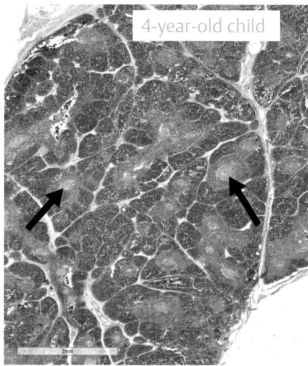

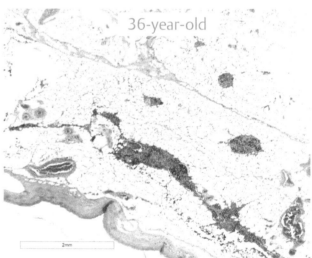

Fig. 21.9 Thymus at different stages of development: infant, age 4 years, age 17 years, age 36 years. Arrows indicate Hassel's corpuscles.

21.4 Chapter Review

Formed elements of the blood have a limited lifespan and, therefore, must be produced continuously. The bone marrow is the site of production of these cells. As the name implies, this tissue is located within bones, and its highly cellular nature underscores its function in cell production. In newborns, most of the bone marrow is red marrow, which is actively involved in blood cell production (hematopoiesis). As a person matures, some red marrow is replaced by adipose to form yellow marrow, which may be called upon to become active red marrow in crisis or pathological conditions. Most formed elements are released from the bone marrow as mature, or nearly mature, cells. The exception is T lymphocytes, which must complete their maturation in the thymus. The thymus is derived from the oral cavity, and the cells derived in this way are epithelial reticular cells, which assist in T lymphocyte maturation and selection. As the thymus ages, changes occur that result in a decreased lymphocyte number and an increase in Hassall's corpuscles and adipose tissue.

Questions and Answers

An online-only section of questions and answers accompanying this chapter is hosted on Thieme's MedOne Education site: https://medone-education.thieme.com. Use the code on the media page at the front of this book to gain access. An institutional license to the site is required to access these questions in an interactive format, and individual users are required to register for an individual account to track results.

22   Diffuse Lymphoid Tissue

After completing this chapter, you should be able to:
— Identify, at the light microscope level, each of the following:
  • Diffuse lymphoid tissue
  • Palatine tonsils
    ○ Stratified squamous epithelium
    ○ Connective tissue septa
    ○ Crypts
    ○ Nodules
      ▪ Primary
      ▪ Secondary
        – Germinal centers
        – Corona
    ○ Cell types
      ▪ Blast forms of lymphocytes
      ▪ Mitotic figures
      ▪ Macrophages (tingible macrophages)
      ▪ Reticular or dendritic cells
      ▪ Plasma cells
  • Pharyngeal tonsils
    ○ Same as palatine tonsil, except covered with stratified squamous epithelium and pseudostratified ciliated columnar epithelium with goblet cells
— Evaluate the distribution of T and B cells in lymphoid tissue using immunocytochemistry
— Outline the function of each cell type or structure listed

22.1   Overview of Lymphoid Tissues

The previous chapters described the production and maturation of white blood cells in the bone marrow and thymus. Mature white blood cells are released into the bloodstream; many of these cells move into tissues, where they are involved in immune responses. White blood cells perform these functions throughout the body, but there are some locations where this response is robust. It is these locations, highlighted by an increased number of white blood cells histologically, that will be the focus of the next several chapters.

This chapter will focus on **diffuse lymphoid tissues**. These are collections of white blood cells in tissues and organs that are constantly exposed to external infectious agents (the integumentary [skin], gastrointestinal, and respiratory systems). This discussion will highlight featured structures in which diffuse lymphoid tissues are abundant: the palatine and pharyngeal tonsils. Subsequent chapters will discuss the histology of other lymphoid tissue, namely lymph nodes and the spleen.

22.2   Diffuse Lymphoid Tissue

Recall that organs that are exposed to the outside world (either directly or indirectly) are lined with an epithelium, which separates spaces of the outside world from underlying connective tissues. This is the case for the skin, digestive tract, respiratory tract, and urinary and reproductive systems. The epithelia play a role in keeping pathogenic agents from accessing the underlying connective tissues. When an epithelium is breached, white blood cells migrate to the area in large numbers, creating a site of **inflammation**.

Fig. 22.1 is a scanning view of skin with an area of inflammation that was used in previous chapters to show connective tissues and white blood cells in tissues. The epithelium is at the bottom of the image. The area of inflammation has an increased number of white blood cells, giving that region a basophilia that can be appreciated even at low magnification.

Fig. 22.2 is an image from the same tissue in **Fig. 22.1**, focusing on a region in which the epithelium is intact. Even in areas where an epithelium is not visibly breached, collections of white blood cells can be seen in the underlying connective tissue. White blood cells are scattered throughout the connective tissue, but certain regions (outlined) have a higher density of white blood cells, seen as an increased number of nuclei. These regions are referred to as **diffuse lymphoid tissue**.

Fig. 22.3 is an image of the epithelium and underlying connective tissue from the esophagus. Here diffuse lymphoid tissue can be seen both within and surrounding the outlined region. Within the outlined region, the white blood cells have become more aggregated, forming a round structure referred to as a **lymphoid nodule** (or **follicle**). Histologists refer to this as a **primary nodule** because the density of the white blood cells is relatively consistent throughout the nodule.

> **Helpful Hint**
>
> Many of the cells in these nodules are lymphocytes, which are mostly nucleus with a thin rim of cytoplasm. When lymphocytes crowd together like this, the large number of nuclei gives the region an overall basophilic appearance compared to the surrounding connective tissue.

It is important to note that diffuse lymphoid tissue is transient. It is likely that the regions shown in these images were not infiltrated by white blood cells a day or two ago (more or less), and the white blood cells seen here would either perish or leave

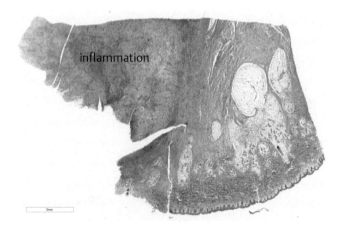

Fig. 22.1   Scanning view of skin with inflammation.

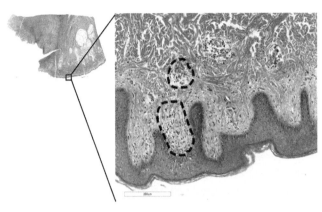

Fig. 22.2 **Skin with intact epithelium showing diffuse lymphoid tissue (outlined).**

the area soon. However, a tissue such as skin or intestines that is exposed to the outside world will always have some diffuse lymphoid tissue.

Diffuse lymphoid tissue can be compared to ants on a sidewalk. The sidewalk represents tissue (stomach, piece of skin), the ants are lymphocytes, and bread crumbs are infectious agents.

For the most part, the sidewalk is clean, so there are only a few stray ants most of the time. However, there will be places where a bread crumb has been dropped on the sidewalk. Ants will migrate to that area and be numerous in that spot. Such a spot is similar to a nodule, in which lymphocytes leave the bloodstream and move into the connective tissue in response to some stimulus.

In a day or two, the crumb will be gone, and so will the ants. However, another bread crumb may have been dropped in another location, and that region will show a similar-looking cluster of hungry ants. After some time, that one will go away too.

So, a view of the sidewalk today will reveal scattered ants, with a few places where there are many of them gathered. Three days from now, there will still be scattered ants, including the places where there were clusters of ants previously. However, new locations of numerous ants will be present. Any day will demonstrate scattered ants with some areas of more numerous ants. The same is true of any organ exposed to the outside world. Sections of these organs will reveal scattered lymphocytes and areas of more lymphocytes representing more activity in that region at the time the tissue was prepared.

Video 22.1 Diffuse lymphoid tissue in the esophagus

Be able to identify:
— Diffuse lymphoid tissue
— Nodules (primary)
https://www.thieme.de/de/q.htm?p=opn/tp/308390101/978-1-62623-414-7_c022_v001&t=video

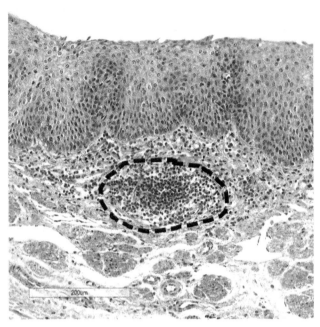

Fig. 22.3 **Diffuse lymphoid tissue, showing a lymphoid nodule (outlined) in the esophagus.**

22.3 Specialized Diffuse Lymphoid Tissue

As mentioned in the preceding section, even though individual nodules come and go, in certain regions of the body, notably the digestive tract, there are areas that consistently contain high numbers of nodules. These structures include the **tonsils** of the pharynx, Peyer's patches in the ileum, and the **appendix**. **Peyer's patches** and the appendix will be discussed in **Chapter 29** on the intestines. This chapter will focus on the **palatine** and **pharyngeal tonsils** of the pharynx.

22.4 Tonsils

The pharynx, the common tube for the digestive and respiratory tracts, is "guarded" by a ring of tonsils, called the **pharyngeal lymphoid ring** or the tonsillar ring of Waldeyer (**Fig. 22.4**). These structures are strategically placed to initiate an immune response to pathogens entering the body. The major features of this ring are the singular **pharyngeal** and **lingual tonsils** and the paired **palatine tonsils**. **Fig. 22.5** shows a clinical view of the palatine tonsils (black arrows). The surface of these tonsils has many small openings that may be visible to the unaided eye in some individuals.

22.4.1 Palatine Tonsils

The inner lining of the digestive tract is a **mucosa**, which consists of an epithelium and underlying connective tissue. As part of the lining of the digestive tract, the tonsils are essentially a mucosa populated by abundant diffuse lymphoid tissue and numerous lymphoid nodules. Because the epithelium of the oral cavity is stratified squamous nonkeratinized, the epithelium of the palatine tonsils is also stratified squamous nonkeratinized.

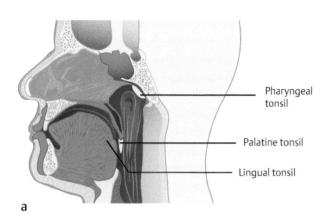

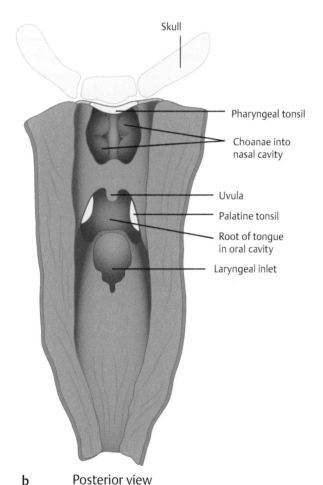

b   Posterior view

Fig. 22.4   **Anatomy of the tonsils (Waldeyer tonsillar ring). (a) Sagittal view of the head. (b) Posterior view of the pharynx, with the posterior wall opened to show the oral and nasal cavities and larynx.**

Fig. 22.6 shows a scanning view of a palatine tonsil. For orientation, the lumen of the oral cavity is to the bottom right of this tissue; at this low magnification the epithelium lining the oral cavity can be seen. The connective tissue side of this tonsil is the left and top portions of this image.

As mentioned, the surface of the tonsils has many openings or pits. These deep invaginations of the epithelium are called

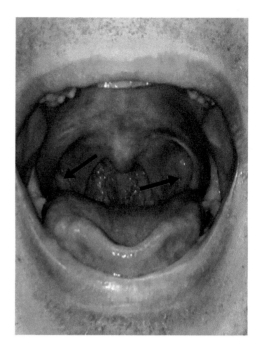

Fig. 22.5   **Palatine tonsils, clinical view (arrows). Image taken by Laura Garrison.**

tonsillar crypts (green arrows), which, like the oral cavity and surface of the palatine tonsil, are lined by stratified squamous epithelium that is thinner (i.e., less stratified) than the epithelium of the oral cavity or esophagus. Tonsillar crypts are connected to the lumen of the oral cavity; because of sectioning, some may appear embedded within the tonsil, but they are nonetheless connected to the oral cavity in a different plane of section. Connective tissue **septa** (black arrows) partition the tonsil from the deeper aspect.

Fig. 22.7 is an image taken at higher magnification, showing both a tonsillar crypt (yellow arrows) and a septum (green arrows). The crypt has a lumen that is continuous with the oral

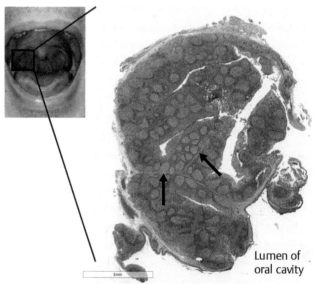

Fig. 22.6   **Palatine tonsil, scanning view. Green arrows indicate tonsillar crypts (pits), which are continuous with the oral cavity. Connective tissue septa (black arrows) support the tonsillar tissue.**

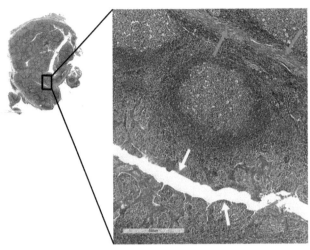

Fig. 22.7   **Palatine tonsil, low to medium magnification, showing a tonsillar crypt (yellow arrows) and a connective tissue septum (green arrows).**

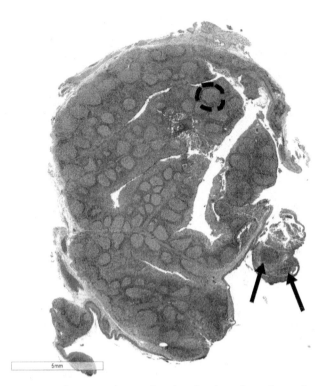

Fig. 22.8   **Palatine tonsils, scanning view showing primary (arrows) and secondary (outlined) nodules.**

cavity and, as mentioned, is lined by a thinner stratified squamous epithelium, which appears fairly disrupted in many places as a result of tissue preparation. The septum is composed of dense irregular connective tissue.

Video 22.2   Palatine tonsil showing orientation, crypts, and septa

Be able to identify:
— Palatine tonsil
— Crypts
— Septa

https://www.thieme.de/de/q.htm?p=opn/tp/308390101/978-1-62623-414-7_c022_v002&t=video

Video 22.3   Palatine tonsil showing nodules

Be able to identify:
— Palatine tonsil
— Primary nodules
— Secondary nodules
   • Germinal center
   • Corona

https://www.thieme.de/de/q.htm?p=opn/tp/308390101/978-1-62623-414-7_c022_v003&t=video

The main feature of tonsils is the abundance of lymphoid nodules (**Fig. 22.8**). Most of the nodules in the tonsils (one is outlined) have a pale central region, called a **germinal center**, surrounded by a thin darker rim. Nodules with germinal centers are called **secondary nodules**. **Primary nodules** (i.e., those lacking germinal centers; black arrows) may be seen, though it is possible that these are secondary nodules cut through the darker outer layers.

Primary nodules consist of unstimulated lymphocytes. Because these "resting" cells are small, they are closely packed; thus the dark appearance of these nodules. Stimulation of lymphocytes by antigen causes them to proliferate. Dividing lymphocytes are larger than their unstimulated counterparts, and, therefore, germinal centers are lighter because the nuclei in these regions are farther apart.

Fig. 22.9 is a higher-magnification image of a secondary nodule (black outline). The darker region surrounding the pale germinal center is typically thicker on one side of the nodule; this region is referred to as the **corona** (yellow outline).

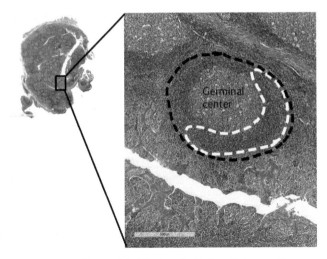

Fig. 22.9   **Secondary nodule (black outline) of a palatine tonsil showing pale germinal center and darker corona (yellow outline).**

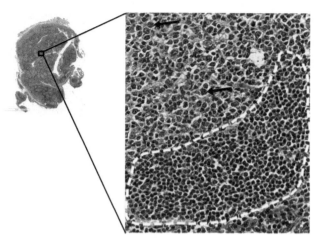

Fig. 22.10 Portion of a secondary nodule, high magnification, showing corona (yellow outline) and stimulated lymphocytes in the germinal center (black arrows).

Fig. 22.10 is a higher-magnification image of a secondary nodule. The outer region of the nodule (corona, outlined) is filled with small unstimulated ("resting") lymphocytes, each demonstrating a condensed, heterochromatic nucleus and a thin rim of cytoplasm. In contrast, many lymphocytes in the germinal center (upper left) have been stimulated to proliferate. Although many of these cells are enlarged, the cells that demonstrate the largest nuclei (arrows) are dividing cells referred to as **blast cells**. Again, the overall increase in size of the cells in the germinal center gives this region a pale appearance relative to the surrounding corona.

Fig. 22.11 is an even higher-magnification image of the germinal center from **Fig. 22.10**. Blast cells (yellow arrows) demonstrate large euchromatic nuclei, often with a visible nucleolus. A **macrophage** is indicated (black outline) for comparison; note the very euchromatic nucleus and prominent nucleolus in the macrophage, as well as the pale eosinophilic cytoplasm that is more substantial than that in the blast lymphocytes.

As mentioned, blast cells are dividing cells. Therefore, it is not surprising that close examination of a germinal center will demonstrate **mitotic figures** (**Fig. 22.12**, yellow outlines).

Recall that macrophages are large cells, with more abundant cytoplasm than in lymphocytes (see **Fig. 22.11**). In the context of a lymphoid nodule, they occupy a space relatively devoid of lymphocytes. Therefore, under low or medium magnification (**Fig. 22.13**), the location of the macrophages appears pale (black arrows) when compared to the packed-in lymphocytes (even paler than the germinal center itself).

The pale macrophages scattered against the darker background staining of the nodule created by the densely packed lymphocyte nuclei has been described as having a "starry sky" appearance, similar to a famous painting.

Finally, tapered cells with relatively flattened nuclei can also be seen in lymphoid nodules (**Fig. 22.14**, yellow arrows). These belong to one of several different cell types:

1. **Reticular cells**: fibroblastlike cells that synthesize the collagen framework
2. **Dendritic cells**: cells that process antigens and present them to lymphocytes
3. **Follicular dendritic cells**: cells that trap and present antigens to lymphocytes

In routine H & E-stained sections, it is not possible to distinguish definitively between these cell types.

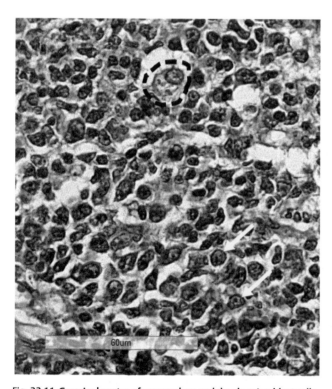

Fig. 22.11 Germinal center of a secondary nodule, showing blast cells (yellow arrows) and a macrophage (outlined).

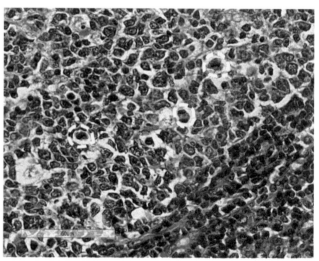

Fig. 22.12 Edge of a germinal center showing mitotic figures (outlined).

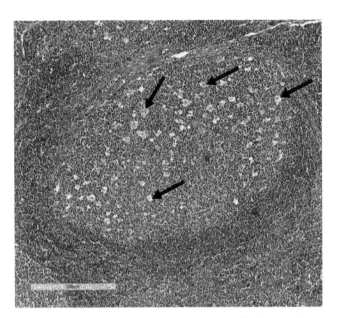

Fig. 22.13 **Germinal center showing macrophages (black arrows).**

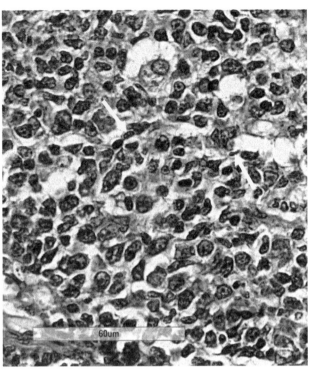

Fig. 22.14 **Germinal center of a secondary nodule, showing tapered cells (arrows).**

Video 22.4   Palatine tonsil showing cell types

Be able to identify:
— Palatine tonsil
— Small lymphocytes
— Blast cells
— Macrophages
— Reticular and dendritic cells (you do not need to distinguish them from each other, but they can be distinguished from lymphocytes and macrophages)
https://www.thieme.de/de/q.htm?p=opn/tp/308390101/978-1-62623-414-7_c022_v004&t=video

Video 22.5   Pharyngeal tonsil

Be able to identify:
— Pharyngeal tonsil
— Respiratory epithelium (pseudostratified ciliated columnar)
— All other structures same as palatine tonsils
https://www.thieme.de/de/q.htm?p=opn/tp/308390101/978-1-62623-414-7_c022_v005&t=video

22.4.2 Pharyngeal Tonsil

As mentioned, the oral cavity and pharynx are lined by stratified squamous nonkeratinized epithelium, which helps to resist friction from passing food. The nasal cavity is lined by respiratory epithelium, namely pseudostratified ciliated columnar epithelium with goblet cells. This epithelium traps and removes particulate matter in inspired air. The **pharyngeal tonsil** (sometimes called **adenoid**) is situated in the transition zone between the nasal cavity and the pharynx (see **Fig. 22.4**). It is histologically similar to the palatine tonsils, with one major exception: the lower portion of the pharyngeal tonsil (facing the oral cavity) is lined by stratified squamous nonkeratinized epithelium like the palatine tonsil, while the upper portion (facing the nasal cavity) is lined by pseudostratified ciliated columnar epithelium. Also, the spaces corresponding to the crypts of the palatine tonsils are wider in the pharyngeal tonsil, so the term "crypts" is typically not used for the pharyngeal tonsil.

Clinical Correlate

Inflammation of the tonsils is called **tonsillitis**, which can be caused by bacterial or viral infections. The patient's throat is red, painful, and tender. Other symptoms such as loss of appetite and fever may be associated with tonsillitis. Treatment typically targets the cause of the inflammation (e.g., antibiotics for a bacterial infection). Repeated tonsillitis in children, or severe cases that cause obstruction of the airways or swallowing, may require **tonsillectomy** (removal of the tonsils).

22.5 T and B Cell Localization in Diffuse Lymphoid Tissue

In tonsils and other tissues and organs that contain lymphoid nodules, **B lymphocytes** are more numerous within the nodules,

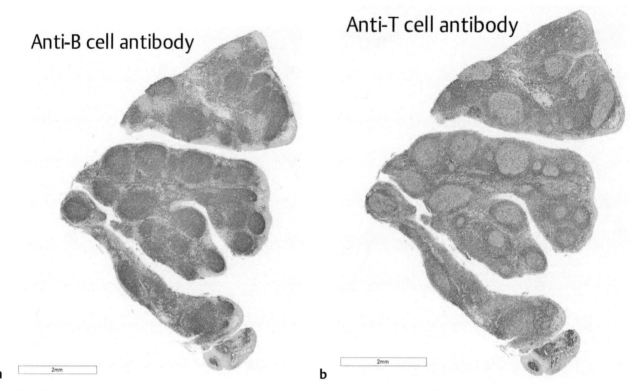

a   2mm   b   2mm

Fig. 22.15 Section of palatine tonsil stained with immunocytochemistry to show the distribution of (a) B lymphocytes and (b) T lymphocytes.

while **T lymphocytes** are more prominent in the regions between the nodules. In standard H & E sections, this is not apparent because B and T cells are indistinguishable. However, the distribution of B and T lymphocytes can be visualized using immunocytochemistry. **Fig. 22.15** shows images of sections of a palatine tonsil stained by immunochemistry using antibodies specific to B cells (**Fig. 22.15a**) or T cells (**Fig. 22.15b**), confirming that indeed B cells are localized to nodules and T cells localize to the region between the nodules, also called the paranodular region. Note that this localizaiton is not exclusive: some B cells are found between nodules, and some T cells with nodules.

Video 22.6   Palatine tonsil immunocytochemistry

Be able to identify:
— Localization of B and T lymphocytes using immunocytochemistry

https://www.thieme.de/de/q.htm?p=opn/tp/308390101/978-1-62623-414-7_c022_v006&t=video

diffuse lymphoid tissue. Round or oval regions of concentrated white blood cells are called nodules and presumably signify an immune response to the presence of a pathogen or other stimulus in that particular region. Since many of the cells in nodules are lymphocytes, which have little cytoplasm, these nodules are recognized even at low magnification as regions of increased basophilia against the eosinophilic background characteristic of the protein-rich connective tissue matrix. Some locations, such as the tonsils of the pharynx, contain numerous lymphoid nodules. Many of these nodules have pale germinal centers and are called secondary nodules. Within these nodules are resting lymphocytes, stimulated lymphocytes (blast cells), macrophages, antigen-presenting dendritic cells, and fibroblast-like reticular cells. Palatine and pharyngeal tonsils can be distinguished from one another by the epithelium that covers their surface; palatine tonsils are covered entirely by stratified squamous epithelium, while the pharyngeal tonsil is covered by respiratory (pseudostratified, ciliated) epithelium facing the nasal cavity and stratified squamous epithelium facing the oral cavity. B and T lymphocyte distribution in lymphoid tissue can be visualized by immunocytochemistry; B lymphocytes are numerous in the nodules, while T lymphocytes populate the tissue between nodules.

22.6   Chapter Review

White blood cells are found in most tissues and organs of the body. However, there are many locations in which white blood cells are numerous. These locations include tissues and organs that are exposed to the outside world, such as the skin and the digestive and respiratory tracts. In these locations, a region of increased numbers of white blood cells is referred to as

Questions and Answers

An online-only section of questions and answers accompanying this chapter is hosted on Thieme's MedOne Education site: https://medone-education.thieme.com. Use the code on the media page at the front of this book to gain access. An institutional license to the site is required to access these questions in an interactive format, and individual users are required to register for an individual account to track results.

23 Lymph Nodes

After completing this chapter, you should be able to:
— Identify, at the light microscope level, each of the following:
  • Lymph node
    ○ Hilus
    ○ Capsule
    ○ Trabeculae
    ○ Cortex
      ▪ Subcapsular sinus
      ▪ Trabecular sinus
      ▪ Nodules (including primary and secondary)
      ▪ Paracortical zone
        – High endothelial venules
    ○ Medulla
      ▪ Medullary cords
      ▪ Medullary sinuses
    ○ Afferent lymphatic vessels
    ○ Efferent lymphatic vessels
— Evaluate the distribution of cell types in lymph nodes
— Outline the function of each cell type and structure listed
— Draw the flow of lymph through a lymph node
— Outline the immune response that occurs in a lymph node
— Correlate the role of lymph nodes in the immune system with the evaluation of nodes on physical and diagnostic exams

23.1 Overview of Lymphoid Organs

Previous chapters looked at the sites of blood cell development and maturation (bone marrow and thymus) as well as locations in the body where the immune response to pathogens is particularly robust (diffuse lymphoid tissues). The next two chapters focus on two specific organs that are involved in filtration of body fluids and stimulating an immune response to pathogens in those fluids: lymph nodes, which are associated with lymphatic fluid and channels, and the spleen, which filters blood.

23.2 Fluid Flow in the Body

Because **lymph nodes** filter lymphatic fluid (lymph), it is useful to consider the source and composition of this fluid before describing the histology of lymph nodes.

Blood flows away from the heart through arteries; the smallest arteries are arterioles. Blood flows from arterioles into capillaries, the vessels where molecular exchange occurs, and then returns to the heart via venules and veins (**Fig. 23.1**). Although there is bidirectional molecular exchange between the blood and tissues, there is usually a net efflux (outflow) of fluid from the lumen of the capillaries into the tissues (**Fig. 23.1**, black arrows). This excess tissue fluid enters lymphatic channels, which return this lymph back into the bloodstream, draining into veins of the upper thorax (**Fig. 23.2**). When tissues are damaged, pathogens and debris are introduced into the tissues/interstitial fluid. These flow into lymphatic channels as part of the lymph.

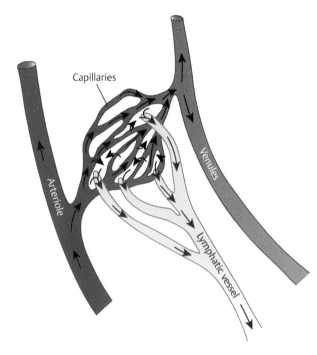

Fig. 23.1 **Blood and lymphatic fluid flow.**

Clinical Correlate

An imbalance in fluid flow at the tissue level can result in accumulation of excess tissue fluid, a condition called **edema**. Edema can be the result of disruption of lymphatic channels (a potential sequela of surgery) or through ion imbalance or protein deficiencies, which result in excess fluid leaving the capillaries.

23.3 Overview of Lymph Nodes

Lymph nodes are in-line filters for the lymphatic fluid that is returning to the bloodstream (**Fig. 23.2**). In this regard, lymphatic fluid flows *through* a lymph node. All lymphatic fluid passes through at least one lymph node before returning to the circulation. This ensures that any debris or organisms that gain access to the lymphatic fluid from tissues are removed before entering the general circulation.

Fig. 23.3 is a schematic drawing of a lymph node; the black arrows represent lymphatic fluid flow through a lymph node. **Afferent lymphatic vessels** bring lymphatic fluid to the lymph node (i.e., these vessels are usually anatomically peripheral to the node), while **efferent lymphatic vessels** carry fluid away from

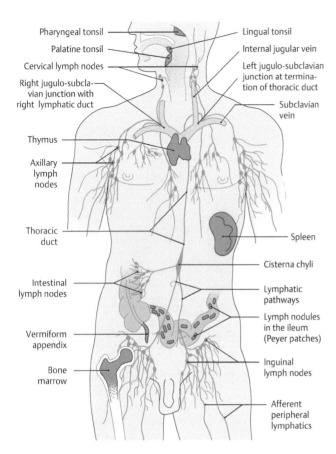

Fig. 23.2 **Lymphatic system.**

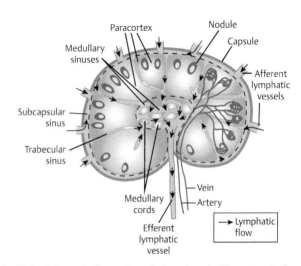

Fig. 23.3 **Schematic illustration of a lymph node. The cortex is the outermost region of the lymph node, bounded by the dotted outline. The medulla is the inner portion, consisting of sinuses and cords.**

the node (i.e., efferent vessels are anatomically proximal to the node). Note that because lymph often flows through more than one lymph node, an efferent lymphatic vessel of one node may be an afferent vessel of another node downstream. Within each lymph node, lymph flows through a series of specialized capillaries called **sinuses** (described subsequently).

A lymph node also has a blood supply, consisting of an artery and vein that enter and leave, respectively, at the same location as the efferent lymphatic vessel and supply and drain capillary beds within the organ. The indentation where the artery enters the organ and the vein and efferent lymphatic vessels leave is referred to as the **hilus**. A lymph node is supported by a connective tissue **capsule**, which projects into the substance of the organ as trabeculae (not shown).

Fig. 23.4 shows a scanning image of a lymph node. The hilus is indicated, and contains arteries, veins, and efferent lymphatic vessels. The cortex can be identified by the numerous nodules (black arrows) and the fact that it is a relatively "solid" tissue. Contrast this with the medulla (a portion of which is outlined); the pale regions within the medulla are **medullary sinuses**.

Video 23.1   Lymph node overview

Be able to identify:
— Lymph node
— Capsule
— Trabecula
— Hilus
— Cortex
— Medulla

https://www.thieme.de/de/q.htm?p=opn/tp/308390101/978-1-62623-414-7_c023_v001&t=video

Fig. 23.5 is a scanning image of a lymph node that has been sectioned mostly through the cortex. Because this is a section through the cortex, nodules are visible not only in the periphery but also in the center of the section.

> **Helpful Hint**
>
> Many other organs as well as lymph nodes have a hilus, such as the kidneys, the spleen, and the lungs.

Like many other organs, lymph nodes have a **cortex** (**Fig. 23.3**, black outlined region) and **medulla** (central region not outlined). These regions are typically less distinct in lymph nodes than in other organs.

> **Helpful Hint**
>
> Note that the indention at the hilus may create slides where these regions are not initially intuitive; for example, cortical tissue may be in the middle of a slide created from a horizontal section near the bottom of the lymph node in **Fig. 23.3**.

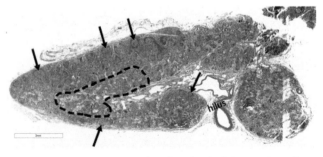

Fig. 23.4 **Scanning image of a lymph node. The hilus is indicated. The cortex consists of numerous nodules (arrows). A portion of the medulla is outlined.**

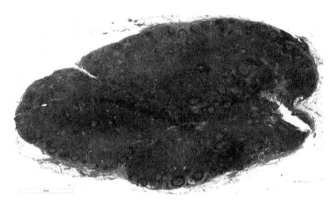

Fig. 23.5   **Lymph node sectioned through the cortex.**

Video 23.2   Lymph node overview

Be able to identify:
— Lymph node
— Capsule
— Trabecula
— (Hilus)
— Cortex
— (Medulla)
https://www.thieme.de/de/q.htm?p=opn/tp/308390101/978-1-62623-414-7_c023_v002&t=video

23.4   Lymphatic Flow through Lymph Nodes

As mentioned, lymph flows through a lymph node (**Fig. 23.3**, black arrows), entering and leaving the lymph node via afferent and efferent lymphatic vessels, respectively. Within the lymph node, lymph flows through sinuses with intuitive names based on position, so that the direction of flow is:

Afferent lymphatic vessels → **subcapsular sinuses** → **trabecular sinuses** → **medullary sinuses** → efferent lymphatic vessel

Fig. 23.6 is an image of a lymph node taken at low-medium magnification. In this image, the approximate locations (or actual examples) of the lymphatic channels are indicated by the arrows.

These lymph node sinuses are similar to capillaries but have a wide diameter, a very porous wall, and supporting cells within the lumen. Structurally, all sinuses in the lymph node are essentially the same; however, the subcapsular and trabecular sinuses are longer and straighter, while the medullary sinuses are wider and more convoluted.

Fig. 23.7 is a closer view of the outer region of the cortex. The capsule (black arrows) surrounds the entire lymph node; just deep to the capsule is the subcapsular sinus (blue brackets). Thin trabeculae (orange arrows) extend from the cortex at right angles into the substance of the lymph node. Trabecular sinuses (green brackets) branch from the subcapsular sinus at right angles and follow the trabeculae toward the medulla.

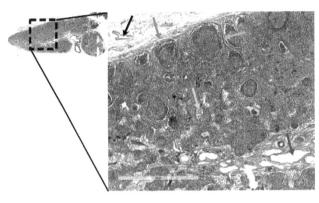

Fig. 23.6   **Lymph node showing lymph flow: from afferent lymphatic vessel (black arrow) to subcapsular sinus (blue arrow) to trabecular sinus (green arrow) to medullary sinus (orange arrow) to efferent lymphatic vessel (red arrow).**

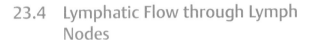

Numerous immune cells are found throughout the lymph node, both in the lumina of the sinuses and in the substance of the node. In addition, the walls of the sinuses are thin and porous. Therefore, it is often challenging to see the exact border of the sinuses.

In the medulla, the medullary sinuses (**Fig. 23.8**, orange arrows) are wider than the subcapsular and trabecular sinuses. The tissue of the medulla (i.e., between the sinuses), which is filled with lymphocytes but contains no nodules, is referred to as **medullary cords** (the nodules in the upper right and lower left are in the cortex; remember sectioning).

Helpful Hint

There are fewer cells in the medullary sinuses than in the subcapsular or trabecular sinuses, and they are wider, so they are more readily identified.

Fig. 23.9 is an image at the junction of the medulla and connective tissue in the hilus, showing a medullary sinus (orange arrows) emptying into a space (black arrows) that eventually connects to efferent lymphatic vessels (red arrows).

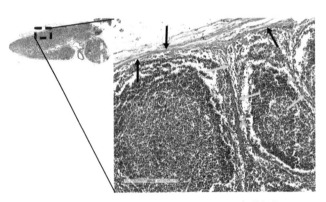

Fig. 23.7   **Cortex of a lymph node showing the capsule (black arrows), trabecula (orange arrows), subcapsular sinus (blue brackets), and trabecular sinuses (green brackets).**

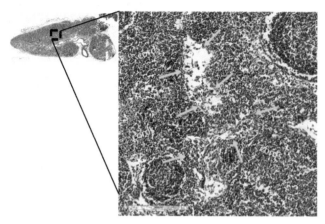

Fig. 23.8   Medulla of a lymph node. A medullary sinus is the pale region in the center; the outer boundary of this sinus is bounded by the orange arrows. The medullary cords are indicated.

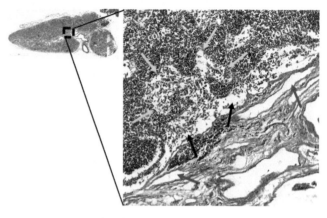

Fig. 23.9   Junction of medulla and hilus of a lymph node showing the medullary sinuses (bounded by orange arrows), medullary cords, and an unnamed lymphatic channel (black arrows) that will connect to efferent lymphatic vessels (red arrows).

Video 23.3   Lymph node sinuses—1

https://www.thieme.de/de/q.htm?p=opn/
tp/308390101/978-1-62623-414-7_c023_
v003&t=video

Video 23.4   Lymph node sinuses—2

Be able to identify:
— Lymph node
— Afferent lymphatic vessels
— Subcapsular sinus
— Trabecular sinus
— Medullary sinus
— Medullary cords
— Efferent lymphatic vessels

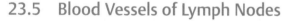

https://www.thieme.de/de/q.htm?p=opn/tp/308390101/978-1-62623-414-7_c023_v004&t=video

23.5   Blood Vessels of Lymph Nodes

As is the case with most organs, an artery enters the lymph node, and a vein leaves it in the same location (blood flowing in opposite directions). The entrance point for these vessels is the hilus. **Fig. 23.10** is from the region of the hilus and shows the artery (A) and vein (V) supplying the lymph node. Note the thicker, more muscular wall in the artery compared to the vein.

Video 23.5   Lymph node vessels

Be able to identify:
— Lymph node
— Artery
— Vein
— Efferent lymphatic vessels

https://www.thieme.de/de/q.htm?p=opn/tp/308390101/978-1-62623-414-7_c023_v005&t=video

Within the lymph node, the artery and vein branch together, with the arteries giving rise to capillary beds in the substance of the lymph node. One specialized feature of the lymph node, called **high endothelial venules** (HEVs), are vessels in which white blood cells move from the bloodstream, through the vessel wall, and into the substance of the lymph node. The process by which a white blood cell moves through a vessel wall in this manner is called **diapedesis** and occurs in many locations.

Fig. 23.11 is a high-magnification image of the cortex of a lymph node, showing an HEV (yellow outline). As the name implies, HEVs are recognized because their endothelial cells are slightly taller than most endothelial cells, which are typically squamous. Close examination reveals that the nuclei lining the lumen of this vessel are rounder instead of flat.

Video 23.6   High endothelial venules

Be able to identify:
— Lymph node
— High endothelial venules

https://www.thieme.de/de/q.htm?p=opn/
tp/308390101/978-1-62623-414-7_c023_v006&t=video

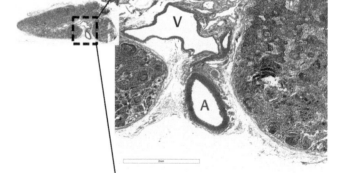

Fig. 23.10 Hilus of a lymph node showing the artery (A) and vein (V) supplying the lymph node.

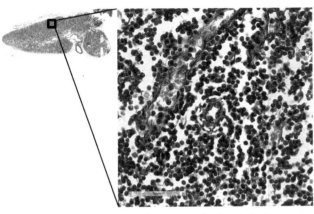

Fig. 23.11 **Cortex of a lymph node showing a high endothelial venule (outlined).**

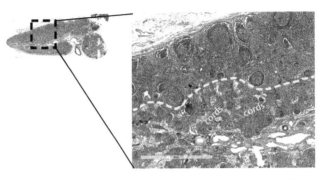

Fig. 23.12 **A portion of a lymph node under low magnification. The dotted line indicates the approximate border of the cortex (above) and medulla (below). Medullary cords are indicated.**

Helpful Hint

In most routine H & E sections, definitive identification of HEVs is not possible, and being able to find them is certainly not high yield. This example is shown because they are often brought up in discussions of immunology. It is important to note that immune cells can arrive at lymph nodes in two ways: through afferent lymphatic vessels and via the bloodstream.

Video 23.7   Lymph node substance

Be able to identify:
— Lymph node
— Cortex
  • Nodules
  • Paracortical zone
— Medulla
  • Medullary cords

https://www.thieme.de/de/q.htm?p=opn/tp/308390101/978-1-62623-414-7_c023_v007&t=video

23.6   Substance of Lymph Nodes

The darker regions of a lymph node (i.e., between the sinuses) will be called here the *substance* of the organ (see **Fig. 23.4**). These regions contain numerous white blood cells, supported by a network of very loose connective tissue laid down by resident fibroblasts and follicular cells.

Fig. 23.12 is a low-power image of a portion of a lymph node. The approximate border between the cortex and medulla is indicated by a yellow dashed line. In the medulla, the medullary cords previously discussed are indicated and are part of the substance of the lymph node. The cortex contains numerous **nodules (follicles)**; most are **secondary nodules** with **germinal centers**. As in other lymphoid tissues (e.g., tonsils), the nodules are rich in **B lymphocytes** but also contain **T lymphocytes**, macrophages, follicular cells, dendritic reticular cells, and fibroblasts. The area of the cortex between the nodules is called the **paracortical zone**, or **deep cortex**, because most of this region is closer to the medulla (most nodes are close to the capsule). The paracortical zone contains mostly T cells (as well as B cells and the other cells mentioned).

Helpful Hint

The border drawn between the cortex and medulla in **Fig. 23.12** is imperfect due to sectioning, as nodules are visible below the line, in what appears to be medulla. The line was drawn largely based on the upper border of the medullary cords and sinuses.

23.7   Cells of Lymph Nodes

Many types of immune and connective tissue cells are found in lymph nodes. Within the lumen of the subcapsular and trabecular sinuses, **lymphocytes** (**Fig. 23.13**, green arrow) are numerous. Cells with flat nuclei and thin cell processes are **reticular cells** (yellow arrow), and **macrophages** (black arrows) can be identified due to their large, euchromatic nuclei. The reticular cells are similar to fibroblasts in that they secrete (and wrap around) the type III collagen fibers that support the lymph node. They also may play a role in the immune response by secreting

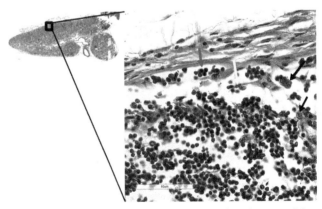

Fig. 23.13 **Cells in the subcapsular sinus of a lymph node. Most of the cells are lymphocytes (green arrow indicates a cluster of five or more of them). Reticular cells have flat nuclei (yellow arrows). Black arrows indicate the much larger macrophages.**

substances that attract lymphocytes and other immune cells. Macrophages are large cells; in lymph nodes they have either a very eosinophilic (upper cell) or "foamy" cytoplasm (lower cell). Macrophages are involved in phagocytosis and antigen presentation.

Fig. 23.14 is an image taken at high magnification of the cortex. A portion of a nodule is to the upper left of the dashed line, and the paracortical zone is to the lower right of the line. As in tonsils, both regions contain abundant lymphocytes; the nodules contain mostly **B lymphocytes**, while **T lymphocytes** dominate the paracortical zone. Macrophages are present in both regions (arrows). Reticular, dendritic, and follicular dendritic cells are more challenging to find because of the abundance of lymphocytes.

In the medulla of the lymph node, many cells are similar to those in the cortex. Of particular note are **plasma cells** (**Fig. 23.15**, yellow arrow), which are abundant in the medullary cords but rarely found in the cortex. Note the cytoplasmic basophilia and off-centered nucleus. Plasma cells residing here most likely differentiated from B cells that were stimulated in the cortex. These plasma cells release antibodies into the medullary sinuses to flow out of the lymph node via the efferent lymphatic vessel.

Video 23.8   Lymph node cells

Be able to identify:
— Lymph node
— Cortex
   • Lymphocytes
   • Macrophages
   • Reticular cells
— Medulla
   • Plasma cells

https://www.thieme.de/de/q.htm?p=opn/tp/308390101/978-1-62623-414-7_c023_v008&t=video

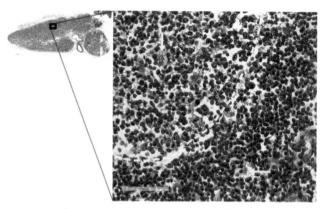

Fig. 23.14 Cells in the cortex of a lymph node. The border between a nodule (upper left) and paracortical zone (lower right) is indicated by the dotted line. Most of the cells in both zones are lymphocytes; macrophages are indicated by the yellow arrows.

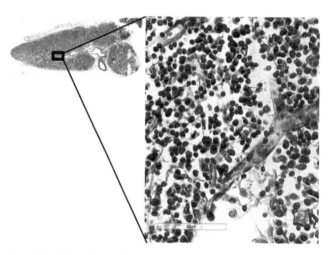

Fig. 23.15 Cells in the medulla of a lymph node showing a plasma cell (yellow arrow).

23.8   Functional Overview of Lymph Nodes

The immune response in lymph nodes (and in general) is very complicated and beyond the scope of this textbook. Here, an overview is provided to place the structures and cells within lymph nodes into context.

Immune cells reach lymph nodes via lymphatic channels or the bloodstream (via high endothelial venules) and reside within the sinuses or the substance of the lymph node. Pathogens and their antigens in tissue fluid are brought to lymph nodes via afferent lymphatic vessels. Lymphatic fluid containing these pathogens flows through the sinuses of lymph nodes. Because the walls of the sinuses are very permeable, lymph flows freely through the substance of the lymph node.

In the germinal centers and paracortical region, macrophages and dendritic cells trap and present antigens from the lymph to B and T lymphocytes, initiating an immune response. Stimulated B cells leave the cortex and migrate to the medulla, where they become resident plasma cells, which actively secrete antibodies into the medullary sinuses. Other stimulated B and T cells can leave the lymph node via the efferent lymphatic vessel to populate sites of infection, where they work to destroy pathogens.

Clinical Correlate

When a person gets a cut or is sick, infectious agents flowing in lymph enter lymph nodes, stimulating T and B lymphocytes. Stimulated T and B lymphocytes divide, increasing the size of the lymph node. These enlarged lymph nodes can be palpated on physical exam and are called **swollen lymph nodes**. The commonly heard term **"swollen glands"** is a misnomer, because lymph nodes are not glands.

Metastatic cancers can spread through the lymphatic system and are often found in lymph nodes that filter lymph draining from the primary cancer. The first nodes that cancer cells spread to are referred to as **sentinel nodes**. Biopsy and assessment of these nodes helps determine the likelihood of metastatic spread from the primary cancer site.

23.9 Chapter Review

There is a net flow of water out of blood capillaries into the surrounding tissue fluid. The tissue fluid is recaptured by lymphatic vessels and returned to the bloodstream. The fluid in lymphatic vessels is called lymph and consists of this tissue fluid plus numerous white blood cells. Before being returned to the bloodstream, lymph passes through at least one lymph node, which functions to filter the lymph and stimulate an immune response to pathogens in the lymph. Lymph arrives at the lymph node via afferent lymphatic vessels and flows through a series of sinuses (subcapsular, trabecular, medullary) before exiting the lymph node via an efferent lymphatic vessel. Blood supply to the lymph node brings additional immune cells via high endothelial vessels. The cortex of a lymph node contains lymphoid nodules like those in tonsils, populated by B lymphocytes, some T lymphocytes, and macrophages and other antigen-presenting cells. Between the nodules is the paracortical zone, which contains the same cell types, but

T lymphocytes predominate over B lymphocytes. The medulla of a lymph node consists of medullary cords and sinuses and has many of these immune cells, as well as plasma cells, which release antibodies into the medullary sinuses to flow out the efferent lymphatic vessel. As lymph flows through a lymph node, immune cells within the node are stimulated by the presence of pathogens in the lymph, becoming cells active in fighting the infection.

Questions and Answers

An online-only section of questions and answers accompanying this chapter is hosted on Thieme's MedOne Education site: https://medone-education.thieme.com. Use the code on the media page at the front of this book to gain access. An institutional license to the site is required to access these questions in an interactive format, and individual users are required to register for an individual account to track results.

24   Spleen

After completing this chapter, you should be able to:
— Identify, at the light microscope level, each of the following:
  • Spleen
    ◦ Hilus
    ◦ Capsule
    ◦ Trabeculae
      ▪ Trabecular arteries and veins
    ◦ White pulp
      ▪ Nodules (including primary and secondary)
      ▪ Central arteries
        – Periarteriolar lymphoid sheath (PALS)
      ▪ Penicillar arteries
    ◦ Red pulp
      ▪ Splenic cords
      ▪ Splenic sinusoids (venous sinusoids)
      ▪ Pulp veins
— Evaluate the distribution of cell types in the spleen
— Outline the function of each cell type and structures listed
— Draw the flow of blood through the spleen
— Indicate conditions that cause splenomegaly and side effects of splenectomy

24.1   Overview of the Spleen

The major functions of the **spleen** include:
1. Filtration of blood and initiation of an immune response to blood-borne pathogens. This is similar to the function of lymph nodes with regard to lymphatic fluid and is largely the function of the region of the spleen known as the **white pulp**.
2. Destruction of aged red blood cells, which is mainly carried out by the **red pulp** of the spleen.

The spleen also serves as a storage reservoir for **platelets**, but this is not readily apparent on histologic slides.

The spleen is located in the upper left abdominal quadrant and supplied by the splenic artery and vein, which pierce the medial aspect of the spleen at its **hilus** (**Fig. 24.1**).

Fig. 24.2 is a scanning image of a portion of the spleen. The spleen is supported by a relatively thick connective tissue **capsule** (blue arrows), which projects into the substance of the organ as **trabeculae** (black arrows). H & E staining clearly demonstrates the two major regions of the spleen: the eosinophilic red pulp and the basophilic white pulp.

Helpful Hint

White pulp is so named because it appears white on fresh (unstained) spleens. Numerous lymphocytes in the white pulp impart these regions with basophilia in H & E sections. The nodules in white pulp are similar to nodules seen in other lymphoid tissues.

Splenic vessels enter the spleen at the hilus, and branches penetrate the **spleen** within the trabeculae as **trabecular arteries** and **veins** (**Fig. 24.3**). Even at low magnification, the artery clearly demonstrates a thicker, more muscular wall than the vein.

Helpful Hint

Note that, due to sectioning, not all trabeculae on a slide will include an artery and vein: some will appear to have only one or the other, while some will appear to have neither.

The spleen filters blood, not lymph, so it does not have afferent lymphatic vessels, and it has only sparse efferent lymphatic vessels (all organs and tissues have efferent lymphatics except the central nervous system). Therefore, identification of lymphatic vessels in the spleen is not necessary.

Video 24.1   Spleen overview

Be able to identify:
— Spleen
— Capsule
— Trabeculae
— Trabecular arteries
— Trabecular veins
— White pulp
— Red pulp
https://www.thieme.de/de/q.htm?p=opn/tp/308390101/978-1-62623-414-7_c024_v001&t=video

24.2   Blood Flow of the Spleen

Understanding the vasculature of the spleen is key to understanding its structure and function (**Fig. 24.4**). Blood enters the spleen through the aforementioned trabecular arteries, which branch into **central arteries (central arterioles)**. These central arteries are within the white pulp of the spleen. The region immediately surrounding central arteries is rich in T cells and is called the **periarterial lymphatic sheath** (PALS). The remainder of the white pulp consists of **nodules** dominated by B cells. The central arterioles give rise to **penicillar arterioles**, which bring blood to the red pulp, ending in specialized **sheathed capillaries**. According to one model, the sheathed capillaries drain directly into **splenic sinusoids (venous sinusoids)** of the red pulp (closed circulation); according to another, they empty into the **splenic cords** of the red pulp, from which blood filters into the sinusoids (open circulation). Either way, the splenic sinusoids of the red pulp collect blood and carry it to **pulp veins**, which drain into trabecular veins.

Helpful Hint

The red pulp of the spleen contains splenic sinusoids and splenic cords. This structure is similar to the medulla of the lymph node; splenic sinusoids are vessels (though here they contain blood), while the splenic cords are the tissue of the spleen.

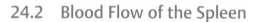

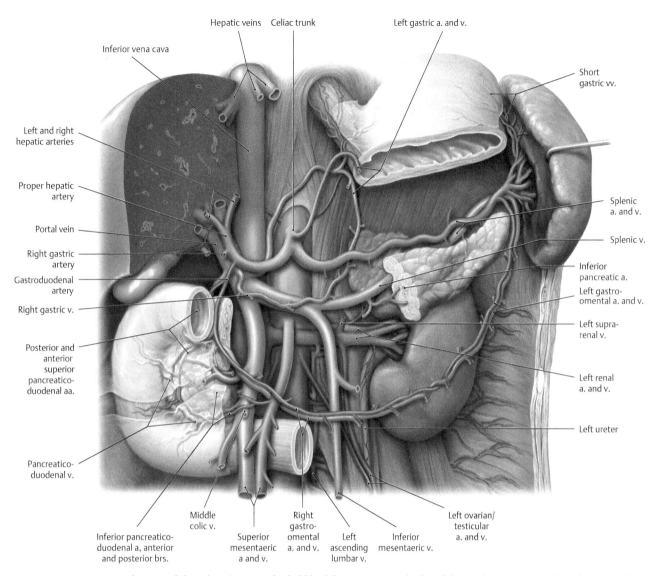

Hepatic veins   Celiac trunk

Inferior vena cava

Left gastric a. and v.

Short gastric vv.

Left and right hepatic arteries

Proper hepatic artery

Portal vein

Right gastric artery

Gastroduodenal artery

Right gastric v.

Posterior and anterior superior pancreatico-duodenal aa.

Pancreatico-duodenal v.

Splenic a. and v.

Splenic v.

Inferior pancreatic a.

Left gastro-omental a. and v.

Left supra-renal v.

Left renal a. and v.

Left ureter

Inferior pancreatico-duodenal a, anterior and posterior brs.

Middle colic v.

Superior mesentaeric a and v.

Right gastro-omental a. and v.

Left ascending lumbar v.

Inferior mesentaeric v.

Left ovarian/testicular a. and v.

Fig. 24.1   Gross anatomic drawing of the spleen (upper right, held back by retractor) and other abdominal organs. From Schuenke M, Schulte E, Schumacher U. *THIEME Atlas of Anatomy. Internal Organs*. Illustrations by Voll M and Wesker K. Second Edition. New York: Thieme Medical Publishers; 2016.

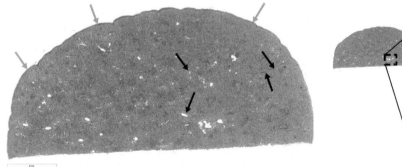

Fig. 24.2   Scanning image of the spleen, showing the capsule (blue arrows) and trabeculae (black arrows).

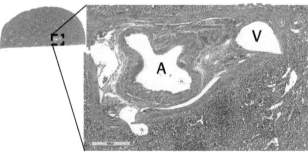

Fig. 24.3   A splenic trabecula (outlined) containing a trabecular artery (A) and vein (V).

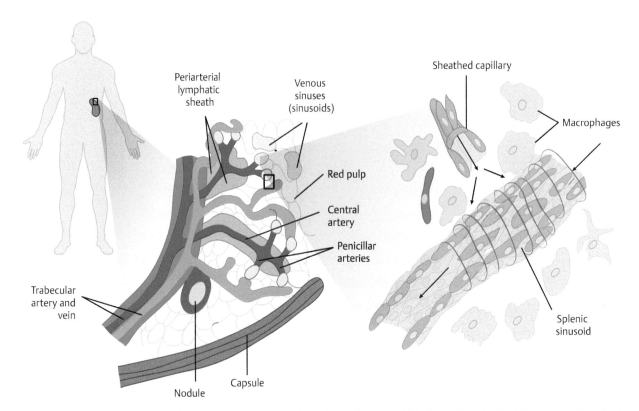

Fig. 24.4   **Central arteries arise from the trabecular arteries at right angles, and course within the white pulp. Penicillar arteries branch at right angles from the central arteries, and enter the surrounding red pulp. Terminal branches of the central arteries form sheathed capillaries, which either connect directly to the venous sinuses (splenic sinusoids; closed circulation), or empty into the red pulp (open circulation). Blood returns via the splenic sinusoids, which ultimately drain back to trabecular veins.**

24.3   White Pulp of the Spleen

White pulp provides the main immune function of the spleen. **Fig. 24.5** shows an area of white pulp. The outlined area is a nodule dominated by lymphocytes. The vessel that is in the center of the nodule is a central artery (central arteriole, arrow). The lymphocytes immediately surrounding the central arteriole are T lymphocytes of the PALS (approximately within the brackets). Lymphocytes in the nodule peripheral to the PALS are mostly B cells.

As shown in **Fig. 24.4**, penicillar arterioles branch at right angles from central arterioles. **Fig. 24.6** shows a nodule with a central arteriole (black arrow) cut at a slightly oblique angle. Smaller vessels in the periphery of the nodule or within the surrounding red pulp are penicillar arterioles (green arrow), which are branches of the central arteriole bringing blood to the red pulp.

When B cells in a nodule are stimulated, they proliferate. Because only one or a few B cells in the nodule are stimulated in this way, this creates nonsymmetrical growth of the white pulp surrounding the central arteriole, so that this artery is seen in the periphery of the nodule (**Fig. 24.7**, arrow). In fact, many central **arterioles** are off-center, like this one, but are recognized as central **arterioles** because they are the largest artery within the nodule. Some nodules, such as the one shown in **Fig 24.8**, develop into secondary nodules with a germinal center. Again, asymmetric proliferation of the lymphocytes has caused the central arteriole (arrow) to cease to occupy the center of the nodule.

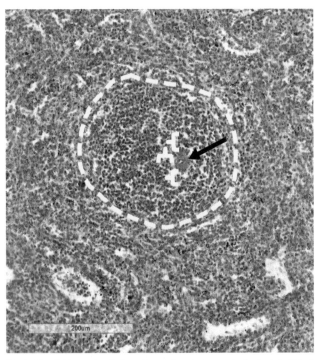

Fig. 24.5   **White pulp of the spleen, showing a central arteriole (black arrow). T lymphocytes immediately surrounding the central arteriole make up the periarterial lymphatic sheath (PALS, yellow brackets). The remainder of the outlined area is a lymphoid nodule rich in B lymphocytes.**

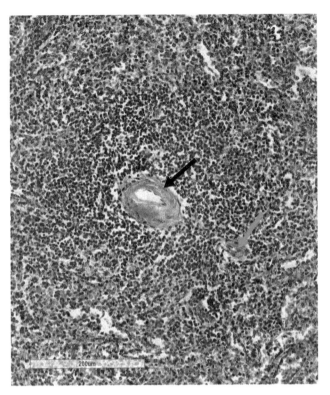

Fig. 24.6   **White pulp of the spleen showing a central arteriole (black arrow) and a penicillar arteriole (green arrow).**

Video 24.2   Spleen white pulp

Be able to identify:
— Spleen
— White pulp
— Central artery (arteriole)
— Penicillar arteriole
— Periarterial lymphatic sheath (PALS)
— Nodule
https://www.thieme.de/de/q.htm?p=opn/tp/308390101/978-1-62623-414-7_c024_v002&t=video

Helpful Hint

The terminal branches of the penicillar arteries are sheathed capillaries, which drain into the splenic sinuses or cords of the red pulp. Sheathed capillaries are surrounded by macrophages that play an important role in filtration of blood. However, they are challenging to find and are not high-yield structures to identify histologically.

24.4   Red Pulp of the Spleen

A major function of the red pulp of the spleen is to filter out aged red blood cells. Therefore, on fresh tissue, this region is red, and in H & E sections these regions are eosinophilic. **Fig. 24.9** is a region of the spleen showing red pulp; a nodule of white pulp is outlined. The red pulp contains splenic sinusoids (SS, venous sinusoids), between which is splenic tissue called splenic cords (of Bilroth, SC).

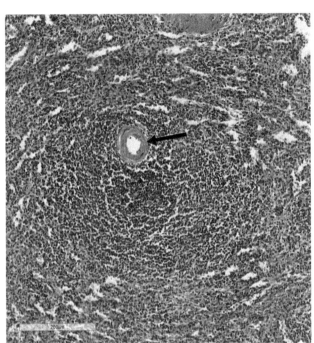

Fig. 24.7   **White pulp of the spleen showing a central arteriole (black arrow), which is off-center due to growth in the nodule.**

Fig. 24.10 is an image of red pulp taken at higher magnification, showing the splenic sinusoids (SS) and splenic cords (SC). The pink lines (green arrows) that form the wall of the splenic sinusoids represent the squamous portion of the endothelial cells and the basement membrane. The nuclei of endothelial cells of the sinusoids bulge into the lumen (black arrows).

The splenic sinusoids coalesce and are tributaries to pulp veins (**Fig. 24.11**, PV), which contain little connective tissue and empty directly into trabecular veins (TV).

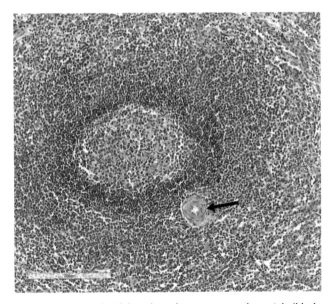

Fig. 24.8   **White pulp of the spleen showing a central arteriole (black arrow), which is off center due to growth in the nodule, which has become a secondary nodule.**

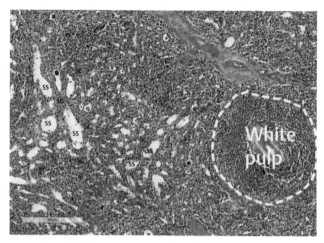

Fig. 24.9   Red pulp of the spleen, low-medium magnification. A nodule of white pulp is indicated. Splenic sinusoids (SS) are the predominant vessels in this region; the pulp tissue here consists of splenic cords (of Bilroth, SC).

Video 24.3   Spleen red pulp

Be able to identify:
— Spleen
— Red pulp
— Splenic sinuses (venous sinusoids)
— Splenic cords (of Bilroth)
— Pulp veins

https://www.thieme.de/de/q.htm?p=opn/tp/308390101/978-1-62623-414-7_c024_v003&t=video

The splenic sinusoids have a unique structure that relates directly to the function of red pulp (see **Fig. 24.4**). In this schematic drawing of a splenic sinusoid, note that the endothelial cells of the splenic sinusoids are very elongated, with slitlike gaps between the cells. The basement membrane (brown rings) of the sinusoids is also incomplete and is organized into rings that encircle the vessel at right angles to the endothelial cells.

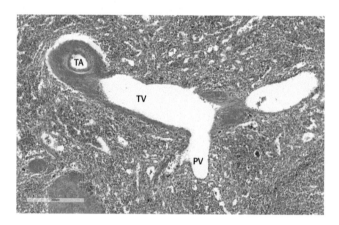

Fig. 24.11 Pulp vein (PV) connected to a trabecular vein (TV). A trabecular artery (TA) is also shown.

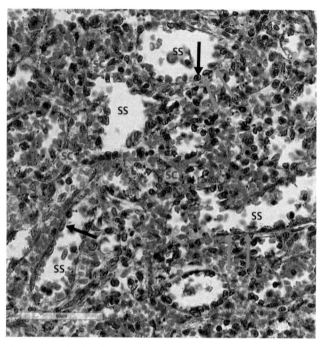

Fig. 24.10 Red pulp of the spleen, high magnification, showing splenic sinusoids (SS) and splenic cords (SC). Endothelial cell nuclei (black arrows) and the basement membrane (green arrows) of the splenic sinusoids are indicated.

Helpful Hint

Many liken the organization of the splenic sinusoids to a leaky barrel. The endothelial cells are similar to the wooden staves, and the basement membrane similar to the metal hoops.

Although the gaps between the endothelial cells are difficult to see in routine H & E-stained tissues, special stains can be used to highlight the reticular fibers of the basement membrane of the spleen, which show up as thin, black threads (**Fig. 24.12**). Splenic sinusoids (SS) and splenic cords (SC) are indicated for orientation. In this image, the basement membrane of the splenic sinusoids demonstrates gaps, large enough to allow flexible cells to pass through.

Video 24.4   Spleen red pulp, reticular stain

Be able to identify:
— Spleen
— Red pulp
— Reticular fibers
— Splenic sinuses (venous sinusoids)
— Splenic cords (of Bilroth)

https://www.thieme.de/de/q.htm?p=opn/tp/308390101/978-1-62623-414-7_c024_v004&t=video

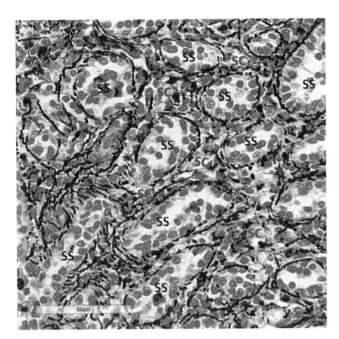

Fig. 24.12 **Red pulp of the spleen, stained for reticular fibers. Splenic sinusoids (SS) and splenic cords (SC) are indicated. The reticular fibers of the basement membrane are highlighted in black with this stain; note the gaps in the basement membrane.**

24.5 Functional Overview of the Spleen

In a very broad sense, the two regions of the spleen—the white and red pulp—perform two major functions: immunity to blood-borne pathogens and red blood cell turnover, respectively (see **Fig. 24.4**). To accomplish this, incoming blood flows through the central arterioles, which are surrounded by T and B cells in the white pulp, stimulating an immune response to pathogens and antigens. Blood then flows through penicillar arteries and sheathed capillaries to the red pulp. Here, there are two theories of splenic circulation. In the **open model**, the sheathed capillaries are not connected to the splenic sinusoids. Blood spills into the splenic cords, and healthy cells maneuver their way through the gaps in the wall of splenic sinusoids to return to the general circulation (**Fig. 24.4**). Aged red blood cells that are unable to pass through the gaps in the splenic sinusoids are recycled by macrophages. In the **closed model**, the sheathed capillaries directly connect to the splenic sinusoids, and the intimate relationship between macrophages in the cords and the splenic sinusoids enables them to remove aged red blood cells. It is likely that the splenic vasculature includes both the open and closed models, such that only a portion of the blood flow to the spleen is filtered by the splenic cords. In either case, aged red blood cells are removed from the circulation, destroyed, and recycled.

24.6 Chapter Review

The spleen is involved in filtering blood, as well as turnover of aged red blood cells and storage of platelets. A fresh sectioned (unstained) spleen shows that it consists of white pulp and red pulp. Because the white pulp is composed of numerous lymphocytes, it appears basophilic in H & E-stained tissues. Understanding the circulation of the spleen is essential to understanding its histology and function. The splenic artery enters the hilus of the spleen and branches into trabecular arteries that penetrate the spleen. Central arteries (central arterioles) branch from trabecular arteries and are surrounded by nodules of the white pulp of the spleen. Pathogens and antigens stimulate an immune response in the nodules of the white pulp, which consist of a periarterial lymphatic sheath of T lymphocytes, surrounded by nodular B lymphocytes. Penicillar arterioles carry blood from the central arterioles to the red pulp, which flows through sheathed capillaries. The red pulp of the spleen consists of splenic sinusoids and splenic cords, which are the vessels and tissue of the red pulp, respectively. The splenic sinusoids are specialized vessels with gaps between the endothelial cells and through the basement membrane. It is here that aged red blood cells are removed from the circulation and destroyed. Blood returns to the circulation via pulp veins, trabecular veins, and the splenic vein.

25   Vessels

After completing this chapter, you should be able to:
— Identify, at the light microscope level, each of the following:
  • Structure of typical vessel
    ◦ Tunics
      ▪ Tunica intima
      ▪ Tunica media
      ▪ Tunica externa (adventitia)
    ◦ Elastic laminae
      ▪ Internal elastic lamina
      ▪ External elastic lamina
    ◦ Cell types
      ▪ Fibroblasts
      ▪ Smooth muscle cells
      ▪ Endothelial cells
  • Arteries
    ◦ Elastic (large) arteries
    ◦ Muscular (medium) arteries
    ◦ Arterioles
  • Veins
    ◦ Venules
    ◦ Medium veins
    ◦ Large veins
  • Capillaries
  • Lymphatic channels
— Identify, at the electron microscope level, each of the following:
  • Capillaries
    ◦ Types
      ▪ Continuous
      ▪ Fenestrated
      ▪ Discontinuous
  • Cells
    ◦ Endothelial cells
    ◦ Pericytes
— Correlate structures visible in electron micrographs with structures in light micrographs, and vice versa
— Outline the function of each cell, structure, and vessel type listed
— Correlate types of vessels with some pathologic conditions

25.1   Overview

The initial chapter in this sequence, **Chapter 16** (Cardiovascular Overview), described the function of the cardiovascular and lymphatic systems and discussed the basic structure of vessels. In addition, the differences between arteries, capillaries, veins, and lymphatic vessels were introduced.

This chapter begins with a quick review of that introductory chapter, integrating new images and features. The remainder of the chapter delves deeper into the types of arteries, veins, and capillaries.

Recall that the major function of the vascular systems is distribution of nutrients, waste products, hormones, and other substances throughout the body. The two components of the vascular system are the **cardiovascular system**, which transports blood, and the **lymphatic system**, which returns tissue fluid (lymph) from the tissues back to the cardiovascular system (**Fig. 25.1**).

25.2   Review of the Basic Features of Vessels

Recall that vessels have three basic components (from inside to outside, **Fig. 25.2**):
1. **Tunica intima** (green double arrow): a simple squamous epithelium, called the **endothelium** (brown arrow), with underlying loose connective tissue
2. **Tunica media** (black double arrow): a thicker layer that consists mostly of smooth muscle and elastic fibers
3. **Tunica externa** (adventitia, blue double arrow): dense irregular connective tissue

In addition, some vessels have elastic laminae, such that the **internal elastic lamina** (yellow dotted line) is situated between the intima and media, and the **external elastic lamina** is between the media and externa.

Video 25.1   Vessel layers

Be able to identify:
— Blood vessel
  • Tunica intima
    ◦ Endothelial cells
  • Tunica media
  • Tunica externa (adventitia)
  • Internal elastic lamina
  • External elastic lamina (position of)
https://www.thieme.de/de/q.htm?p=opn/tp/308390101/978-1-62623-414-7_c025_v001&t=video

Also recall the types of vessels. **Arteries** (arterioles, black outline in **Fig. 25.3**) have thicker walls, due to more developed muscle in the tunica media, compared to **veins** (venules, yellow outline) and **lymphatic vessels** (green outline). Veins typically have more connective tissue than lymphatic vessels, while small lymphatic vessels have numerous valves (not shown) and numerous white blood cells in the lumen. Finally, **capillaries** (arrow) are the smallest vessels, being composed of a single layer of endothelial cells with no tunica media or externa.

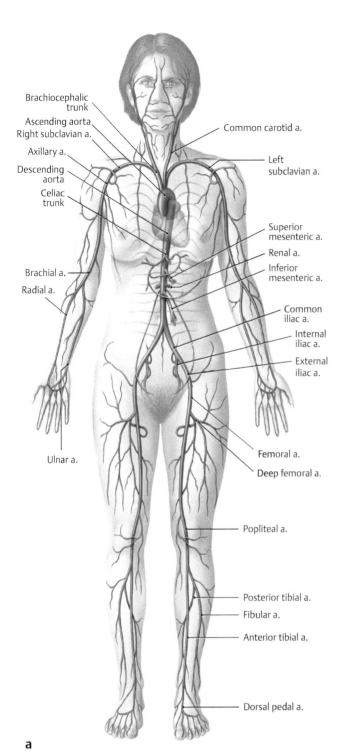

Brachiocephalic trunk
Ascending aorta
Right subclavian a.
Axillary a.
Descending aorta
Celiac trunk
Brachial a.
Radial a.
Ulnar a.

Common carotid a.
Left subclavian a.
Superior mesenteric a.
Renal a.
Inferior mesenteric a.
Common iliac a.
Internal iliac a.
External iliac a.
Femoral a.
Deep femoral a.
Popliteal a.
Posterior tibial a.
Fibular a.
Anterior tibial a.
Dorsal pedal a.

a

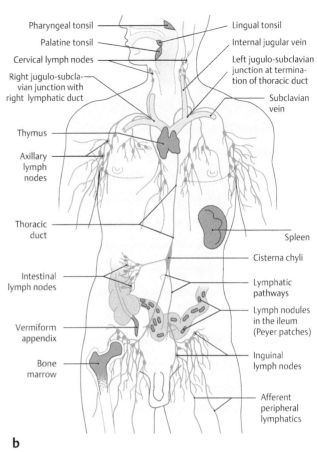

Pharyngeal tonsil
Palatine tonsil
Cervical lymph nodes
Right jugulo-subcla-vian junction with right lymphatic duct
Thymus
Axillary lymph nodes
Thoracic duct
Intestinal lymph nodes
Vermiform appendix
Bone marrow

Lingual tonsil
Internal jugular vein
Left jugulo-subclavian junction at termina-tion of thoracic duct
Subclavian vein
Spleen
Cisterna chyli
Lymphatic pathways
Lymph nodules in the ileum (Peyer patches)
Inguinal lymph nodes
Afferent peripheral lymphatics

b

Fig. 25.1 **(a) Cardiovascular and (b) lymphatic systems. From Schuenke M, Schulte E, Schumacher U.** *THIEME Atlas of Anatomy. Internal Organs.* **Illustrations by Voll M and Wesker K. Second Edition. New York: Thieme Medical Publishers; 2016**

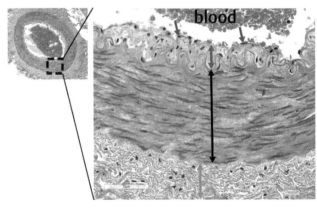

Fig. 25.2 **Structure of a typical blood vessel (artery). Blood in the lumen is indicated. The double arrows indicate the extent of the layers: green, tunica intima; black, tunica media; blue, tunica externa. The brown arrows indicate nuclei of endothelial cells. The wavy dotted line is over a portion of the internal elastic lamina.**

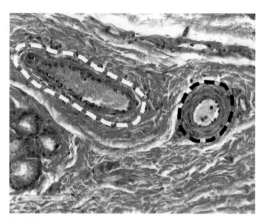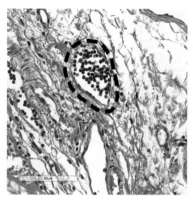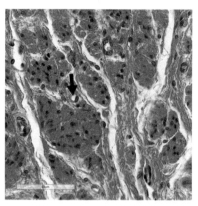

Fig. 25.3 Comparison of types of vessels, showing a vein (venule, yellow outline), artery (arteriole, black outline), lymphatic vessel (green outline), and capillary (arrow).

Video 25.2   Esophagus showing blood vessels

Be able to identify:
— Artery/arteriole
— Vein/venule
— Capillary

https://www.thieme.de/de/q.htm?p=opn/tp/308390101/978-1-62623-414-7_c025_v002&t=video

Video 25.3   Lymph node showing lymphatic vessels

Be able to identify:
— Lymphatic vessel

https://www.thieme.de/de/q.htm?p=opn/tp/308390101/978-1-62623-414-7_c025_v003&t=video

this region (outlined), which mainly consists of elastic fibers with some collagen.

The tunica externa (adventitia) is dense irregular connective tissue and mostly consists of collagen (**Fig. 25.4**, green arrows), with some elastic fibers. Like other connective tissues, these matrix fibers are secreted by resident fibroblasts, which account for most of the nuclei in this region.

As mentioned, in many vessels, there are elastic sheets that separate the layers of the blood vessel wall:
1. Internal elastic lamina (**Fig. 25.4**, purple arrows) between the tunica intima and tunica media
2. External elastic lamina (**Fig. 25.4**, blue arrows, barely visible) between the tunica media and tunica externa

Following are some rules of thumb regarding the elastic laminae:
1. They are more commonly found in arteries than in veins.
2. They are more often present in larger vessels than in smaller ones.
3. The external elastic lamina is not common, but the internal elastic lamina can be seen in many vessels.

25.3   Details on the Structure of Vessels

The tunica intima has three components. The brown arrows in **Fig. 25.4** indicate **endothelial cells**, simple squamous cells that line the lumen. The loose connective tissue (marked with X's) below the endothelial cells is called the **subendothelial layer**. The **basement membrane** between these two cannot be seen.

Fig. 25.5 is an electron micrograph showing part of an endothelial cell, with a small portion of a second. Endothelial cells are simple squamous; the nuclei of these cells are outside the plane of section. A characteristic feature of endothelial cells (and smooth muscle cells) are numerous **caveolae** (2, **pinocytotic vesicles**), which form vesicles (3) that transport material from the vascular lumen (8) to the connective tissue of the subendothelial layer (9) and vice versa. The label 6 indicates the gap between the two endothelial cells, which extends up and then to the right.

The tunica media in vessels is predominantly made up of smooth muscle cells (especially in arteries), whose nuclei are atypically elongated in the vessel in **Fig. 25.4** (black arrows). The smooth muscle cells secrete most of the extracellular material in

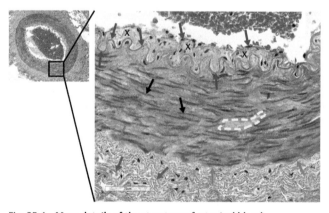

Fig. 25.4 More details of the structure of a typical blood vessel (artery). Brown arrows mark endothelial cells; X's mark subendothelial layer; black arrows indicate smooth muscle cells; yellow outline encloses extracellular material in tunica media; green arrows mark collagen fibers in tunica externa; purple arrows indicate internal elastic lamina; blue arrows mark external elastic lamina.

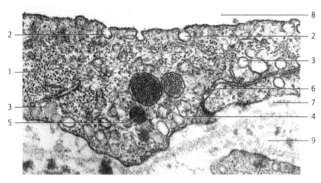

Fig, 25.5 **Electron micrograph of endothelial cell. (1) intermediate filaments; (2) caveolae (pinocytotic vesicles); (3) transport vesicles; (4) Weibel-Palade body (involved in clotting); (5) lysosomes; (6) gap between two endothelial cells; (7) basement membrane; (8) lumen of vessel; (9) connective tissue of subendothelial layer.**

Video 25.4   Details of vessel walls—1

https://www.thieme.de/de/q.htm?p=opn/ tp/308390101/978-1-62623-414-7_c025_ v004&t=video

Video 25.5   Details of vessel walls—2

Be able to identify:
— Tunica intima
  • Endothelial cells
  • Subendothelial layer
— Tunica media
  • Smooth muscle cells
  • Connective tissue
— Tunica externa (adventitia)
  • Fibroblasts
  • Elastic lamina
— Internal elastic lamina
— External elastic lamina
https://www.thieme.de/de/q.htm?p=opn/tp/308390101/978-1-62623-414-7_c025_v005&t=video

A final note on the structure of vessels relates with regards to the blood supply to the cells in the vessel wall. Because diffusion is inefficient over large distances, blood in the lumen of a vessel can provide oxygen and nutrients only to the tunica intima and possibly the inner portion of the tunica media. However, cells in the outer layers of a vessel require nutrients. There are small vessels in the wall of a vessel, called the **vasa vasorum**, that supply cells in the outer regions of the blood vessel; they are derived from branches of the vessel itself in the case of an artery, or from a nearby artery in the case of a vein.

Helpful Hint

Vasa vasorum are not critical to identify but are mentioned because they may be referred to in some instances. The term literally means "vessels of the vessels": small blood vessels within the wall of larger vessels.

25.4   Types of Blood Vessels

Arteries and veins can be categorized into three types each (**Fig. 25.6**). These distinctions are not based purely on size but on histologic features as well. In terms of blood flow, for arteries distributing blood away from the heart, the types of vessels are **elastic (large) arteries**, **muscular (medium) arteries** (in **Fig. 25.6** labeled "Small artery distant from the heart"), and **arterioles**. For veins returning to the heart, the types are **venules**, **medium veins**, and **large veins**.

Helpful Hint

This categorization is convenient. However, the transition between the different types of vessels is gradual; many vessels have histologic features that are "between" categories (e.g., a vessel may have characteristics of both a large elastic and muscular artery).

In addition, there are three types of capillaries; each type has histologic features that reflect its permeability. These are **continuous**, **fenestrated**, and **discontinuous capillaries** (not shown in **Fig. 25.6**, see later image).

From a histologic standpoint, it is easiest to begin with the vessels used in the general description just given: the muscular (medium) artery and its corresponding medium vein. From here, the discussion will proceed to other vessels.

25.4.1   Muscular (Medium) Arteries and Medium Veins

Fig. 25.7 is an image capturing a portion of the wall of a muscular (medium) artery and medium vein where they are adjacent. The lumen of each vessel is indicated, as are the tunicae (double

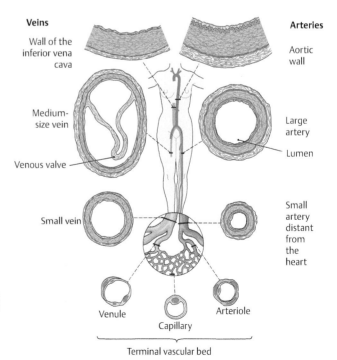

Fig. 25.6   **Types of vessels. From Schuenke M, Schulte E, Schumacher U.** *THIEME Atlas of Anatomy. Internal Organs.* **Illustrations by Voll M and Wesker K. Second Edition. New York: Thieme Medical Publishers; 2016.**

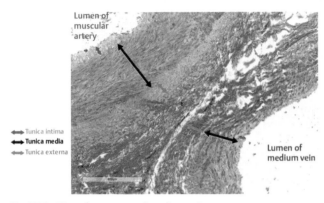

Lumen of
muscular
artery

Tunica intima
Tunica media
Tunica externa

Lumen of
medium vein

Fig. 25.7   **Muscular artery and medium vein.**

arrows). Again, note that the tunica media of the muscular artery contains substantially more smooth muscle than the medium vein, both in thickness of the entire media and in density of muscle cells relative to connective tissue in that layer. The internal elastic lamina is also more prominent in the artery. Typically, the tunica externa of a vein is considered to be more substantial than in an artery, but this is not obvious on this slide.

Video 25.6   Muscular (medium) artery and medium vein

Be able to identify:
— Muscular (medium) artery
— Medium vein
— All regions and structures previously mentioned
https://www.thieme.de/de/q.htm?p=opn/tp/308390101/978-1-62623-414-7_c025_v006&t=video

Fig. 25.8 is an electron micrograph of part of the wall of a muscular artery. The smooth muscle in the tunica media is about four cells thick (labeled "media" with double arrows); one myocyte is indicated (3), and the nucleus of another is labeled (6). The endothelium (1), internal elastic lamina (2), external elastic lamina (4), and adventitia (5) are shown.

25.4.2   Arterioles and Venules

Histologically, arterioles are simply smaller muscular arteries, and venules are smaller medium veins. **Fig. 25.9** shows an arteriole (yellow outline) and venule (blue outline). Note that the arteriole has a more muscular wall than the venule and is rounder. The shape of the venule is irregular, it has a wider lumen, and it has less smooth muscle.

Helpful Hint

Texts differentiate muscular arteries and arterioles based on the number of layers of smooth muscle cells in the tunica media; for example, arterioles have one or two layers of smooth muscle, but muscular arteries have 3–40 layers. Unfortunately, the numbers used by different sources vary, and some add "small arteries" as a category. Therefore, in some cases, as seen with the central artery/ arteriole of the spleen, both terms can be used to describe vessels near these cutoffs. The same is true for venules and medium veins.

Helpful Hint

Remember: when identifying arteries versus veins, or arterioles versus venules, it is best to choose pairs so that you can make a proper comparison. Also, keep in mind that, in smaller vessels, it becomes more challenging to distinguish arterioles from venules because the total thickness of the tunica media is smaller.

Video 25.7   Muscular (medium) artery and vein to arterioles and venules

Be able to identify:
— Muscular artery
— Medium vein
— Arteriole
— Venule
https://www.thieme.de/de/q.htm?p=opn/tp/308390101/978-1-62623-414-7_c025_v007&t=video

Fig. 25.10 is an electron micrograph of part of the wall of an arteriole. This arteriole is very similar to a muscular artery, except that the smooth muscle in the tunica media here (3) is only one cell thick.

Basic Science Correlate: Physiology

Histologically, arterioles are basically smaller muscular arteries. However, physiologically, the difference between arterioles and muscular arteries is substantial.

The diameter of blood vessels is controlled largely by the state of contraction of the smooth muscle in the tunica media. Naturally, smaller vessels have both a smaller lumen and a less substantial total amount of smooth muscle. However, *proportionally*, arterioles have a higher smooth muscle/lumen ratio than muscular arteries, even if this distinction is subtle histologically. Therefore, contraction of smooth muscle in arterioles has a more significant impact on vessel diameter, making arterioles the vessels that have a larger impact on regulation of blood flow.

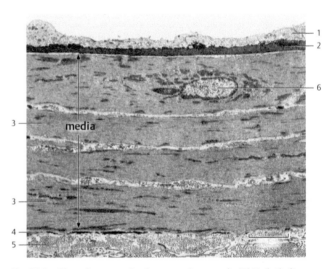

media

Fig. 25.8   **Muscular artery in electron micrograph. (1) Endothelium; (2) internal elastic lamina; (3) smooth muscle cell in tunica media; (4) external elastic lamina; (5) tunica externa (adventitia); (6) nucleus of smooth muscle cell.**

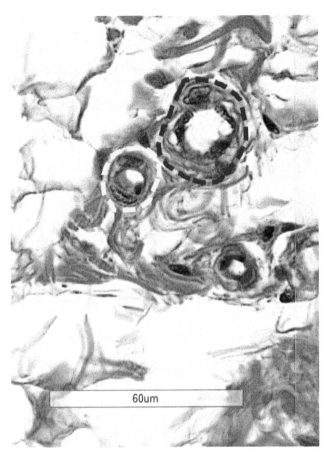

Fig. 25.9 Arteriole (yellow outline) and venule (blue outline).

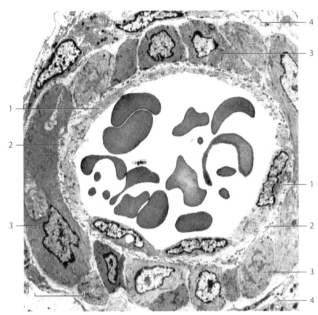

Fig. 25.10 Arteriole in electron micrograph. (1) Endothelium; (2) subendothelial connective tissue; (3) smooth muscle cell in tunica media; (4) tunica externa (adventitia).

Video 25.8 Elastic artery

Be able to identify:
— Elastic artery
https://www.thieme.de/de/q.htm?p=opn/
tp/308390101/978-1-62623-414-7_c025_
v008&t=video

25.4.3 Elastic Arteries

It is not surprising that elastic (large) arteries are vessels that contain abundant elastic tissue, in the form of tubes of elastin between layers of smooth muscle cells within the tunica media. **Fig. 25.11** shows an example of an elastic artery, focusing on the elastic fibers (yellow arrows) that are prominent in the tunica media. Most of the nuclei in the media belong to smooth muscle cells, which are largely responsible for secreting the elastic fibers.

Elastic arteries are vessels that receive blood from the ventricles, such as the aorta, pulmonary trunk, proximal portions of the brachiocephalic artery, left common carotid, and left subclavian arteries.

Basic Science Correlate: Physiology

Physiologically, elastic arteries serve two purposes:
— They expand during ventricular systole (contraction), accepting the bolus of ejected blood.
— They recoil during diastole (ventricular relaxation), propelling blood forward.
So, although they do not "contract" to create a propulsive force, they do assist the ventricles in maintaining blood flow during diastole (when the ventricles are not contracting).

Fig. 25.12 is a similar elastic artery stained with a special stain called **resorcin**, which highlights the elastic fibers within this vessel (yellow arrows in inset indicate elastic fibers in the tunica media). Recall that the large dark bands (orange arrows) are artifacts caused by folding of the vessel during tissue preparation (see **Chapter 1**).

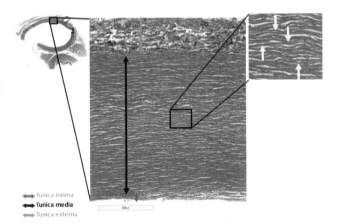

Tunica intima
Tunica media
Tunica externa

Fig. 25.11 Elastic (large) artery. The three tunics are indicated. The tunica media is dominated by large sheets of elastic fibers (yellow arrows in enlarged region to the right).

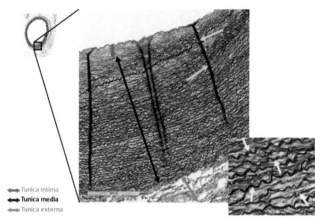

→ Tunica intima
→ **Tunica media**
→ Tunica externa

Fig. 25.12 **Elastic (large) artery, stained for elastic fibers (resorcin stain). The three tunics are indicated. The tunica media is dominated by large sheets of elastic fibers (yellow arrows in enlarged region to the right). The large dark bands (thick orange arrows) are artifacts.**

Video 25.9   Elastic artery—elastic stain

Be able to identify:
— Elastic artery
https://www.thieme.de/de/q.htm?p=opn/
tp/308390101/978-1-62623-414-7_c025_
v009&t=video

25.4.4   Large Veins

Large veins have a unique characteristic relative to all other vessels. In addition to the circularly arranged smooth muscle in the tunica media, they have numerous, *longitudinally* oriented bundles of smooth muscle in the *tunica externa (adventitia)*.

The purpose of this substantial amount of extra smooth muscle is unclear. It is possible that these muscle bundles are involved in contraction similar to gut peristalsis, assisting venous return to the atria under low pressures.

Helpful Hint

Therefore, in a cross section of a large vein, the smooth muscle in the tunica media is cut longitudinally, while the smooth muscle in the tunica adventitia is cut in cross section. In a longitudinal section of a large vein, these orientations are reversed.

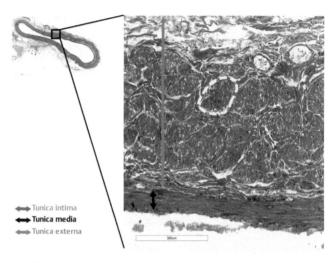

→ Tunica intima
→ **Tunica media**
→ Tunica externa

Fig. 25.13 **Large vein in cross section (the vein is collapsed). The three tunics are indicated. Large bundles of longitudinally oriented smooth muscle appear in cross section in the tunica externa (yellow outline is one bundle).**

Fig. 25.13 is a cross section of a large vein (not a longitudinal section); it is thin-walled, so it is collapsed. The predominant feature of large veins is the numerous bundles of smooth muscle (one bundle outlined) in the tunica externa. Note that, like all vessels except capillaries, this vessel still has circularly arranged smooth muscle in the tunica media.

Video 25.10 Large vein

Be able to identify:
— Large vein
https://www.thieme.de/de/q.htm?p=opn/
tp/308390101/978-1-62623-414-7_c025_v010&t=video

25.4.5   Capillaries

Capillaries are the smallest vessels (see **Fig. 25.6**) and consist of only endothelial cells and supporting basement membrane. The thin wall of these vessels maximizes diffusion for efficient nutrient and waste exchange between the blood and surrounding tissues.

Another cell type associated with capillaries is the **pericyte**. Pericytes lie outside the endothelial lining but form an incomplete layer of cells. They share characteristics with both endothelial cells and smooth muscle cells and are thought to be stem cells for vessel cells and other cell types such as osteoblasts and adipocytes.

Fig. 25.14 shows a capillary (arrow) within a bundle of smooth muscle. In H & E-stained tissues, capillaries are recognized as almost perfectly round rings, with a thin wall representing the cytoplasm of the endothelial cell. The diameter of the lumen is typically the size of a red blood cell. As shown in this capillary, an endothelial cell nucleus is commonly seen that bulges into the lumen of the capillary.

There are three types of capillaries. The classification of capillaries is based on their ultrastructural characteristics, which relate to the permeability of the vessel. These types, listed in order of increasing permeability, include (**Fig. 25.15**):

1. **Continuous capillaries** are lined with endothelial cells with tight junctions and a complete basement membrane.
2. **Fenestrated capillaries** have endothelial cells with tight junctions and a complete basement membrane, but the endothelial cells have **fenestrations** (pores) in them.
3. **Discontinuous capillaries** (or **sinusoids**) have endothelial cells with fenestrations and gaps between the cells and an incomplete basement membrane (having gaps).

Continuous Capillaries

Continuous capillaries (**Fig. 25.16**) consist of endothelial cells (1, 4) joined by tight junctions and a complete basement membrane (basal lamina, 2). Typically, endothelial cells in continuous capillaries have numerous **caveoli/pinocytotic vesicles** and **transport vesicles** (transport vesicles labeled at 7) that carry molecules across the endothelium by transcytosis. A pericyte (3) is shown, recognized because it shares the basement membrane with the endothelial cells; note near 2 that the basement membrane of the endothelial cells splits to pass on either side of the pericyte.

> **Helpful Hint**
>
> Pericytes form an *incomplete* layer of cells that share a basement membrane with endothelial cells. If this were an arteriole, the cells in the position of the pericyte would be smooth muscle of the tunica media. However, smooth muscle cells of the tunica media form a complete layer around the endothelial cells and have a basement membrane not shared with the endothelial cell.

Although all types of capillaries are very permeable, continuous capillaries are the least permeable of the three types of capillaries. Continuous capillaries are located in tissues such as skeletal muscle, bone, cartilage, and generic connective tissues.

Fenestrated Capillaries

Fig. 25.17 shows a portion of the wall of a fenestrated capillary. As in continuous capillaries, fenestrated capillaries are lined by a complete layer of endothelial cells (2) joined by tight junctions and a complete basement membrane (red arrows). The distinguishing feature between fenestrated and continuous capillaries is that the endothelial cells of fenestrated capillaries have numerous **fenestrations** (black arrows), which are pores through the endothelial cell. In most

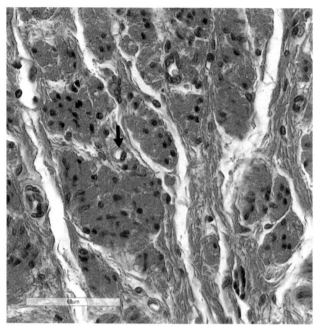

Fig. 25.14 **Capillary (arrow).**

organs with fenestrated capillaries (except the kidney), a **diaphragm** spans the gap of the fenestrations, seen here as a thin line. A fenestrated capillary from the kidney is shown in **Fig. 25.18**; note the fenestrations without diaphragms (black arrows). Fenestrated capillaries typically have fewer pinocytotic vesicles than continuous capillaries do.

Fenestrated capillaries are more permeable than continuous capillaries and are located in organs that require more robust exchange, or exchange of larger molecules, such as endocrine organs and some organs of the digestive tract.

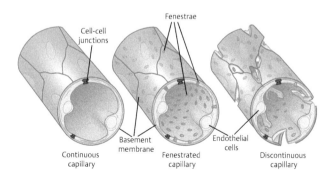

Fig. 25.15 **Types of capillaries.**

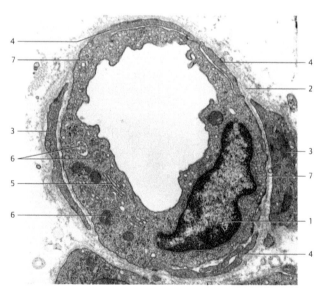

Fig. 25.16 **Continuous capillary in electron micrograph. (1) Endothelial cell nucleus; (2) basement membrane (basal lamina); (3) pericytes; (4) endothelial cell; (5) Golgi apparatus; (6) Weibel-Palade bodies; (7) transport vesicles.**

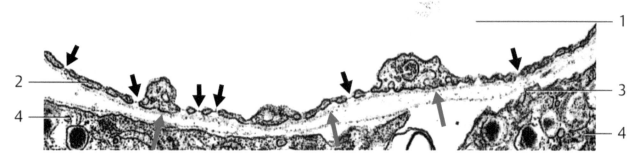

Fig. 25.17 **Fenestrated capillary in electron micrograph. (1) Capillary lumen; (2) endothelial cell; (3) cell membrane of endocrine gland cell; (4) cytoplasm of endocrine gland cell. Black arrows point to fenestrations (note the dark line [diaphram] spanning the fenestration); red arrows point to the basement membrane (basal lamina).**

Discontinuous Capillaries

Fig. 25.19 shows a portion of the wall of a discontinuous capillary. Discontinuous capillaries, also known as discontinuous sinusoids, sinusoidal capillaries, or simply sinusoids, consist of fenestrated endothelial cells (2) without diaphragms, with large gaps between the cells (arrows), and an incomplete or absent basement membrane (basal lamina, not visible in this image).

Discontinuous capillaries are the most permeable capillaries; the large gaps and fenestrations in these vessels permit everything except the formed elements (red blood cells, white blood cells, platelets) to pass through. The result is that the plasma membranes of cells supplied by these capillaries (such as the hepatocytes in **Fig. 25.19**) are essentially bathed in plasma.

Discontinuous sinusoids are found in the liver, which will be discussed later (see **Chapter 33**). Vessels with similar structure to discontinuous sinusoids are the venous sinuses of the spleen (splenic sinusoids; **Chapter 24**) and the sinuses of lymph nodes (**Chapter 23**).

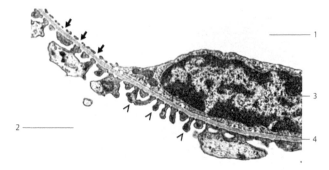

Fig. 25.18 **Fenestrated capillary of the kidney in electron micrograph. (1) Capillary lumen; (2) urinary (Bowman) space; (3) endothelial cell nucleus; (4) basement membrane. Black arrows indicate fenestrations; arrowheads point to podocyte foot processes (see Chapter 36 for discussion of podocytes and the urinary space).**

Strictly speaking, the terms "sinus" and "sinusoids" refer to vessels with large diameters. Most discontinuous capillaries have a wide diameter, as in the liver, so many histologists simply say "sinusoids" when referring to discontinuous capillaries. However, some capillaries with a continuous endothelial structure have a wide diameter and are also called sinuses or sinusoids (e.g., bone marrow). In addition, these terms are used to describe some veins as well. And, of course, there are the air sinuses in the skull. Therefore, when describing the histology and resulting permeability of capillaries, the terms "discontinuous" or "discontinuous capillary" or "discontinuous sinusoids" are preferred over simply "sinusoids."

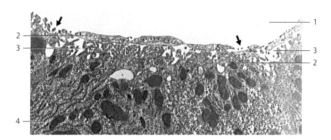

Fig. 25.19 **Discontinuous capillary of the liver in electron micrograph. (1) Capillary lumen; (2) endothelial cell; (3) space of Disse; (4) liver cell (hepatocyte). Arrows indicate gaps.**

Capillaries form extensive networks called **capillary beds** (**Fig. 25.20**). A single arteriole can give rise to hundreds of capillaries in a capillary bed. This increases surface area for extensive molecular exchange between the blood and tissues supplied by the capillary network.

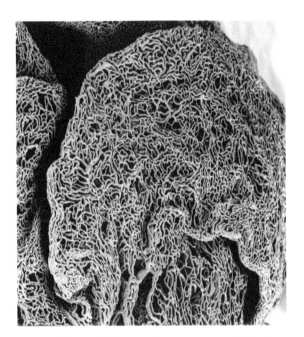

Fig. 25.20 Capillary bed. This image is a cast, created by injecting a resin into a capillary network and allowing that resin to harden, then removing the tissues, leaving the hardened resin, which represents the lumina of the vessels. Nearly all the vessels in this image are capillaries.

25.5 Chapter Review

Vessels carry fluid (blood or lymph) around the body. Arteries carry blood away from the heart, which flows into capillaries, the site of gas exchange. Blood from capillaries flows back to the heart via veins, and lymphatic vessels carry tissue fluid that leaks from capillaries and brings it back to the circulatory system. Vessels are composed of three layers: tunica intima, tunica media, and tunica adventitia. Of note are the endothelial cells of the tunica intima, which form the inner lining of vessels, and the smooth muscle in the tunica media. Arteries and veins can be differentiated because arteries have thicker walls than veins. Lymphatic channels have thinner walls than veins, have valves in the smallest lymphatic vessels, and typically have numerous white blood cells in the lumen. Capillaries are small and consist of only endothelial cells. There are different types of arteries, veins, and capillaries. Muscular arteries are characterized by a thick tunica media. Arterioles are similar to muscular arteries but are much smaller and regulate blood flow to tissues. Elastic arteries feature abundant elastic fibers in the tunica media that allow them to accept boluses of blood ejected from the heart; elastic recoil propels that blood forward during diastole. Venules are smaller veins, while large veins are characterized by large bundles of smooth muscle oriented longitudinally in the tunica externa. There are three types of capillaries. Continuous capillaries consist of endothelial cells without fenestrations, have a complete basement membrane, and are the least permeable. Fenestrated capillaries have fenestrations in the endothelial cells and are more permeable than continuous capillaries. Discontinuous capillaries are the most permeable because the endothelial cells have large fenestrations, large gaps between the cells, and an incomplete basement membrane. Capillary networks are extensive and are called capillary beds.

Questions and Answers

An online-only section of questions and answers accompanying this chapter is hosted on Thieme's MedOne Education site: https://medone-education.thieme.com. Use the code on the media page at the front of this book to gain access. An institutional license to the site is required to access these questions in an interactive format, and individual users are required to register for an individual account to track results.

26   Heart

After completing this chapter, you should be able to:
— Identify, at the light microscope level, each of the following:
  • Cardiac muscle tissue
    ◦ Intercalated disks
  • Layers of the heart
    ◦ Endocardium
    ◦ Myocardium
    ◦ Epicardium
  • Ventricles
  • Atria
  • Valves
    ◦ Atrioventricular
    ◦ Semilunar
      ▪ Annulus fibrosus
      ▪ Purkinje fibers
— Outline the function of each structure listed
— Outline the conduction system of the heart and the role of the anulus fibrosus in this system
— Draw the flow of blood through the circulatory system

26.1   Review of Cardiac Muscle

This chapter focuses on the wall of the heart and its associated structures (e.g., valves). Because a major component of the heart is **cardiac muscle**, it is useful to review the histology of cardiac muscle.

Fig. 26.1 is an image of cardiac muscle in longitudinal section. Recall from **Chapter 14** that cardiac muscle is composed of large, branched muscle cells, which are connected to each other by **intercalated disks**. These intercalated disks (arrow), which are unique to cardiac muscle tissue, include **adherent junctions** for cell-cell strength as well as **gap junctions** to allow electrical synchrony. Like skeletal muscle, cardiac muscle fibers are packed with myofibrils that are in-register and give the tissue a striated appearance in longitudinal section. In contrast to skeletal muscle, each cardiac muscle cell has a single nucleus that is centrally located.

In cross section (**Fig. 26.2**), cardiac muscle is characterized by cells with a significant amount of highly eosinophilic cytoplasm surrounding the centrally located nucleus. Because the cells do not taper, most cells are the approximately the same size, regardless of whether the cell is cut through the nucleus or not. Irregularly shaped cells signify branch points.

Video 26.1   Cardiac muscle

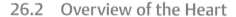

Be able to identify:
— Cardiac muscle
— Intercalated disks
https://www.thieme.de/de/q.htm?p=opn/tp/308390101/978-1-62623-414-7_c026_v001&t=video

26.2   Overview of the Heart

The **heart** is an in-line pump for the cardiovascular system, continuous with the veins and arteries that are attached to it (vena cava, pulmonary veins, pulmonary artery, and aorta). The heart has four chambers: **right atrium**, **left atrium**, **right ventricle**, and **left ventricle**. Atrioventricular valves (right and left) separate the atria from the ventricles. The **right atrioventricular valve** is also referred to as the **tricuspid valve**, and the **left atrioventricular valve** is called the **bicuspid** or **mitral valve**. Semilunar valves (**pulmonary** and **aortic**) separate the ventricles from the arteries into which they discharge: the **pulmonary artery** and **aorta**.

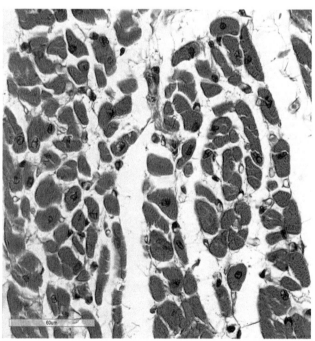

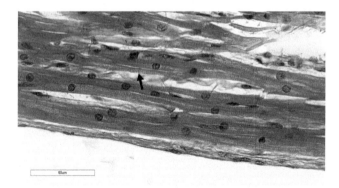

Fig. 26.1   **Cardiac muscle in longitudinal section. The arrow indicates an intercalated disk.**

Fig. 26.2   **Cardiac muscle in cross section.**

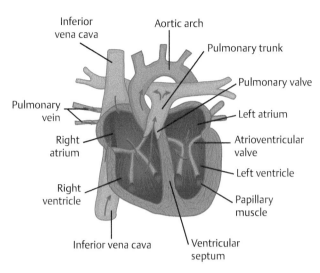

Fig. 26.3 **Anatomy of the heart. Green arrows represent the direction of blood flow.**

Fig. 26.3 is a drawing of the internal anatomy of the heart; arrows represent blood flow through the heart. Deoxygenated blood from the tissues returns to the right atrium via the **venae cavae** and **coronary sinus** (not shown). The right atrium pumps blood to the right ventricle, which propels blood through the pulmonary artery to the **lungs** for oxygenation. Blood returns from the lungs via **pulmonary veins**, which drain into the left atrium. The left atrium pumps blood to the left ventricle, which propels blood to the tissues via the aorta (note that the arrow leading from the left ventricle to the aorta passes behind the pulmonary artery).

26.3 Wall of the Heart

Like the vessels, the wall of the heart is organized into three layers (**Fig. 26.4**):

1. **Endocardium** consists of a simple squamous endothelium (plus basement membrane) with an underlying subendo-cardial region consisting of connective tissue, with some smooth muscle and nerves.
2. **Myocardium** is cardiac muscle with connective tissue elements.

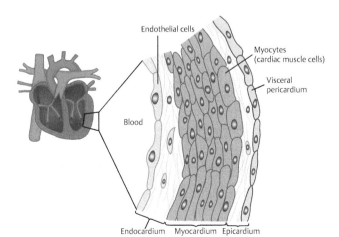

Fig. 26.4 **Layers of the wall of the heart.**

3. **Epicardium** is mostly adipose tissue, with an outer **visceral pericardium**, a simple squamous epithelium covering the outer surface of the heart.

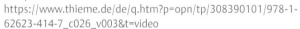

Helpful Hint

Note the similarities between the wall of the heart and blood vessels. The major differences are that the muscle in the myocardium is cardiac muscle, and the epicardium is covered by a simple squamous epithelium (visceral pericardium).

Fig. 26.5 is a scanning view of a section through the wall of a ventricle; the lumen and pericardial cavity are indicated. The three layers of the wall are readily seen. The endocardium is thin, so it is barely visible at this magnification.

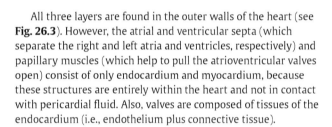

Video 26.2 Heart wall layers

Be able to identify:
— Endocardium
— Myocardium
— Epicardium

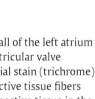

https://www.thieme.de/de/q.htm?p=opn/tp/308390101/978-1-62623-414-7_c026_v003&t=video

All three layers are found in the outer walls of the heart (see **Fig. 26.3**). However, the atrial and ventricular septa (which separate the right and left atria and ventricles, respectively) and papillary muscles (which help to pull the atrioventricular valves open) consist of only endocardium and myocardium, because these structures are entirely within the heart and not in contact with pericardial fluid. Also, valves are composed of tissues of the endocardium (i.e., endothelium plus connective tissue).

26.4 Heart Chambers

Fig. 26.6 is a scanning image showing the wall of the left atrium and ventricle, and a cusp of the left atrioventricular valve (arrows). This slide was stained using a special stain (trichrome) that is similar to H & E but also stains connective tissue fibers an "aqua" color. This staining highlights connective tissue in the endocardium and valve.

Note that:
1. The myocardium in the ventricle is thicker than in the atrium.
2. The endocardium is thicker in the atrium than in the ventricle.
3. There are vessels in the epicardium: the coronary arteries and cardiac veins that supply the heart

Video 26.3 Atrium and ventricle

Be able to identify:
— Atrium
— Ventricle
— Atrioventricular valve
— Layers of each chamber

https://www.thieme.de/de/q.htm?p=opn/tp/308390101/978-1-62623-414-7_c026_v004&t=video

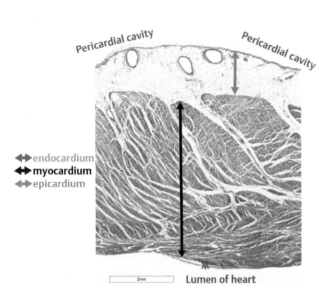

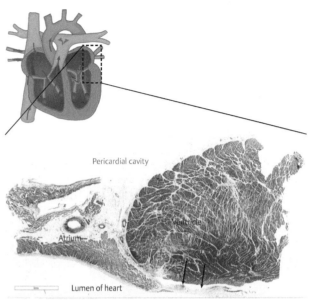

Fig. 26.5   Layers of the wall of the heart in scanning view. The lumen of the heart (containing blood) and the pericardial cavity (containing pericardial fluid) are indicated. The three layers of the heart wall are shown.

Fig. 26.6   Scanning view of the left atrium, left ventricle, and intervening cusp of the left atrioventricular valve (arrows; valve lies in what would be the "open" position). The lumen of the heart and pericardial cavity are indicated. The larger image is rotated 90 degrees counterclockwise relative to the orientation drawing.

Clinical Correlate

The vessels in the epicardium supply the cardiac muscle cells in the myocardium. **Atherosclerotic plaques** in the coronary arteries are common and are a contributing factor to **coronary artery disease**. Plaque rupture stimulates clot formation, which causes obstruction of the affected vessel (**coronary thrombosis**). Cardiac muscle cells supplied by the obstructed vessel become ischemic (**myocardial ischemia**, experienced as **angina pectoris**) and may die (**myocardial infarction**, or **heart attack**).

Fig. 26.7 is a scanning view of the anterior wall of the right ventricle and pulmonary artery (yellow line), as well as the pulmonary semilunar valve (arrows). The myocardium of the right ventricle is not as thick as the myocardium of the left

ventricle. The characteristic features of the pulmonary artery (elastic artery) are challenging to appreciate in longitudinal section, but its position connected to the ventricle allows proper identification.

Video 26.4   Right ventricle and pulmonary artery

Be able to identify:
— Ventricle
— Elastic artery
— Semilunar valve
— Layers of each chamber
https://www.thieme.de/de/q.htm?p=opn/tp/308390101/978-1-62623-414-7_c026_v005&t=video

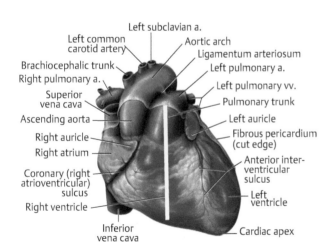

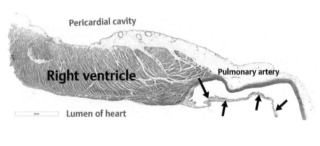

Fig. 26.7a, b   Scanning view of the anterior wall of the right ventricle and pulmonary artery and intervening pulmonary valve (arrows; valve lies in what would be the "open" position), sectioned as shown by the yellow line in the anatomic drawing. From Schuenke M, Schulte E, Schumacher U. *THIEME Atlas of Anatomy. Internal Organs*. Illustrations by Voll M and Wesker K. Second Edition. New York: Thieme Medical Publishers; 2016.

Fig. 26.8 is a scanning image that is difficult to visualize, but is shown by the dotted line in the anatomical drawing. The aorta passes posterior to the pulmonary artery. This section is through the anterior wall of the left ventricle, aorta, and aortic valve (arrows), but it also includes the posterior wall of the pulmonary artery as well as the connective tissue that is shared between these great vessels.

Video 26.5 Left ventricle, aorta, and pulmonary artery

Be able to identify:
— Ventricle
— Elastic artery
— Semilunar valve
— Layers of each chamber
https://www.thieme.de/de/q.htm?p=opn/tp/308390101/978-1-62623-414-7_c026_v006&t=video

26.5 Heart Valves

Valves in the heart prevent backflow of blood. **Fig. 26.9** is a medium-power view of a valve, showing that it has a core of connective tissue, covered by endothelial cells (arrows). These endothelial cells are continuous with the endothelium lining the chambers of the heart.

Fig. 26.10 is a similar image, taken from the base of the valve. In this region, there is a thickening of connective tissue called the **anulus fibrosus** (outlined; sometimes spelled annulus fibrosus, and sometimes with **cordis** added to distinguish it from the anulus fibrosus of an intervertebral disk).

Video 26.6 Valves and anulus fibrosus

Be able to identify:
— Valve
— Anulus fibrosus
https://www.thieme.de/de/q.htm?p=opn/tp/308390101/978-1-62623-414-7_c026_v007&t=video

Helpful Hint

In the setting of a gross anatomy lab or in patients, it is necessary to distinguish between the right and left sides of the heart, including differentiating between the right and left chambers and valves and between the aorta and pulmonary artery. In histologic slides and images, however, the exact source of the tissue is not always provided. The thickness of the ventricles can sometimes be of assistance, because the myocardium of the left ventricle is much thicker than the myocardium of the right ventricle. However, in a single slide or image in which comparison is not possible, it is often sufficient to identify structures without indicating which side (e.g., ventricle, atrioventricular valve, elastic artery).

Basic Science Correlate: Physiology

The four valves of the heart are in approximately the same plane (see dotted lines in **Fig. 26.11**). More specifically, it is the base of the valves that are in this same plane, at the location of the anulus fibrosus of each valve.

Fig. 26.12 is a superior view of the heart with the atria, aorta, and pulmonary artery removed. The base of each valve is a ring, the anulus fibrosus ("fibrous anulus" in **Fig. 26.12**). Each ring is connected to adjacent rings (by tissue called "trigones" in the figure), forming a set of four rings and connecting tissues, all composed of dense fibroelastic connective tissue.

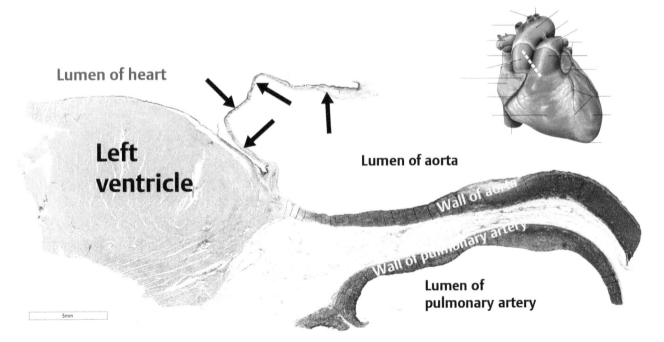

Fig. 26.8 **Scanning view of the anterior wall of the left ventricle and aorta and intervening aortic valve (arrows; valve lies in what would be the "closed" position), as well as a portion of the pulmonary artery. This tissue was sectioned as shown by the dashed yellow line in the anatomic drawing; note that the lower portion of the dotted line passes behind the pulmonary artery. Therefore, the section includes the anterior wall of the aorta and left ventricle and the posterior wall of the pulmonary artery.** Inset from Schuenke M, Schulte E, Schumacher U. *THIEME Atlas of Anatomy. Internal Organs.* **Illustrations by Voll M and Wesker K. Second Edition. New York: Thieme Medical Publishers; 2016.**

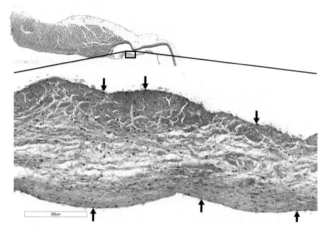

Fig. 26.9   Heart valve (pulmonary valve) consists of a core of connective tissue covered by an endothelium (arrows).

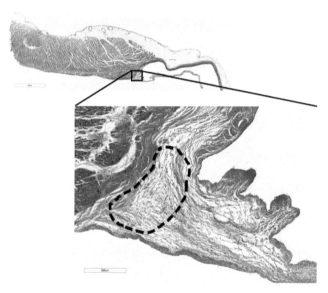

Fig. 26.10 Heart valve (pulmonary valve) at the base of the valve, showing the anulus fibrosus (outlined).

Structurally, the anulus fibrosus and interconnecting fibrous tissues provide a central anchor for the heart valves as well as for the heart muscle of the atria and ventricles. Functionally, this dense sheet of connective tissue electrically separates the atria from the ventricles so that they can beat as separate units (the atria and ventricles do not contract at the same time). Note there is an opening in this connective tissue sheet for the **bundle of His** (see following section).

26.6   Conducting System of the Heart

The conducting system of the heart transmits electrical stimuli to cardiac muscle in a systematic fashion to accomplish directional pumping of blood.

The stimulus is initiated by the **sinoatrial (SA) node**, located near the superior vena cava. Because cardiac muscle cells are connected by gap junctions, the impulse from the SA node spreads through the atria toward the ventricles. This causes a contraction wave in the atria that propels blood through the atrioventricular valves. However, the electrical impulse does not pass directly to the ventricles because the fibrous tissue of the anulus fibrosus, which does not conduct, separates the ventricles from the atria.

Impulses from the atria reach the **atrioventricular (AV) node**, which passes the impulse through the anulus fibrosus via the bundle of His (see **Fig. 26.13**), down the ventricular septum via the **right** and **left bundle branches**, and finally into the remainder of the ventricular wall via **Purkinje fibers**. In this manner, ventricular contraction spreads as a wave down the septum, and then from the apex toward the great arteries, propelling blood superiorly toward the arteries.

Fig. 26.14 is a medium- to high-magnification image of the endocardium of a ventricle. The cells in the outlined region are Purkinje fibers, modified cardiac muscle cells. They are easily identified because they have striations and intercalated disks like cardiac muscle cells in the myocardium, but the cytoplasm near the nucleus contains glycogen, which, in many cells, does not stain well.

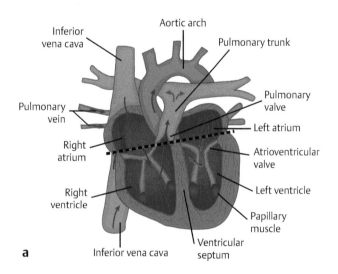

a

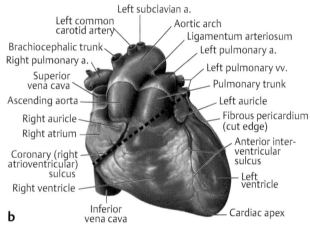

b

Fig. 26.11a, b   Position of the heart valves (dotted lines). Note that all four valves are approximately in the same plane. Fig. 26.11b from Schuenke M, Schulte E, Schumacher U. *THIEME Atlas of Anatomy. Internal Organs.* Illustrations by Voll M and Wesker K. Second Edition. New York: Thieme Medical Publishers; 2016.

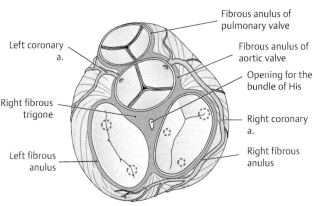

Fig. 26.12 **Superior view of the heart with the atria, aorta, and pulmonary artery removed, showing the four heart valves. The anuli fibrosi of the valves are connected together to make up a sheet of connective tissue between the atria and ventricles (tan region). Gilroy A, Atlas of Anatomy, based on the work of Schünke M, Schulte E, Schumacher U. Illustrations by M. Voll and K. Wesker.**

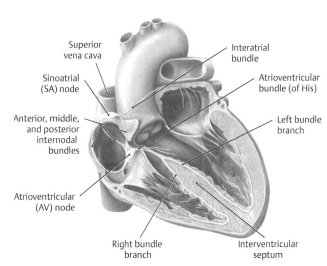

Fig. 26.13 **The conducting system of the heart. Gilroy A, Atlas of Anatomy, based on the work of Schünke M, Schulte E, Schumacher U. *THIEME Atlas of Anatomy. Internal Organs.* Illustrations by M. Voll and K. Wesker. Second Edition. New York: Thieme Medical Publishers; 2016.**

Video 26.7   Purkinje fibers

Be able to identify:
— Purkinje fibers
https://www.thieme.de/de/q.htm?p=opn/
tp/308390101/978-1-62623-414-7_c026_
v008&t=video

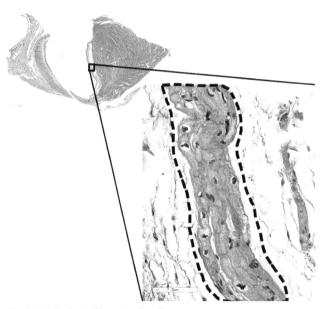

Fig. 26.14 **Purkinje fibers (outlined).**

26.7 Blood Flow through the Circulatory System

Now that all the structures of the circulatory system have been described, the path of blood flow can be discussed (see **Fig. 26.3** and **Fig. 25.5**). There are two circuits in the circulatory system:

- The **pulmonary circuit**, driven by the right side of the heart, pumps deoxygenated blood to the lungs for oxygenation; this blood returns to the left side of the heart.

- The **systemic circuit**, driven by the left side of the heart, pumps oxygenated blood to the tissues to deliver oxygen and other nutrients; this blood returns to the right side of the heart.

Blood flow in each circuit is through the system of vessels shown in **Fig. 25.5**:

Elastic artery → muscular artery → arteriole → capillary → venule → medium vein → large vein

Putting it all together, deoxygenated blood returns to the heart via large veins (venae cavae) and is collected by the right atrium. The right atrium pumps blood to the right ventricle, which pumps blood out to the pulmonary artery. The pulmonary artery branches into smaller arteries, arterioles, and then capillaries in the lungs, which are the vessels that enable diffusion of oxygen into the blood and carbon dioxide out of it. After the blood picks up oxygen, the capillaries in the lungs converge to form venules and then pulmonary veins, which bring oxygenated blood to the left side of the heart, namely the left atrium. Blood from the left atrium is pumped to the left ventricle, which pumps

blood out to the aorta. Branches of the aorta include muscular arteries, which branch to form smaller arteries and arterioles. Arterioles lead to tissue capillaries. The tissue capillaries are where oxygen and nutrients are delivered to tissues and carbon dioxide and wastes are collected from them. Tissue capillaries converge to form venules, which are tributaries to small and medium veins and, ultimately, large veins (the venae cavae), which bring blood back to the right atrium.

26.8 Chapter Review

The major tissue type in the heart is cardiac muscle, which is striated muscle. Cardiac muscle is composed of long, large cells that are joined end to end by intercalated disks, which function to adhere cells together so that their forces add up and to connect them electrically so that they contract at the same time. Like vessels, the heart wall is composed of three layers, called the endocardium, myocardium, and epicardium. The major differences between these layers in the heart and those in vessels is that the myocardium is composed of cardiac and not smooth muscle, and the outer epicardium is covered by a visceral layer of pericardium. The heart has four chambers: right atrium, right ventricle, left atrium, and left ventricle. The ventricles have a thicker myocardium than the atria, while the endocardium in the atria is thicker than in the ventricles. The valves of the heart are composed of a core of connective tissue covered by endothelium continuous with the endothelium that forms the inner lining of the chambers. At the base of the valves, the connective tissue core is thicker, forming the anulus fibrosus, which supports the valves and electrically separates the atria from the ventricles. The conduction system of the heart creates spontaneous contractions that are coordinated to maximize blood flow. Purkinje fibers in the ventricular endocardium are recognized as cells with striations and intercalated disks but with glycogen near the nucleus.

Questions and Answers

An online-only section of questions and answers accompanying this chapter is hosted on Thieme's MedOne Education site: https://medone-education.thieme.com. Use the code on the media page at the front of this book to gain access. An institutional license to the site is required to access these questions in an interactive format, and individual users are required to register for an individual account to track results.

27   Integument

After completing this exercise, be able to:
— Identify, at the light microscope level, each of the following:
* Layers of skin
    ◦ Epidermis
        ▪ Stratum basale
        ▪ Stratum spinosum
        ▪ Stratum granulosum
        ▪ Stratum lucidum (thick skin only)
        ▪ Stratum corneum
    ◦ Dermis
        ▪ Papillary layer
        ▪ Reticular layer
        ▪ Dermal papilla and epidermal pegs
    ◦ Hypodermis
* Accessory structures
    ◦ Hair
        ▪ Follicle
        ▪ Shaft
        ▪ Matrix
        ▪ Dermal papilla
    ◦ Arrector pili muscle
    ◦ Glands
        ▪ Sebaceous glands
        ▪ Cells of sweat glands
            – Secretory cells
            – Myoepithelial cells
            – Fibroblasts
        ▪ Sweat glands
            – Eccrine
            – Apocrine
            – Ducts
    ◦ Specialized sensory receptors
        ▪ Meissner corpuscles
        ▪ Pacinian corpuscles
— Distinguish between thick and thin skin
— Ascertain the source of a sample of skin based on histologic features:
* Typical skin (e.g., forearm)
* Scalp
* Palms of hands/soles of feet
* Axilla/groin
— Outline the function of each cell, structure, and vessel type listed
— Predict the phenotype of integument in patients with mutations in critical skin structures

27.1   Functions of the Integument

The **integument** (**skin**) is the largest organ of the body, covering almost the entire outer surface. Its main function is to protect the underlying tissues from trauma and infectious agents. The function of the integument in preventing infections is underscored by the fact that infections in intact skin are not common, but they invariably happen when the epithelium of the skin is breached. In addition, the integument is involved in sensation through receptors in the skin, as well as excretion via sweat glands. Temperature regulation occurs via **sweat glands**, as well as through regulation of blood flow, which causes skin to turn red when overheated or pale when cold. Finally, adipose storage occurs in the skin, and vitamin D_3 synthesis occurs in the integument as well.

27.2   Overview of the Integument

The integument consists of three regions (**Fig. 27.1**, from superficial to deep):
— **Epidermis**: stratified squamous keratinized epithelium
— **Dermis**: loose and dense irregular connective tissue
— **Hypodermis** (subcutaneous layer): mostly adipose

> **Basic Science Correlate: Gross Anatomy**
>
> The hypodermis is the **superficial fascia** in gross anatomy. Many authors do not include the subcutaneous layer (hypodermis) as part of the integument; it will be discussed here for the sake of completeness.

Fig. 27.2 is a scanning image taken from the skin of the sole of the foot. The epidermis (black bracket), dermis (green bracket), and hypodermis (purple bracket) are indicated. The space at the bottom of the image represents the outside world; underlying/deeper tissues and organs (e.g., muscles) would be located at the top of the image. Even at this low magnification, it may be possible to appreciate that the epidermis is stratified squamous keratinized epithelium, the dermis is connective tissue, and the hypodermis is mostly adipose tissue. These regions are examined in detail in later sections.

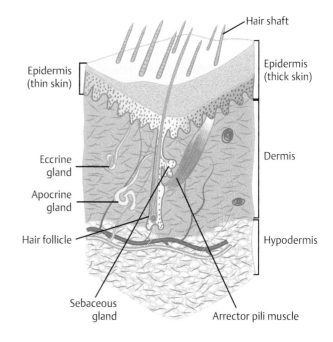

Fig. 27.1   **Integument.**

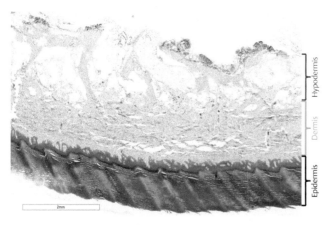

Fig. 27.2   **Scanning image of the skin from the sole of the foot. The superficial portion is down. Epidermis (black bracket), dermis (green bracket), and hypodermis (purple bracket) are indicated.**

As shown in **Fig. 27.3**, the epidermis can be divided into four to five regions (strata). One of these layers, the stratum lucidum, is present only in thick skin and is not visible in many images and slides. The dermis can be divided into two layers. The papillary layer adjacent to the epidermis is composed of loose connective tissue, while the reticular layer is made up of dense irregular connective tissue.

27.3   Epidermis

Fig. 27.4 shows the **epidermis** of the sole of the foot. The epidermis (black bracket) is a stratified squamous keratinized epithelium. Recall that the keratinized layer of this type of epithelium consists of packed cells full of keratin, but without nuclei. In the sole of the foot, the keratinized layer (**Fig. 27.4**, red bracket) is very thick. This layer of dead cells in the skin is called the **stratum corneum** (see **Fig. 27.3**).

As shown in **Fig. 27.3**, the living portion of the epidermis is composed of three or four layers, depending on skin thickness.

Therefore, the epidermis is composed of four or five total layers (**Fig. 27.5**, from deep to superficial):

- **Stratum basale** (**stratum germinativum**) (brown bracket and arrows): single layer of cuboidal stem cells
- **Stratum spinosum** (green bracket): cuboidal cells, some cell division, spinous connections between cells via desmosomes

- **Stratum granulosum** (blue bracket): cells becoming flattened and containing dense **keratohyalin granules**, which impart a dark staining to the cells in this region
- **Stratum lucidum** (in region of orange bracket): in thick skin only, cells clear (not visible in **Fig. 27.5**; bracket indicates approximate location)
- **Stratum corneum** (red bracket): cells that have lost organelles and are filled with keratin

Video 27.1   Layers of the epidermis in thick skin

Be able to identify:
— Stratum basale
— Stratum spinosum
— Stratum germinativum
— (Stratum lucidum—know where this should be)
— Stratum corneum
https://www.thieme.de/de/q.htm?p=opn/tp/308390101/978-1-62623-414-7_c027_v001&t=video

The previous images were taken from the sole of the foot, which is covered by **thick skin**. As shown in **Fig. 27.5**, thick skin is characterized by a thick stratum corneum. The other prominent place covered with thick skin is the palms of the hands.

The remainder of the body is covered by **thin skin**. **Fig. 27.6** is an image taken of the skin covering the ear. As the name implies, in thin skin, many of the layers are thinner, but this is especially true in the stratum corneum (keratinized layer, red bracket). In addition, the elusive stratum lucidum is not present in thin skin. The stratum basale (stratum germinativum, brown bracket), being one cell thick, does not change, and the stratum spinosum (green bracket) remains fairly substantial. However, the stratum granulosum (blue bracket) is very thin; its presence is shown by cells with small dense purple granules just deep to the stratum corneum (blue arrow).

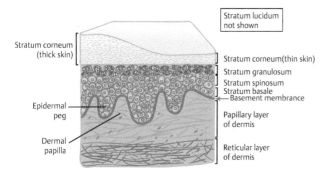

Fig. 27.3   **Layers (strata) of the epidermis.**

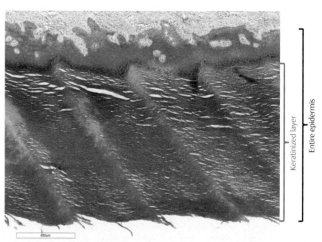

Fig. 27.4   **Epidermis of the sole of the foot, low magnification. The epidermis is stratified squamous keratinized epithelium. The entire epidermis is indicated by the black bracket; the keratinized layer (red bracket) is thick on the sole of the foot.**

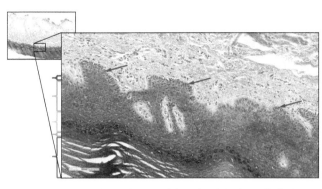

Fig. 27.5   **Layers of the epidermis of the sole of the foot (thick skin): stratum basale (brown bracket and brown arrows); stratum spinosum (green bracket); stratum granulosum (blue bracket); stratum lucidum (orange bracket); stratum corneum (red bracket).**

Video 27.2   Layers of the epidermis in thin skin

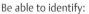

Be able to identify:
— Stratum basale
— Stratum spinosum
— Stratum germinativum
— Stratum corneum
https://www.thieme.de/de/q.htm?p=opn/tp/308390101/978-1-62623-414-7_c027_v002&t=video

27.4   Cells of the Epidermis

The epidermis consists of several cell types, including keratinocytes and melanocytes, discussed in detail in the following paragraphs. Other cells that are not seen in routinely stained slides of the epidermis include **Merkel cells**, which provide a sensory function, and **Langerhans cells**, which are related to macrophages and provide an immune function.

27.4.1   Keratinocytes

Keratinocytes are the most prominent cell type in the epidermis. Indeed, most of the nuclei seen in histologic sections of the epidermis belong to keratinocytes. Keratinocytes in the stratum basale divide, providing cells that progress superficially through the epidermis toward the stratum corneum. As they progress, they express **keratin tonofilaments** (intermediate filaments), which interact with **desmosomes** that form strong cell-cell junctions. The combination of keratin and desmosomes makes the epidermis resistant to shear stress.

Recall from **Chapter 5** that desmosomes are cell-cell junctions common in epithelia and other tissues. The stratum spinosum of the epidermis got its name because the cells are joined by desmosomes. During tissue preparation, cell shrinkage causes epithelial cells to pull apart from each other, but they remain attached at the desmosomes, creating spinous **intercellular bridges** of cytoplasm (**Fig. 27.7**, 1) that join adjacent cells.

Fig. 27.8 is an electron micrograph of the basal aspect of the epidermis, showing keratin tonofilaments within cells of the stratum basale (4) and cells of the stratum spinosum (3). The underlying dermis (1) is just deep to cells of the stratum

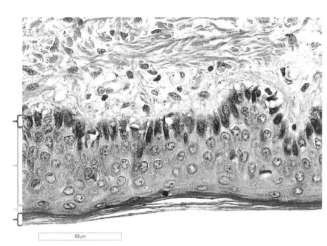

Fig. 27.6   **Layers of the epidermis of ear (thin skin): stratum basale (brown bracket); stratum spinosum (green bracket); stratum granulosum (blue bracket and blue arrow); stratum corneum (red bracket).**

basale; the basement membrane between these layers is not well preserved. The keratinocytes have abundant thick keratin tonofilaments (4) in the cytoplasm and are joined by desmosomes (2).

As the keratinocytes progress toward the surface, they accumulate dense keratohyalin granules. These granules contain proteins that bundle keratin filaments and form the granulated appearance characteristic of cells of the stratum granulosum. This layer is readily seen in sections of thick skin as a basophilic band two to three cells thick (see **Fig. 27.5**, blue bracket). In thin skin, where this layer is one to two cells thick, cells with obvious keratohyalin granules are more challenging to find (see **Fig. 27.6**, blue arrow). The cells in the stratum granulosum also take on a more squamous appearance. The transition to the stratum corneum includes loss of the nucleus and other organelles and a definitive squamous morphology. Ultimately, the keratinocytes become nothing more than a plasma membrane filled with keratin, and they pack together into the keratinized layer characteristic of skin.

Clinical Correlate

Mutations in keratins and desmosomes give rise to skin-blistering diseases. For example, **epidermolysis bullosa simplex** is caused by mutations in keratin genes. The skin in these patients is fragile, and blisters form under minimal stress. These are typically diagnosed early, as childbirth often results in blister formation.

27.4.2   Melanocytes

Melanocytes produce pigment (**melanin**), which is packaged into vesicles called **melanosomes**, which are transferred to keratinocytes. Melanin protects the keratinocyte DNA from damage caused by ultraviolet rays from the sun.

Fig. 27.9 is a drawing of a melanocyte, showing its location in the basal aspect of the epidermis. Melanocytes have numerous processes that extend between the keratinocytes, enabling transfer of melanosomes to multiple cells.

Because melanosomes are transferred to keratinocytes as they are produced by the melanocyte, melanocytes themselves do not normally store melanin. Therefore, in **Fig. 27.10**, the

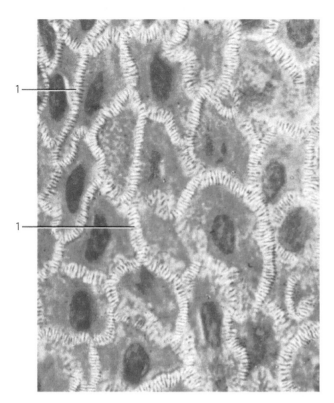

Fig. 27.7   **Keratinocytes in the stratum spinosum of the epidermis. Cells of the stratum spinosum are joined by desmosomes. During tissue preparation, cell shrinkage causes cells to pull apart from each other, but they remain connected where they are joined by desmosomes. This leaves spiny processes, called cytoplasmic bridges (1), between the cells, marking the location of desmosomes.**

cells containing brown pigment (arrows) are keratinocytes, not melanocytes. The melanocytes are indeed present, near the basal layer, but are generally not seen in routine H & E.

Clinical Correlate

Albinism is a decrease or absence of activity of tyrosinase, an enzyme critical for melanin production. Patients with this condition are susceptible to sunburn and skin cancer.

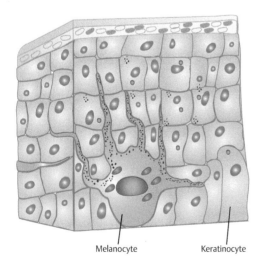

Melanocyte   Keratinocyte

Fig. 27.9   **Melanocyte.**

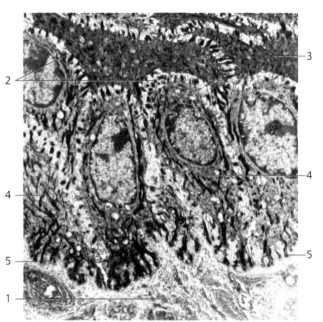

Fig. 27.8   **Basal aspect of the epidermis. (1) Dermis; (2) desmosomes, (3) cell of the stratum spinosum, (4) keratin tonofilaments within cells of the stratum basale; (5) spinous processes connecting keratinocyte to the basement membrane.**

27.5   Dermis and Hypodermis

The **dermis** is composed of two layers (**Fig. 27.11**):
- **Papillary layer** (green bracket): loose connective tissue
- **Reticular layer** (blue bracket): dense irregular connective tissue

Fig. 27.12 is an image of the dermal-epidermal junction, showing that the papillary layer is indeed loose connective tissue. This is richly vascularized to supply the overlying epidermis, which lacks blood vessels. The dense irregular connective tissue in the reticular layer contains abundant type I collagen fibers (to provide resistance to shear forces) and elastic fibers (to allow the tissue to stretch and return to its original shape).

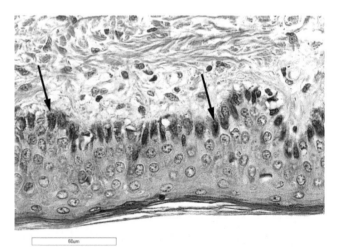

60um

Fig. 27.10 **Epidermis of the skin showing keratinocytes containing melanin. This tissue was stained with H & E; the brown seen here is pigment in the cells, not due to staining. Because melanocytes do not store pigment, they are not easily identified in routine H & E-stained sections.**

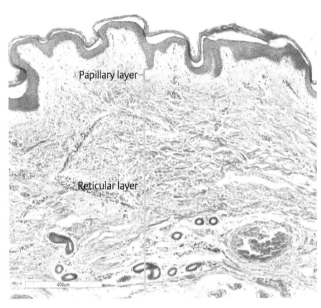

Fig. 27.11 **Dermis of the skin, low magnification, showing the papillary layer (green bracket) and reticular layer (blue bracket).**

Also of note is that the dermal-epidermal junction undulates (**Fig. 27.13**), creating fingerlike projections of the dermis, called **dermal papillae** (black arrows) and corresponding **epidermal pegs** (**epidermal ridges**, green arrows). These provide resistance to shear forces, reducing the risk of the epidermis "slipping" over the dermis. It is not surprising that these features are more extensive in tissues subject to high stress such as the sole of the foot (**Fig. 27.13b**).

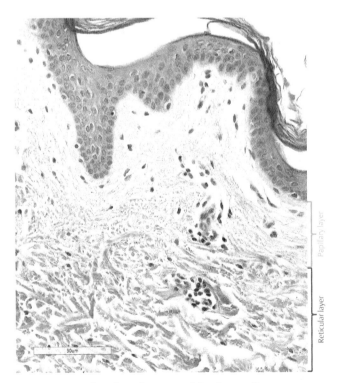

Fig. 27.12 **Dermal-epidermal junction of the skin, medium magnification, showing the papillary layer (green bracket) and reticular layer (blue bracket).**

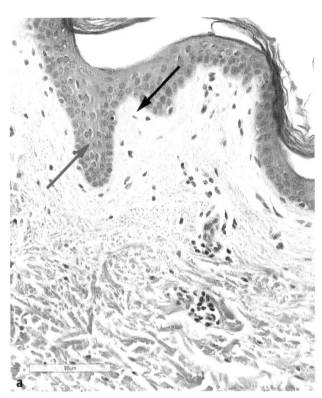

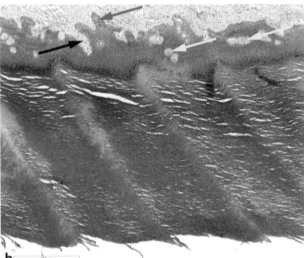

Fig. 27.13 **Undulations of the dermal-epidermal junction in (a) thin skin and (b) thick skin. The fingerlike projections of the dermis are called dermal papillae (black arrows), and complementary extensions of the epidermis are called epidermal pegs (green arrows). Due to sectioning, portions of dermal papillae may appear to be within the epidermis (yellow arrows).**

Helpful Hint

There are regions of dermis that appear to be within the epidermis (yellow arrow, **Fig. 27.13b**). These represent the upper portions of dermal papillae cut in cross section.

As previously mentioned, skin-blistering disorders can occur from mutations in keratins or desmosomes in the epidermis. Also in this class of skin-blistering diseases are mutations of proteins of the basement membrane (**junctional epidermolysis bullosa**) or collagens (**dystrophic epidermolysis bullosa**). The entire spectrum of these blistering diseases varies from mild to severe.

As mentioned in the beginning of this section, the **hypodermis** is the deepest layer of the integument (see **Fig. 27.2**, purple bracket) and is largely composed of unilocular adipose tissue. The thickness of this layer depends on the region of the body from which it was taken and body habitus.

Video 27.3   Layers of the epidermis in thin skin

Be able to identify:
— Dermis
— Papillary layer
— Reticular layer
— Epidermal ridges and dermal papilla
— Hypodermis

https://www.thieme.de/de/q.htm?p=opn/tp/308390101/978-1-62623-414-7_c027_v003&t=video

27.6   Accessory Structures of the Skin

Accessory structures of the skin are modifications of the epidermis and dermis that perform a variety of functions, including protection and thermoregulation.

Accessory structures of the skin include:
- Hair and hair follicles
- Arrector pili muscles
- Exocrine glands: sebaceous, eccrine, and apocrine

27.6.1   Hair and Hair Follicle

The **hair follicle**, which produces a **hair**, develops through a complex set of interactions similar to the formation of glands (**Fig. 27.14**). Epithelial cells of the epidermis proliferate and then project into the underlying connective tissue of the dermis. At the deepest part of the hair follicle, a **dermal papilla** develops and protrudes into the follicle. During this process, the basement membrane remains faithful to the epithelial-connective tissue border. The **matrix** is a region of specialized epithelial stem cells that form around the dermal papilla and contributes to the formation and growth of the hair.

Fig. 27.15 is an image taken from the scalp showing several hair follicles, mostly in longitudinal section. **Hair shafts** (blue arrows) are readily seen in the centers of several hair follicles. The hair follicles (red arrows) have epithelial cells similar to the surface epidermis, but with fewer layers of cells. At the base of the follicle (top in this image), the dermal papilla (orange arrow) projects into the base of the follicle; the epithelial cells surrounding the dermal papilla form the matrix (green arrow).

Hair growth follows a similar progression as that of epidermal cells. Like cells of the stratum basale, keratinocytes in the matrix

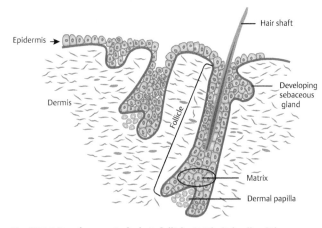

Fig. 27.14 **Development of a hair follicle. Epithelial cells of the epidermis proliferate and project into the underlying dermis. Note that the basement membrane (dark, undulating line) maintains its position between the epithelium and connective tissue (between epidermis and dermis). The epidermal growth then forms the hair follicle; cells in the matrix will proliferate and contribute to the hair. The dermal papilla is part of the dermis that provides blood supply to the follicle, especially the matrix cells.**

proliferate. As the cells mature, they accumulate keratins (hard keratins), lose their nuclei, and are added to the base of the shaft. In this way, the hair is pushed outward, accounting for growth of the hair. Melanocytes in the matrix produce pigment, which is transferred to the keratinocytes before they are added to the hair shaft.

Video 27.4   Hair

Be able to identify:
— Hair shaft
— Hair follicle
— Dermal (hair) papilla
— Matrix

https://www.thieme.de/de/q.htm?p=opn/tp/308390101/978-1-62623-414-7_c027_v004&t=video

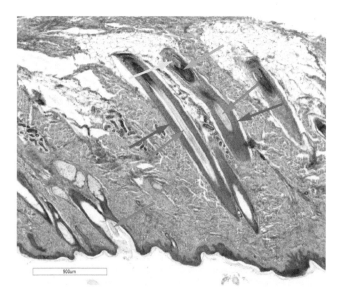

Fig. 27.15 **Scalp in scanning view, showing hair shafts (blue arrows), hair follicles (red arrows), dermal papilla (orange arrow), and matrix (green arrow).**

27.6.2 Arrector Pili Muscles

An **arrector pili muscle** (**Fig. 27.16**, outlined) is associated with each hair follicle. The arrector pili muscle is smooth muscle that attaches to the hair follicle near its base and to the dermis near the epidermis. When exposed to cold temperatures, this muscle contracts, erecting the hair. In furry animals, this provides insulation, but it is not very important in humans.

The end of the arrector pili muscle that attaches to the dermis pulls downward during contraction, creating a depression in the skin. When this happens, areas of skin adjacent to these attachment points appear to rise up, so-called "goose pimples" or "goose bumps."

27.6.3 Sebaceous Glands

Fig. 27.17 is a low-magnification image of the scalp, showing **sebaceous glands** (outlined), associated with hair follicles. These glands are found adjacent to the hair follicle to which they are attached, about one-third of the way down the follicle from the surface epithelium. **Fig. 27.18** shows a closer view of a sebaceous gland. Sebaceous glands secrete by **holocrine secretion**. In this process, cells at the base of the gland (black arrows) proliferate. Like the surface epithelial cells, the progeny then progress toward the lumen in the center of the gland (not in the plane of section). During this process, the cells enlarge as they accumulate secretory product in their cytoplasm. The secretory product washes out during tissue preparation, giving the cytoplasm a pale appearance, with central nuclei. Mature cells near the ducts break open, releasing secretory contents: an oily product called **sebum**, which coats the surface of the hair shaft, providing the hair and skin with lubrication and waterproofing.

Video 27.5   Sebaceous gland and arrector pili muscle

Be able to identify:
— Sebaceous gland
— Arrector pili muscle
https://www.thieme.de/de/q.htm?p=opn/tp/308390101/978-1-62623-414-7_c027_v005&t=video

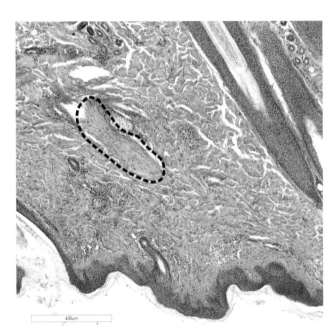

Fig. 27.16 **Scalp at low to medium magnification, showing arrector pili muscle (outline).**

Clinical Correlate

Sloughing of cells in sebaceous glands and hair follicles is a continuous process. **Acne** occurs when hair follicles become clogged with dead cells. The result is an accumulation of oily secretions from sebaceous glands, forming skin blemishes of various types (pimples, whiteheads, blackheads). Because testosterone increases the size and oiliness of sebaceous gland secretions, acne is typically most severe during puberty. Other conditions, such as pregnancy and use of anabolic steroids, may also cause acne.

27.6.4 Sweat Glands

The **sweat glands** of the skin include **eccrine** and **apocrine sweat glands**, which are exocrine glands (as is the sebaceous gland). Formation of exocrine glands in epithelia was discussed in **Chapter 6** (see **Fig. 6.3**). Gland formation begins when epithelial cells proliferate and subsequently invaginate into the underlying connective tissue. Of note, the basement membrane remains faithful to the basal side of the epithelium during this process, separating the epithelial cells of the gland from the connective tissue. Exocrine glands form when a lumen appears within the invaginated epithelium. When fully developed, the epithelial cells of glands release their secretory product apically into the lumen via secretory vesicles, a process termed **merocrine secretion**.

Helpful Hint

Recall that in holocrine secretion, a secretory cell fills with its product, and then the whole cell ruptures. Therefore, cell renewal is a main feature of glands that secrete via this method, such as sebaceous glands. Eccrine and apocrine glands secrete product by the merocrine pathway, in which the product is released by exocytosis of the contents of secretory vesicles. Therefore, cell turnover in these glands is not extensive.

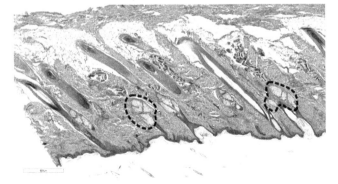

Fig. 27.17 **Scalp at low to medium magnification showing sebaceous glands (outlined).**

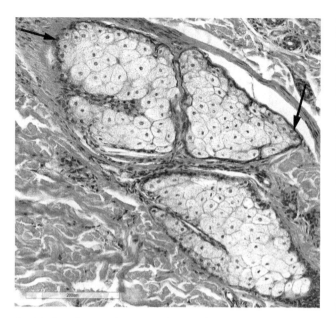

Fig. 27.18 **Scalp at medium magnification showing sebaceous gland. The arrows indicate basal cells of the gland.**

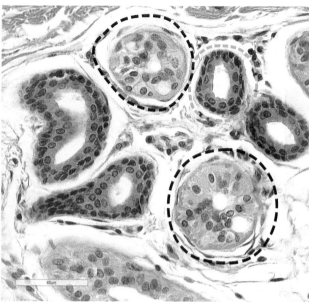

Fig. 27.19 **Eccrine sweat glands (black outlines) and ducts (green outline).**

Eccrine Sweat Glands

Eccrine sweat glands are found in most locations of the body. The sweat produced by eccrine sweat glands is more dilute than plasma and is involved in temperature regulation. **Fig. 27.19** shows eccrine sweat glands (black outlines) in the dermis. Though the staggered nuclei give the appearance of a pseudostratified epithelium, the epithelium is simple columnar. The cells have a pale eosinophilic cytoplasm, and the lumen is small but distinct (if in the plane of section).

Apocrine Sweat Glands

Apocrine sweat glands (**Fig. 27.20**, outlined) are found in select locations, notably the axilla and pubic regions (also the areola of the breast and the circumanal region). Secretions from apocrine sweat glands contain organic components, designed to provide lubrication to these regions. Although these secretions are not naturally odoriferous, they are metabolized by surface bacteria, which generate the odor characteristic of these regions. Like eccrine glands, apocrine glands are composed of a simple epithelium. However, they are larger glands, with a wider lumen. The cells of apocrine glands have an irregular apical border, and their cytoplasm is highly eosinophilic.

Myoepithelial Cells

Closer examination of both eccrine and apocrine glands reveals flattened nuclei near the basal aspect, against the basement membrane (**Fig. 27.20**, black arrows). These cells are **myoepithelial cells**, which are frequently found in glands such as these sweat glands as well as mammary glands. Myoepithelial cells contain contractile proteins and are thought to assist in glandular secretion. Note that myoepithelial cells are epithelial and located on the epithelial side of the basement membrane. Other flattened nuclei on the connective tissue side of the basement membrane (green arrow) are most likely fibroblasts.

Sweat Gland Ducts

Ducts (see **Fig. 27.19**, green outline) for both eccrine and apocrine glands are similar in size to eccrine glands (outlined in black). Ducts have a narrow and distinct lumen (though typically wider than the lumen of an eccrine gland) and are composed of a stratified cuboidal/columnar epithelium in which the cells have a cytoplasm more eosinophilic than that of eccrine glands. In a single image such as this, one cannot distinguish whether ducts belong to eccrine or apocrine glands.

Video 27.6   Eccrine glands, apocrine glands, and sweat gland ducts

Be able to identify:
— Sweat gland cells
  • Secretory cells
  • Myoepithelial cells
  • Fibroblasts
— Eccrine sweat glands
— Apocrine sweat glands
— Sweat gland ducts
https://www.thieme.de/de/q.htm?p=opn/tp/308390101/978-1-62623-414-7_c027_v006&t=video

27.7   Sensory Receptors in Skin

There are a number of types of sensory receptors in skin that detect sensations of light touch, pressure, heat, cold, and other stimuli (**Fig. 27.21**). There are two types of receptors that are readily visible on routine H & E-stained slides: Meissner corpuscles and pacinian corpuscles.

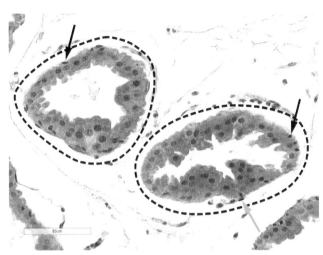

Fig. 27.20 **Apocrine sweat glands (outlined). Myoepithelial cells (black arrows) and a fibroblast (green arrow) are shown.**

27.7.1   Meissner's Corpuscles

Meissner's corpuscles are touch receptors found in dermal papillae. They are composed of an unmyelinated nerve ending, with flattened supportive cells (**Fig. 27.22**). The nerve ending forms a characteristic spiral, similar to that shown in **Fig. 27.22a**. The supportive cells are all oriented along the axis of the nerve (i.e., "horizontal"). Therefore, Meissner corpuscles stand out as oval structures in dermal papillae because most of the nuclei, which belong to supporting cells, are in the same (horizontal) orientation (**Fig. 27.22b**).

27.7.2   Pacinian Corpuscles

Pacinian corpuscles are pressure receptors found in the deep dermis and hypodermis. They are very large and can be seen on tissue

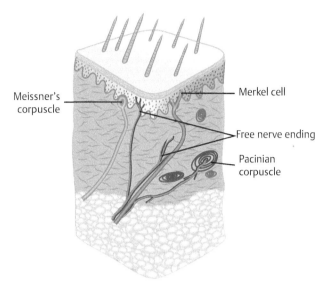

Meissner's corpuscle

Merkel cell

Free nerve ending

Pacinian corpuscle

Fig. 27.21 **Sensory receptors in the skin.**

slides with the unaided eye (or at very low power, as outlined in **Fig. 27.23a**). They are composed of an unmyelinated nerve ending covered with multiple layers of connective tissue, forming a structure with the appearance of a cut onion (**Fig. 27.23b**).

Video 27.7   Meissner's and pacinian corpuscles

Be able to identify:
— Pacinian corpuscles
— Meissner corpuscles

https://www.thieme.de/de/q.htm?p=opn/tp/308390101/978-1-62623-414-7_c027_v007&t=video

27.8   Identifying the Location of a Skin Sample Using Histologic Features

Finally, the location of the body from which a sample of skin was taken can be ascertained based on the characteristic features of a skin sample. The following provides a summary of the features and structures of the skin, and where on the body they are found:

• Thick skin (see **Fig. 27.2**): palms of the hands, soles of the feet
• Thin skin (see **Fig. 27.6**): everywhere except palms of the hands and soles of the feet
• Hair (see **Fig. 27.15**): on most regions of the body except thick skin
• Sebaceous glands (see **Fig. 27.18**): found where hair is located and in some places that lack hair
• Eccrine sweat glands (see **Fig. 27.19**): on most regions of the body
• Apocrine sweat glands (see **Fig. 27.20**): axilla, pubic region, nipple, circumanal region

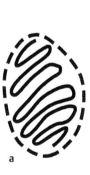

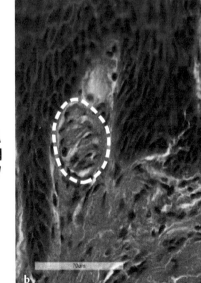

a

b

Fig. 27.22 **Meissner's corpuscle. (a) Shape of the nerve ending that forms the core of the corpuscle. (b) Histologic image of the dermal-epidermal junction showing a Meissner's corpuscle (blue outline) within a dermal papilla.**

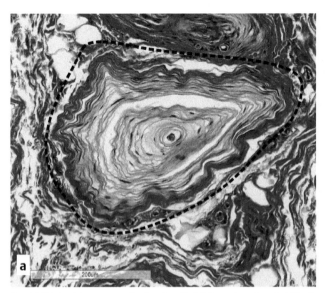 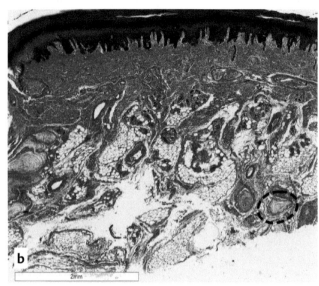

Fig. 27.23 **Pacinian corpuscles (outlined). (a) Scanning view. (b) Medium magnification.**

27.9   Chapter Review

The integument (skin) is the largest organ of the body and serves many functions. It is composed of three layers: the epidermis, dermis, and hypodermis.

The epidermis is a stratified squamous keratinized epithelium, the degree of keratinization in different locations in the body varies from thick to thin skin. There are five layers of the epidermis: stratum basale, stratum spinosum, stratum granulosum, stratum lucidum (thick skin only), and stratum corneum. Keratinocytes are the most prominent cell in the epidermis and are mitotically active in the stratum basale. These cells synthesize keratins and desmosomes for shear strength. They flatten as they move toward the surface, where they lose their nuclei and make up the protective keratin layer until they are sloughed off. Melanocytes produce the pigment melanin, packaging it into specialized organelles called melanosomes, which are transferred to keratinocytes. Melanin protects the DNA of keratinocytes from ultraviolet damage.

The dermis is composed of two regions: the papillary layer is a loose connective tissue, and the reticular layer is dense irregular connective tissue. The hypodermis is mostly unilocular adipose tissue.

Accessory structures of the skin include hair follicles, arrector pili muscles, sweat glands, and sensory receptors. Hair follicles generate hairs and are associated with arrector pili muscles that erect the hairs. Sebaceous glands produce an oily secretion that lubricates hairs and skin. There are two types of sweat glands. Eccrine sweat glands are found throughout the body and produce a watery secretion for temperature regulation. Eccrine glands have cells with a smooth apical surface and pale cytoplasmic eosinophilia. Apocrine sweat glands are found in the axilla, the groin, and a few other locations and produce a secretion that includes an organic component. Apocrine glands are larger than eccrine glands, with cells that have an irregular apical surface and more eosinophilic cytoplasm. Sweat gland ducts are stratified; the cells have a regular apical surface and an eosinophilic cytoplasm. Meissner's corpuscles are coil-like structures that transmit fine touch sensation in dermal papillae, while pacinian corpuscles are large structures in the dermal-hypodermal junction that transmit pressure and vibration and have the appearance of a sectioned onion. The location of the body from which a section of skin was taken can be determined based on its histologic features.

Questions and Answers

An online-only section of questions and answers accompanying this chapter is hosted on Thieme's MedOne Education site: https://medone-education.thieme.com. Use the code on the media page at the front of this book to gain access. An institutional license to the site is required to access these questions in an interactive format, and individual users are required to register for an individual account to track results.

28 Overview of the Gastrointestinal System

Learning Objectives

After completing this chapter, you should be able to:
— Describe the general organization of the gastrointestinal system
  • Main pathway
  • Accessory organs
— Outline the development of the gastrointestinal system, and correlate embryonic structures with structures of the gastro-intestinal tract
— Identify, at the light microscope level, each of the following:
  • Layers of the gastrointestinal tract
    ○ Mucosa
      ▪ Epithelium
      ▪ Lamina propria
      ▪ Muscularis mucosa
    ○ Submucosa
    ○ Muscularis
      ▪ Inner circular layer
      ▪ Outer longitudinal layer
    ○ Adventitia/serosa
  • Elaborations of the gastrointestinal tract that increase surface area
    ○ Plicae circulares
    ○ Villi
    ○ Microvilli (brush border)
  • Neural and endocrine structures of the gastrointestinal tract
    ○ Enteric nervous system
      ▪ Myenteric plexus
      ▪ Submucosal plexus
    ○ Enteroendocrine cells (with special staining)
— Outline the function of each of the layers, structures, and cells listed

28.1 Organization of the Gastrointestinal System

The **gastrointestinal (GI) system** (**Fig. 28.1**), also known as the **alimentary system** or **digestive system**, is a tube designed to break down and absorb ingested nutrients. The inner space of the GI tract, the **lumen**, is the location where large organic molecules in food are broken down into smaller molecules that can be absorbed. The inner lining of the GI tract is an epithelium, and substances enter the body by crossing that epithelium into the underlying connective tissue. Substances that do not cross this epithelial barrier (e.g., dietary fiber) are released in the feces; therefore, they simply pass through a hole in the body.
The main tube (**gut tube, GI tract, alimentary canal**) of the GI system consists of several organs. From cranial to caudal, these are the oral cavity, pharynx, esophagus, stomach, small intestine (duodenum, jejunum, ileum), and large intestine (colon). Food passes through these organs during the process of digestion.

Accessory organs (salivary glands, pancreas, liver, gallbladder) develop from the GI tract and secrete fluids into the lumen of the gut tube to aid in digestion.
This first chapter in this series on the GI system discusses the basic structure of the gut tube. This provides a foundation for subsequent chapters, which look at specific organs of the GI system in greater detail.

28.2 Development of the Gastrointestinal System

In order to understand the overall organization of the GI system, it is useful to describe its development briefly. **Fig. 28.2** shows cross sections of an embryo between weeks 3 and 6 of development. Initially, the embryo is a disk-shaped structure consisting of three layers: **ectoderm**, **mesoderm**, and **endoderm** (**Fig. 28.2a**). During weeks 3 through 6, the embryo folds (**Fig. 28.2b-e**) to produce the tube-shaped body plan of the newborn and adult. During this embryonic folding, the endoderm is folded to form the inner lining of the gut tube. A body cavity called the **intraembryonic coelom** develops within the mesoderm, so that the mesoderm splits into **splanchnic** and **somatic mesoderm**. The splanchnic mesoderm is associated with the endoderm

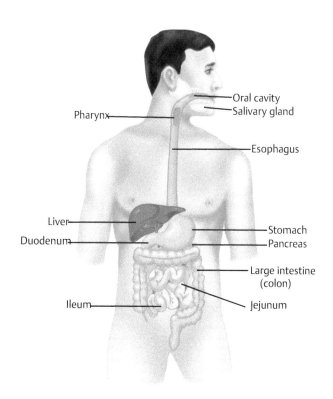

Fig. 28.1 **The gastrointestinal (GI) system.**

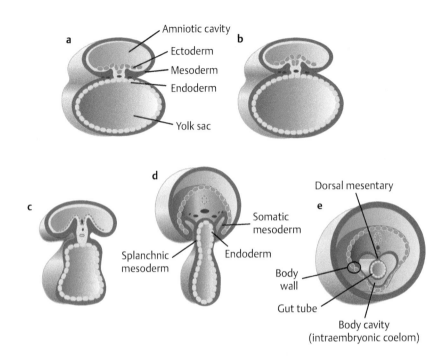

Fig. 28.2   **Development of the GI system; transverse views through the abdominal region. (a) At the beginning of week 3. (b) 19 days. (c) 20 days. (d) 22 days. (e) Week 6.**

and forms the remainder of the wall of the gut tube, while the somatic mesoderm is associated with ectoderm and forms the inner lining of the body wall.

The resulting gut tube is just that, a tube, with a space in the middle, the lumen, through which ingested food passes and is digested. The components of the wall of the gut tube are (**Fig. 28.3**):

1. Endoderm, which forms an epithelium, and is the inner lining of the gut tube; the type of epithelium varies in different parts of the tube
2. Splanchnic mesoderm, which forms two tissues:
   - The bulk is **mesenchyme**, which is embryonic connective tissue that will form connective tissue, vessels, and smooth muscle that make up the wall of the gut tube.
   - The outer layer is a **mesothelium** (epithelium derived from mesoderm). Usually this is simple squamous and provides a smooth outer surface called the **visceral peritoneum** to enable **peristalsis** (movement).

Basic Science Correlate: Gross Anatomy

The inner lining of the body wall is made of somatic mesoderm. The innermost layer of somatic mesoderm forms a mesothelium, becoming the **parietal peritoneum**. The intraembryonic coelom in this region forms the **peritoneal cavity**.

The gut tube is connected to the dorsal body wall by a structure called the **dorsal mesentery**; vessels and nerves access the gut tube via the dorsal mesentery.

Fig. 28.4 is a scanning view of a cross section through the colon, which will serve as one model in this overview of the GI system. As mentioned, the GI system is a tube, with a lumen in the center. The inner lining of the tube is an epithelium derived from endoderm (**Fig. 28.4**, yellow arrows), which is in contact with GI tract contents (at this point, feces). The outer layer is an epithelium (mesothelium) derived from splanchnic mesoderm (**Fig. 28.4**, red arrows) and is in contact with peritoneal fluid. The remainder of the wall (**Fig. 28.4**, black brackets) mostly consists of connective tissue and muscle derived from splanchnic mesoderm (mesenchyme).

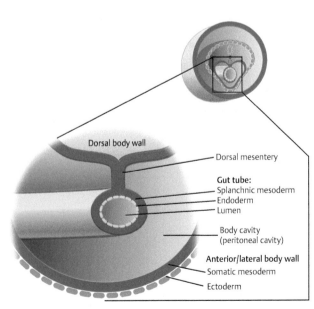

Fig. 28.3   **Detailed view of the newly formed gut tube.**

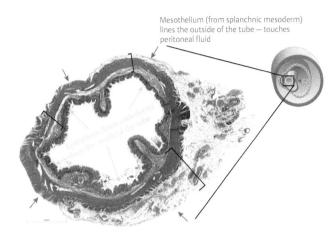

Fig. 28.4   Embryonic origin of GI tissues. The tissues derived from endoderm and mesothelium are indicated by the arrows. Tissues derived from mesenchyme are indicated by the brackets.

Video 28.1   Colon showing basic origin of GI system

Be able to:
— Describe the embryonic origin of the GI system
https://www.thieme.de/de/q.htm?p=opn/
tp/308390101/978-1-62623-414-7_c028_v001&t=video

In many cases (as in the colon in **Fig. 28.4**), the border between the epithelium and underlying connective tissue (i.e., the basement membrane) undulates extensively. In other locations, such as the esophagus (**Fig. 28.5**) the epithelium has fewer undulations, so the border between it and the underlying connective tissue is more apparent (dotted line).

It is also important to note that the esophagus and some other parts of the gut tube are not suspended by dorsal mesentery but are embedded in the dorsal body wall (the esophagus is posterior to the heart and lungs). This is shown in **Fig. 28.6**, a drawing of the embryo in the thoracic region. In this location, the gut tube (esophagus) is not covered by a mesothelium on the outer surface. This concept will be discussed later in this chapter.

28.3   Glands of the Gastrointestinal System

In numerous locations, the epithelium of the digestive tract forms simple **glands** in which the surface epithelial cells invaginate into the underlying connective tissue. Where present, these glands are numerous, which obscures the overall structure. **Fig. 28.7** is a region of the colon showing glands cut in longitudinal section (one gland is in the rectangle), demonstrating that colonic glands form a simple tubular shape.

Fig. 28.8 is a high-magnification image of two colonic glands. Many of the cells in this gland are mucus-secreting goblet cells, which do not stain well. The epithelium at the surface (1) extends down into the connective tissue (2–4) and then back to the surface again (5–7). A lumen is also visible within the gland. The basement membrane (orange arrows) is a pink band that follows the epithelium faithfully, separating it from the underlying (surrounding) connective tissue. The dark purple structures at the bases of the cells are nuclei; because this slide is overstained, the

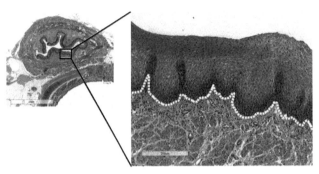

Fig. 28.5   Esophagus showing location of the basement membrane (yellow dotted line).

individual nuclei appear to merge into a single, purple band. In the colon, the connective tissue is very cellular because of large numbers of white blood cells.

Helpful Hint

Just below the gland with the numbers, there is a dark-staining oval region. This is a gland in which the plane of section passes through the base or side of a gland, so only a cluster of nuclei is seen.

Fig. 28.9 is from a region of the colon in which the glands are cut in cross section. The lumen is visible in many glands (yellow arrows), and the basement membrane (orange arrows) separates the epithelium from the surrounding connective tissue.

Video 28.2   Colon showing basic GI system glands

Be able to:
— Identify simple tubular glands
https://www.thieme.de/de/q.htm?p=opn/
tp/308390101/978-1-62623-414-7_c028_v002&t=video

During the formation of glands of the GI system, the depth of invagination of the epithelium varies. Some glands are shorter, as in the colon, while others grow into the deeper regions of the

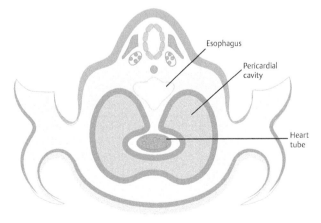

Fig. 28.6   Drawing of the developing embryo in the thoracic region showing the esophagus in the dorsal body wall.

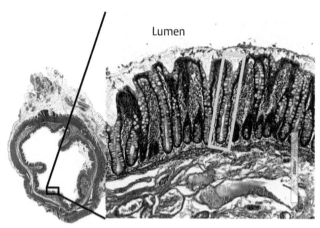

Lumen

Fig. 28.7   Epithelium of the colon showing a gland in longitudinal section (rectangle).

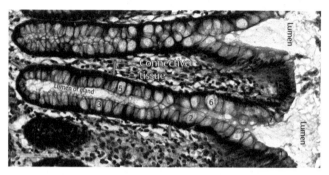

Fig. 28.8   Detailed image of two colonic glands. The main lumen of the colon and the gland are indicated. The sequence of numbers 1 through 7 indicate the invagination of the epithelium of the gland. The basement membrane (orange arrows) is between the epithelium and connective tissue.

digestive tract wall. Still others extend out from the wall of the digestive tract to form separate organs: the salivary glands, liver and gallbladder, and pancreas (**Fig. 28.10**). For the most part, these organs are large outgrowths of the gut tube, composed of epithelial cells, supported by connective tissue, and are connected to the main GI tract by ducts. These will be described in more detail in later chapters.

28.4   Basic Structure of the Gastrointestinal Tract

The wall of the digestive tract in most regions is composed of four layers. Some of these layers have subcomponents (**Fig. 28.11**):

1. **Mucosa**
   i. **Epithelium**: exact type varies depending on location
   ii. **Lamina propria**: loose connective tissue with vessels, nerves, lymphatics, glands
   iii. **Muscularis mucosae**: smooth muscle
2. **Submucosa**: dense irregular connective tissue with larger vessels, nerves, lymphatics, glands
3. **Muscularis externa**: composed of smooth or skeletal muscle:
   i.   Inner circular layer
   ii. Outer longitudinal layer
4. **Serosa** (if suspended by dorsal mesentery) or **adventitia** (if in the dorsal body wall)

Fig. 28.12 is a low-magnification image of the colon, showing these four regions: mucosa (black bracket), submucosa (blue bracket), muscularis externa (green bracket), and serosa (red bracket).

Video 28.3   Colon showing basic GI system structure

Be able to identify:
— Mucosa
— Submucosa
— Muscularis externa
— Serosa/adventitia
https://www.thieme.de/de/q.htm?p=opn/tp/308390101/978-1-62623-414-7_c028_v003&t=video

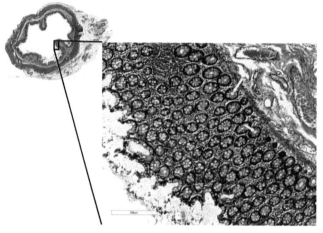

Fig. 28.9   Colonic glands in cross section. The lumen of the glands (yellow arrows) and the location of the basement membrane (orange arrows) are indicated.

28.4.1   Mucosa and Submucosa

Fig. 28.13 shows the two innermost layers of the GI tract: the mucosa and submucosa. These two layers are separated by the muscularis mucosae (yellow arrows), a thin layer of smooth muscle that provides some movement to the mucosal tissue.

- The mucosa (**Fig. 28.13**, black bracket) is composed of an epithelium, loose connective tissue called lamina propria, and the muscularis mucosae. The loose connective tissue in the lamina propria is populated by numerous white blood cells.
- The submucosa (**Fig. 28.13**, blue bracket) is dense irregular connective tissue.

The lamina propria and submucosa are well vascularized, with numerous lymphatic vessels, both of which are important for distributing absorbed nutrients to the body.

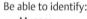

Video 28.4   Colon showing the mucosa and submucosa

Be able to identify:
— Mucosa
   • Epithelium
   • Lamina propria
   • Muscularis mucosae
— Submucosa
https://www.thieme.de/de/q.htm?p=opn/tp/308390101/978-1-62623-414-7_c028_v004&t=video

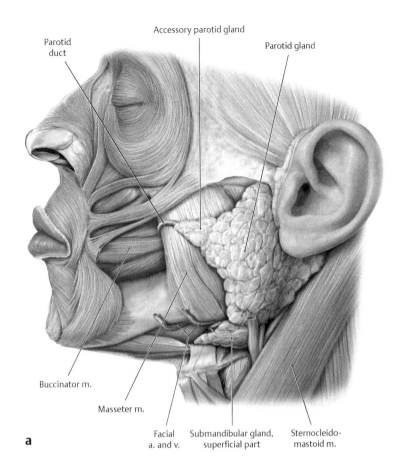

Parotid
duct

Accessory parotid gland

Parotid gland

Buccinator m.

Masseter m.

Facial
a. and v.

Submandibular gland,
superficial part

Sternocleido-
mastoid m.

a

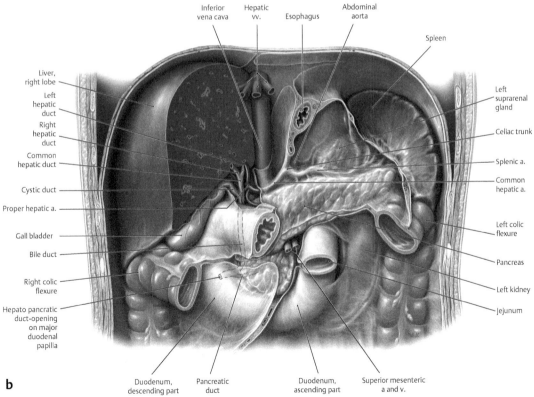

Inferior
vena cava

Hepatic
vv.

Esophagus

Abdominal
aorta

Spleen

Liver,
right lobe

Left
hepatic
duct

Right
hepatic
duct

Common
hepatic duct

Cystic duct

Proper hepatic a.

Gall bladder

Bile duct

Right colic
flexure

Hepato pancreatic
duct-opening
on major
duodenal
papilla

Left
suprarenal
gland

Celiac trunk

Splenic a.

Common
hepatic a.

Left colic
flexure

Pancreas

Left kidney

Jejunum

Duodenum,
descending part

Pancreatic
duct

Duodenum,
ascending part

Superior mesenteric
a and v.

b

Fig. 28.10 **Named glands of the digestive tract.** (a) Salivary glands; (b) liver, pancreas, and gallbladder. Fig. 28.10a from Schuenke M, Schulte E, Schumacher U. *THIEME Atlas of Anatomy. Head, Neck, and Neuroanatomy.* Illustrations by Voll M and Wesker K. Second Edition. New York: Thieme Medical Publishers; 2016 Fig. 28.10b from Schuenke M, Schulte E, Schumacher U. *THIEME Atlas of Anatomy. Internal Organs.* Illustrations by Voll M and Wesker K. Second Edition. New York: Thieme Medical Publishers; 2016.

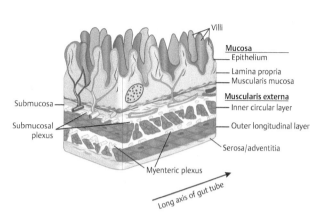

Fig. 28.11 Histology of the GI tract (drawing) showing the basic four layered structure of the wall of the gut tube: mucosa, submucosa, muscularis externa, and serosa (or adventitia).

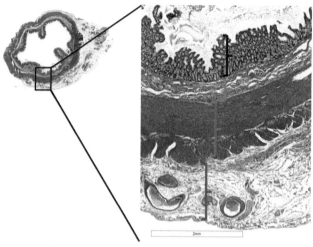

Fig. 28.12 Histology of the GI tract (image). Mucosa (black bracket), submucosa (blue bracket), muscularis externa (green bracket) serosa (red bracket).

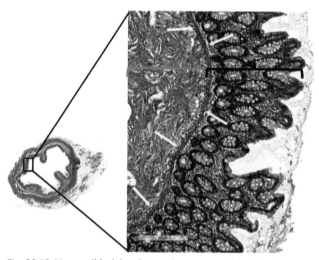

Fig. 28.13 Mucosa (black bracket) and submucosa (blue bracket) of the GI tract, separated by the muscularis mucosae (yellow arrows).

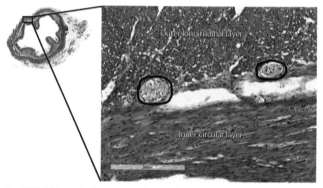

Fig. 28.14 Muscularis externa of the colon in cross section; two ganglia are outlined.

28.4.2 Muscularis Externa

The muscularis externa is a thick layer of muscle responsible for large peristaltic waves of contraction. In most organs (stomach, intestines), it is composed of smooth muscle, but it is composed of skeletal muscle in the very uppermost portion of the GI tract (upper esophagus), where the movement is mostly under voluntary control.

The muscularis externa has two parts:
- An inner circular layer, in which the muscle cells are oriented perpendicular to the direction of the tube (i.e., they "wrap around" the tube)
- An outer longitudinal layer, in which the muscle cells are oriented along the tube

Fig. 28.14 shows a section of the muscularis externa cut in cross section. In this orientation, the inner circular layer of smooth muscle shows a longitudinal view, while the outer longitudinal layer shows smooth muscle in cross section. The outlined structures are autonomic ganglia that innervate these muscles, which will be discussed later in this chapter.

Video 28.5   Colon showing the muscularis externa

Be able to identify:
- Muscularis externa
  - Inner circular layer
  - Outer longitudinal layer
- Autonomic ganglia

https://www.thieme.de/de/q.htm?p=opn/tp/308390101/978-1-62623-414-7_c028_v005&t=video

Fig. 28.15 shows a section of the small intestine cut longitudinally. Because this section is perpendicular to the orientation of the colon from **Fig. 28.14**, the orientation of the smooth muscle layers in the muscularis externa is switched: the inner circular layer shows cross-sectional profiles of smooth muscle, while the outer longitudinal layer shows longitudinal profiles.

Helpful Hint

Because **Fig. 28.15** shows only a portion of the wall of the small intestine, not an entire cross section, the orientation of the tissue may not be obvious if it is not provided in the slide description. A useful rule of thumb is that the orientation of the section taken from the gut is the same as the orientation of the outer longitudinal layer of the muscularis externa in that section.

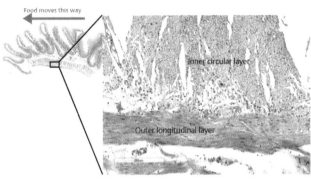

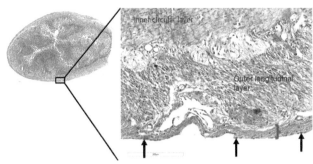

Fig. 28.15 **Muscularis externa of the small intestine in longitudinal section.**

Fig. 28.16 **Serosa of the small intestine (red bracket). The mesothelial cells on the outer surface are indicated (black arrows).**

28.4.3   Adventitia or Serosa

The outer layer of the GI tract is a thin layer called either an adventitia or a serosa, based on either the absence or presence, respectively, of the visceral peritoneum. An adventitia is composed of connective tissue, whereas a serosa is connective tissue plus a mesothelium (the visceral peritoneum).

Fig. 28.16 shows the outer layers of the ileum, part of the small intestine, which is covered by visceral peritoneum and suspended by a dorsal mesentery. The two parts of the muscularis externa are labeled. Here, the outer connective tissue of the gut tube (red bracket) is covered by a simple squamous mesothelium (black arrows), so it is a serosa.

Video 28.6   Ileum showing serosa

Be able to identify:
— Serosa
https://www.thieme.de/de/q.htm?p=opn/
tp/308390101/978-1-62623-414-7_c028_
v006&t=video

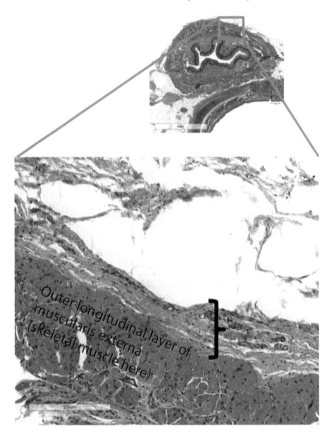

As mentioned, the esophagus and other parts of the gut tube are not suspended by dorsal mesentery but are embedded within the dorsal body wall (see **Fig. 28.6**). Therefore, as shown in **Fig. 28.17**, these regions of the gut tube are not covered by a mesothelium, so the outer surface is an adventitia (marked by the bracket).

Video 28.7   Esophagus showing adventitia

Be able to identify:
— Adventitia
https://www.thieme.de/de/q.htm?p=opn/
tp/308390101/978-1-62623-414-7_c028_
v007&t=video

Fig. 28.17 **Adventitia of the esophagus (black bracket).**

Helpful Hint

In many cases, the mesothelium of a serosa will not be well preserved on a particular slide, or the connective tissue of an adventitia might appear smooth as if it were covered with epithelium. For most histologic studies, the distinction between a serosa and an adventitia is not critical. The differences are pointed out here because these terms are often used, and because they provide an understanding of the gross anatomy and embryology of the GI tract (e.g., gross anatomy terms such as intraperitoneal vs. retroperitoneal).

28.5   Surface Modifications of the Gastrointestinal Tract

The primary function of the GI tract is to break down organic molecules from food in the lumen and absorb these products of

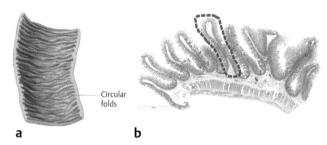

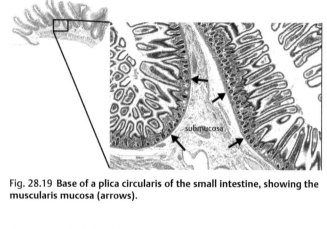

Fig. 28.18 Plicae circulares of the small intestine. (a) Gross view of the internal surface of the intestine. (b) Scanning magnification of the intestine with one plica outlined. From Schuenke M, Schulte E, Schumacher U. *THIEME Atlas of Anatomy. Internal Organs.* Illustrations by Voll M and Wesker K. Second Edition. New York: Thieme Medical Publishers; 2016.

Fig. 28.19 Base of a plica circularis of the small intestine, showing the muscularis mucosa (arrows).

digestion as well as vitamins, minerals, electrolytes, and water. This largely occurs at the apical plasma membrane of the epithelial cells of the mucosa, a process that is enhanced by surface modifications that increase surface area.

The increase in surface area occurs at three levels:

1. Plicae circulares (gross level)
2. Villi (microscopic level)
3. Microvilli (cellular level)

These mucosal modifications are most elaborate in the small intestine, where chemical breakdown and absorption are robust. Organs of the tract that are not involved in chemical breakdown or absorption, such as the esophagus, do not require such an elaborate mucosal morphology.

28.5.1   Plicae Circulares

Plicae circulares (also called valves of Kerckring) are circular folds that extend about one-half to two-thirds of the way around the inner surface of the intestine (**Fig. 28.18a**). These permanent folds are small, but visible grossly. In tissues sectioned and magnified, plicae appear as large structures (**Fig. 28.18b**, one plica circularis is outlined). As shown in **Fig. 28.19**, plicae are large undulations of

the mucosa, including the muscularis mucosae (arrows), so that the core of a plica is connective tissue of the submucosa.

28.5.2   Villi

Villi (**Fig. 28.20**; one is outlined in black) are undulations of the epithelium of the mucosa; there are hundreds of villi on one plica circularis. At the base of the villi, the epithelium extends down into the lamina propria to form glands (**Fig. 28.20**, yellow outline). **Fig. 28.21** is a higher-magnification image of the base of several villi, showing that the core of each villus is lamina propria. A thin wisp of muscularis mucosae (**Fig. 28.21**, yellow arrows) extends at right angles from the main layer of the muscularis mucosae (black arrows) into the center of each villus.

28.5.3   Microvilli

As described in **Chapter 5**, **microvilli** are fingerlike surface modifications of the plasma membrane supported by a core of microfilaments. In light micrographs (**Fig. 28.22**), individual

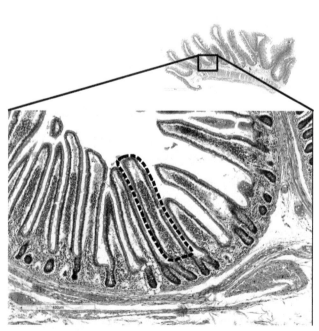

Fig. 28.20 Villi of the small intestine. A villus is outlined in black; a gland is outlined in yellow.

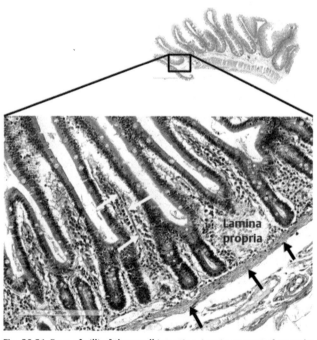

Fig. 28.21 Base of villi of the small intestine. Lamina propria forms the core of each villus. The muscularis mucosa is shown (black arrows). An extension of the muscularis mucosa is in the center of each villus (yellow arrows).

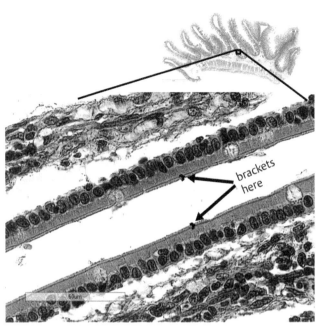

Fig. 28.22 **Microvilli of the intestine in light microscopy (black brackets).**

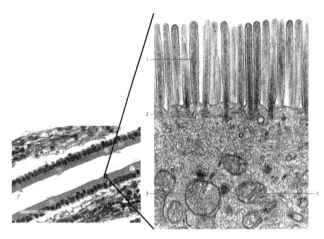

Fig. 28.23 **Microvilli of the intestine in electron microscopy: (1) microvillus; (2) terminal web; (3) mitochondria.**

microvilli cannot be seen; however, collectively they are visible on the apical surface of epithelial cells of the small intestine (**Fig. 28.22**, brackets) and are often referred to as the brush border. **Fig. 28.23** is an electron micrograph of the apical membrane of the epithelial cells, showing microvilli (1).

Video 28.8 Jejunum showing surface modifications

Be able to identify:
— Plicae circulares
— Villi
— Microvilli
https://www.thieme.de/de/q.htm?p=opn/tp/308390101/978-1-62623-414-7_c028_v008&t=video

28.6 Innervation of the Gastrointestinal Tract

Since the GI tract is mostly visceral, it is innervated by the autonomic nervous system. A review of the anatomy of the autonomic nervous system reveals that neural structures within the wall of the GI tract include (**Fig. 28.24**):
• Postganglionic sympathetic axons
• Preganglionic parasympathetic axons
• Parasympathetic ganglia
• Postganglionic parasympathetic axons
• Afferent fibers

Sympathetic ganglia are located outside the target organ, whereas parasympathetic ganglia of the intestine are in the wall of the target organ.

Although smooth muscle contraction (peristalsis) and glandular secretion in the GI tract are controlled to some extent by the central nervous system, there is a system of short-loop reflexes in which afferent neurons that respond to chemicals and stretch

directly stimulate postganglionic neurons in autonomic ganglia. Since these ganglia belong predominantly to the parasympathetic system, these short-loop circuits (consisting of afferent sensory nerves, interneurons in the parasympathetic ganglia, and the postganglionic parasympathetic neurons) are entirely within the wall of the GI tract. This gives rise to the concept of an **enteric nervous system**, a system of neurons entirely within the digestive tract that can function independently from the central nervous system.

Although these neural structures can be found everywhere in the wall of the GI tract, the ganglia are organized into two main locations:
• The **myenteric plexus** (the **Auerbach plexus**, **Fig. 28.25**, black arrows) is between the inner circular and outer longitudinal layers of the muscularis externa.
• The **submucosal plexus** (the **Meissner plexus**) is in the submucosal layer.

Fig. 28.26 is a higher-magnification view of a ganglion of the myenteric plexus (solid yellow outline). Three or four neuronal cell bodies can be seen in the upper right portion of this ganglion (dotted yellow outline). Ganglia of the submucosal plexus are much more challenging to find; one is shown in **Fig. 28.27** (solid yellow outline).

Video 28.9 Colon showing the enteric nervous system

Be able to identify:
— Enteric nervous system
  • Myenteric plexus
  • Submucosal plexus
https://www.thieme.de/de/q.htm?p=opn/tp/308390101/978-1-62623-414-7_c028_v009&t=video

Clinical Correlate

Neurons of the enteric nervous system are derived from **neural crest cells**, which arise from ectoderm and migrate into the gut tube. Absence of these cells results in decreased motility in that portion of the gastrointestinal tract. This condition, called **congenital megacolon** or **Hirschsprung disease**, typically affects regions of the colon (large intestine).

Somatic afferent (sensory)
Somatic efferent (motor)
Sympathetic, preganglionic
Sympathetic, postganglionic
Parasympathetic, preganglionic
Parasympathetic, postganglionic
Visceral afferent (sensory)

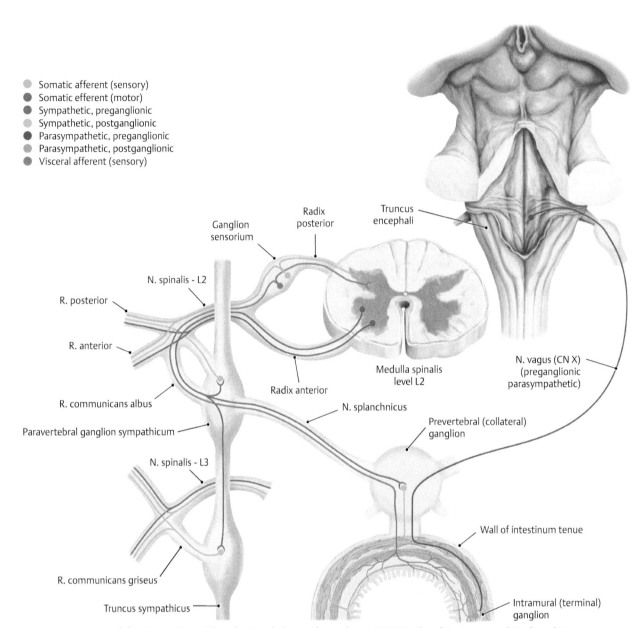

Ganglion sensorium

Radix posterior

Truncus encephali

N. spinalis - L2

R. posterior

R. anterior

Medulla spinalis level L2

N. vagus (CN X) (preganglionic parasympathetic)

R. communicans albus

Radix anterior

N. splanchnicus

Paravertebral ganglion sympathicum

Prevertebral (collateral) ganglion

N. spinalis - L3

Wall of intestinum tenue

R. communicans griseus

Truncus sympathicus

Intramural (terminal) ganglion

Fig. 28.24 Innervation of the GI tract. From Schuenke M, Schulte E, Schumacher U. *THIEME Atlas of Anatomy. Head, Neck, and Neuroanatomy.* Illustrations by Voll M and Wesker K. Second Edition. New York: Thieme Medical Publishers; 2016.

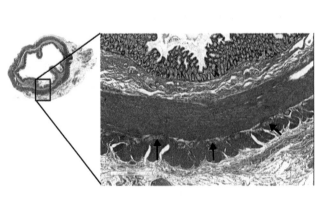

Fig. 28.25 Myenteric plexus of the GI tract (arrows) located between the inner circular and outer longitudinal layers of the muscularis externa..

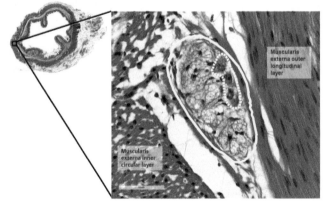

Muscularis externa outer longitudinal layer

Muscularis externa inner circular layer

Fig. 28.26 A single ganglion of the myenteric plexus of the GI tract (solid outline). Three neuronal cell bodies can be seen within this ganglion (dotted outline).

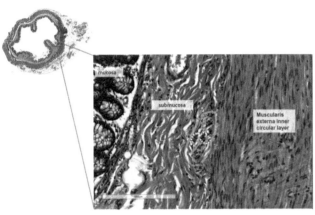

Fig. 28.27 **A single ganglion of the submucosal plexus of the GI tract (solid outline). Neuronal cell bodies can be seen within this ganglion (dotted outline).**

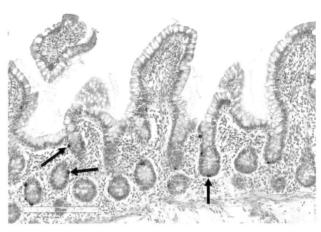

Fig. 28.28 **Ileum stained with silver, showing enteroendocrine cells (arrows).**

28.7   Endocrine Secretions of the Gastrointestinal Tract

Not only does the GI tract respond to neural stimulation, but it also secretes, and responds to, endocrine signals. The epithelial cells in the GI tract that release these hormones are called **enteroendocrine cells**. These hormones are released into the underlying connective tissue and either act locally on glands and smooth muscle or diffuse into the bloodstream to be carried to other organs.

Enteroendocrine cells cannot be distinguished from other cell types of the epithelium with routine H & E staining. However, the secretory granules of these cells react with special silver stains, as seen in **Fig. 28.28** (arrows). Note that the staining is on the basal aspect of these cells; the secretory granules in these cells are adjacent to the basal plasma membrane, to be released into the connective tissue and bloodstream.

Video 28.10 Ileum showing enteroendocrine cells

Be able to identify:
— Enteroendocrine cells
https://www.thieme.de/de/q.htm?p=opn/
tp/308390101/978-1-62623-414-7_c028_v010&t=video

28.8   Chapter Review

The gastrointestinal (GI) tract is a tube that extends from the cranial to the caudal end of the body and through which ingested food passes and is digested and absorbed. It is derived from embryonic endoderm, which forms the inner epithelial cells, and splanchnic mesoderm, which forms the remainder of the tissues. The epithelial cells of the gastrointestinal tract form glands, including single cells (goblet cells) among the surface epithelium, multicellular glands that invaginate into the underlying tissues to form smaller glands within the gut tube, and larger organs such as salivary glands, the liver, and the pancreas that connect to the GI tract through ducts. The wall of the GI tract has a four-layered structure; mucosa, submucosa, muscularis externa, and an outer layer that is either adventitia or serosa. The mucosal layer consists of an epithelium, lamina propria, and muscularis mucosae. The muscularis externa has an inner circular and an outer longitudinal layer. The inner surface of the GI tract has surface modifications at three levels: plicae circulares, villi, and microvilli. These modifications increase surface area for enzymatic digestion and absorption of nutrients. To stimulate glandular secretion and muscular action, the GI system has nerves (enteric plexus) and enteroendocrine cells that act locally but also influence other organs in the GI system. Subsequent chapters will discuss the organs of the GI tract in greater detail.

Questions and Answers

An online-only section of questions and answers accompanying this chapter is hosted on Thieme's MedOne Education site: https://medone-education.thieme.com. Use the code on the media page at the front of this book to gain access. An institutional license to the site is required to access these questions in an interactive format, and individual users are required to register for an individual account to track results.

29   Intestines

After completing this chapter, you should be able to:
— Identify, at the light microscope level, each of the following:
- Small intestine
  - Structures
    - Plicae, villi, microvilli (review)
    - Intestinal crypts (of Lieberkühn)
  - Cells
    - Enterocytes (intestinal absorptive cells)
    - Goblet cells
    - Paneth cells
    - Enteroendocrine cells (review, covered in **Chapter 28**)
  - Regions
    - Duodenum
      - Submucosal (Brunner) glands
      - Ampulla of Vater
    - Jejunum
    - Ileum
      - Peyer's patches
- Large intestine
  - Structures
    - Intestinal crypts (of Lieberkühn)
    - Taeniae coli
  - Cells
    - Enterocytes (intestinal absorptive cells)
    - Goblet cells
— Outline the function of each organ, structure, or cell type listed
— Predict the result of a defect in the organ, structure, or cell type listed

29.1   Overview of the Small and Large Intestines

The previous chapter overviewed the main features of the gastro-intestinal (GI) system. This and the next four chapters discuss the organs of the GI system in greater detail. Although many texts begin with the oral cavity and proceed toward the anal canal (which is perfectly logical), this first organ chapter will cover the **small** and **large intestines** (**Fig. 29.1**). This is because the function of the GI tract is to break down and absorb nutrients, and, since the intestines are largely involved in the process of absorption, it makes sense to begin here (or at least is a reasonable option). In addition, **Chapter 28** used the intestines as a model organ to describe the basic features of the GI tract, so this is a nice transition.

The **small intestine** receives **chyme**, a fluid that consists of partially digested food and digestive secretions from the oral cavity and stomach. The small intestine is the primary site for chemical breakdown of organic molecules and absorption of these organic molecules, as well as vitamins, minerals, ions, and water. There are three regions of the small intestine (**Fig. 29.1**):

1. The **duodenum** is a C-shaped segment about 12 inches long (from which it gets its name), connected to the lower end of the stomach. The duodenum receives chyme from

the stomach as well as bile produced by the liver and digestive enzymes and buffers released from the pancreas.
2. The **jejunum** is a convoluted tube that has greatly enhanced inner surface area and is involved in chemical breakdown and absorption of nutrients.
3. The **ileum** is a continuation of the jejunum that completes nutrient absorption.

The terminal portion of the small intestine, the ileum, connects to the **large intestine** (**colon**). The large intestine has different named parts based on location or shape (ascending, transverse, descending, sigmoid); most of the large intestine functions to absorb water and vitamins. The final product of the GI tract, the feces, is stored in the **rectum** and is passed out through the anal canal in a bowel movement.

29.2   Small Intestine

Because the previous chapter presented the general structure of the GI tract, only a reminder here is necessary to describe many of the main features of the small intestine. **Fig. 29.2** shows a scanning view of the jejunum. Recall that the wall of the GI tract has four regions:

1. The **mucosa** is the innermost layer consisting of an epithelium (simple columnar in the intestines), underlying connective tissue called **lamina propria**, and the **muscularis mucosae**, composed of smooth muscle.
2. The **submucosa** contains denser connective tissue.

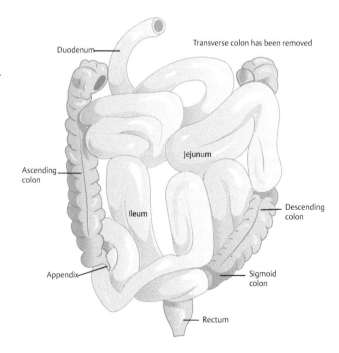

Fig. 29.1   **Small and large intestines.**

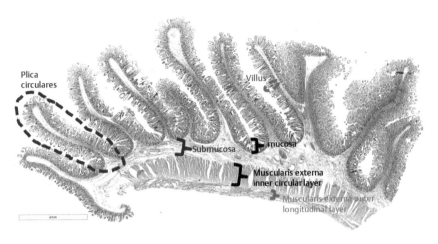

Fig. 29.2 Jejunum in longitudinal section, showing the four-layered structure typical of the gastrointestinal (GI) tract. A plica circularis (blue outline) and a villus (red outline) are also shown.

3. The **muscularis externa** has an inner circular and an outer longitudinal layer; in the intestines these layers are entirely smooth muscle.
4. The thin outer connective tissue layer is called **serosa** where it is covered by an epithelium and **adventitia** where it is not.

Also recall that the small intestine, and in particular the jejunum, has an inner surface that is covered with projections that greatly increase the surface area available for digestion and absorption. **Fig. 29.2** shows two of these features that increase surface area: a **plica circularis** and a **villus**, visible to the unaided eye and with the light microscope, respectively. The third feature, **microvilli**, are projections of the plasma membrane, less than 2 μm long (see **Fig. 28.23**) that provide abundant plasma membrane area in which digestive enzymes and transport pumps are placed to assist in digestion and absorption.

> ### Clinical Correlate
>
> **Celiac disease** (**celiac sprue**) is an autoimmune disorder caused by a reaction to ingested gluten. In most cases, the inflammatory reaction results in loss of the villus and microvillus structures of the small intestine. This decreases digestion and absorption efficiency, and nutrients remaining in the fecal material cause abdominal cramping, diarrhea, and foul-smelling stools. Treatment is to remove gluten from the diet.

Also note that, as discussed in the preceding chapter, epithelial invaginations at the base of the villi form **glands** (**Fig. 29.3**, yellow outline). In the small and large intestine, these glands are specifically referred to as **intestinal crypts** (of Lieberkühn).

29.3 Epithelial Cell Types of the Small Intestine

Many of the cells and structures of the small intestine (e.g., smooth muscle, vessels) have been discussed in previous chapters and do not require further discussion. However, the epithelium of the small intestine, both the surface epithelium and the epithelium that forms the intestinal crypts, is specialized for digestion and absorption. The cells of this simple columnar epithelium are as follows:

- **Enterocytes** or **intestinal absorptive cells** (**Fig. 29.4**; two are outlined) are the most numerous cell type seen in the epithelium of the small intestine. These cells have elaborate microvilli, express digestive enzymes in the brush border, and absorb nutrients. They have basally located nuclei and eosinophilic cytoplasm.
- **Goblet cells** (**Fig. 29.4**, arrows) are recognized because their numerous mucus-containing secretory granules do not stain well on routine H & E preparations.
- **Stem cells** divide to replace cells lost cells during continuous epithelial turnover. These cells are located in the junction of the villi and crypts but are not seen in H & E sections.
- **Enteroendocrine cells** release hormones basally and have already been discussed in the preceding chapter.
- **Paneth cells** are most readily seen at the base of the crypts (**Fig. 29.5**, outlined regions). They produce antibacterial proteins such as lysozymes and alpha-defensins, which are released into the lumen of the intestinal tract. Their secretory

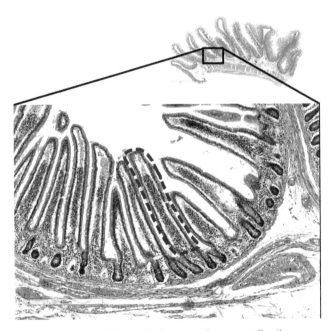

Fig. 29.3 Jejunum in longitudinal section, showing a villus (brown outline) and gland or intestinal crypt (yellow outline).

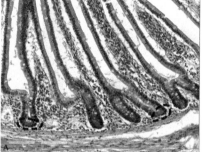
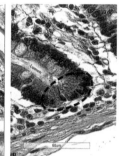

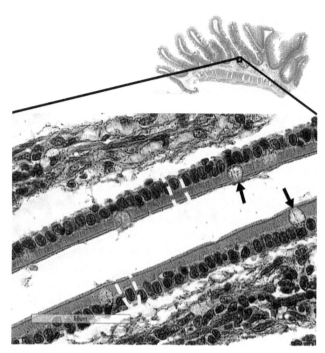

Fig. 29.4   **Epithelium of the jejunum, showing enterocytes (outlines) and goblet cells (arrows).**

Fig. 29.5   **Jejunum, showing Paneth cells (outlined) at the base of the intestinal crypts. (a) Medium magnification. (b) Base of the intestinal crypt at high magnification.**

29.4   Regions of the Small Intestine

As mentioned earlier, the small intestine has three regions: duodenum, jejunum, and ileum, listed in order of passage of food. Each performs a slightly different function and has histologic features consistent with these functions. They are described in the following sections not in the order in which food passes through them but in the order that makes the most sense histologically.

29.4.1   Jejunum

Because the jejunum has been a model for the structure of the gastrointestinal tract and epithelial cell types, and because it is the most "generic," it is useful to describe it first. Indeed, the jejunum is characterized because it has all the main features previously described: elaborate surface modifications (plicae, villi), intestinal crypts, simple columnar epithelium with microvilli and goblet cells, and numerous Paneth cells (see **Figs 29.2** through **Fig. 29.5**). In addition, it lacks features specific to the duodenum and ileum (described subsequently).

granules are highly eosinophilic on H & E-stained sections and are located in the apical aspect of the cytoplasm (**Fig. 29.5b**). These cells are numerous in the small intestine, especially the cranial portion (closest to the stomach), become less numerous distally, and are rare in the large intestine.

- **M cells** transport antigen from the lumen of the digestive tract to T lymphocytes in the lamina propria and, therefore, assist in immunity. M cells are not distinguishable on routine H & E-stained slides.

Basic Science Correlate: Cell Biology

Paneth cells secrete their product apically, into the lumen of the intestine. Therefore, secretory granules in these cells are stored apical to the nucleus (see eosinophilic staining in **Fig. 29.5b**). On the other hand, enteroendocrine cells secrete their product basally, into the connective tissue and bloodstream. Recall that the latter cells must be visualized by a special (silver) stain and that their secretory granules are basally located (see **Fig. 28.28**).

Video 29.1   Intestinal epithelium cell types

Be able to identify:
— Small intestine
  - Enterocytes (intestinal absorptive cells)
  - Goblet cells
  - Paneth cells
https://www.thieme.de/de/q.htm?p=opn/tp/308390101/978-1-62623-414-7_c029_v001&t=video

Video 29.2   Jejunum—H & E

https://www.thieme.de/de/q.htm?p=opn/tp/308390101/978-1-62623-414-7_c029_v002&t=video

Video 29.3   Jejunum—PAS

Be able to identify:
— Jejunum
https://www.thieme.de/de/q.htm?p=opn/tp/308390101/978-1-62623-414-7_c029_v003&t=video

29.4.2   Ileum

The ileum includes all the features of the small intestine just described, plus large regions of diffuse lymphoid tissue called **Peyer's patches**. These are large nodules, seen even at low magnification (**Fig. 29.6**), located on the antimesenteric side of the ileum (the side opposite the mesentery).

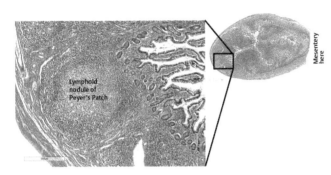

Fig. 29.6   Ileum showing lymphoid nodules (Peyer's patches).

Video 29.4   Ileum

Be able to identify:
— Ileum
  • Peyer's patches
https://www.thieme.de/de/q.htm?p=opn/
tp/308390101/978-1-62623-414-7_c029_v004&t=video

29.4.3 Duodenum

The duodenum is the initial portion of the small intestine and receives chyme from the stomach, bile from the liver, and pancreatic secretions. It is C-shaped (**Fig. 29.7**); the **pancreas** is nestled against its concave side. **Fig. 29.8** shows a scanning view of the duodenum, rotated so that its orientation is similar to that of the drawing. Note that only a portion of the wall of the duodenum is shown (the anatomic left side adjacent to the pancreas).

Because the duodenum receives acidic chyme from the stomach and digestive secretions from the pancreas and liver, it secretes a tremendous amount of mucus for protection. Although goblet cells of the surface epithelium play some role here, **submucosal glands (Brunner glands)** within the duodenum provide the bulk of this mucus (**Fig. 29.9**).

Video 29.5   Duodenum

Be able to identify:
— Duodenum
  • Submucosal (Brunner) glands
https://www.thieme.de/de/q.htm?p=opn/tp/308390101/978-1-62623-414-7_c029_v005&t=video

In or near the wall of the duodenum, the **pancreatic duct** and **bile duct** meet to form a dilated duct, the **ampulla of Vater**, which drains into the lumen of the duodenum (**Fig. 29.7**). The presence of the ampulla of Vater is marked by an elevation on the inner surface of the duodenum called the **greater duodenal papilla**, which is visible to the unaided eye on gross specimens. Release of liver and pancreatic secretions into the duodenum is controlled by the **sphincter of Oddi**, a specialization of the inner circular layer of the muscularis externa near the opening of the ampulla of Vater.

Basic Science Correlate: Physiology

The sphincter of Oddi is relaxed by **cholecystokinin**, which is released by the duodenum in response to fatty acids in a meal. This relaxation allows bile and pancreatic secretions to enter the duodenum.

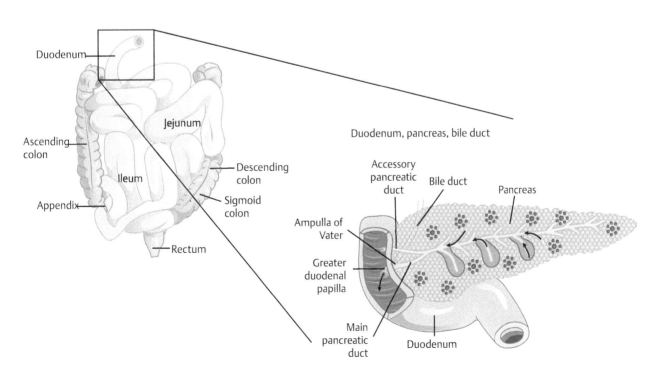

Fig. 29.7   **Drawing of the duodenum and pancreas. The pancreatic duct carrying secretions from the pancreas and bile duct from the liver join to form a wider duct called the ampulla of Vater, which passes through the wall of the duodenum. The presence of the ampulla forms an elevation in the inner surface of the duodenum, the greater duodenal papilla.**

Fig. 29.8   Scanning view of part of the wall of the duodenum near the greater duodenal papilla, including part of the pancreas adjacent to the duodenum.

Fig. 29.10 is the scanning view of the duodenum, showing the ampulla of Vater (arrows) and the major (greater) duodenal papilla (outlined). The sphincter of Oddi is not readily seen on this slide.

Video 29.6   Duodenum showing the ampulla of Vater

Be able to identify:
— Duodenum
   • Ampulla of Vater
https://www.thieme.de/de/q.htm?p=opn/tp/308390101/978-1-62623-414-7_c029_v006&t=video

29.5   Large Intestine

The ileum empties into the large intestine in the lower right abdominal quadrant (**Fig. 29.1**). The large intestine has several parts: ascending (beginning with the caecum), transverse (not shown), descending, sigmoid, rectum. Histologically, all these regions of the large intestine are similar to the small intestine, except that the large intestine has numerous goblet cells and lacks villi (**Fig. 29.11**).

The function of the large intestine is to absorb water and some vitamins. Therefore, it is the site of transition of undigested material from a liquid state to a solid state. Mucus from goblet cells provides lubrication for the passage of the solid mass. Enterocytes are present but are greatly outnumbered by goblet cells.

In the large intestine, the outer longitudinal layer of the muscularis externa is thick in some regions and very thin in others. The thickened regions are called **taeniae coli**. Typically, three are present, but in **Fig. 29.12**, one is obvious (outlined) and the other two are more ill defined. It is likely that the later two are fused together to make one larger structure (arrows).

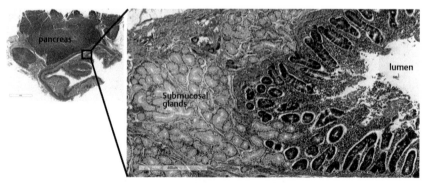

Fig. 29.9   Duodenum showing abundant mucus glands in the submucosa. Note the lumen of the duodenum to the right; the surface epithelium is not well preserved.

Duodenum, pancreas, bile duct

Accessory
pancreatic
duct   Bile duct
                              Pancreas
Ampulla of
Vater
Greater
duodenal
papilla
Main
pancreatic   Duodenum
duct

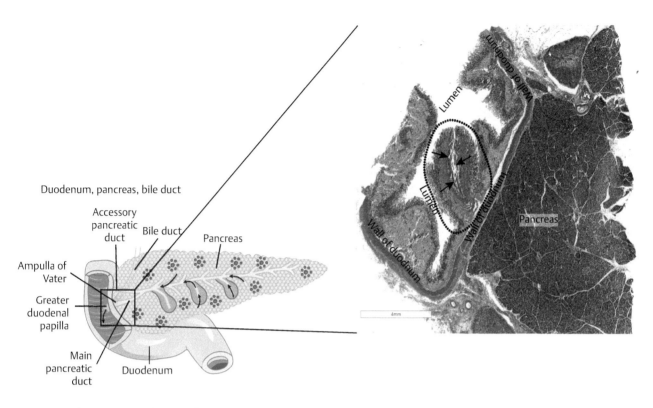

Fig. 29.10 **Duodenum showing the ampulla of Vater (arrows) within the greater duodenal papilla (outlined).**

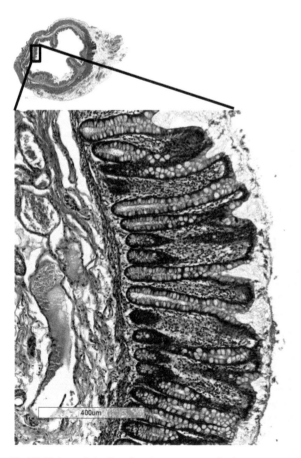

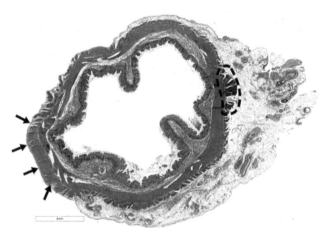

Fig. 29.12 **Scanning view of the large intestine showing taeniae coli (outlined and arrows).**

Fig. 29.11 **Large intestine showing mucosa and submucosa.**

Video 29.7   Large intestine

Be able to identify:
— Large intestine (colon)
https://www.thieme.de/de/q.htm?p=opn/
tp/308390101/978-1-62623-414-7_c029_
v007&t=video

Finally, the **appendix** is a modified portion of the large intestine, about the size of a pinky finger, located in the lower right abdominal quadrant (see **Fig. 29.1**). The histology of the appendix is similar to that of the rest of the large intestine, except that it has numerous lymphoid nodules.

Clinical Correlate

Although the function of the appendix is unclear, it is a common source of pathologic inflammation (appendicitis). The appendix houses colonic bacteria, and rupture of the appendix can cause generalized **peritonitis** (inflammation of the abdominal visceral organs), which may be life threatening. Treatment for appendicitis is surgical removal.

29.6   Chapter Review

The small intestine is the major site for chemical breakdown and absorption of nutrients. It has all the basic features of the gastrointestinal tract, including a four-layered structure (mucosa, submucosa, muscularis externa, adventitia/serosa), as well as glands (called intestinal crypts) and modifications (plicae, villi, microvilli) that increase surface area. The epithelium of the intestine includes several cell types, including enterocytes, goblet cells, stem cells, enteroendocrine cells, and M cells. There are three parts of the small intestine. The duodenum has large numbers of mucus-secreting glands that protect it from acidic chyme from the stomach. The duodenum also receives bile from the liver and pancreatic secretions. The jejunum has the most elaborate surface modifications and is the main site for nutrient breakdown and absorption. The ileum can be identified by the presence of large lymphoid nodules called Peyer patches. The main function of the large intestine is to absorb water, converting fecal material from liquid to solid. It has histologic features similar to the small intestine but lacks villi, has few Paneth cells, and has abundant goblet cells.

Questions and Answers

An online-only section of questions and answers accompanying this chapter is hosted on Thieme's MedOne Education site: https://medone-education.thieme.com. Use the code on the media page at the front of this book to gain access. An institutional license to the site is required to access these questions in an interactive format, and individual users are required to register for an individual account to track results.

30 Oral Cavity, Tongue, and Salivary Glands

After completing this chapter, you should be able to:
— Identify, at the light microscope level, each of the following:
- Tongue
  - Papilla
    - Filiform
    - Fungiform
    - Circumvallate
      - Serous glands
  - Taste buds
- Salivary glands
  - Structures in each gland
    - Acini
      - Serous acini
      - Mucus acini
      - Serous demilunes
    - Ducts
      - Intercalated
      - Striated
      - Excretory
  - Types of salivary glands
    - Parotid
    - Submandibular
    - Sublingual
— Outline the function of each structure listed

30.1 Introduction

This chapter will focus on some of the main structures of the oral cavity. The histology of the tongue will be discussed, including its papillae and taste buds. This will be followed by a more in-depth look at the salivary glands, which were initially presented in **Chapter 6**. This will include a review of glandular secretion and then contrast the histologic features of the three salivary glands.

30.2 Tongue

In a typical view of the **tongue** (i.e., on physical exam), only the anterior aspects are visible (**Fig. 30.1**). However, much of the tongue is in the posterior aspect of the oral cavity. The dorsum is the upper surface; the ventral surface is the "bottom" of the tongue. Most of the main features of the tongue, including papillae and taste buds, are found on the dorsal surface (**Fig. 30.2**).

Fig. 30.3 shows a scanning view of a section through the tongue. The core of the tongue is thick skeletal muscle, the fibers of which are oriented in all directions. The surface mucosa consists of a stratified squamous epithelium and a dense irregular connective tissue. Mixed mucous and serous glands are found within the connective tissue but also extend into the muscle.

Video 30.1 Tongue overview

Be able to identify:
— Tongue
https://www.thieme.de/de/q.htm?p=opn/
tp/308390101/978-1-62623-414-7_c030_
v001&t=video

The dorsal surface of the tongue features projections called **papillae**. There are four types of papillae (see **Fig. 30.2**):
1. **Filiform papillae** (not labeled) are conical projections, scattered throughout the anterior two-thirds of the tongue.
2. **Fungiform papillae** are mushroom-shaped, scattered throughout the anterior two-thirds of the tongue.
3. **Foliate papillae** are ridge-shaped and are found on the lateral side of the tongue. These are underdeveloped in humans, so they are not discussed here.
4. **Circumvallate papillae** are large, about 12 to 15 of these form a V-shape that divides the anterior two-thirds of the tongue from the posterior one-third of the tongue.

30.2.1 Filiform and Fungiform Papillae

Closer examination of the dorsal surface of the anterior two-thirds of the tongue at higher magnification reveals that it contains filiform and fungiform papillae.

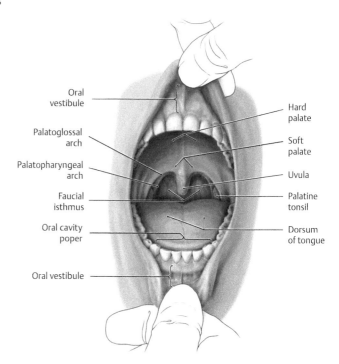

Fig. 30.1 **Oral cavity, clinical view.**

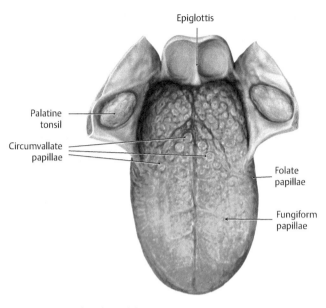

Fig. 30.2   **Dorsal surface of the tongue, showing location of papillae.**

Filiform papillae (**Fig. 30.4**, arrows) are conical projections of the epithelium; these are lightly keratinized and lack taste buds.

Fungiform papillae (**Fig. 30.5**, outlined) are mushroom-shaped, have a core of connective tissue, and are lightly keratinized. These papillae do have taste buds, but they are not seen in this image.

Video 30.2   Tongue filiform and fungiform papillae

Be able to identify:
— Tongue
  • Filiform papillae
  • Fungiform papillae
https://www.thieme.de/de/q.htm?p=opn/tp/308390101/978-1-62623-414-7_c030_v002&t=video

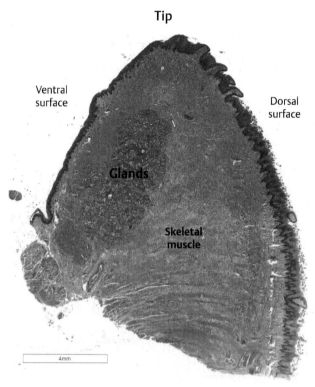

Fig. 30.3   **Sagittal section through tongue, scanning magnification.**

Video 30.3   Base of the tongue showing circumvallate papillae

Be able to identify:
— Tongue
  • Circumvallate papilla
    ○ Serous glands (Von Ebner's glands)
https://www.thieme.de/de/q.htm?p=opn/tp/308390101/978-1-62623-414-7_c030_v003&t=video

30.2.2   Circumvallate Papilla

Circumvallate papillae (**Fig. 30.6**, black outline) are large, with a core of connective tissue. They are lightly keratinized and have many taste buds. They are surrounded by a deep trench (space). Serous glands (**Fig. 30.6**, yellow outline), sometimes called Von Ebner's glands, secrete into the trench.

Taste buds (**Fig. 30.7**, outlined) are found on all papillae except filiform papillae. However, they are best seen on circumvallate papillae. They are tulip-shaped modifications of the epithelium and contain several cell types, including sensory cells, supportive cells, and stem cells. Receptors on the sensory cells bind to ingested molecules and relay the signal to a peripheral nerve that transmits the signal to the central nervous system for recognition and processing.

Helpful Hint

Individual cell types of taste buds are difficult to see on routine H & E; recognizing a taste bud on these slides is usually sufficient.

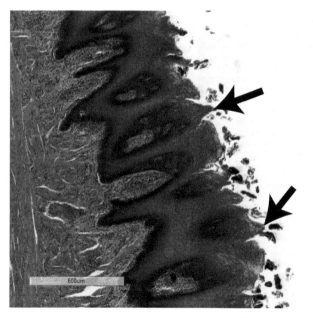

Fig. 30.4   **Filiform papillae on the dorsal surface of the tongue.**

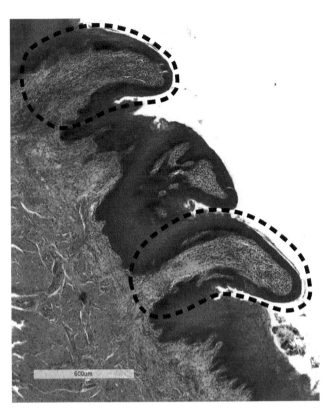

CHAPTER 30

Fig. 30.5 **Fungiform papillae on the dorsal surface of the tongue (outlined).**

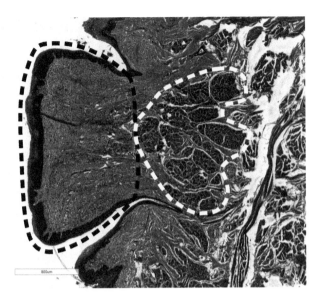

Fig. 30.6 **Circumvallate papilla on the dorsal surface of the tongue (black outline), with serous acini (Von Ebner's glands, yellow outline).**

Clinical Correlate

Although defining lobes and lobules in organs in histologic specimens is not precise, they do have clinical significance. For example, if a tumor is isolated to one lobule in the lung (i.e., one bronchopulmonary segment; see **Chapter 39**), that single lobule can be removed as a unit, without disturbing the function of the remaining lobules.

30.3 Salivary Glands

Saliva is composed of water, mucus, ions, buffers, antibodies (immunoglobulin A [IgA]), and some digestive enzymes. There are three paired salivary glands (**Fig. 30.8**):

- **Parotid gland**
- **Submandibular gland**
- **Sublingual gland**

Fig. 30.9 is a scanning view of a section through the parotid gland. Glandular organs, including the salivary glands, can be divided into **lobes** (**Fig. 30.9**, black outline) and **lobules** (**Fig. 30.9**, blue outline). Lobes and lobules are defined based on branching during development. A lobule contains one common duct into which the secretory elements (described in the next subsection) drain; ducts from adjacent lobules combine to form a larger duct that drains all lobules in the lobe.

Helpful Tip

In sections of salivary glands, identifying the precise outline of a lobe or lobule is not necessarily an exact science. In any given image or section, histologists may define lobes or lobules slightly differently, so it is not high yield to worry too much about this.

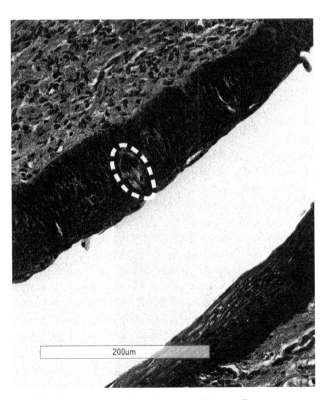

Fig. 30.7 **Taste bud on surface of circumvallate papilla.**

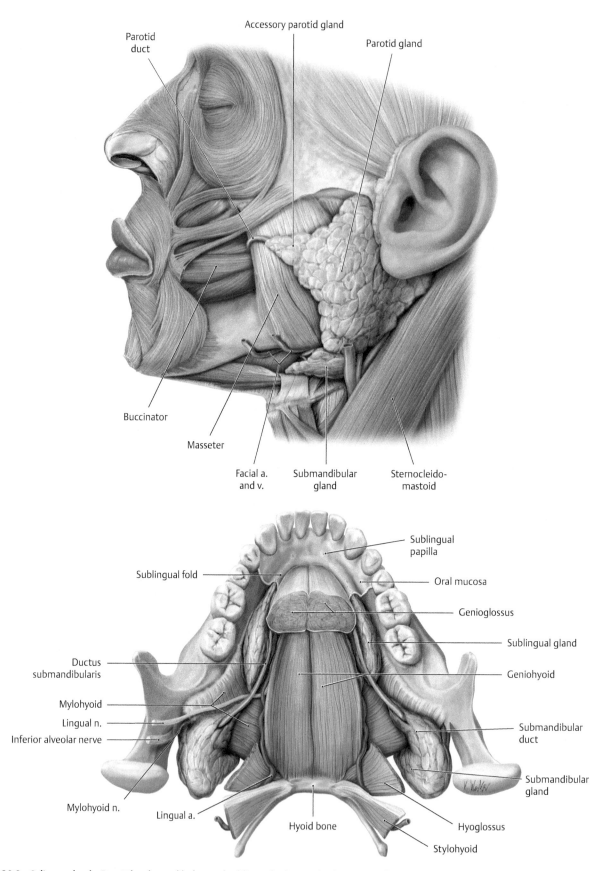

Fig. 30.8   **Salivary glands. Parotid, submandibular, and sublingual salivary glands are paired organs with ducts leading to the oral cavity.**

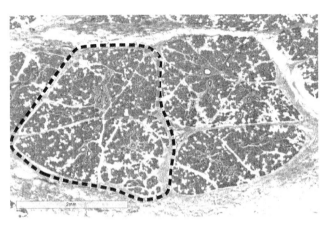

Fig. 30.9 **Parotid gland, showing lobe (black outline) and lobule (blue outline).**

30.3.1 Acini

Fig. 30.10 illustrates the secretory end pieces of a salivary gland. The secretory cells are organized into **acini** (or possibly tubules), which surround a lumen. Recall that the apical side of the cell faces the lumen, while the basement membrane (basal lamina) is on the basal side of the acinar cells.

The secretory cells are either **serous** (produce a watery secretion) or **mucous** (produce a carbohydrate-rich secretion that is sticky). In many cases, each acinus consists of all serous or all mucus-secreting cells. In some acini, there are a few serous cells associated with a mucous acinus; these serous cells are referred to as **serous demilunes**.

In **Fig. 30.11**, two acini are outlined. Note that acini vary in size to some extent, but much of this can be attributed to the plane of sectioning. The lumen of each acinus is usually not visible, though a lumen can be seen in the acinus outlined in yellow. Each acinus has around 6 to 12 or more cells; cell borders can be seen in some cases, especially in the lower right region of the acinus outlined in black, and in the acinus outlined in yellow.

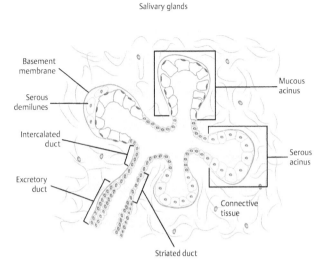

Fig. 30.10 **Secretory end piece of a typical salivary gland.**

In many cases, individual cells are not easily distinguished. The nucleus of some cells is not in the plane of section.

Recall that glandular cells are epithelial. Loose (**Fig. 30.11**, black arrow) and dense (**Fig.30.11**, green arrow) irregular connective tissue is located between the acini. The row of red blood cells in the center of the image, between the two acini, indicates a capillary.

Also recall that there are two types of acini: serous and mucous. **Serous acini** (**Fig. 30.11**, black outline) secrete a protein-rich, watery solution and are characterized by pink cytoplasm, some cytoplasmic basophilia due to protein production, and round nuclei in the basal aspect of the cell. **Mucous acini** (**Fig. 30.11**, yellow outline) have pale cytoplasm due to granules that stain poorly in routine preparations, and their nuclei are flattened against the basal membrane of the cell.

Also recall that individual acini can be mixed. In **Fig. 30.12**, some of the mucous acini have clusters of serous secreting cells, called **serous demilunes** (**Fig. 30.12**, yellow outlines).

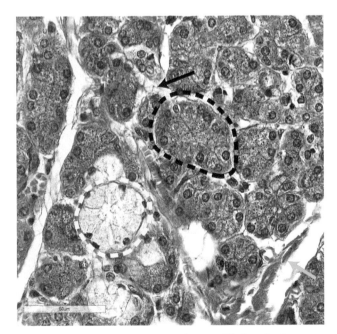

Fig. 30.11 **Mucous (yellow outline) and serous (black outline) acini, surrounded by loose (black arrow) and dense irregular connective tissue (green arrow).**

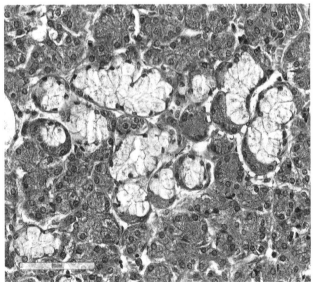

Fig. 30.12 **Serous demilunes (yellow outline).**

Video 30.4   Submandibular gland showing
serous and mucous acini

Be able to identify:
— Acini
  • Serous acini
  • Mucous acini
  • Serous demilunes

https://www.thieme.de/de/q.htm?p=opn/tp/308390101/978-1-
62623-414-7_c030_v004&t=video

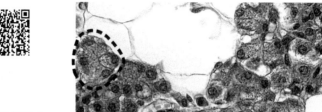

30.3.2 Ducts

In salivary glands, **ducts** transmit fluid to the oral cavity. In
addition, the ducts closer to the secretory end pieces (acini) are
also involved in modification of the salivary content as it passes
through them. The ducts in salivary glands are (listed in order of
flow of saliva) **intercalated ducts**, **striated ducts**, and **excretory
ducts** (see **Fig. 30.10**):

Intercalated ducts (**Fig. 30.13**, green outline) are typically
narrower than acinar units and composed of a simple cuboidal
epithelium. The minimal cytoplasm of the cells of intercalated
ducts underscores the fact that activity in these ducts is minimal.
A small amount of loose connective tissue provides support.

> **Helpful Hint**
>
> **Fig. 30.13** is a nice image of an intercalated duct, but the acini are
> not well represented here. One acinus is outlined in black to pro-
> vide a sense of the size of the intercalated duct. Intercalated ducts
> are short, so they are challenging to find in histologic specimens.

**Fig. 30.13 Intercalated duct (green outline), and serous acinus for
comparison (black outline).**

Most **striated ducts** (**Fig. 30.14a**, **b**, outlined) are approximately the same diameter as the secretory units (acini), but some
are larger. They are composed of a simple, tall columnar epithelium. These ducts are very active in ion transport, so the cells
lining them have eosinophilic cytoplasm and elaborate **basolateral infoldings** of the plasma membrane to provide surface area
for ion pumps. These infoldings are barely visible as striations
in the basal aspect of the cell (**Fig. 30.14b**, upper left and upper
right portion of the duct). The nucleus is located in the center of
the cell to allow room for these basolateral infoldings.

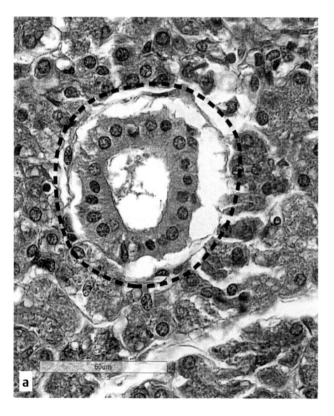

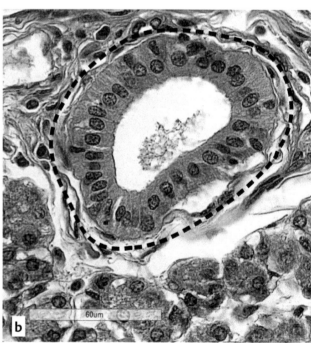

Fig. 30.14 (a, b) Striated ducts (outlined).

The basolateral infoldings in these cells are fairly elaborate; unfortunately, they are challenging to see, even in a good light micrograph. Therefore, to identify striated ducts, it is easiest to look for nuclei that are centrally located, unusual for epithelial cells that line a tube (nuclei are usually basally located in acini and other ducts).

Also note that in the smaller duct in **Fig. 30.14a**, the epithelial cells pull away from the surrounding connective tissue during fixation. This artifact is characteristic of many striated ducts but is not always observable (as in **Fig. 30.14b**).

Fig. 30.15 is actually from the kidney, but it shows basolateral infoldings of the plasma membrane (2). The basolateral cell membrane undulates to create more plasma membrane to place ion pumps and channels. Cells that do this are actively involved in moving ions or water across the membrane, so they require large numbers of mitochondria (3).

Fig. 30.16 shows a fortuitous image of acini and ducts in continuity, together with a drawing (**Fig. 30.16b**) for comparison. In **Fig. 30.16a** (labeled, **Fig. 30.16c** is an unlabeled version of the same image), acini (black outlines) are shown connected to intercalated ducts (yellow dotted lines), which lead into a striated duct (green line).

Finally, **excretory ducts** (**Fig. 30.17**, outlined) are conduits to the oral cavity (i.e., they are not involved in ion or water transport across the epithelium). They can be intralobular (within a lobule), interlobular (between lobules), or interlobar (between lobes); however, this distinction is not critical. Smaller ducts are lined by a simple columnar epithelium, which becomes stratified cuboidal and then stratified columnar in sections of the duct that are progressively larger and closer to the oral cavity. The thickness of the supporting connective tissue also increases with increasing duct size. In **Fig. 30.17**, a striated duct is to the right for direct comparison (i.e., on the right edge of the image, just above the excretory duct circled to the right).

Video 30.5   Parotid gland showing ducts

Be able to identify:
— Ducts
  • Intercalated
  • Striated
  • Excretory
https://www.thieme.de/de/q.htm?p=opn/tp/308390101/978-1-62623-414-7_c030_v005&t=video

30.3.3   Identification of Salivary Glands

As mentioned earlier, there are three pairs of salivary glands. The easiest way to distinguish specimens from the three salivary glands is to compare the ratio of serous to mucous glands:
• The **parotid gland** is all serous acini (**Fig. 30.18a**).
• The **submandibular gland** is mostly serous acini, with some mucous acini (**Fig. 30.18b**).
• The **sublingual gland** is mostly mucous acini, with a few serous acini (**Fig. 30.18c**).

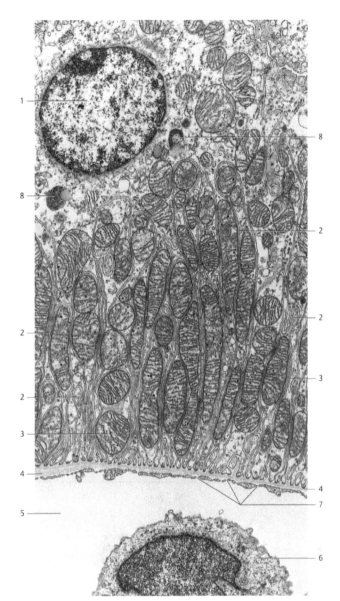

Fig. 30.15 Basolateral infoldings from a proximal convoluted tubule in the kidney of a rat; this tissue has similar features to striated ducts: (1) nucleus; (2) basolateral infoldings; (3) mitochondria; (4) basal lamina; (5) lumen of capillary; (6) endothelial cell; (7). fenestrated endothelium; (8) lysosomes.

There are other helpful tips here:
— In the parotid gland, unilocular adipose tissue is interspersed among the acini. This is pretty reliable; however, be careful not to confuse unilocular adipose cells with mucous glands.
— The parotid gland has longer intercalated ducts, but these are challenging to find.
— The sublingual ducts are short, so ducts within the sublingual gland are fewer.
All that said, the easiest way to distinguish these three salivary glands is to look at the serous/mucous ratio.

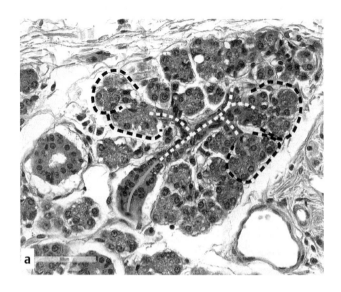

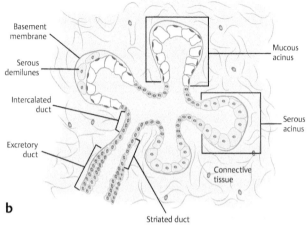

Basement
membrane

Serous
demilunes

Intercalated
duct

Excretory
duct

Mucous
acinus

Serous
acinus

Connective
tissue

Striated duct

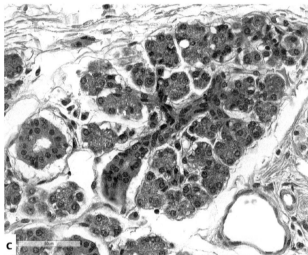

Fig. 30.16 A secretory end piece of a salivary gland, showing (a) light micrograph with labels, (b) drawing depicting the general structure of the light micrograph, and (c) the light micrograph without lablels. Serous acini (black outlines), intercalated duct (yellow dotted line) and striated duct (green solid line) are indicated in (a).

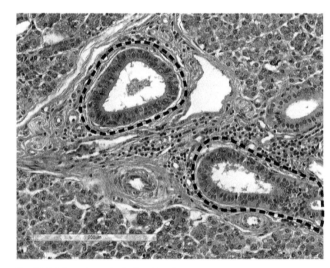

Fig. 30.17 Excretory ducts (outlined).

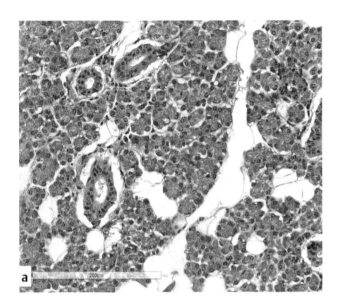

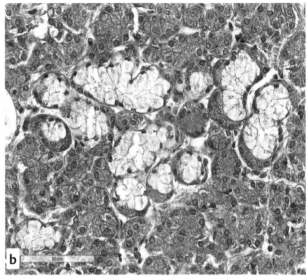

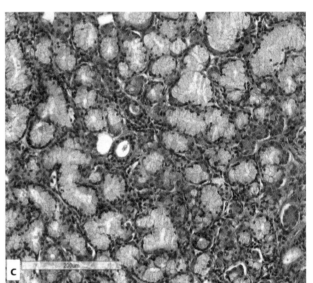

Fig. 30.18 **Comparison of salivary glands: (a) parotid gland; (b) submandibular gland; (c) sublingual gland.**

Video 30.6a Parotid gland—SL091

https://www.thieme.de/de/q.htm?p=opn/tp/308390101/978-1-62623-414-7_c030_v006a&t=video

Video 30.6b Submandibular gland—SL092

https://www.thieme.de/de/q.htm?p=opn/tp/308390101/978-1-62623-414-7_c030_v006b&t=video

Video 30.6c Sublingual gland—SL093

https://www.thieme.de/de/q.htm?p=opn/tp/308390101/978-1-62623-414-7_c030_v006c&t=video

Be able to identify:
— Parotid gland
— Submandibular gland
— Sublingual gland

30.4 Chapter Review

The oral cavity features a number of structures involved in ingesting food and initiating the process of digestion. The tongue has a very thick core of skeletal muscle oriented in multiple directions, covered by a mucosa that features filiform, fungiform, and circumvallate papillae. Salivary glands contain serous and mucous acini that produce watery, protein-rich and thick, carbo-hydrate-rich fluids, respectively, which together make up saliva; these secretions are modified by the ducts (mostly the striated ducts) that lead to the oral cavity. The three types of salivary glands (parotid, submandibular, and sublingual) can be distin-guished by the relative ratio of serous and mucous acini.

Questions and Answers

An online-only section of questions and answers accompanying this chapter is hosted on Thieme's MedOne Education site: https://medone-education.thieme.com. Use the code on the media page at the front of this book to gain access. An institutional license to the site is required to access these questions in an interactive format, and individual users are required to register for an individual account to track results.

31   Pharynx, Esophagus, and Stomach

After completing this chapter, you should be able to:
— Identify, at the light microscope level, each of the following:
   • Pharynx (oropharynx)
   • Esophagus
     ○ Upper
     ○ Middle
     ○ Lower
   • Stomach
     ○ Cardiac and pyloric regions
       ▪ Junctions
         – Esophageal-cardiac junction
         – Pyloric-duodenal (gastroduodenal) junction
           ◊ Pyloric sphincter
     ○ Body and fundus
       ▪ Gastric pits
         – Surface mucous cells
       ▪ Gastric glands
         – Mucous neck cells
         – Parietal cells
         – Chief cells
— Identify, at the electron microscope level, each of the following:
   • Stomach
     ○ Chief cells
       ▪ Zymogen granules
     ○ Parietal cells
       ▪ Canaliculi
       ▪ Tubulovesicles
— Outline the function of each organ or structure and cell type listed
— Correlate the appearance of each structure or cell in light micrographs with its appearance in electron micrographs and vice versa

31.1   Overview of the Pharynx, Esophagus, and Stomach

This chapter covers the remainder of the upper part of the gastrointestinal (GI) system; that is, the pharynx, esophagus, and stomach (oral cavity was discussed in a previous chapter) (see **Fig. 31.1**). The pharynx and esophagus are muscular tubes that serve to carry ingested material from the oral cavity to the stomach. The stomach can store large meals and pass partially digested food slowly to the duodenum of the small intestine. The stomach has an acidic environment and digestive enzymes that liquefy ingested material.

31.2   Pharynx

The **pharynx** is the common pathway of the respiratory and digestive systems. It has three parts, each named for the structure that is anterior to that part (**Fig. 31.2**):
  1. **Nasopharynx** (purple brace) is posterior to the nasal cavity.
  2. **Oropharynx** (black brace) is posterior to the oral cavity.

3. **Laryngopharynx** (yellow brace) is posterior to the larynx. The landmarks to demarcate these are the soft palate (black arrow) and epiglottis (yellow arrow).

Although swallowing is a reflex action, the muscles within the wall of the pharynx are skeletal muscle (**Fig. 31.3**). Being the conduit for boluses of food, the inner lining of the pharynx consists of stratified squamous nonkeratinized epithelium, and the wall of the pharynx has substantial elastic tissue for expansion.

The features of the pharynx seen in a low-magnification image include (**Fig. 31.4**):
  1. Stratified squamous nonkeratinized **epithelium** (black arrows)
  2. **Lamina propria** (black brace), including a dense band of elastic fibers (green brace)
  3. **Muscularis** (purple brace) consisting of skeletal muscle

Note: There is no muscularis mucosae in the pharynx, so there is no submucosa.

Many of the histologic features of the pharynx, such as stratified squamous nonkeratinized epithelium and skeletal muscle, are pretty straightforward, so higher magnification is not necessary. The unique feature of the pharynx is that the lamina propria (**Fig. 31.5**, black brace) includes a thick band of elastic tissue (green brace) in the deeper aspect, adjacent to the muscular layer.

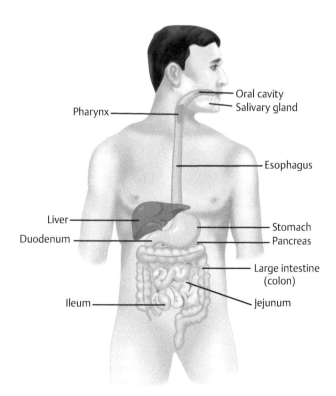

Fig. 31.1   **Gastrointestinal system.**

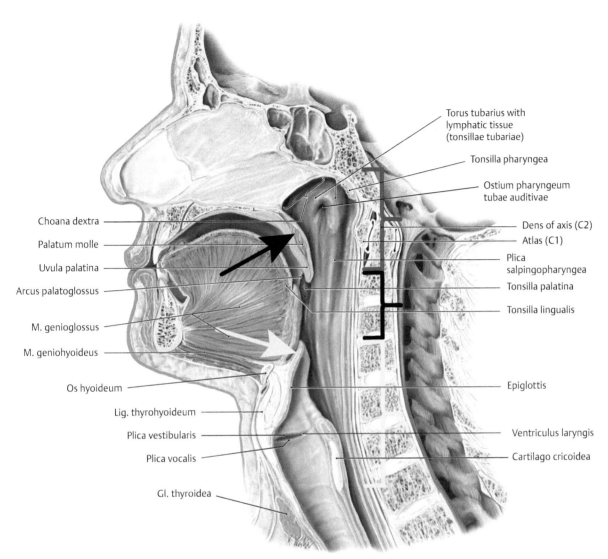

Torus tubarius with lymphatic tissue (tonsillae tubariae)

Tonsilla pharyngea

Ostium pharyngeum tubae auditivae

Choana dextra

Palatum molle

Uvula palatina

Arcus palatoglossus

M. genioglossus

M. geniohyoideus

Os hyoideum

Lig. thyrohyoideum

Plica vestibularis

Plica vocalis

Gl. thyroidea

Dens of axis (C2)

Atlas (C1)

Plica salpingopharyngea

Tonsilla palatina

Tonsilla lingualis

Epiglottis

Ventriculus laryngis

Cartilago cricoidea

Fig. 31.2   Sagittal section of the head and neck showing the pharynx. The regions of the pharynx are indicated by the brackets: nasopharynx (purple), oropharynx (black), and laryngopharynx (yellow). The soft palate (black arrow) and epiglottis (yellow arrow) are landmarks that separate these regions of the pharynx.

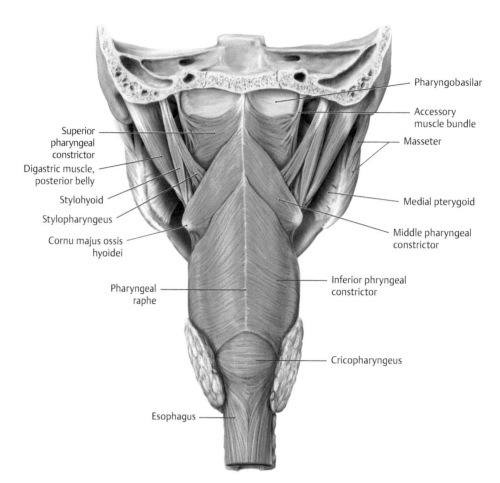

Pharyngobasilar

Accessory
muscle bundle

Masseter

Superior
pharyngeal
constrictor

Digastric muscle,
posterior belly

Stylohyoid

Stylopharyngeus

Cornu majus ossis
hyoidei

Medial pterygoid

Middle pharyngeal
constrictor

Pharyngeal
raphe

Inferior phryngeal
constrictor

Cricopharyngeus

Esophagus

Fig. 31.3   **Posterior view of the pharynx.**

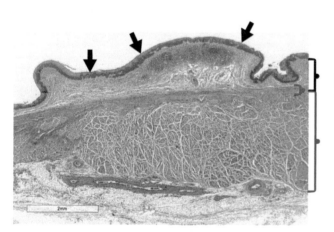

Fig. 31.4   **Pharynx, scanning view. The histological layers are indicated by the brackets: mucosa (black), including an elastic layer (green) which is part of the mucosa, and muscularis (purple). The stratified squamous epithelium is indicated by the black arrows.**

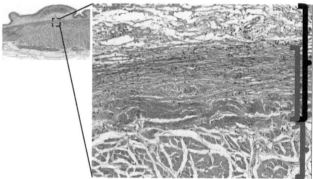

Fig. 31.5   **Pharynx at high magnification showing the elastic band (green bracket). The mucosa (black bracket) and muscularis (purple bracket) are also indicated.**

31.3 Esophagus

The **esophagus** is a muscular tube that connects the pharynx to the stomach. It is the first portion of the digestive tract that has the four-layered organization mentioned in **Chapter 28**: mucosa, submucosa, muscularis (externa), **adventitia**.

The characteristic features of the esophagus relate to its function (see **Fig. 31.6**):

- Epithelium is stratified squamous, nonkeratinized, providing a moist surface resistant to friction, conducive to movement of swallowed boluses to the stomach.

- Muscularis externa transitions from skeletal muscle (upper portion) to smooth muscle (middle and lower segments); this is a gradual transition, so the upper middle region contains a mixture of skeletal and smooth muscle.

- There is a thick **muscularis mucosae**.

- **Esophageal glands** provide lubrication.

The esophagus is in the posterior wall of the thorax, so its outer layer is an adventitia and not a serosa (i.e., it is not covered by visceral peritoneum).

Enlargement of the mucosa shows a stratified squamous nonkeratinized epithelium and a thick muscularis mucosae (**Fig. 31.7**, braces). Esophageal glands are not readily apparent in this image.

Despite the nodule seen on the left side of this image, diffuse lymphoid tissue is not as prominent in the esophagus as in the rest of the GI tract, likely because exposure to food is transient in this region.

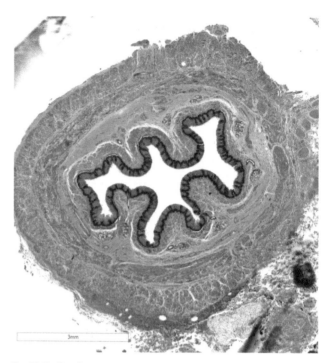

Fig. 31.6 **Esophagus scanning view.**

The upper portion of the esophagus, being continuous with the pharynx, contains skeletal muscle in the muscularis externa. Partway (about one-third of the way) down the esophagus, smooth muscle (**Fig. 31.8**, black outlines) is interspersed with the skeletal muscle (**Fig. 31.8**, yellow outlines) in the muscularis

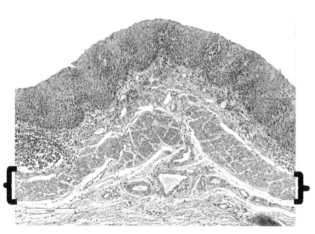

Fig. 31.7 **Esophagus showing muscularis mucosae (black braces).**

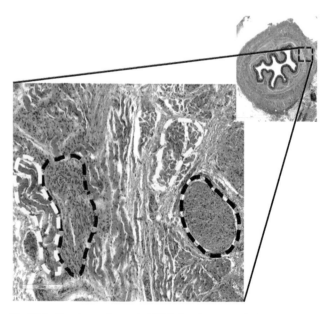

Fig. 31.8 **Esophagus (upper/middle) showing muscularis externa. Skeletal muscle (yellow) and smooth muscle (black) are outlined.**

externa. This creates a nice comparison of smooth and skeletal muscle, discussed in **Chapters 13** and **14**. By about the middle of the esophagus, the muscularis externa has transitioned completely into smooth muscle (**Fig. 31.9**). The remainder of the digestive tract has smooth muscle in the muscularis externa.

The muscularis mucosae has no such transition; it is always smooth muscle, from the cranial esophagus to the colon.

Video 31.3a Middle esophagus

https://www.thieme.de/de/q.htm?p=opn/tp/308390101/978-1-62623-414-7_c031_v003a&t=video

Video 31.3b Lower esophagus

Be able to identify:
— Esophagus
   • Upper
   • Middle
   • Lower
https://www.thieme.de/de/q.htm?p=opn/tp/308390101/978-1-62623-414-7_c031_v003b&t=video

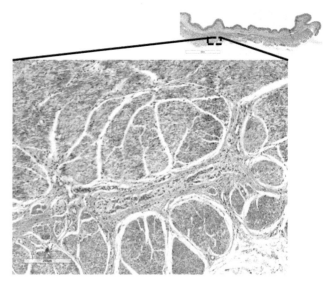

Fig. 31.9   **Esophagus (lower) showing muscularis externa.**

More specific regions include the pyloric antrum, pyloric canal, and so forth. These are gross anatomic distinctions not relevant to routine histologic discussions.

31.4   Stomach

The **stomach** is a dilated portion of the gastrointestinal tract that accepts food from a meal and slowly releases it into the duodenum (**Fig. 31.10**). It is involved in food breakdown, produces pepsin and hydrochloric acid, and has abundant mucous cells to protect the mucosal lining from these harsh agents.

The stomach can be divided into four major regions:
• Cardia
• Fundus
• Body
• Pylorus

Histologically, the stomach can be divided into three parts:
1. Cardia
2. Fundus and body
3. Pylorus

These are demarcated by the dotted lines in **Fig. 31.11**.

The cardia and the pylorus are similar to each other, as are the body and fundus. The cardia and pylorus will be discussed first, along with their adjacent organs: the esophagus and duodenum, respectively. This will be followed by a detailed examination of the histologic features of the fundus and body.

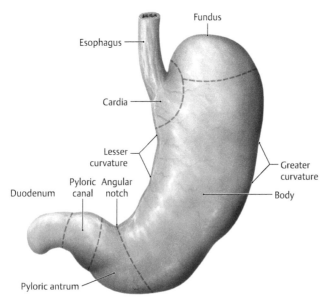

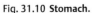

Fig. 31.10 **Stomach.**

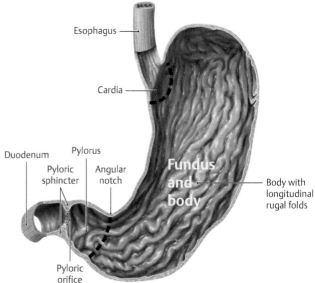

Fig. 31.11 **Stomach inner surface showing regions.**

Like the esophagus and intestines, the wall of the stomach has the four-layered structure characteristic of the GI tract. Features unique to the stomach include:

- **Rugae** are internal folds in an empty stomach that are not present when distended. These are very large and not readily apparent on histologic slides (i.e., too big to be appreciated).

- The muscularis externa consists of three layers of smooth muscle: an inner circular layer, an outer longitudinal layer, and an **oblique layer**. This organization is often not obvious on histologic slides.

- The mucosa has a unique structure because the epithelium undulates. Although the inner surface of the stomach is relatively smooth (i.e., it lacks villi), there are openings that lead to deep holes called **gastric pits** (**Fig. 31.12**). The deep portion of each pit narrows to form a **neck**, from which two or more **gastric glands** extend.

The glands are tightly packed, with little lamina propria between them; this often distorts the visualization of these glands on histologic section.

Three images of the stomach taken at low magnification are shown in **Fig. 31.13a–c**. All are sectioned so that the pits are cut in longitudinal section. The approximate extent of the pits (yellow braces) and glands (blue braces) is indicated in each image. The lumen is indicated for each image, as is the muscularis mucosae (arrows). The pits are fewer and wider than glands; this can be helpful to determine the transition point between the two, where the structures become narrower and more numerous.

Fig. 31.14 shows an oblique section through the mucosa so that the pits are mostly cut in cross section (muscularis mucosae indicated by the arrows). Although pits and glands are easier to visualize in longitudinal views as shown in **Fig. 31.13**, the diameter of the lumen may also be used to determine the transition from pits to glands in **Fig. 31.14** (dotted line).

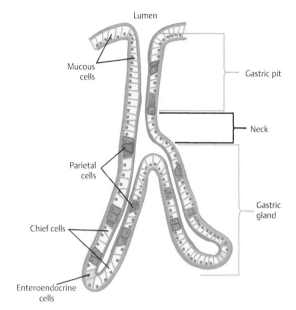

Fig. 31.12 **Stomach histology showing epithelial modifications.**

Video 31.4c Overview of the stomach—pylorus of stomach and duodenum

https://www.thieme.de/de/q.htm?p=opn/tp/308390101/978-1-62623-414-7_c031_v004c&t=video

Be able to identify:
— Stomach
  • Pits
  • Glands

31.4.1 Cardia and Pylorus

The cardia and pylorus regions of the stomach are quite similar (**Fig. 31.15a, b**). Apart from stem cells and **enteroendocrine cells** (which are not seen on routine H & E stain anyway), the epithelium of the surface, pits, and glands in these regions consists of mucus-secreting cells. This can be appreciated even in these low-magnification images, where the entire pits and all the glands consist of tall columnar cells with pale, eosinophilic

Video 31.4a Overview of the stomach—body of stomach

https://www.thieme.de/de/q.htm?p=opn/tp/308390101/978-1-62623-414-7_c031_v004a&t=video

Video 31.4b Overview of the stomach—cardia of stomach and esophagus

https://www.thieme.de/de/q.htm?p=opn/tp/308390101/978-1-62623-414-7_c031_v004b&t=video

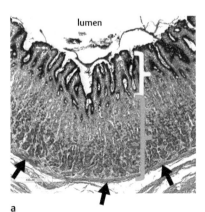
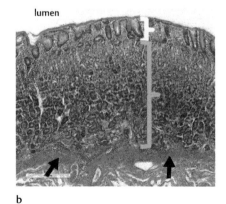
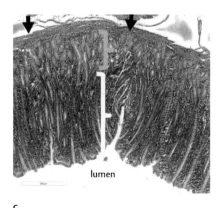

a   b   c

Fig. 31.13 **Regions of the gastric mucosa. (a) Body of stomach, PAS stained. (b) Body of stomach, H & E stained. (c) Pylorus. Mucosal structures are indicated: pits (yellow brackets), glands (blue brackets), and muscularis mucosa (black arrows).**

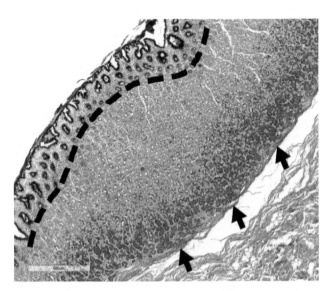

Fig. 31.14 Regions of the gastric mucosa in an oblique section. The muscularis mucosae (black arrows) is indicated. The dotted line represents the approximate border between the pits and glands.

cytoplasm. These mucus-secreting cells in the stomach (as well as in the gallbladder and pancreatic ducts) are more eosinophilic than goblet cells or the mucus-secreting cells of salivary glands.

> **Helpful Hint**
>
> Subtle histology note: The pylorus and cardia of the stomach can be differentiated by comparing the heights of the pits and glands (i.e., pit-to-gland ratio). The cardia has shorter pits than the pylorus (see **Fig. 31.13c** to appreciate how long the pits in the pylorus can be).

Video 31.5a Esophageal-cardiac junction #1

https://www.thieme.de/de/q.htm?p=opn/
tp/308390101/978-1-62623-414-7_c031_
v005a&t=video

Video 31.5b Esophageal-cardiac junction #2

https://www.thieme.de/de/q.htm?p=opn/
tp/308390101/978-1-62623-414-7_c031_
v005b&t=video
Be able to identify:
— Esophageal-cardiac junction

Video 31.6   Pylorus-duodenum junction

Be able to identify:
— Pylorus-duodenum junction
https://www.thieme.de/de/q.htm?p=opn/
tp/308390101/978-1-62623-414-7_c031_
v006&t=video

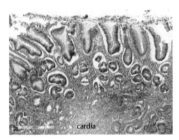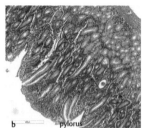

Fig. 31.15 Gastric mucosa of (a) the cardia and (b) the pylorus.

31.4.2   Fundus and Body

The mucosa of the fundus and body of the stomach produce products that aid in digestion (see **Fig. 31.11**). Like the rest of the gastrointestinal tract, these regions have stem cells and enteroendocrine cells. The following features are unique about these regions:

- The mucus-secreting cells cover the surface and line the pits (**surface mucous cells**), and some extend into the neck region of the glands (**mucous neck cells**).
- Two new cell types are within the glands:
  1. **Chief cells** secrete pepsinogen, an inactive protease that is converted to an active form (pepsin) by hydrochloric acid in the stomach lumen. Chief cells are more numerous in the base of the glands.
  2. **Parietal cells** secrete hydrochloric acid and gastric intrinsic factor. Hydrochloric acid activates pepsinogen and is bacteriostatic. Intrinsic factor significantly increases the absorption of vitamin B_{12}, which is necessary for red blood cell production. Parietal cells are more numerous in the upper portion of the glands.

> **Helpful Hint**
>
> So, basically, as compared to the cardia and pylorus, which have mucus-secreting cells throughout the pits and glands, the fundus and body have two additional cells that can be found in the glands.

It is helpful to look at drawings and electron micrographs of chief and parietal cells to understand their function first; this will help explain their histologic features on H & E-stained sections.

Chief Cells

Chief cells are protein-secreting cells, which have been discussed previously. They have abundant rough endoplasmic reticulum (RER) in the basal aspect of the cell; a prominent Golgi apparatus; and numerous secretory granules, called **zymogen granules**, in the apical region of the cell (**Fig. 31.16**).

Fig. 31.17 is an electron micrograph from a gastric gland showing a chief cell, with portions of adjacent cells, surrounding the lumen of a gastric gland. Note the elaborate RER in the basal aspect of the cell and secretory granules (zymogen granules) in the apical half of the cell. Several profiles of the Golgi apparatus are also evident.

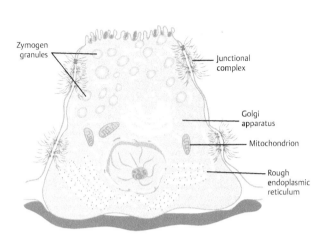

Fig. 31.16 **Chief cell illustration.**

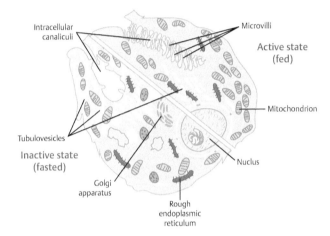

Fig. 31.18 **Parietal cell illustration. This drawing is of one parietal cell, with half the cell showing the fasted state, the other half showing the fed state. In fact, the entire cells is either in the fasted or inactive state, the cell has been divided here to highlight the differences.**

Helpful Hint

In H & E sections, the RER will give the chief cell cytoplasmic basophilia on its basal aspect, and the secretory granules will stain eosinophilic at the apical end of the cell.

Parietal Cells

Parietal cells secrete hydrochloric acid via membrane-bound transport proteins (pumps) located in the apical plasma membrane, which is elaborated to form an **intracellular canaliculus** that contains numerous microvilli. **Fig. 31.18** shows a drawing of a single parietal cell, conceptually divided to show the cell in its inactive state (lower left) and active state (upper right). Parietal cells produce proton and chloride pumps and sequester them in **tubulovesicles** (tube-shaped secretory vesicles) near the apical membrane of the cell when the cell is inactive. Therefore, when the cell is inactive, it contains many of these tubulovesicles, and its intracellular canaliculus and microvilli are not well developed.

As food enters the stomach, requiring acid secretion, the tubulovesicles containing the membrane-bound transport proteins fuse with the apical plasma membrane. This greatly enhances the

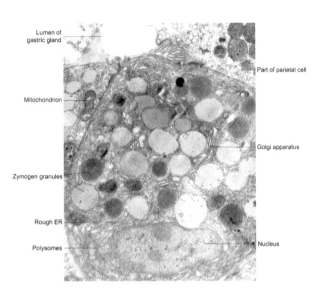

Fig. 31.17 **Chief cell, electron micrograph. Image ccourtesy of Michael Hortsch, University of Michigan, © 2005 The Regents of the University of Michigan.**

depth of the intracellular canaliculus and the number of associated microvilli (with a decrease in the number of tubulovesicles).

Helpful Hint

The transport channels are made "ahead of time" and stored in tubulovesicles when the cell is inactive, so parietal cells do not display elaborate RER. These cells have numerous mitochondria to support the energy requirements of these transport channels (pumps).

Fig. 31.19, an electron micrograph from a gastric gland, shows an active parietal cell. The lumen of the gland is not obvious but is toward the top of the image. Note the intracellular canaliculus with elaborate microvilli. Tubulovesicles are minimal, as most or all have fused with the canalicular network in this active cell. There are regions of ribosomes (polysomes) and a small Golgi apparatus, less developed than in the chief cell.

Helpful Hint

In H & E sections, the numerous mitochondria and tubulovesicles will impart cytoplasmic eosinophilia onto the parietal cell, and the cell will be large and round, with a centrally located nucleus.

Cells of the Fundus and Body in Light Micrographs

To examine these cells on glass slides, it is easier to start with a PAS-stained image counterstained with eosin and azure (azure shows basophilia). In **Fig. 31.20**, the muscularis mucosae is to the upper right, and the lumen is to the left. Note:

1. Mucus-secreting cells (white outline) are PAS positive.
2. Parietal cells (green outlines) are large, with a central nucleus and pale eosinophilic cytoplasm.
3. Chief cells (thin yellow outlines) have basophilia in their basal aspects and eosinophilia in their apical aspects.

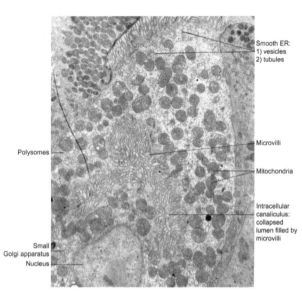

Fig. 31.19 Parietal cell, electron micrograph. Image courtesy of Michael Hortsch, University of Michigan, © 2005 The Regents of the University of Michigan.

Helpful Hint

Parietal cells are eosinophilic and are more numerous in the upper gland, while chief cells are basophilic and are more numerous in the base of the glands. Therefore, at low power the top of the gland is more eosinophilic, while the base is more basophilic.

Fig. 31.21 is a gastric gland at higher magnification, showing many chief cells (**Fig. 31.21b**, black outline); an individual chief cell is indicated (yellow outline). Note the intense cytoplasmic basophilia in these cells, especially in their basal aspect. Parietal cells (arrows) are also evident, demonstrating pale cytoplasmic eosinophilia and a central nucleus.

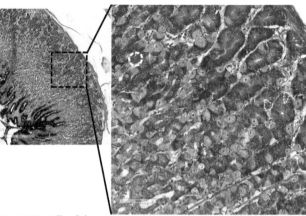

Fig. 31.20 Cells of the gastric mucosa, medium magnification, PAS stain, showing mucus-secreting cell (white), parietal cells (green), chief cells (yellow).

Video 31.7   Fundus and body PAS stain

Be able to identify:
— Fundus/body of stomach
   • Mucus-secreting cells
      ○ Surface mucous cells
      ○ Mucous neck cells
   • Parietal cells
   • Chief cells

https://www.thieme.de/de/q.htm?p=opn/tp/308390101/978-1-62623-414-7_c031_v007&t=video

Fig. 31.22 is from an H & E-stained slide, which is much more challenging because the staining differences are more subtle. A part of the muscularis mucosae is in the upper right. The lumen is toward the bottom of the slide, the base of the glands at the top. Note the cell types in the gastric glands:
• Mucus-secreting cells (green arrows)
• Parietal cells (black arrows)
• Chief cells (yellow arrows)

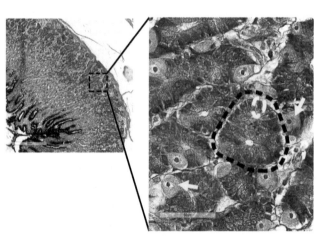

Fig. 31.21 Gastric glands, high magnification, showing a single gland (black outline), parietal cells (yellow arrows) and a chief cell (yellow outline).

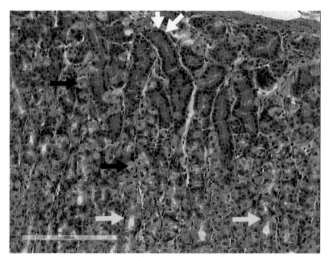

Fig. 31.22 Cells of the gastric mucosa, H & E stain. Mucus-secreting cells (green arrows), parietal cells (black arrows) and chief cells (yellow arrows) are shown.

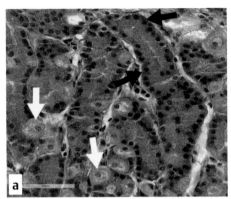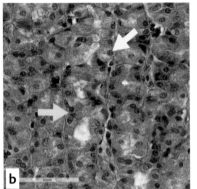

Fig. 31.23 Cells of the gastric glands, H & E stain. (a) Base of gland. (b) Neck of gland. Mucus-secreting cells (green arrows), parietal cells (yellow arrows) and chief cells (black arrows) are shown.

The parietal cells are readily identified by their large size, round shape, and pale eosinophilic cytoplasm. The difference between chief cells and mucous neck cells is more subtle here. However, note that chief cells are closer to the base of the gland (top of slide), while the mucous neck cells are near the neck. The chief cells also demonstrate more intense cytoplasmic basophilia.

High-magnification images better demonstrate these cell types. **Fig. 31.23a** is from the base of the gland, while **Fig. 31.23b** was taken from the neck. Here, the cytoplasmic basophilia in the basal aspect of the chief cells (black arrows) is easier to appreciate, while the surface mucous cells (green arrow) have apical eosinophilia but less basophilia. Parietal cells (yellow arrows) are large, round, with a centrally located nucleus and pale eosinophilic cytoplasm.

Helpful Hint

Recognizing chief and parietal cells in both electron and light micrographs is much more high yield than identifying mucous neck cells.

Many histologists and pathologists say that parietal cells look like fried eggs.

Video 31.8   Fundus and body H & E stain

Be able to identify:
— Fundus/body of stomach
  • Mucus-secreting cells
    ◦ Surface mucous cells
    ◦ Mucous neck cells
  • Parietal cells
  • Chief cells

https://www.thieme.de/de/q.htm?p=opn/tp/308390101/978-1-62623-414-7_c031_v008&t=video

31.5   Chapter Review

The pharynx and esophagus serve as conduits, transporting food from the oral cavity to the stomach. The histologic features of these organs serve this function, highlighted by an inner lining of stratified squamous nonkeratinized epithelium that resists friction from swallowed food; both smooth and skeletal muscle to propel food toward the stomach; and, especially in the pharynx, elastic fibers to allow expansion.

The stomach provides storage for large meals, and it slowly releases its contents into the duodenum in liquid form. Its histologic architecture includes undulations of the surface epithelium (pits and glands) to increase surface area, as well as muscular layers to mix food mechanically with digestive secretions. Parietal cells and chief cells work together to produce digestive secretions. Parietal cells secrete hydrochloric acid and are eosinophilic, while chief cells secrete pepsinogen and feature cytoplasmic basophilia. To protect the surface epithelia from these harsh digestive components, the surface and neck regions are composed of mucous cells: tall columnar cells with a pale eosinophilic cytoplasm. The entire stomach (cardia, fundus, body, pylorus) contains these mucous cells, while parietal and chief cells are found in the glands of the fundus and body of the stomach.

Questions and Answers

An online-only section of questions and answers accompanying this chapter is hosted on Thieme's MedOne Education site: https://medone-education.thieme.com. Use the code on the media page at the front of this book to gain access. An institutional license to the site is required to access these questions in an interactive format, and individual users are required to register for an individual account to track results.

32   Pancreas

After completing this chapter, you should be able to:
— Identify, at the light microscope level, each of the following:
  • Pancreas
    ◦ Serous acini
    ◦ Ducts
      ▪ Intercalated ducts
        – Centroacinar cells
      ▪ Excretory ducts
    ◦ Pancreatic islets (of Langerhans)
— Identify, at the electron microscope level, each of the following:
  • Pancreas
    ◦ Exocrine cells
    ◦ Endocrine cells
— Outline the function of each organ or structure and cell type listed
— Correlate the appearance of each structure or cell in light micrographs with their appearance in electron micrographs, and vice versa
— Compare type 1 and type 2 diabetes mellitus

32.1   Development of the Pancreas, Liver, and Gallbladder

The previous chapters focused on the gastrointestinal (GI) tract, as well as the salivary glands. This chapter and the next address the accessory organs of the GI system in the abdomen, namely the **pancreas**, **liver**, and **gallbladder**.

Fig. 32.1 is a drawing of early development of the GI tract in the region of the stomach and duodenum. Recall that the early gut tube has an inner lining of endoderm (an epithelium, yellow in this drawing), surrounded by splanchnic mesenchyme (embryonic connective tissue, red). The gut tube is suspended from the body wall by mesenteries, which are composed of mesenchyme.

The pancreas, liver, and gallbladder are glands and, therefore, are evaginations of the endoderm into the mesenchyme of the duodenum. These organs grow out of the duodenal wall and into the connective tissue of the mesentery. The pancreas and liver are large endodermal outgrowths, so they are largely composed of epithelial cells, with sparse connective tissue.

Because the liver and pancreas are glands, a review of the histology of gland development discussed in **Chapter 6** is beneficial. The gallbladder develops in a similar manner. Glands in the body develop through an interaction of an epithelium and underlying connective tissue (**Fig. 32.2**). Epithelial cells that line the inner surface of a lumen (such as the duodenum in the case of the pancreas, liver, and gallbladder) proliferate and then evaginate into the surrounding splanchnic connective tissue (**Fig. 32.2a–c**). Note that the basement membrane evaginates with the epithelium. From here, two things can occur:

1. For **endocrine gland** formation (**Fig. 32.2d**), the secretory cells lose their connection with the original epithelium, forming clusters of cells that secrete product basally (across the basement membrane) into the connective tissue and, eventually, the bloodstream (blue arrows).

2. For **exocrine gland** formation (**Fig. 32.2e**), a lumen develops, and the deeper cells secrete product out their apical side (blue arrows) into a duct that carries the secretions to the surface of the original epithelium (i.e., the lumen of the duodenum).

In the pancreas, some cells become exocrine, while others become endocrine. In the liver, there is a single set of cells (hepatocytes) that remain structurally exocrine but perform both exocrine and endocrine functions.

32.2   Pancreas

Fig. 32.3 is a drawing of the pancreas and associated duct system that leads to the duodenum. Within the substance of the pancreas, the glandular cells are either exocrine (acinar) or endocrine (**islets of Langerhans**). The exocrine cells form **acini**, which remain connected to the duct system. These cells release their product apically, ultimately to be released into the lumen of the duodenum (**Fig. 32.3**, black arrows). Endocrine cells separate from the ducts, forming clusters of cells that secrete their products basally into the connective tissue and ultimately to the bloodstream (**Fig. 32.3**, black arrows).

32.2.1   Exocrine Pancreas

The exocrine portion of the pancreas secretes a large amount of digestive enzymes in the form of inactive enzyme precursors that become activated in the duodenum. **Fig. 32.4** is an image from the pancreas. In general, the features of the exocrine pancreas are similar to features of salivary glands: cells organized into acini (in **Fig. 32.4**, two acini are outlined), with nuclei in the basal aspect of the cell. These cells produce large amounts of protein (enzymes), so these cells demonstrate very intense cytoplasmic basophilia around the nucleus due to abundant rough endoplasmic reticulum (RER). In addition, these inactive enzymes are stored in granules in the apical aspect of the cells, which stain eosinophilic (not very obvious in this image).

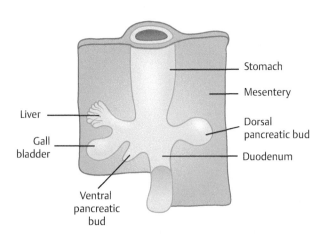

Fig. 32.1   **Development of the pancreas, liver, and gallbladder from the duodenum of the gastrointestinal tract.**

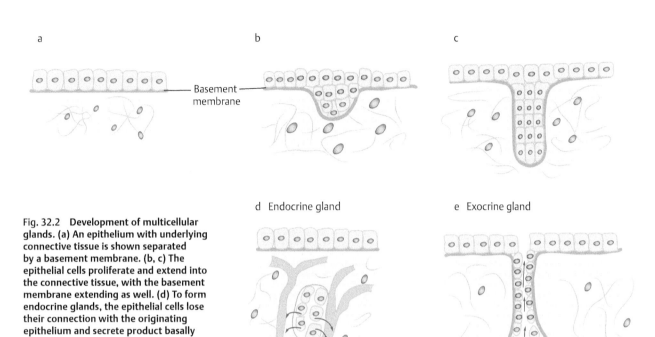

Fig. 32.2 Development of multicellular glands. (a) An epithelium with underlying connective tissue is shown separated by a basement membrane. (b, c) The epithelial cells proliferate and extend into the connective tissue, with the basement membrane extending as well. (d) To form endocrine glands, the epithelial cells lose their connection with the originating epithelium and secrete product basally into the connective tissue (blue arrows). (e) In exocrine glands, the epithelial cells maintain connection to the surface; the deeper cells form the gland that produces secretory product, which is carried to the surface via ducts.

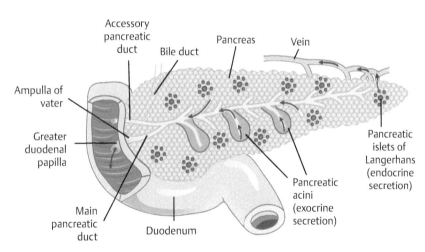

Fig. 32.3 Structure of the pancreas. Cells in pancreatic acini remain connected to the duodenum via ducts, and secrete digestive enzyme precursors. Pancreatic islets of Langerhans secrete insulin and glucagon into the bloodstream.

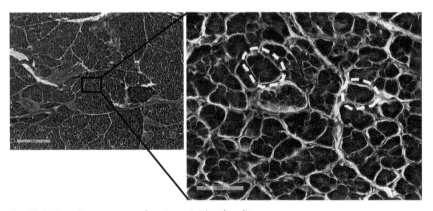

Fig. 32.4 Exocrine pancreas, showing acini (outlined).

Staining in the pancreas is much more intense than in salivary glands; this is because the pancreas is producing much larger quantities of proteins.

Fig. 32.5 is from a different preparation of the pancreas. The acinar organization in this image is less obvious; one acinus is outlined. In this image, the apical regions of the acinar cells are more intensely eosinophilic, underscoring the fact that these cells contain numerous secretory granules in their apical aspect. Cytoplasmic basophilia is still visible in most cells.

Video 32.1   Pancreatic acini—1

https://www.thieme.de/de/q.htm?p=opn/
tp/308390101/978-1-62623-414-7_c032_
v001&t=video

Video 32.2   Pancreatic acini—2

https://www.thieme.de/de/q.htm?p=opn/
tp/308390101/978-1-62623-414-7_c032_
v002&t=video

Be able to identify:
— Exocrine pancreas (serous acini)

Like serous cells in the salivary glands and chief cells of the stomach, acinar cells of the pancreas have the characteristic features of protein-secreting cells. **Fig. 32.6** is an electron micrograph of a single acinus in the pancreas, showing about a half-dozen acinar cells surrounding a lumen (1). A loose connective tissue surrounds the acinus, which contains blood vessels (3). The acinar cells have robust RER in the basal aspect of the cells (2) and a large number of electron-dense granules apically.

The presence of RER, Golgi, and secretory granules is characteristic of all cells that are involved in regulated protein secretion. Here, these pancreatic acinar cells produce lots of protein, so RER is prominent, and granules are numerous. Unfortunately, this is also true for many other cell types (e.g., chief cells from the stomach). The obvious question is how to tell these cell types apart from one another.

In many cases, the location of the secretory granules is a clue. For example, granules at the apical aspect of the cell eliminates enteroendocrine cells, which demonstrate granules on their basal aspect. In other cases, clues to which organ is the source tissue are apparent. For example, in the stomach a chief cell is often next to a parietal cell, a unique feature that indicates the image is from the stomach, and not the pancreas. Unfortunately, cells such as these pancreatic acinar cells have a similar appearance to acinar cells of salivary glands. Even though pancreatic acinar cells have more RER and secretory granules than salivary gland cells do, this may be hard to tell for sure in an isolated image. In cases such as this, the source tissue is often indicated to avoid confusion.

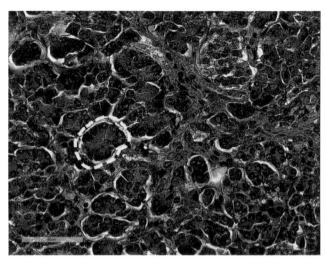

Fig. 32.5   **Exocrine pancreas, showing acinus (outlined).**

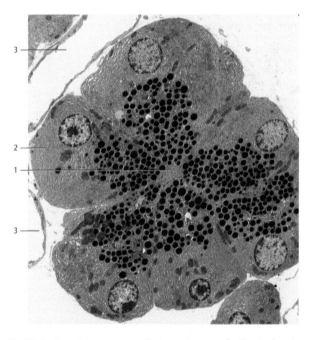

Fig. 32.6   **Exocrine pancreas, electron micrograph of a single acinus showing approximately six acinar cells: (1) lumen of the acinus; (2) rough endoplasmic reticulum (RER); (3) capillaries in the surrounding connective tissue.**

32.2.2   Ducts of the Exocrine Pancreas

Before considering the ducts of the pancreas, a quick review of salivary gland ducts is useful. Recall that the duct system in salivary glands consist of (**Fig. 32.7**):
1. **Intercalated ducts**, which are simple conduits for fluid
2. **Striated ducts**, which have epithelial cells with numerous basolateral infoldings for ion transport and concentrate saliva
3. **Excretory ducts**, in which the epithelium becomes stratified and the surrounding connective tissue is more prominent

Fig. 32.8 is a drawing of the duct system of the exocrine pancreas. The features specific to the ducts of the exocrine pancreas include:

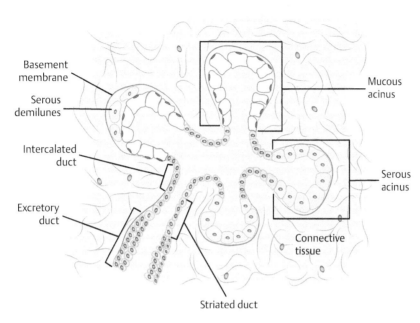

Fig. 32.7 **Drawing of salivary gland acini and ducts.**

1. The intercalated ducts begin *within* the acinus; duct cells of this initial portion are referred to as **centroacinar cells**. The intercalated ducts of the pancreas (including the centroacinar cells) are not mere conduits of fluid; they also release a bicarbonate secretion that helps neutralize acidic chyme from the stomach.
2. There are no striated ducts in the pancreas.
3. The epithelium of the excretory ducts (labeled "intralobular duct" in **Fig. 32.8**) remains simple throughout, all the way to the duodenum. (This is also true of the gallbladder and bile ducts.)

Fig. 32.9 shows the ducts of the exocrine pancreas. In this image, several pancreatic acini are outlined in black, and the intercalated ducts that they empty into are indicated by the dotted yellow lines. Centroacinar cells (arrows) can be identified as nuclei in the center of an acinus, near the duct, with pale cytoplasm against the background of acinar cells with intense cytoplasmic basophilia.

Fig. 32.10 is another image of centroacinar cells and an intercalated duct. Two adjacent acini (outlined by blue dashed semicircles) appear to have intercalated ducts connecting them. Some centroacinar cell nuclei (arrows) are indicated. The structure outlined in yellow is likely a cross section of an intercalated duct. Note that the cells lining the intercalated ducts are very low cuboidal and do not stain as intensely as the acinar cells.

Exocrine pancreas

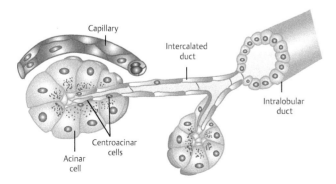

Fig. 32.8 **Drawing of acini and ducts of the exocrine pancreas.**

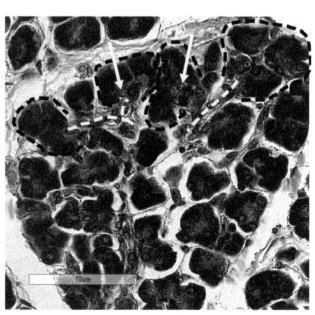

Fig. 32.9 **Initial duct system of the exocrine pancreas. Four acini are outlined in black. Intercalated ducts from three of these are indicated by the dotted yellow lines. Centroacinar cells are indicated by the yellow arrows.**

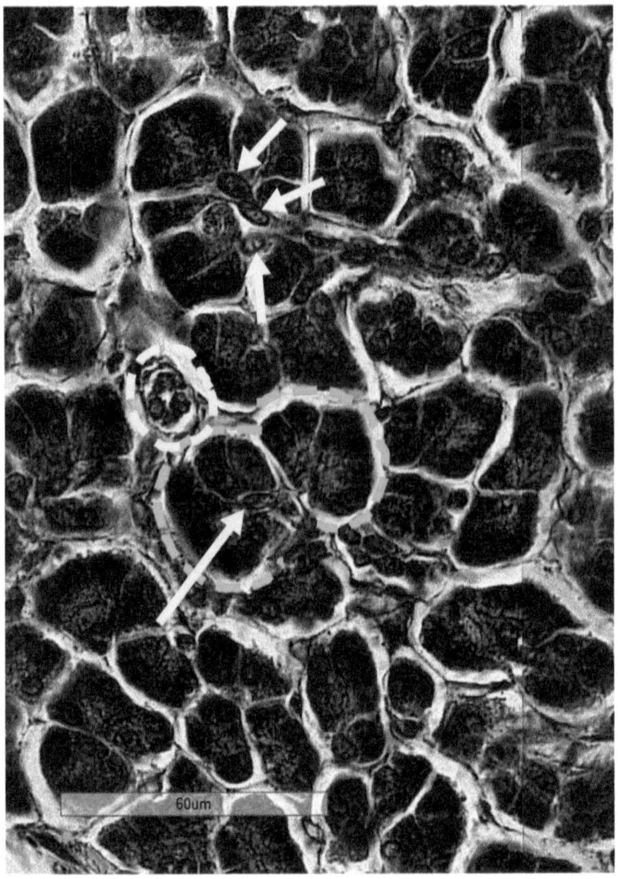

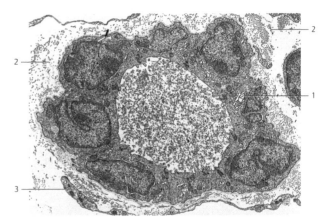

Fig. 32.10 Centroacinar cells and intercalated ducts of the exocrine pancreas. Two adjacent acini are outlined in blue. Centroacinar cells are indicated by the arrows. An intercalated duct is outlined in yellow.

Helpful Hint

Cells of intercalated ducts, including centroacinar cells, secrete a bicarbonate-rich product. Since they are not major protein-secreting cells, it makes sense that these cells are pale, especially in comparison to the intensely stained acinar cells.

Fig. 32.11 is an electron micrograph of an intercalated duct. These ducts secrete bicarbonate, so they exhibit some organelles of active cells (e.g., Golgi apparatus at 1), but lack the extensive RER seen in acinar cells. The duct is surrounded by loose connective tissue, including collagen fibers (2) and part of a fibroblast (3).

The larger excretory ducts of the pancreas (and liver) are lined by a simple epithelium throughout. This is in contrast to excretory ducts in salivary glands, which are lined by a stratified epithelium. **Fig. 32.12** shows an excretory duct from the pancreas (outlined). Despite the substantial connective tissue support, the epithelium is simple columnar. The epithelial cells demonstrate pale eosinophilia.

Video 32.3   Pancreatic ducts

Be able to identify:
— Intercalated ducts
   • Centroacinar cells
— Excretory ducts
https://www.thieme.de/de/q.htm?p=opn/tp/308390101/978-1-62623-414-7_c032_v003&t=video

Fig. 32.11 Intercalated duct in the pancreas on electron micrograph. (1) Golgi apparatus; (2) collagen fibers; (3) fibroblast.

As mentioned in **Chapter 29**, the ultimate destination of the **pancreatic duct** and **bile duct** is the duodenum. These two ducts join together to form the **hepatopancreatic ampulla (of Vater)**, which passes through the duodenal wall. The presence of the ampulla creates a nipplelike projection on the inner wall of the duodenum called the **greater duodenal papilla** (see **Fig. 29.10** and associated text for review). **Fig. 32.13** is a high-magnification image of the inner lining of the ampulla of Vater. Although the epithelium is sloughed off in many places, places where the epithelium remains demonstrate that it is simple columnar.

Video 32.4   Ampulla of Vater

Be able to identify:
— Hepatopancreatic ampulla (of Vater)
https://www.thieme.de/de/q.htm?p=opn/tp/308390101/978-1-62623-414-7_c032_v004&t=video

Basic Science Correlate: Physiology

Pancreatic secretions are stimulated by the release of chyme from the stomach into the duodenum. Secretin stimulates duct cells to release bicarbonate, while cholecystokinin stimulates secretion of digestive enzyme precursors from acinar cells.

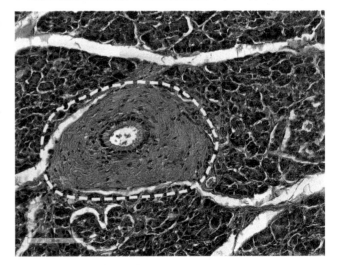

Fig. 32.12 Excretory duct of the pancreas (outlined).

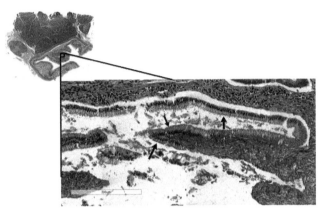

Fig. 32.13 **Duodenum and pancreas showing the ampulla of Vater. Epithelial cells lining the ampulla are indicated by the black arrows.**

32.2.3 Endocrine Pancreas

The endocrine portion of the pancreas, the **pancreatic islets of Langerhans**, secretes hormones, principally insulin and glucagon, that regulate glucose levels in the bloodstream. **Fig. 32.14** shows two pancreatic islets (yellow outlines). Although the cells within the islets secrete protein hormones and, therefore, exhibit cytoplasmic basophilia and eosinophilia, their staining is not as intense as that of the surrounding exocrine acinar cells.

> **Helpful Hint**
>
> Protein hormone production in islet cells requires RER, Golgi, and secretory vesicles; therefore, they exhibit some cytoplasmic basophilia and eosinophilia. However, only a small amount of a hormone is necessary to elicit an appropriate response in target cells. In contrast, large amounts of digestive enzymes are needed to digest large meals daily (especially on holidays). Therefore, the exocrine acinar cells that secrete those enzymes contain much more RER, Golgi, and secretory vesicles than islet cells do and, therefore, stain much more intensely.

Video 32.5 Pancreatic islets of Langerhans

Be able to identify:
— Pancreatic islets of Langerhans
https://www.thieme.de/de/q.htm?p=opn/tp/308390101/978-1-62623-414-7_c032_v005&t=video

To underscore the difference between exocrine and endocrine pancreatic cells with regard to protein-synthesizing activity, **Fig. 32.15** shows a specially prepared tissue in which DNA is stained red and RNA is stained blue. Although the cytoplasm of the pancreatic islet cells (outlined) do exhibit some RNA staining, the exocrine acinar cells stain much more intensely for RNA. This demonstrates that acinar cells contain more RER than islet cells. Also, this image more clearly demonstrates centroacinar cells (yellow arrows). At least one intercalated duct (black arrows) is also visible as a double row of nuclei (stained red in this image).

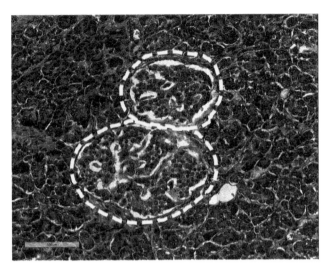

Fig. 32.14 **Pancreatic islets of Langerhans (two are outlined).**

Video 32.6 Pancreas RNA stain

Be able to identify:
— Serous acini
— Intercalated ducts
— Centroacinar cells
— Pancreatic islets (islets of Langerhans)
https://www.thieme.de/de/q.htm?p=opn/tp/308390101/978-1-62623-414-7_c032_v006&t=video

Pancreatic islets of Langerhans consist of more than one cell type, which are not distinguished in routine H & E-stained tissues. However, special stains can be used to identify these cells.

Fig. 32.16 is an image from a specially stained preparation of pancreas, highlighting specific cells in the pancreatic islets of Langerhans:
- Alpha cells (stained red) secrete glucagon.
- Beta cells (stained blue) secrete insulin.
- Delta cells (and other islet cells), not specially stained here, release somatostatin.

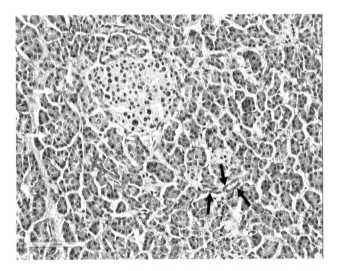

Fig. 32.15 **Pancreas, special stain (azure B and basic fuchsin) in which DNA is red, RNA is blue. A pancreatic islet of Langerhans is outlined, surrounded by excretory acini. Centroacinar cells (arrows) and an intercalated duct (black arrows) are indicated.**

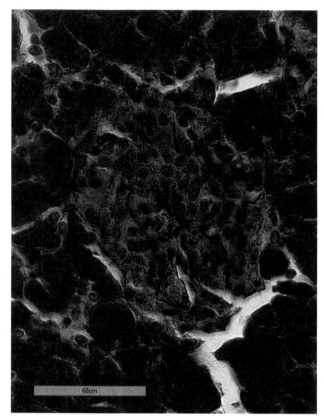

Fig. 32.16 **Pancreatic islet of Langerhans surrounded by acini. This tissue was prepared with a special stain to show alpha cells (red) and beta cells (blue).**

Video 32.7   Pancreatic islets of Langerhans, special stain

Be able to identify:
— Pancreatic islets of Langerhans
https://www.thieme.de/de/q.htm?p=opn/
tp/308390101/978-1-62623-414-7_c032_v007&t=video

Clinical Correlate

Type 1 diabetes mellitus is caused by a decrease in insulin production or release. **Type 2 diabetes mellitus** occurs when cells have a reduced response to insulin secreted by the pancreas. Patients with either condition have elevated blood sugar, which causes a multitude of clinical sequelae, such as damage to peripheral vessels and the kidneys. Treatment depends on the type and severity. Typically, type 1 diabetes is treated with insulin replacement, while type 2 diabetes is managed in a variety of ways including lifestyle (dietary) changes and drugs that decrease blood sugar through various mechanisms.

Fig. 32.17 is an electron micrograph of a cell in a pancreatic islet of Langerhans. This image demonstrates that cells from the islets have the protein machinery expected of cells with regulated secretion, including numerous secretory granules (2). Note that there is no lumen, so the granules are distributed throughout the cell (not apically). Profiles of RER are not easily seen in this image; compare to the amount of RER seen in acinar cells (see **Fig. 32.6**).

For most purposes, it is not necessary to identify specific cell types of the pancreatic islets, on either light or electron micrographs.

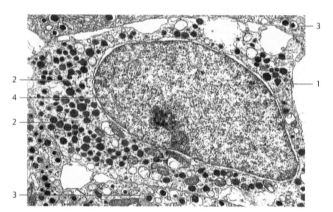

Fig. 32.17 **Pancreatic islet of Langerhans in electron micrograph: (1) delta cell, (2) secretory granule; (3) beta cell; (4) nucleus.**

32.3 Chapter Review

The pancreas is derived from endoderm and surrounding mesenchyme of the gastrointestinal tract, growing out of the duodenal wall to create a distinct organ that remains connected to the duodenum by the pancreatic duct. The epithelial cells that form the pancreas either remain attached to the duct system, forming the exocrine pancreas, or detach from the ducts to form the endocrine pancreas. The secretory end pieces of the exocrine pancreas, the acini, produce digestive enzymes. Acinar cells have all the characteristic features of protein-secreting cells, including abundant rough endoplasmic reticulum (RER) in the basal aspect of the cells, a prominent Golgi apparatus, and numerous secretory granules in the apical cytoplasm near the lumen. In light micrographs, these acinar cells have cytoplasmic basophilia basally and eosinophilia apically. The ducts of the exocrine pancreas are lined by a simple epithelium and ultimately connect to the ampulla of Vater. Of note, the intercalated ducts and centroacinar cells secrete a product rich in bicarbonate that helps to buffer acidic secretions from the stomach. The endocrine portion of the pancreas, consisting of the pancreatic islets of Langerhans, also secretes proteins (insulin, glucagon), but its overall level of protein synthesis is less than that of acinar cells. Therefore, pancreatic islets demonstrate paler staining than acinar cells do. In electron micrographs, pancreatic islet cells have secretory granules distributed throughout the cells. Specific cell types in the pancreatic islets can be demonstrated with special stains.

Questions and Answers

An online-only section of questions and answers accompanying this chapter is hosted on Thieme's MedOne Education site: https://medone-education.thieme.com. Use the code on the media page at the front of this book to gain access. An institutional license to the site is required to access these questions in an interactive format, and individual users are required to register for an individual account to track results.

33   Liver and Gallbladder

After completing this chapter, you should be able to:
— Identify, at the light microscope level, each of the following:
  • Liver
    ○ Lobule (classic liver lobule)
      ▪ Central vein (terminal hepatic venule)
      ▪ Portal triad
        – Hepatic artery
        – Hepatic portal vein
        – Intrahepatic bile duct
      ▪ Hepatocytes
      ▪ Liver macrophages (Kupffer cells)
      ▪ Sinusoids
      ▪ Endothelial cells
    ○ Veins
      ▪ Central vein
      ▪ Sublobular vein
      ▪ Hepatic vein
  • Gall bladder
    ○ Extrahepatic bile duct
    ○ Hepatopancreatic ampulla (of Vater)
— Identify, at the electron microscope level, each of the following:
  • Liver
    ○ Hepatocyte
    ○ Sinusoid
    ○ Endothelial cell
    ○ Space of Disse (perisinusoidal space)
    ○ Bile canaliculus
— Outline the function of each organ or structure and cell type listed
— Correlate the appearance of each structure or cell in light micrographs with its appearance in electron micrographs, and vice versa
— Predict the histology of disease states of the liver

33.1   Overview of the Liver

The **liver** is the largest internal organ in the body. It is located in the upper right quadrant of the abdomen (**Fig. 33.1**). The outer portion of the liver is a thick connective tissue capsule (of Glisson), which is covered in places by visceral peritoneum. Cells of the liver, **hepatocytes**, are involved in a wide variety of metabolic functions, including storage of organic molecules absorbed from a meal, production of most plasma proteins, and detoxification. The liver also produces **bile**, which is secreted into a **canalicular system** that ultimately drains into the duodenum via **bile ducts**.

As mentioned in the previous chapter, the liver is a gland; therefore, hepatocytes are epithelial in origin. The liver receives a dual blood supply. Oxygenated blood is delivered by a **proper hepatic artery**. In addition, the liver receives blood that has passed through capillaries of the intestines and is brought to the liver via the **hepatic portal vein**. This blood is oxygen-poor but nutrient-rich. Both blood supplies drain into the capillaries of

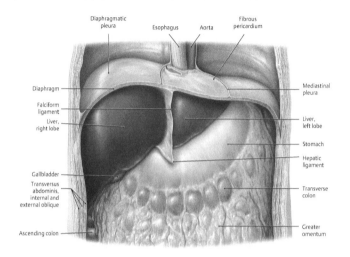

Fig. 33.1   **Contents of the upper abdomen.**

the liver, called **sinusoids**, which drain via **hepatic veins** into the **inferior vena cava**.

Because of its dual blood supply and bile duct system, the histologic organization of the liver is quite complicated. Furthermore, although hepatocytes remain connected to a duct system (i.e., they are **anatomically** similar to exocrine glands), they are not organized into easily recognizable acini such as those that are the hallmark of the pancreas and salivary glands. Furthermore, hepatocytes are both exocrine and endocrine cells, so discussion of the liver must cover both of these functions.

This chapter begins with individual hepatocyte structure and function. This is followed by a discussion of the organization of hepatocytes into liver lobules (classic and portal). From here, the exocrine function of the liver is presented, focusing on the bile ducts that carry bile to the duodenum. This is followed by a consideration of endocrine function in the liver, which focuses on blood flow, including the dual blood supply into the liver, the liver capillaries (sinusoids), and blood flow away from the liver. Finally, liver macrophages, called **Kupffer cells**, are discussed.

33.2   Hepatocytes

From a cellular standpoint, hepatocytes are incredibly dynamic, involved in metabolic regulation, production of plasma proteins, bile production, and degradation of toxins. Because of this, hepatocytes are ideal for studying cellular architecture because they contain excellent examples of most cellular organelles. **Fig. 33.2** and **Fig. 33.3** are electron micrographs of the cytoplasm of hepatocytes. Note the abundant rough endoplasmic reticulum (RER) for synthesis of plasma proteins and smooth endoplasmic reticulum (SER) for degradation of toxins and glycogen metabolism. Hepatocytes store carbohydrate in the form of glycogen, which can be in the form of larger clumps (**Fig. 33.2**, outlined), but also interspersed among the SER (**Fig. 33.3**, arrows).

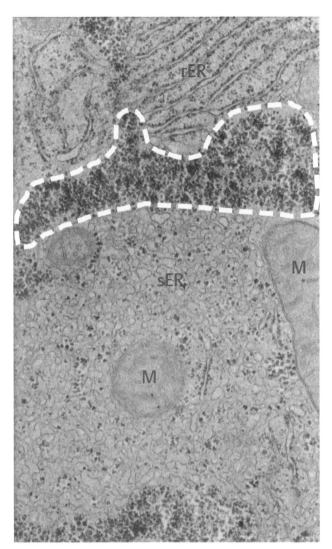

Fig. 33.2 Hepatocyte cytoplasm in electron micrograph, high magnification. Glycogen is outlined; rough and smooth endoplasmic reticulum are shown (rER and sER, respectively), as well as two mitochondria (M). Image courtesy of Robert and Emma Lou Cardell.

Hepatocytes also have numerous peroxisomes and lysosomes (not shown).

Hepatocytes are cuboidal or hexagonal in shape (**Fig. 33.4**, outlined in red). The nucleus (yellow outline) is very euchromatic with a prominent nucleolus, underscoring the fact that hepatocytes are very active cells.

These cellular features produce the characteristic features of hepatocytes seen in light micrographs. **Fig. 33.5** is an image of liver tissue in which the hepatocytes have been artifactually separated from each other, allowing better visualization of individual cells. Again, hepatocytes are cuboidal or polygonal-shaped cells, with a central euchromatic nucleus containing a prominent nucleolus. Note that some cells are binucleate (black arrows). The hepatocyte cytoplasm is eosinophilic because of numerous mitochondria and cellular proteins. The presence of RER creates regions of cytoplasmic basophilia in some cells, but this is not as localized as in the exocrine pancreas or chief cells of the stomach (i.e., the RER in hepatocytes is dispersed throughout the cell).

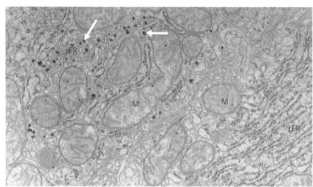

Fig. 33.3 Hepatocyte cytoplasm in electron micrograph, medium magnification. Glycogen is indicated by the arrows; rough and smooth endoplasmic reticulum are shown (rER and sER), as well as two mitochondria (M). Image courtesy of Robert and Emma Lou Cardell.

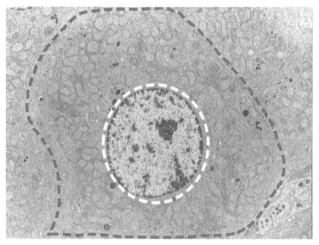

Fig. 33.4 Hepatocyte in electron micrograph, low magnification. A single hepatocyte (red outline) and parts of a few others are shown. The nucleus is outlined in yellow. Image courtesy of Robert and Emma Lou Cardell.

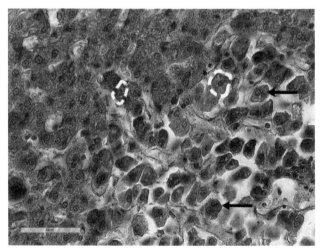

Fig. 33.5 Liver showing hepatocytes (outlined). Some hepatocytes are binucleate (black arrows).

Glycogen does not stain well in routine H & E; therefore, many hepatocytes exhibit clear areas.

33.3   The Classic Liver Lobule

Now that the basic features of hepatocytes have been discussed, the organization and function of the liver can be addressed. **Fig. 33.6** is a low-magnification light micrograph of the liver, showing that hepatocytes are grouped together into polygon-shaped **lobules** (yellow line) containing hundreds of hepatocytes. These are referred to as **classic liver lobules**, which share connective tissue "walls" with adjacent liver lobules. The connective tissue that bounds each lobule is relatively sparse, so the outer borders of lobules are sometimes difficult to see. Each corner of the lobule contains a **portal canal** (**portal triad**, in regions of black circles in **Fig. 33.6**), which contains vascular structures and bile ducts within more substantial connective tissue support. These portal canals help to visualize the boundaries of the lobule. In the center of the lobule is a **central vein** (arrow). Hepatocytes within each lobule are organized into plates that radiate from (toward) the central vein.

Video 33.1   Overview of the liver and classic liver lobule

Be able to identify:
— Liver
   • Lobule
https://www.thieme.de/de/q.htm?p=opn/tp/308390101/978-1-62623-414-7_c033_v001&t=video

Since the liver is a gland, it may be tempting to think that a liver lobule is a single secretory end piece that drains into a single bile duct. However, this is not the case. Each classic liver lobule is derived from numerous secretory end pieces, so that several bile ducts drain a single lobule. **Fig. 33.7** is a drawing of the organization of a liver lobule. The bile ducts are at the "corners" of the polygon, in the portal canals. The liver secretory units are end pieces composed of hepatocytes organized into

tubular glands, often called **plates** by pathologists. Only several glands of this lobule are shown for simplicity. The "blind end" of each gland is near the center of the classic lobule (adjacent to the central vein). The lumen of each gland (i.e., the space between the hepatocytes) is called a **bile canaliculus**, which is lined by the plasma membrane of the hepatocytes. Liver excretory product—bile—is released into bile canaliculi, in which it flows toward the periphery of the lobule. The hepatocytes adjacent to the wall of the lobule are continuous with duct cells that line **bile ductules**, which are small ducts that lead to larger **intrahepatic bile ducts** located in the portal triads.

Basic Science Correlate: Gross Anatomy

Note that, in gross anatomy, as the small bile ducts described here join together to form larger ducts, the larger ducts have specific names, including hepatic duct, (common) bile duct, and so forth. The term "bile duct" here is generic and is the term used histologically to describe any duct carrying bile. Some histologists distinguish bile ducts within the liver (intrahepatic bile ducts) from those outside the liver (extrahepatic, discussed later).

33.4   The Portal Liver Lobule

The classic liver lobule just described is defined by the connective tissue that surrounds the lobule. In this classic liver lobule, the bile duct is situated in the portal canals at the "corners" of the lobule, with a central vein in the center of each lobule (**Fig. 33.8**, yellow shaded region in A).

On the other hand, the organization of the liver can be described in a way that considers all the hepatocytes that drain into a single bile duct. In this way, the portal canal, with its bile duct, is at the center of a **portal lobule**, which is a

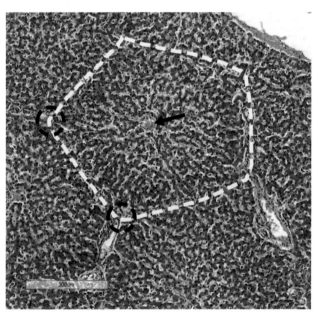

Fig. 33.6   **Liver at low magnification, showing a classic liver lobule (yellow outline), portal canals (black outlines) and central vein (arrow).**

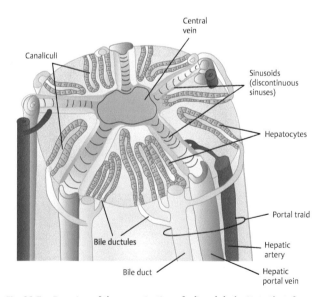

Fig. 33.7   **Drawing of the organization of a liver lobule. Note that, for simplicity, only several glands (plates) of hepatocytes are shown in this drawing. Actual liver lobules are packed with hepatocytes (see Fig. 33.6). Note the relative size of structures is not representative; for example, the central vein here is drawn larger than it's actual relative size.**

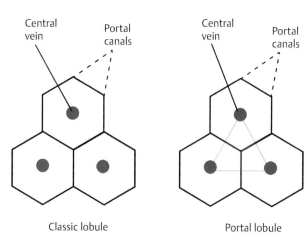

Fig. 33.8 **Lobules of the liver.**

Classic lobule   Portal lobule

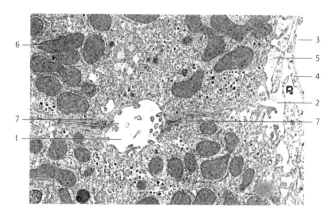

Fig. 33.9 **Electron micrograph of the liver showing (1) a canaliculus (1); (2) perisinusoidal space of Disse; (3) lumen of sinusoid; (4) endothelial cell; (5) reticular fibers; (6) mitochondrion; (7) area near junctional complex.**

triangle-shaped region with central veins at the corners (**Fig. 33.8**, yellow shaded region in B). All hepatocytes within a portal lobule ultimately developed from the bile duct within the portal canal in the center of the portal lobule, into which they excrete their bile. Each classic liver lobule drains into several bile ducts.

33.5 Exocrine Liver

The liver is both an exocrine and an endocrine gland. The exocrine secretory product of the liver is bile. As mentioned above, the lumen into which bile is first secreted by the hepatocytes is called a canaliculus (see **Fig. 33.7**), which is formed by the plasma membranes of the hepatocytes.

Helpful Hint

Canaliculi are similar to the lumen of an acinus in the salivary gland or the lumen of gastric glands in the stomach; they are lined by the apical plasma membranes of hepatocytes.

Canaliculi are too small to see in light micrographs. (The spaces between plates of hepatocytes in **Fig. 33.6** are capillaries known as sinusoids, which will be discussed later.) However, canaliculi can be seen in electron micrographs. In **Fig. 33.9**, two adjacent hepatocytes are shown, one above the other. Between them is the lumen of a bile canaliculus (1). Note that the wall of the canaliculus is formed by the plasma membranes of the hepatocytes (i.e., there are no endothelial cells or other cells that line the lumen). A few hepatocyte microvilli project into the lumen of the canaliculus. Near the canaliculus, tight junctions are formed between the two cells (near 7), sealing the canaliculus.

At the wall of the classic liver lobule, the hepatocytes are continuous with bile ductules and bile ducts, which are lined by a simple cuboidal epithelium (see **Fig. 33.7**). **Fig. 33.10** shows two bile ducts (outlined in yellow), recognized as small tubes lined by simple cuboidal epithelium within the connective tissue of the portal triad (portal triad outlined in black).

Helpful Hint

The other two structures (X and Y) in **Fig. 33.10** are vessels (branches of the hepatic artery and hepatic portal vein) which will be described subsequently. Note that the inner epithelium of the vessels (X and Y) is simple squamous, not cuboidal like the epithelium of the bile ducts. Together, these three structures—artery, portal vein, bile duct—constitute a portal triad.
Also note that this particular triad has two bile ducts. Typically, a triad includes only one of each structure (artery, portal vein, bile duct). It is likely that these two ducts are merging.

Video 33.2 Intrahepatic bile ducts of the liver

Be able to identify:
— Liver
  • Portal triad
  • Intrahepatic bile duct
https://www.thieme.de/de/q.htm?p=opn/tp/308390101/978-1-62623-414-7_c033_v002&t=video

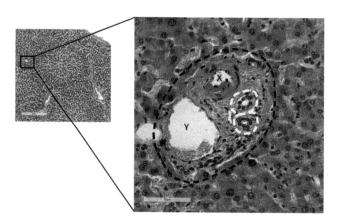

Fig. 33.10 **Components of a portal triad. The triad is outlined in black. Bile ducts are outlined in yellow; X is a branch of a hepatic artery; Y is a branch of the hepatic portal vein.**

The intrahepatic bile ducts within portal triads merge with other similar ducts to form larger ducts. **Fig. 33.11** shows a low-magnification image of a larger intrahepatic bile duct cut in longitudinal section (outlined).

Intrahepatic bile ducts combine into larger ducts, which ultimately exit the inferior aspect of the liver as extrahepatic bile ducts (**Fig. 33.12**, bile duct, cystic duct). **Fig. 33.13** shows the cystic duct (CD, which connects to the gallbladder) and the common hepatic duct (CHD). The enlarged image in **Fig. 33.13** shows that these ducts are lined by a simple columnar epithelium, with an underlying loose connective tissue. The remainder of the wall is dense irregular connective tissue with sparse smooth muscle (not shown). The bile duct (common bile duct, **Fig. 33.12**) is formed by the union of the common hepatic duct and cystic duct and joins with the pancreatic duct to form the ampulla of Vater, transporting bile to the duodenum (see **Chapter 32**).

Video 33.3   Extrahepatic bile duct

https://www.thieme.de/de/q.htm?p=opn/
tp/308390101/978-1-62623-414-7_c033_
v004&t=video

Video 33.4   Extrahepatic bile ducts

Be able to identify:
— Extrahepatic bile duct

https://www.thieme.de/de/q.htm?p=opn/
tp/308390101/978-1-62623-414-7_c033_
v003&t=video

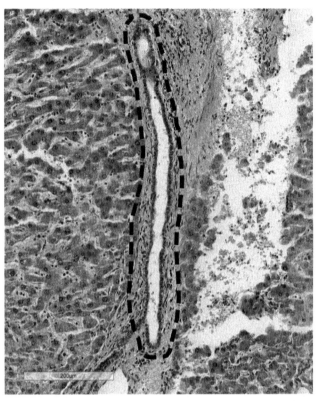

Fig. 33.11 **Large intrahepatic bile duct.**

33.6 Endocrine Liver

The endocrine function of the liver centers around its specialized blood supply. As mentioned previously, the liver receives a dual blood supply (**Fig. 33.12**). Oxygenated blood is supplied by the **proper hepatic artery**, while oxygen-poor but nutrient-rich blood is supplied by the **hepatic portal vein**. Both of these vessels enter the liver via the **porta hepatis**, a region on the inferior aspect of

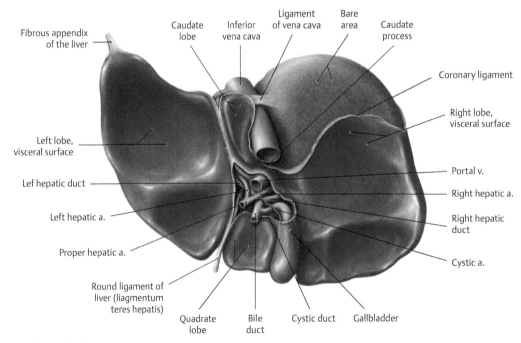

Fig. 33.12 **Inferior view of the liver.**

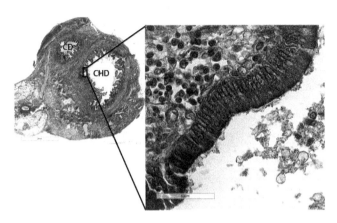

Fig. 33.13 **Extrahepatic ducts of the liver. CD marks the cystic duct; CHD indicates the common hepatic duct (Fig. 33.13).**

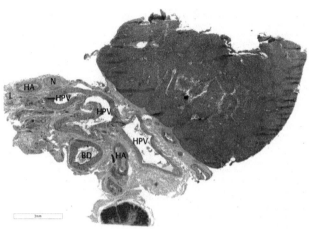

Fig. 33.14 **Section of the liver and porta hepatis. The porta hepatis includes branches of the proper hepatic artery (HA), branches of the hepatic portal vein (HPV), extrahepatic bile duct (BD), autonomic nerves (N), and lymphatic vesssels (L).**

the liver where these vessels enter and the bile ducts exit the liver. Within the liver, the proper hepatic artery and hepatic portal vein branch together in the connective tissue partitions (septa), and then, ultimately, in portal triads of the liver lobules. Here, both of these vessels empty into the capillaries of the liver, the **sinusoids**. Blood flows from the sinusoids through a series of veins and exits via **hepatic veins** on the dorsal surface of the liver; the hepatic veins drain into the **inferior vena cava (Fig. 33.13)**.

33.6.1 Blood Flow to the Liver

A scanning image of a section of liver including the porta hepatis is shown in **Fig. 33.14**. The porta hepatis contains the proper hepatic artery (HA), hepatic portal vein (HPV), extrahepatic bile duct (BD), autonomic nerves (N), and lymphatic vessels (L), supported by dense irregular connective tissue. The hepatic portal vein provides 70–80% of the blood supply to the liver, so it is much larger than the proper hepatic artery.

Helpful Hint

The proper hepatic artery and hepatic portal vein branch as they enter the liver. For simplicity, branches of these structures will simply be called "hepatic arteries" and "hepatic portal veins."

Video 33.5 Porta hepatis

Be able to identify:
— Porta hepatis
  • Extrahepatic bile duct
  • Hepatic artery
  • Hepatic portal vein
  • Autonomic nerves and lymphatic vessels
https://www.thieme.de/de/q.htm?p=opn/tp/308390101/978-1-62623-414-7_c033_v005&t=video

Within the liver, the hepatic artery and hepatic portal vein branch within connective tissue septa, together with the bile ducts exiting the liver. **Fig. 33.15** shows one such connective tissue partition, containing sections through a hepatic artery,

hepatic portal vein, and bile duct. Nerves (arrow) and lymphatic vessels (not shown) may be visible.

Helpful Hint

Because the intrahepatic bile duct has columnar epithelium, it is distinguished from the vessels by the basophilia created by the closely packed nuclei, even at low magnification. The hepatic portal vein is the largest structure in this grouping, and it has thin walls; the hepatic arteries have thick walls typical of arteries and arterioles.

The hepatic arteries and hepatic portal veins continue to branch within the connective tissue of the liver, getting smaller as they do so. As seen in **Fig. 33.10**, at the level of the classic liver lobule, the final branches of the hepatic artery (X) and hepatic portal vein (Y) are within the portal triad. Nerves and lymphatic vessels may be present within the triad but are usually too small to be seen.

Helpful Hint

As mentioned previously, the term "portal triad" refers to the connective tissue and associated structures seen at the corners of a classic liver lobule. This term arises from the fact that these regions typically have three visible structures: hepatic artery, hepatic portal vein, bile duct.

Video 33.6 Portal triad

Be able to identify:
— Portal triad
  • Intrahepatic bile duct
  • Hepatic artery
  • Hepatic portal vein
https://www.thieme.de/de/q.htm?p=opn/tp/308390101/978-1-62623-414-7_c033_v006&t=video

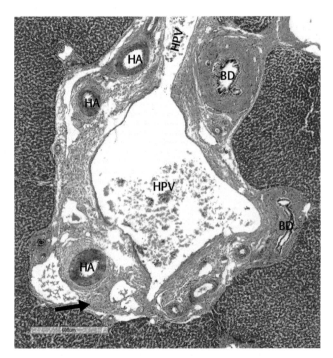

Fig. 33.15 **Connective tissue septum within the liver, showing hepatic arteries (HA), hepatic portal vein (HPV), intrahepatic bile ducts (BD), autonomic nerve (arrow).**

33.6.2 Liver Sinusoids

Fig. 33.16 is a more detailed drawing of a classic liver lobule. The hepatic artery and hepatic portal vein in the triad send small branches into the walls of the classic liver lobule. Both of these types of vessels empty into the capillaries of the liver, the **liver sinusoids**, so they contain mixed blood: oxygenated blood from the hepatic arteries and oxygen-poor but nutrient-rich blood from the hepatic portal veins.

The liver sinusoids are discontinuous capillaries oriented toward the central vein of a classic liver lobule. In H & E images of the liver (**Fig. 33.17**), sinusoids (marked with X) are seen as pale areas between hepatocytes, often with red blood cells in their lumen. Close examination reveals that these vessels are lined with endothelial cells (endothelial cell nuclei are indicated by yellow arrows, endothelial cell cytoplasm by black arrows).

Fig. 33.18 is an enlarged region from **Fig. 33.17**, showing the lumen of the sinusoids (X) and endothelial cells (arrows) more clearly. A space between the endothelial cells and hepatocytes, called the **perisinusoidal space**, better known as the **space of Disse**, is visible (S). In this image, the spaces marked (S) are artifactually enlarged; thinner areas can be seen that are more representative of the true size of these spaces.

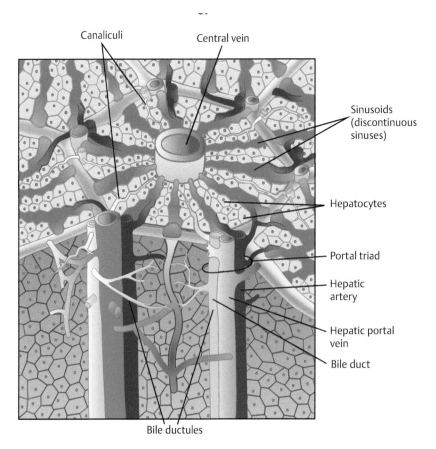

Canaliculi

Central vein

Sinusoids (discontinuous sinuses)

Hepatocytes

Portal triad

Hepatic artery

Hepatic portal vein

Bile duct

Bile ductules

Fig. 33.16 **Detailed drawing of the histology of the liver.**

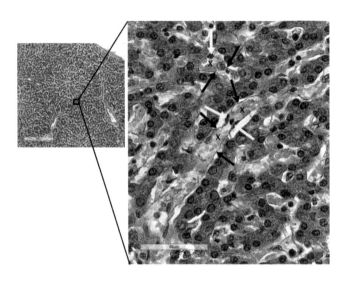

Fig. 33.17 **Liver sinusoids (X), lined by endothelial cells; endothelial cell nuclei are marked with yellow arrows, endothelial cell cytoplasm with black arrows.**

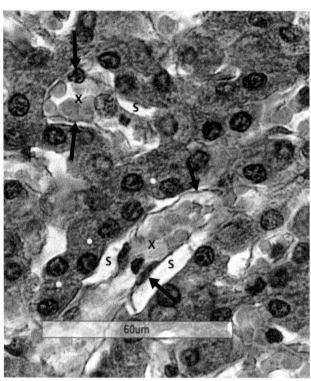

Fig. 33.18 **Liver sinusoids (X) at high magnification, lined by endothelial cells (nuclei and cytoplasm marked with black arrows). Perisinusoidal spaces of Disse (S) are visible. The approximate size and location of canaliculi are indicated by the yellow dots for comparison.**

Helpful Hint

Remember, bile canaliculi are too small to be seen in light micrographs. A few small yellow dots have been added to **Fig. 33.18** to provide a sense of the size and location of the canaliculi relative to sinusoids.

Helpful Hint

Sinusoids are approximately the same size, or slightly larger than, hepatocyte nuclei. For comparison, canaliculi (2 in **Fig. 33.19**; 4 in **Fig. 33.20**) are approximately the size of small mitochondria. Also note that sinusoids are lined by endothelial cells, while canaliculi are lined by hepatocyte plasma membrane.

Video 33.7 Liver sinusoids

Be able to identify:
— Sinusoids
— Endothelial cells

https://www.thieme.de/de/q.htm?p=opn/
tp/308390101/978-1-62623-414-7_c033_v007&t=video

Fig. 33.20 is an electron micrograph taken at slightly higher magnification. Sinusoids (1) can be seen above and to the lower right of the hepatocyte. Portions of endothelial cells (2) line the sinusoids; the gaps in this lining are clearly visible. Hepatocyte microvilli populate the perisinusoidal space of Disse (3). A canaliculus (4) is also present for comparison.

Helpful Hint

Blood vessels are on the basal side of a gland. So the side of the hepatocyte facing the sinusoid can be considered the basal side, and the hepatocyte membrane lining the canaliculus can be considered the apical side. However, hepatocytes are not as obviously polarized as, say, chief cells, so these terms are not often used with regard to hepatocytes. However, thinking about the hepatocyte in this way may be useful to organize the endocrine vs. exocrine function of these cells.

In electron micrographs, liver sinusoids (1 in **Fig. 33.19**) are seen as large-diameter capillaries. They are discontinuous, which means that, although the endothelial cells (black arrows) may form some cell-cell junctions with neighboring endothelial cells, there are large gaps between them. The endothelial cells also have fenestrations without diaphragms, and the basal lamina is discontinuous.

The space between the hepatocyte plasma membrane and the discontinuous endothelial cells is the perisinusoidal space (4 in **Fig. 33.19**; space of Disse), which contains numerous microvilli of the hepatocyte (better seen in **Fig. 33.20** and especially in **Fig. 33.21**). The sinusoids are very permeable; essentially, only formed elements are unable to pass through the endothelial cell gaps. Therefore, plasma is free to enter the space of Disse, bathing the plasma membrane of the hepatocyte.

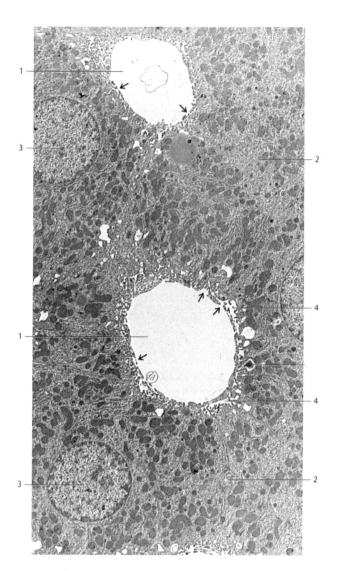

Fig. 33.19 Electron micrograph of the liver showing (1) liver sinusoids; (2) bile canaliculi; (3) hepatocyte nuclei; (4) perisinusoidal space of Disse. Arrows indicate endothelial cells.

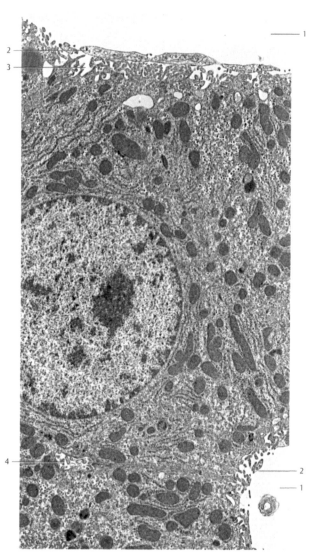

Fig. 33.20 Electron micrograph of a liver hepatocyte and (1) adjacent sinusoids above and to the lower right; (2) endothelial cells; (3) perisinusoidal space of Disse; (4) canaliculus.

Fig. 33.21 is a higher-magnification view of the wall of a sinusoid (1). Because of the high magnification, the endothelial cell (4) lining the sinusoid does not happen to include any of its gaps or fenestrations. Hepatocyte microvilli (2) and reticular fibers (3) are shown within the perisinusoidal space of Disse.

33.6.3   Liver Acinus

As just described, blood flows through the sinusoids from the periphery of a classic liver lobule toward the central vein. Along the way, hepatocytes change the composition of blood. This process includes removal of glucose and other nutrients and secretion of blood proteins and other liver products into the blood. Based on blood flow, the liver can be organized into diamond-shaped **liver acini** (**Fig. 33.22**). The central structure of a liver acinus is the "wall" of a classic liver lobule, and the corners of the diamond are portal canals and central veins.

Hepatocytes are very metabolically active and change the blood composition extensively as it flows through the sinusoids. Because blood flows through the sinusoids from the center of the liver acinus toward the central veins, the hepatocytes in zone 1 of

a liver acinus (in zone 1 of **Fig. 33.22**) are exposed to blood that is quite different from the blood that is bathing the hepatocytes near the central veins (**Fig. 33.22**, zone 3).

33.6.4   Blood Flow Away from the Liver

As just mentioned, all sinusoids within a classic liver lobule drain into a **central vein** (also known as a **terminal hepatic venule**). As shown in **Fig. 33.23**, the central vein is located in the center

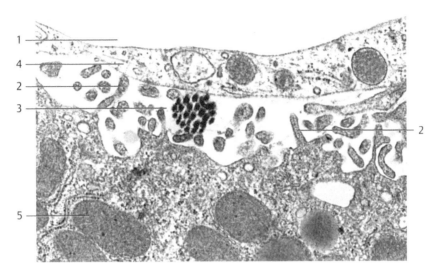

Fig. 33.21 Electron micrograph of (1) a liver sinusoid, showing (1) microvilli and (3) reticular fibers in the perisinusoidal space of Disse; (4) endothelial cell; and (5) mitochondrion.

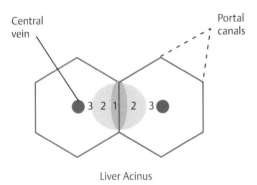

Central vein

Portal canals

Liver Acinus

Fig. 33.22 Liver acinus. Two classic liver lobules are shown (hexagons). The liver acinus is the shaded region; the central structure of a liver acinus is the boundary between two classic liver lobules. As blood flows from the wall toward the central veins, it is modified by hepatocytes, creating zones (1–3). Zone 1 hepatocytes are exposed to more nutrients and oxygen; zone 3 hepatocytes receive less of these.

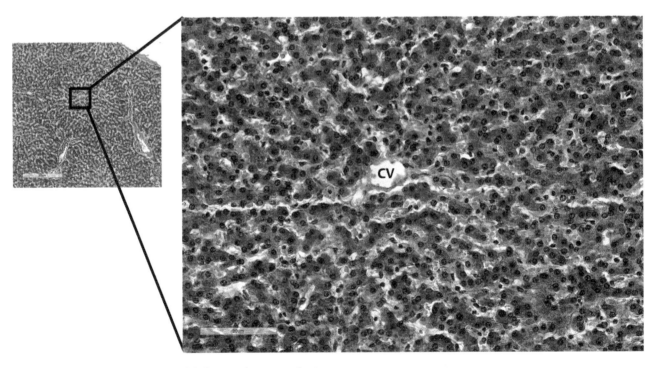

Fig. 33.23 Central vein of a classic liver lobule at medium magnification.

of a classic liver lobule, and sinusoids and plates of hepatocytes radiate toward the central vein. **Fig. 33.24** is a higher-magnification image of a central vein, showing at least two sinusoids connected to it at the 12 o'clock and 4 o'clock positions. Central veins have a structure similar to a small venule and are lined by endothelial cells supported by a very thin layer of loose irregular connective tissue.

The liver is structured such that liver lobules are arranged side by side (**Fig. 33.25**). Central veins are oriented vertically within each liver lobule (relative to the lobule, not necessarily the body). The central veins join at right angles to a **sublobular vein**, which is located along the "bottom" of a series of lobules. Sublobular veins then join at right angles to larger **hepatic veins**, which eventually drain into the inferior vena cava.

As just mentioned, central veins can be identified in the center of a classic liver lobule (**Fig. 33.23** and **Fig. 33.24**). Central, sublobular, and hepatic veins can be identified together by taking advantage of the fact that they join each other at right angles. **Fig. 33.26** shows such a section, in which smaller central veins (black arrows) are connected at right angles to a sublobular vein (yellow arrows), which connects at right angles to a hepatic vein (hepatic vein perpendicular to the plane of section of this image). The green arrows represent another sublobular vein connected to the hepatic vein.

Recall that, as veins become larger, the amount of connective tissue in their walls increases. This is true here as well: the central veins have scant connective tissue, sublobular veins have slightly more, and hepatic veins have thicker connective tissue.

Helpful Hint

Central veins, sublobular veins, and hepatic veins are not bundled together with intrahepatic bile ducts, hepatic arteries, and hepatic portal veins in the triads at the corners of each classic lobule. This is a useful way to differentiate the central, sublobular, and hepatic veins from hepatic portal veins.

Don't forget that hepatic portal veins and hepatic veins are different. The hepatic portal veins carry blood *to* the liver sinusoids, while the hepatic veins drain blood *from* the liver.

Video 33.8   Liver veins

Be able to identify:
— Central veins (terminal hepatic venule)
— Sublobular vein
— Hepatic vein
https://www.thieme.de/de/q.htm?p=opn/tp/308390101/978-1-62623-414-7_c033_v008&t=video

33.7 Kupffer Cells

Resident **liver macrophages** are commonly called **Kupffer cells**. These cells are found in the lining of sinusoids and are involved in breakdown of red blood cells. They are usually not identifiable on routine H & E-stained slides. However, they take up dyes such as trypan blue by phagocytosis, so they can be visualized in animals injected with this dye (**Fig. 33.27**, arrows).

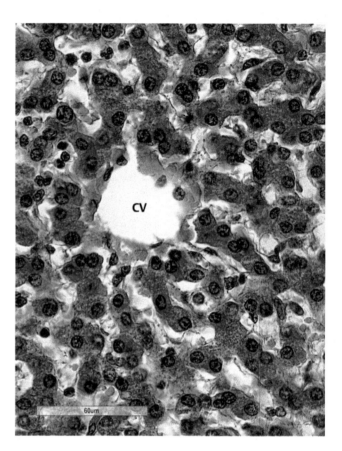

Fig. 33.24 Central vein of a liver lobule at high magnification, showing two sinusoids (at the 12 o'clock and 4 o'clock positions) connected to the central vein.

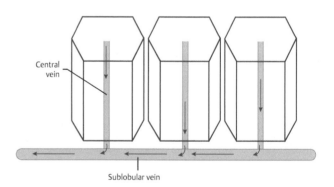

Fig. 33.25 Organization of lobules in the liver. Three classic liver lobules are shown as hexagon-shaped cylinders. A central vein is in the center of each lobule, each receiving blood from the sinusoids within that lobule. A sublobular vein receives blood from several central veins and is oriented at right angles to them.

Video 33.9   Liver macrophages (Kupffer cells)

Be able to identify:
— Liver macrophages (Kupffer cells)
https://www.thieme.de/de/q.htm?p=opn/tp/308390101/978-1-62623-414-7_c033_v009&t=video

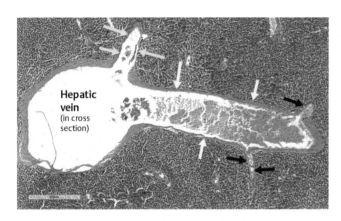

Fig. 33.26 Image of liver showing central veins (black arrows), sublobular veins (green and yellow arrows), and a hepatic vein in cross section.

Clinical Correlate

Because hepatocytes are epithelial, the liver has the capacity to regenerate. However, continued insult, as seen in alcohol abuse and hepatitis, results in increased deposition of connective tissue and disorganization of the lobular architecture of the liver, a condition called **cirrhosis**.

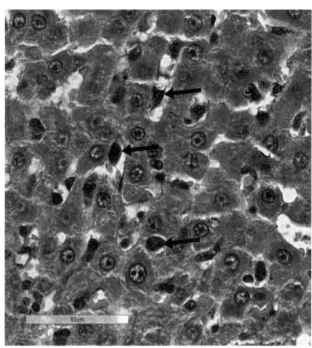

Fig. 33.27 Image of liver showing liver macrophages (Kupffer cells, arrows). Animals were injected with trypan blue, which is taken up by liver macrophages by phagocytosis. The animals were sacrificed and stained with H & E.

33.8 Gallbladder

Bile is produced continuously by hepatocytes. Between meals, this bile is not released into the duodenum. Rather, it flows in a retrograde fashion up the cystic duct to be stored by the **gallbladder** (see **Fig. 33.12**). The epithelial cells of the gallbladder concentrate the bile. Upon arrival of fat from a meal, enteroendocrine cells in the duodenum release hormones that stimulate contraction of smooth muscle in the wall of the gallbladder, releasing stored bile.

The gallbladder lacks a muscularis mucosae. Therefore, it has a three-layered structure (**Fig. 33.28**):

1. Mucosa (black bracket): A simple columnar epithelium plus lamina propria. The epithelial cells are very active in concentrating bile, so they are tall columnar with highly eosinophilic cytoplasm. The mucosa is thrown up into folds, creating the impression of glands (asterisk in **Fig. 33.28**) on histologic section.
2. Muscularis (red bracket): Smooth muscle interspersed with connective tissue. The smooth muscle here is fairly thin.
3. Adventitia or serosa (green bracket): Connective tissue that may be covered by a simple epithelium, depending on whether the section is from the side in contact with the liver (adventitia) or the side covered by visceral peritoneum (serosa; see **Fig. 33.12**).

Video 33.10 Gallbladder

Be able to identify:
— Gallbladder
https://www.thieme.de/de/q.htm?p=opn/
tp/308390101/978-1-62623-414-7_c033_
v010&t=video

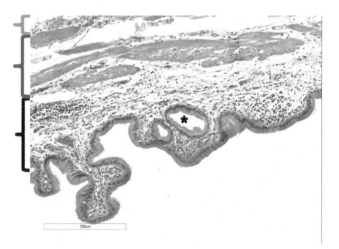

Fig. 33.28 Gallbladder, showing the mucosa (black bracket), muscularis (red bracket), and adventitia/serosa (green bracket). Asterisk (*) indicates a mucosal fold that has the appearance of a gland.

33.9 Chapter Review

Like the pancreas, the liver and gallbladder develop as outgrowths from the gastrointestinal tract. Although the histologic structure of the liver remains exocrine with ducts that connect to the duodenum, the liver cells (hepatocytes) are both endocrine and exocrine in function. Hepatocytes are very active metabolically and exhibit euchromatic nuclei (with nucleoli) and a cytoplasm that is highly eosinophilic with areas of cytoplasmic basophilia due to abundant cellular organelles. Hepatocytes are organized together into classic liver lobules, defined by connective tissue borders in which portal triads are at the corners. The portal triads contain a hepatic artery, hepatic portal vein, and bile duct. Plates of hepatocytes in a classic liver lobule, and the sinusoids between them, radiate toward a central vein.

The exocrine function of hepatocytes is the production of bile, which is initially released into bile canaliculi, which are small channels created between the hepatocytes themselves. At the periphery of a classic liver lobule, in the portal triad, canaliculi connect to bile ducts, which are lined by a cuboidal epithelium. These intrahepatic bile ducts combine to form larger bile ducts, which eventually exit the liver as extrahepatic bile ducts, which have similar features as intrahepatic bile ducts except that they are supported by more substantial connective tissue.. As an alternative way to describe the liver, portal liver lobules feature bile ducts in the portal triad as the central structure. The portal liver lobule is the developmental unit.

The endocrine function of the liver relates to blood flow. This involves the dual blood supply via the hepatic artery and hepatic portal vein, which enter the liver at the porta hepatis, branch in the liver connective tissue, and ultimately are part of the portal triad. These vessels empty into the liver sinusoids, which are very permeable discontinuous capillaries. As another way to describe the structure of the liver, liver acini feature blood flow as the main point of focus, and hepatocytes in different zones are exposed to different contents of blood. Sinusoids drain into a central vein, which joins with a sublobular vein, and then one of the hepatic veins, which exit the liver and empty into the inferior vena cava.

Resident liver macrophages, called Kupffer cells, are involved in red blood cell turnover.

Bile produced by the liver is stored and concentrated in the gallbladder, which has a three-layered structure consisting of a mucosa, muscularis, and adventitia/serosa.

Questions and Answers

An online-only section of questions and answers accompanying this chapter is hosted on Thieme's MedOne Education site: https://medone-education.thieme.com. Use the code on the media page at the front of this book to gain access. An institutional license to the site is required to access these questions in an interactive format, and individual users are required to register for an individual account to track results.

34   Overview of the Kidney

After completing this chapter, you should be able to:
— Identify, at the light microscope level, each of the following:
  • Anatomic features of the kidneys
    ○ Cortex
      ▪ Medullary rays (pars radiata)
      ▪ Pars convoluta
    ○ Medulla
      ▪ Renal pyramid
      ▪ Renal papilla
      ▪ Renal columns
    ○ Hilus (drawings only)
    ○ Sinus
    ○ Urinary structures of the kidney
      ▪ Renal pelvis (drawings only)
      ▪ Major calyces (drawings only)
      ▪ Minor calyces
    ○ Vessels of the kidneys
      ▪ Renal artery and vein
      ▪ Interlobar artery and vein
      ▪ Arcuate artery and vein
      ▪ Interlobular artery and vein
      ▪ Afferent arteriole, glomerulus, efferent arteriole
      ▪ Peritubular capillaries and vasa recta
— Differentiate between cortical and juxtamedullary nephrons
— Recognize and discriminate between renal lobes and renal lobules and between medullary rays and pars convoluta
— Diagram blood circulation through the kidneys
— Outline the function of each cell, structure, and vessel type listed

34.1   Physiology of the Urinary System

Excess or insufficient levels (concentration) of water, ions, buffers, and other molecules in the bloodstream can result in serious pathology affecting all organ systems, especially the nervous system and muscles. In addition, waste products produced by cells must be eliminated, while at the same time useful organic molecules such as glucose must be retained. The main function of the **urinary (excretory) system** (**Fig. 34.1**) is to adjust blood (plasma) levels of these molecules. During this process, excess is removed from the body, forming urine. The functional unit of the kidneys that accomplish this are microscopic tubes called **nephrons**; each kidney is endowed with almost a million nephrons at birth.

The kidneys perform this function by two main mechanisms:
• Actively adjusting levels of these molecules in the plasma
• Secreting hormones (e.g., renin) that are involved in regulation of these molecules

The remainder of the urinary system (i.e., the extrarenal organs: ureters, bladder, and urethra) is involved in transport, storage, and removal of urine.

In this sequence of chapters, the first three will focus on the histology of the kidneys. The extrarenal organs will be discussed in the final chapter.

34.2   Gross Anatomy of the Kidneys

The **kidneys** are retroperitoneal structures, meaning they are positioned behind the gastrointestinal tract, in the posterior abdominal wall (**Fig. 34.2**).

Fig. 34.3 is a drawing of a kidney sectioned in the coronal plane. Note:
• The **medulla** (not labeled) is a region that includes the **medullary (renal) pyramids** (are triangular in longitudinal (coronal) section) and the tissue between these pyramids, the **renal columns**.
• A **renal papilla** is the tip of a renal pyramid.
• Each pyramid/papilla drains into a **minor calyx**. Two or more minor calyces join to form a **major calyx**, and major calyces ultimately join to form the **renal pelvis**, which then narrows to form the **ureter**. The calyces, pelvis, and ureter are part of the extrarenal structures involved in transporting urine to the bladder.
• The **renal sinus** is the space created when the fat between the calyces and renal vessels is dissected away.
• The **renal capsule** is a thin connective tissue covering of the kidney.

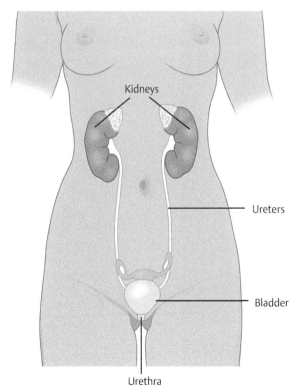

Fig. 34.1   **Urinary system (female).**

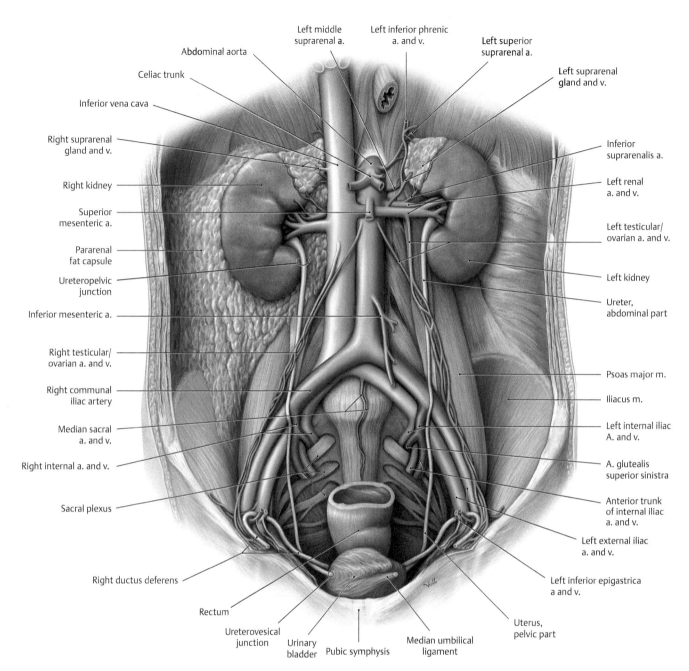

Left middle
suprarenal a.

Left inferior phrenic
a. and v.

Left superior
suprarenal a.

Abdominal aorta

Celiac trunk

Inferior vena cava

Left suprarenal
gland and v.

Right suprarenal
gland and v.

Inferior
suprarenalis a.

Right kidney

Left renal
a. and v.

Superior
mesenteric a.

Left testicular/
ovarian a. and v.

Pararenal
fat capsule

Left kidney

Ureteropelvic
junction

Ureter,
abdominal part

Inferior mesenteric a.

Right testicular/
ovarian a. and v.

Psoas major m.

Right communal
iliac artery

Iliacus m.

Median sacral
a. and v.

Left internal iliac
A. and v.

Right internal a. and v.

A. glutealis
superior sinistra

Sacral plexus

Anterior trunk
of internal iliac
a. and v.

Left external iliac
a. and v.

Right ductus deferens

Left inferior epigastrica
a and v.

Rectum

Ureterovesical
junction

Urinary
bladder

Pubic symphysis

Median umbilical
ligament

Uterus,
pelvic part

Fig. 34.2 **Abdomen with the gastrointestinal organs removed to show kidneys and ureters located in the posterior abdominal wall.**

Like many organs, the kidney can be divided into several lobes: **renal lobes** (**Fig. 34.4**, one lobe is outlined in black). A renal lobe includes a renal pyramid as well as its associated cortex (including portions of the renal columns on either side of the pyramid). Urine produced by the nephrons in a renal lobe drains into the minor calyx associated with that lobe. Human kidneys have 10 to 20 of these lobes, each oriented such that the renal papilla is close to the renal sinus.

Fig. 34.5 is a scanning view of a section through the kidney, similar to the region outlined in red in **Fig. 34.4**. In this scanning view of a portion of the kidney, a nearly complete lobe is outlined in black, including the cortex, medulla (pyramid), and papilla. The cup-shaped space surrounding the papilla is a minor calyx. To the right of this lobe is most of a second lobe (yellow outline), with cortex and medulla, but the papilla and minor calyx are out of the plane of section. Further to the right is part of a third lobe. The bottom of the slide contains adipose tissue of the renal sinus, including blood vessels, which will be examined later. The dotted green line represents the border between the cortex (above) and medulla (below).

Helpful Hint

It is useful to think in three dimensions. **Fig. 34.3** and **Fig. 34.4** show about nine lobes, but more are situated on either side of the plane of section.

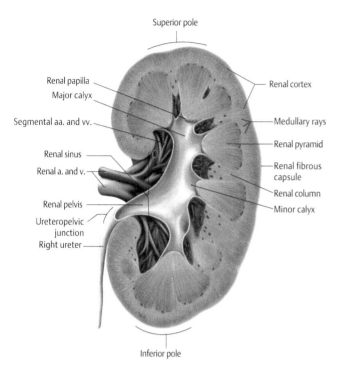

Fig. 34.3 **Kidney in coronal section.**

Video 34.1 Gross anatomy of the kidney

Be able to identify:
— Renal lobe
— Cortex
— Medulla
  • Renal pyramid
  • Renal papilla
  • Renal columns
— Sinus
— Minor calyx

https://www.thieme.de/de/q.htm?p=opn/tp/308390101/978-1-62623-414-7_c034_v001&t=video

34.3 Overview of the Nephron

As mentioned, each kidney contains about 1 million excretory structures called **nephrons**, which adjust plasma levels of molecules. Each nephron ultimately drains its product (urine) into a minor calyx via a collecting duct.

Histologically, the parts of the nephron include (**Fig. 34.6**):

• **Renal corpuscle**
• **Proximal convoluted tubule (PCT)**
• **Loop of Henle**
  • **Thick descending limb**
  • **Thin limb (descending and ascending)**
  • **Thick ascending limb**
• **Distal convoluted tubule (DCT)**
• **Connecting tubule (collecting tubule)**
• **Collecting duct**

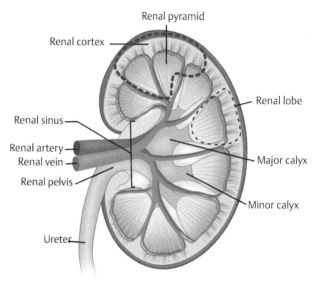

Fig. 34.4 **Kidney in coronal section. One lobe, which includes a renal pyramid and associated cortex, is outlined in black. The region outlined in red, which contains 2+ lobes, indicates a region similar to that shown in Fig. 34.5.**

Basic Science Correlate: Physiology

Blood is filtered by the renal corpuscle to produce **provisional urine** (known as **ultrafiltrate**). This fluid then flows down the tubular system (in the order listed), and the ultrafiltrate is modified by cells of the tubules. The final product, **urine**, flows out the end of the collecting ducts into a minor calyx.

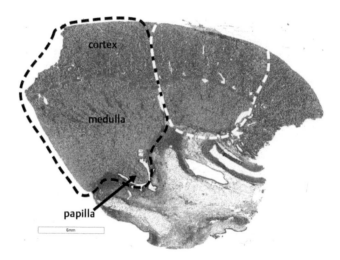

Fig. 34.5 **Part of the kidney in coronal section, corresponding to the region outlined in red in Fig. 34.4, showing one complete lobe (black outline) with the renal papilla in the plane of section, one lobe in which the papilla is not in the plane of section (yellow outline), and one incomplete lobe (to the right of the yellow outline). The green dotted line indicates the border between the cortex and medulla. The region at the bottom of the slide below the lobes is the renal sinus, which contains renal vessels and adipose tissue.**

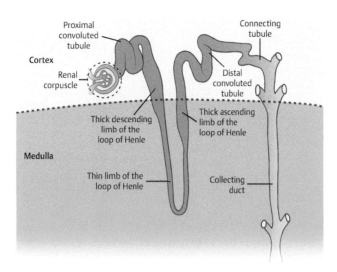

Fig. 34.6   Nephron. The dotted line indicates the border between the cortex (above dotted line) and medulla (below).

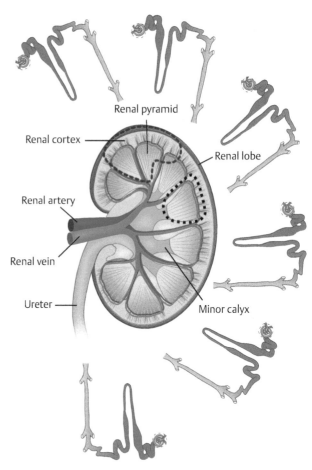

Fig. 34.7   Orientation of nephrons in the kidney.

As mentioned, all renal papillae are directed toward the renal pelvis. The nephrons within the kidney have a similar organization. As shown in **Fig. 34.7**, nephrons in the kidney are oriented so that the tips of the loops of Henle are closest to the minor calyx, and all collecting ducts are directed toward the minor calyx that drains that lobe.

Nephrons are positioned as shown in **Fig. 34.6**, where the dashed red line indicates the approximate border of cortex above the line and medulla below:

- The coiled parts of the nephron (corpuscle and proximal and distal convoluted tubules) are entirely in the cortex.

- The straight parts of the nephron (loop of Henle, collecting ducts) are located in the medulla but extend into the cortex.

34.4   Classification of Nephrons

Nephrons can be classified into two categories based on the position of the corpuscle and the length of the loop of Henle (**Fig. 34.8**):

1. **Cortical nephrons** are almost entirely in the cortex. The renal corpuscle of these nephrons is located in the outer region of the cortex. A very short loop of Henle in these nephrons extends only a short distance into the medulla.
2. **Juxtamedullary nephrons** have a renal corpuscle in the cortex, located adjacent to the medulla. The loops of Henle of juxtamedullary nephrons are long and extend into the deeper portions of the medulla. Juxtamedullary nephrons are important for setting up the concentration gradient in the medulla used in concentration of urine.

34.5   Renal Lobes and Renal Lobules

Recall that a renal lobe consists of a renal pyramid and the cortex associated with it (**Fig. 34.4**, black outline). **Fig. 34.9** is a drawing showing a close-up view of a renal lobe. The cortex of each lobe can be broken down into renal lobules (blue shaded rectangle in enlarged region to the right) such that:

- The core of each lobule is composed of straight portions of the nephron (loops of Henle and collecting ducts) that extend

into the cortex; this region is called the **medullary ray** or **pars radiata** (collection of dark lines within rectangle; one medullary ray is looped).

- The periphery of each lobule (paler pink portion within rectangle but outside the medullary ray) is composed of the coiled parts of the nephron (corpuscle, PCT, DCT) and is called the **pars convoluta** (bracket indicates one pars convoluta).

Helpful Hint

Each lobule shares a border with an adjacent lobule; the exact border between lobules is not easily identified but is about halfway between medullary rays, as shown by the rectangle.

There are many lobules per lobe of the kidney. For simplicity, this drawing shows only five lobules in this lobe.

Fig. 34.10 shows the cortex and outer medulla (border between the two indicated by the dashed black line). The cortex contains medullary rays (above black brackets), seen as collections of tubules oriented in the same direction extending from the corticomedullary junction toward the outer surface (capsule) of the kidney. Note that, due to sectioning, it is unusual to see an entire medullary ray from one end to the other; in this region, most can be seen clearly at the corticomedullary junction but "disappear" about one-third to one-half the way toward the

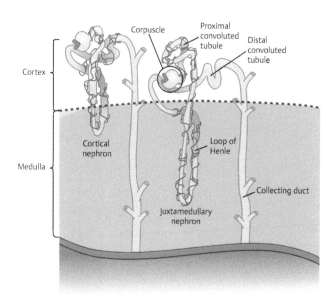
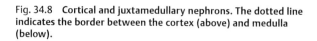

Fig. 34.8 **Cortical and juxtamedullary nephrons. The dotted line indicates the border between the cortex (above) and medulla (below).**

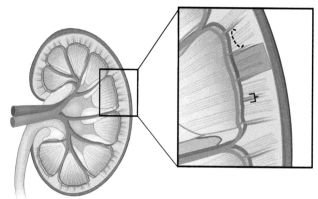

Fig. 34.9 **Close-up of a renal lobe showing renal lobules. One lobule is indicated (shaded box). The central structure of the lobule is a medullary ray (pars radiata, outlined). The pars convoluta is the portion of the cortex not including the medullary rays (i.e., between medullary rays; one is indicated by the bracket).**

capsule. The regions between the medullary rays form the pars convoluta (blue bracket), in which the tubules are in many different orientations.

A lobule (outlined in yellow) is defined as a medullary ray plus the tubules within the adjacent partes convolutae that are connected to (i.e., belong to the same nephrons as) the tubules in that medullary ray. The border between adjacent lobules is about halfway between two medullary rays. In a section such as this, half of each pars convoluta "belongs" to one medullary ray (or lobule), and the other half belongs to the adjacent medullary ray.

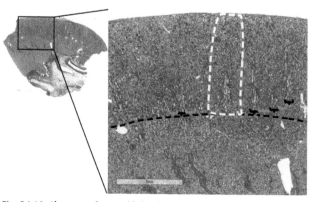

Fig. 34.10 **Close-up of a renal lobe showing a renal lobule (outlined in yellow). Medullary rays (partes radiatae, black brackets) and partes convolutae (blue brackets) are shown. The border between the cortex and medulla is indicated by the black dashed line.**

Video 34.2   Renal lobules—1

https://www.thieme.de/de/q.htm?p=opn/tp/308390101/978-1-62623-414-7_c034_v002&t=video

Video 34.3   Renal lobules—2

Be able to identify:
— Medullary rays (pars radiata)
— Pars convoluta
— Lobule

https://www.thieme.de/de/q.htm?p=opn/tp/308390101/978-1-62623-414-7_c034_v003&t=video

lobules share borders. The central region of each lobule is a medullary ray (outlined in yellow), which can be recognized because all the tubules in this region are cut in cross section in this orientation. Recall that the medullary rays contain straight tubules (i.e., ascending and descending portions of the loops of Henle), and collecting ducts. Peripheral to each medullary ray is the pars convoluta (between yellow and black outlines), in which the tubules (proximal and distal convoluted tubules) are cut in a variety of orientations. Renal corpuscles can also be seen in the pars convoluta (arrows).

Fig. 34.11 shows the drawing of a renal lobe from **Fig. 34.9**, with a black line indicating the plane of section for the next image, **Fig. 34.12**. The arrow reinforces the direction in which the observer will be looking when viewing **Fig. 34.12**.

Fig. 34.12 shows such a tangential cut through the cortex; three adjacent lobules are outlined in black. Note that adjacent

Video 34.4   Renal lobules in tangential cut through the cortex

Be able to identify:
— Medullary ray (pars radiata)
— Pars convoluta
— Lobule

https://www.thieme.de/de/q.htm?p=opn/tp/308390101/978-1-62623-414-7_c034_v004&t=video

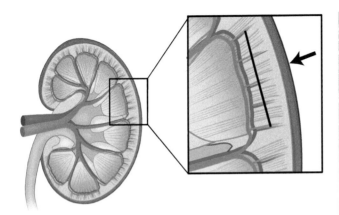

Fig. 34.11 **Close-up of a renal lobe. The black line is the plane of section for a tangential section in Fig. 34.12.**

34.6   Blood Supply of the Kidney

Because the kidneys are involved in filtering plasma, they receive much more blood flow than required for the metabolic needs of the kidney cells. Indeed, the kidneys receive one-fifth of the cardiac output. The renal blood supply is organized to ensure efficient blood flow to each lobule and nephron (**Fig. 34.13**). Renal vessels enter and leave the kidney at the **hilus** (indentation on the medial side of the kidney). The **renal artery** branches into **segmental arteries** within the renal sinus. These segmental arteries give rise to **interlobar arteries**, which run in the renal columns between the renal pyramids (i.e., between the lobes, hence the name). At the junction of the medulla and cortex, the interlobar arteries branch at right angles, forming **arcuate arteries** that are oriented parallel to the capsule, between the cortex and medulla. Branching from the arcuate arteries at right angles are **interlobular arteries**, which run in the cortex toward the capsule (i.e., between the lobules). All these arteries have accompanying veins (arteries are red, veins are blue).

> **Helpful Hint**
>
> The microvasculature of the kidney—afferent and efferent arterioles, glomerulus, peritubular capillaries, and vasa recta—will be discussed in subsequent chapters.

With the structure of the renal vasculature in mind, it helps to reinforce that renal vessels are recognized by their position within the kidney:
- Renal and segmental vessels are in the sinus.
- Interlobar vessels are in the renal columns (between pyramids or lobes).
- Arcuate vessels are between the cortex and medulla.
- Interlobular vessels are in the cortex, between lobules.

> **Helpful Hint**
>
> It cannot be stressed enough here: All the arteries in the kidney look like arteries, and all the veins look like veins. It is true that the arteries get smaller as they branch, and the veins get larger as they return to the renal vein, and this may be useful, but do not lose sight of the fact that the definitive way to identify these vessels is by their position in the context of the kidney.

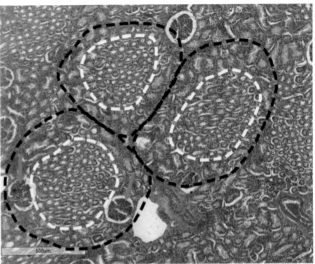

Fig. 34.12 **Tangential section through the renal cortex along the plane indicated by the yellow line in Fig. 34.11. Three lobules are outlined in black. The medullary rays are within the yellow outlines; the partes convolutae are between the yellow and black outlines. Blue arrows indicate renal corpuscles in the pars convoluta.**

Fig. 34.14 is a scanning image of the kidney (the same image from **Fig. 34.5**), showing a nearly complete renal lobe (outlined), a portion of an adjacent lobe, and a small piece of another lobe to the right. Vessels within the sinus (black arrows) are either renal or segmental (they cannot be differentiated in this section). Vessels between the renal pyramids (i.e., between lobes, yellow arrows) are interlobar vessels, while vessels within the corticomedullary junction are arcuate vessels (green arrows).

> **Helpful Hint**
>
> Although many of the vessels shown in **Fig, 34.14** run longitudinally in this orientation (e.g., the arcuate vessels run between the medulla and cortex in an arc shape), in most cases, cross-sectional profiles are seen because the vessels are not exactly parallel to the plane of section. That said, the interlobar vessels in **Fig. 34.14** are cut in longitudinal section and give a pretty good appreciation of the direction and extent of these vessels.

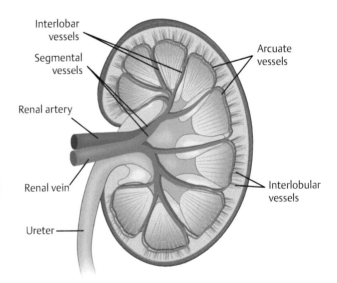

Fig. 34.13 **Renal vessels.**

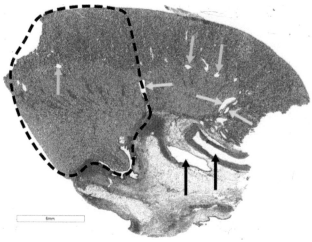

Fig. 34.14 **Scanning view of the kidney showing renal vessels. One lobe is outlined. Black arrows indicate segmental or renal vessels; orange arrows point to interlobar vessels; green arrows mark arcuate vessels.**

Fig. 34.15 is an image of the cortex and outer medulla; the border between the cortex and medulla is indicated by the dotted line. Arcuate vessels (green arrows) can be seen more clearly along the corticomedullary junction. In the medulla, interlobar vessels (orange arrows) are present. In the cortex, small profiles of interlobular vessels can be seen (blue arrows).

Fig. 34.16 is an image of the renal cortex adjacent to the medulla, showing two medullary rays (between brackets). Longitudinal and cross-sectional profiles of interlobular vessels (blue arrows) can be seen in the middle of the pars convoluta (i.e., between lobules). In fact, the presence of these vessels signifies the border between adjacent lobules (thus the name interlobular vessels).

For all of the vessels shown in these figures at low magnification, there are both arteries and veins present. Differentiating between them may be possible at these magnifications but usually requires higher magnification to examine the thickness of the wall, as described in the chapters on vessel morphology.

Video 34.5   Renal vessels—1

https://www.thieme.de/de/q.htm?p=opn/
tp/308390101/978-1-62623-414-7_c034_
v005&t=video

Video 34.6   Renal vessels—2

Be able to identify:
— Renal artery and vein (or segmental artery and vein)
— Interlobar artery and vein
— Arcuate artery and vein
— Interlobular artery and vein
https://www.thieme.de/de/q.htm?p=opn/tp/308390101/978-1-
62623-414-7_c034_v006&t=video

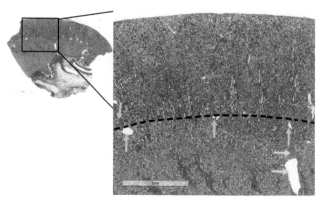

Fig. 34.15 **The cortex and medulla of the kidney showing renal vessels. Orange arrows indicate interlobar vessels; green arrows mark arcuate vessels; blue arrows indicate interlobular vessels.**

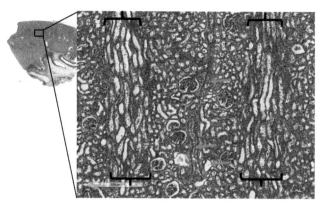

Fig. 34.16 **The cortex of the kidney, adjacent to the medulla, showing medullary rays (black brackets) and interlobular vessels (blue arrows).**

34.7   Chapter Review

The kidney is responsible for regulating the molecular composition of plasma. In this regard, the kidney must remove waste products generated by cells and maintain balance of water, ions, and buffers. The kidney achieves this through the action of nephrons, microscopic structures that filter serum to produce provisional urine (ultrafiltrate, see **Chapter 36**), and then modify that urine. The kidney contains a cortex, a medulla, and a sinus. The sinus includes the urinary structures (calyces, pelvis) as well as renal vessels and adipose tissue. The medulla is divided into renal pyramids; each pyramid and associated cortex form a renal lobe. Within the cortex, each lobe is divided into renal lobules, which include a central medullary ray and peripheral pars convoluta. The blood supply within the kidneys is highly organized and includes renal vessels, segmental vessels, interlobar vessels, arcuate vessels, and interlobular vessels. These vessels are recognized in histologic sections based on their position in the kidney.

Questions and Answers

For further study on this chapter, please see the accompanying Question and Answer material found at http://medone.thieme.com. Code redemption (see inside front cover) required, for personal use only.

35 Tubules of the Kidney

After completing this chapter, you should be able to:
— Identify, at the light microscope level, each of the following:
  • Proximal convoluted tubule
  • Thick descending limb of the loop of Henle
  • Thin limb of the loop of Henle
  • Thick ascending limb of the loop of Henle
  • Distal convoluted tubule
  • Collecting duct (papillary duct)
  • Peritubular capillaries
  • Vasa recta
— Identify, at the electron microscope level, each of the following:
  • Proximal convoluted tubule/thick descending limb of the loop of Henle
  • Thick ascending limb of the loop of Henle/distal convoluted tubule
  • Collecting ducts (papillary ducts)
— Outline the function of each structure and vessel type listed
— Correlate the structural features of renal tubules with their function
— Correlate the appearance of each structure or cell in light micrographs with its appearance in electron micrographs, and vice versa

35.1 Overview of the Nephron

Recall from the previous chapter that each kidney contains nearly 1 million **nephrons (Fig. 35.1)**. As discussed briefly in the previous chapter, these nephrons are responsible for maintaining optimal levels of water, ions, and buffers in the plasma. The first step in this process is the production of an **ultrafiltrate (provisional urine)** through filtration of plasma; this process occurs in the **renal corpuscle**. The ultrafiltrate flows through the tubule of the nephron, where it is modified by **selective reabsorption** (recapture of filtered molecules) and **active secretion** (moving molecules from the blood into the urine) to form the final product, **urine**, which is eliminated from the body.

This chapter will focus on all of the parts of the nephron except for the renal corpuscle, which will be discussed in the next chapter. The portions of the nephron described in this chapter, the different segments of the tubule, are involved in modifying urine as it passes through the lumen. Therefore, the epithelial cells that line the tubule are very active in transport of ions and water across their membranes.

35.2 Microvasculature of the Kidney

Recall that the blood supply to the kidney is well organized (**Fig. 35.2**). Blood flows through a **renal artery**, which divides into **segmental arteries**. Segmental arteries give rise to **interlobar arteries**, which run between the **medullary pyramids** (i.e., between lobes). Interlobar arteries give rise to **arcuate arteries**, located in the corticomedullary junction. **Interlobular arteries** branch from the arcuate arteries at right angles to supply the cortex.

The microvasculature of the kidney includes a portal system, which is defined as two capillary beds in sequence (similar to the hepatic portal vessels in the gastrointestinal system). Here, the first capillary bed is the **glomerulus**, which is the capillary bed in the renal corpuscle (**Fig. 35.3**). The second capillary bed is either the **peritubular plexus of capillaries** (peritubular capillary plexus) or the **vasa recta**.

More specifically, **afferent arterioles** bring blood from the interlobular arteries to the glomeruli, and **efferent arterioles** carry blood away from the glomeruli (**Fig. 35.3**). From here, blood flow takes one of two paths:

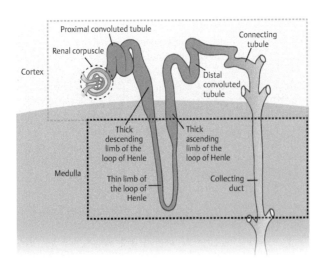

Fig. 35.1   **Nephron. The portions of the nephron are divided in this chapter based on location. Structures within the cortex and outer portion of the medulla are within the yellow rectangle; structures within the black rectangle are located in the deep medulla.**

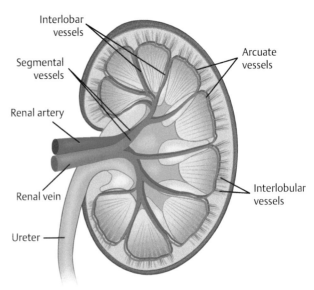

Fig. 35.2   **Renal vessels.**

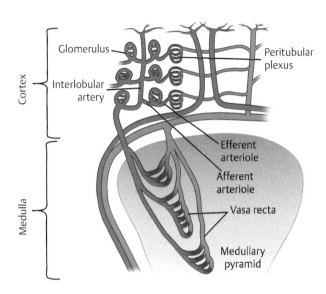

Fig. 35.3   **Microvasculature of the kidney.**

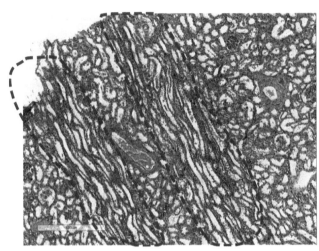

Fig. 35.4   **Renal cortex showing medullary rays (pars radiata, outlined) and pars convoluta (between outlined regions).**

1. Efferent arterioles in the outer regions of the cortex supply the peritubular capillary plexus, which surrounds the tubules in the cortex, mostly the proximal and distal convoluted tubules.
2. Efferent arterioles leaving glomeruli located near the medulla (i.e., from juxtamedullary nephrons) give rise to long vessels called vasa recta that follow the course of the loops of Henle.

This chapter will focus on the tubules, so it will highlight the peritubular capillary plexus and vasa recta. The next chapter, covering the renal corpuscle, will examine the glomerulus as well as the afferent and efferent arterioles.

35.3   Renal Tubules

Recall that the cortex of the kidney consists of two regions (**Fig. 35.4**). The medullary rays (pars radiata, outlined) are characterized by straight tubules aligned in the same orientation. In the pars convoluta (between outlined regions), the tubules are tortuous, so sections seen here are in different orientations. It is important to note that the tubules of the medullary rays are extensions (continuations) of tubules from the outer portion of the medulla, so that the tubules in these medullary rays are the same as those in the outer medulla (described subsequently).

Fig. 35.5 is a high-powered image of the pars convoluta, showing a variety of tubules in cross, longitudinal, and oblique sections (two examples are outlined in yellow). These tubules are lined by a simple cuboidal epithelium, and their lumen contains ultrafiltrate (provisional urine). The basement membrane of the epithelium can be seen in many tubules (just inside the yellow dashed outline). There is sparse connective tissue, with blood vessels, between the tubules. There are several tubule segments that can be distinguished in **Fig. 35.5** (the two outlined tubules are clearly different). Proper identification of these tubule segments is based on specific characteristics of the epithelial cells and is the main focus of this chapter. The round tuft in the bottom center is a renal corpuscle, the topic of the next chapter.

By way of introduction, **Fig. 35.6** is a comparison of a renal tubule in light and electron microscopy. Traditionally, when describing tissues or organs, it is best to begin with

low-magnification light micrographs and then drill down to cellular detail in electron micrographs. The tubules of the kidneys have many light microscopic characteristics (e.g., eosinophilia) that are due to cellular features seen in electron micrographs (numerous mitochondria). Although this is true for many tissues and organs, many of these cellular features are crucial for proper identification of these kidney tubules, so it is more practical to describe them at the electron microscopic level first and then describe how these features affect the appearance of the tubules when viewed with the light microscope.

35.4   Renal Tubules in the Cortex and Outer Medulla

Renal tubule segments located in the cortex and outer medulla are within the yellow rectangle in **Fig. 35.1**. **Table 35.1** shows the location of each of these tubule segments of the nephron.

Tubule segments shown on the same row in **Table 35.1** (e.g., proximal convoluted tubule and descending thick limb) have similar histologic features at both the light and electron microscopic levels. In a light micrograph, the location of these tubules

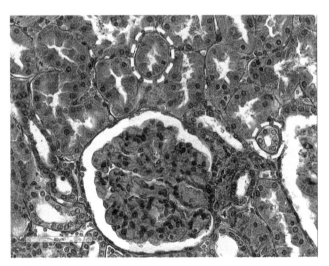

Fig. 35.5   **Pars convoluta of renal cortex showing renal tubules (outlined).**

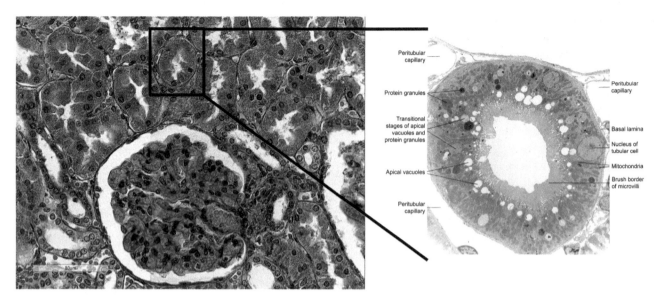

Fig. 35.6   Comparison of a renal tubule in light and electron microscopy (electron micrograph courtesy of Michael Hortsch, University of Michigan, © 2005 The Regents of the University of Michigan).

Table 35.1   Tubule segments in the pars convoluta and their counterparts in the pars radiata or outer medulla

Pars convoluta	Pars radiata and outer medulla
Proximal convoluted tubule	Descending thick limb of the loop of Henle
Distal convoluted tubule	Ascending thick limb of the loop of Henle
Connecting duct	Collecting duct

(i.e., in the pars convoluta or pars radiata) will enable these tubule segments to be distinguished from each other. In electron micrographs, magnification is typically too high to determine whether the image is from the pars convoluta or pars radiata; therefore, differentiating between tubule segments with similar characteristics is not possible. For most purposes, it is not necessary to distinguish between connecting and collecting ducts.

35.4.1   Proximal Convoluted Tubule and Descending Thick Limb of the Loop of Henle

Fig. 35.7 is an electron micrograph of a proximal convoluted tubule.

Characteristics of **proximal convoluted tubules** and **descending thick limbs of the loop of Henle** include:

- Large cells
- Numerous microvilli (brush border)
- Numerous mitochondria
- Numerous basolateral infoldings (see **Fig. 35.8** and following discussion)

Remember, this is an electron micrograph, so, if it were not labeled, the magnification would be too high to determine with confidence whether this tubule is a proximal convoluted tubule in the pars convoluta or the descending thick limb in a medullary ray.

Fig. 35.8a is an electron micrograph from the proximal convoluted tubule. Numerous undulations of the basolateral plasma membrane can be seen, especially on enlargement (**Fig. 35.8b**). These **basolateral infoldings** (2, and red arrows), and the microvilli on the apical surface (see **Fig. 35.7**) increase the surface area of the plasma membrane available for placement of ion pumps and channels, which modify the ultrafiltrate as it flows through the lumen of the tubule.

As mentioned previously, it is useful to consider the cellular features visible on electron micrographs of renal tubules, because these features manifest as features of these tubules in light microscopy. **Table 35.2** shows the characteristics of proximal convoluted tubules and descending thick limbs in electron micrographs and the corresponding features of these tubules in light micrographs.

Table 35.2   Histologic features of proximal convoluted tubules and descending thick limbs of the loop of Henle

Electron microscopic features	Light microscopic characteristics
Large cells	Nuclei spread out, fewer nuclei
Numerous microvilli	Fuzzy apical surface obstructing lumen
Numerous mitochondria	Eosinophilic cytoplasm
Numerous basolateral infoldings	Borders between cells not apparent

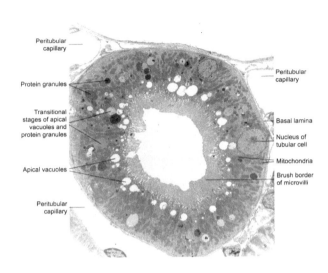

Fig. 35.7   **Electron micrograph of a proximal convoluted tubule. Courtesy of Michael Hortsch, University of Michigan, © 2005 The Regents of the University of Michigan.**

Fig. 35.9 is a light micrograph of the pars convoluta with two proximal convoluted tubules outlined. In fact, most of the tubules in the upper portion of this image are proximal convoluted tubules. The epithelial cells in these tubules have nuclei spaced far apart, fuzzy apical borders, eosinophilic cytoplasm, and no visible borders between cells.

Helpful Hint

Visible borders between cells will be seen as a dark line. These lines will be seen later in the discussion of collecting ducts.

Fig. 35.10 is a light micrograph of a medullary ray (or outer medulla), with descending thick limbs of loops of Henle outlined. The histologic features of the descending thick limbs are the

same as for the proximal convoluted tubule in **Fig. 35.9**. These tubules in **Fig. 35.10** are identified as descending thick limbs and not proximal convoluted tubules based on their location within a medullary ray (or outer medulla).

Helpful Hint

Note that most of the tubules in **Fig. 35.10** surrounding the circled descending thick limbs are in the same orientation (sectioned lengthwise), because this is a medullary ray (or outer cortex). Compare to the tubules in **Fig. 35.9**, which are in different orientations.

Video 35.1   Proximal convoluted tubule and thick descending limb

Be able to identify:
— Proximal convoluted tubule
— Descending thick limb of the loop of Henle

https://www.thieme.de/de/q.htm?p=opn/tp/308390101/978-1-62623-414-7_c035_v001&t=video

Clinical Correlate

Glucose passes through the filtration apparatus of the renal corpuscle and is part of the ultrafiltrate (provisional urine) that enters the tubular system. The proximal convoluted tubule has glucose transporters that remove glucose from the ultrafiltrate and return it to the blood. This is an efficient process; normally, all the glucose is reabsorbed in this way, and little glucose is lost in the urine. In **diabetes mellitus**, excess blood glucose results in excess glucose in the ultrafiltrate, which overwhelms the glucose transporters in the proximal convoluted tubules. This results in glucose in the urine, or **glycosuria**. Diabetes mellitus is quite common. **Renal glycosuria** is due to genetic defects in the genes coding for the glucose transporters and is much less common.

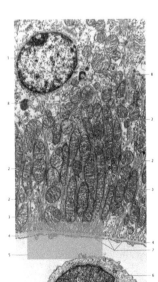

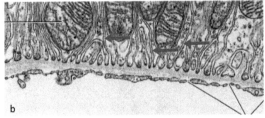

Fig. 35.8   **(a) Electron micrograph of basal aspect of a proximal convoluted tubule epithelial cell, showing (1) nucleus; (2) basolateral infoldings; (3) mitochondria; (4) basal lamina (basement membrane); (5) capillary lumen; (6) endothelial cell, region with nucleus; (7) fenestrated endothelium; (8) lysosomes. (b) Enlargement of shaded region in (a), giving a clearer view of the basolateral infoldings (red arrows).**

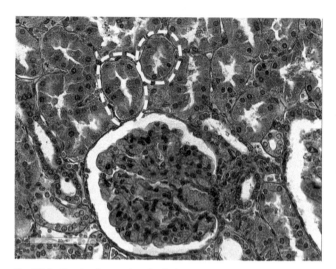

Fig. 35.9 **Proximal convoluted tubules (outlined).**

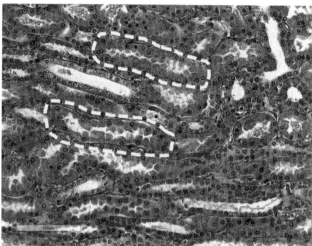

Fig. 35.10 **Descending thick limbs of loops of Henle.**

35.4.2   Distal Convoluted Tubule and Ascending Thick Limb of the Loop of Henle

Fig. 35.11 is an electron micrograph of a distal convoluted tubule.

Characteristics of the **distal convoluted tubule** and **ascending thick limb of the loop of Henle** include:

- Small cells
- Few microvilli
- Numerous mitochondria (in most cells)
- Numerous basolateral infoldings (not visible at this magnification, but similar to those in the proximal convoluted tubule shown in **Fig. 35.8**)

These cellular features translate into characteristics in light micrographs, as indicated in **Table 35.3**.

Fig. 35.12 is a light micrograph of the pars convoluta, showing two distal convoluted tubules (outlined). Note that these tubules have numerous nuclei that are closer together, a sharp apical surface with a wide lumen, eosinophilic cytoplasm, and no apparent borders between the cells. **Fig. 35.12** also shows nice examples of the plexus of capillaries in the pars convoluta: the peritubular capillaries (arrows).

> **Helpful Hint**
>
> Distal convoluted tubules are shorter than proximal convoluted tubules; therefore, there are fewer profiles of distal convoluted tubules than of proximal convoluted tubules in the pars convoluta.

Table 35.3 Histologic features of distal convoluted tubule and ascending thick limb of the loop of Henle

Electron microscopic features	Light microscopic characteristics
Small cells	Nuclei close together, more numerous
Few microvilli	Sharp apical surface, wide lumen
Numerous mitochondria	Eosinophilic cytoplasm
Numerous basolateral infoldings	Borders between cells not apparent

Fig. 35.13 is a light micrograph of a medullary ray (or outer medulla), with ascending thick limbs of loops of Henle outlined. The histologic features of the ascending thick limbs are the same as for the distal convoluted tubule in **Fig. 35.12**. These tubules in **Fig. 35.13** are identified as ascending thick limbs and not distal convoluted tubules based on their location within a medullary ray (or outer medulla).

> **Helpful Hint**
>
> Comparing proximal (**Fig. 35.9**) and distal (**Fig. 35.11**) tubules, and their corresponding thick limbs (**Fig. 35.10** and **Fig. 35.12**, respectively). They both have eosinophilic cytoplasm and no visible borders between the cells. The cells in proximal tubules are larger, so these tubules have fewer nuclei than the distal tubules. The proximal tubules also have more prominent microvilli, so their apical border is more irregular than the border of distal tubules.

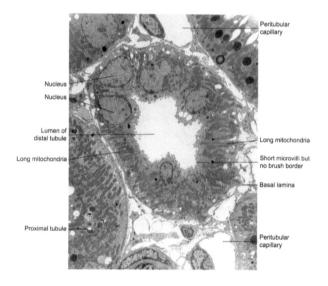

Fig. 35.11 **Electron micrograph of a distal convoluted tubule. Image courtesy of Michael Hortsch, University of Michigan. © 2005 The Regents of the University of Michigan.**

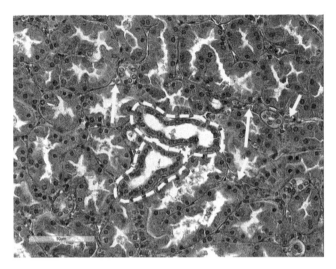

Fig. 35.12 **Distal convoluted tubules (outlined). Peritubular capillaries are indicated by the arrows.**

Video 35.2 Distal convoluted tubule and thick ascending limb

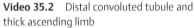

Be able to identify:
— Distal convoluted tubule
— Thick ascending limb of the loop of Henle
https://www.thieme.de/de/q.htm?p=opn/tp/308390101/978-1-62623-414-7_c035_v002&t=video

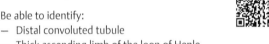

Basic Science Correlate: Physiology

The thick ascending limb of the loop of Henle and the distal convoluted tubule are very active in modifying the ion content of provisional urine. In particular, they are responsible for reuptake of sodium, which results in reuptake of water (both moving from urine back into the blood). Many diuretics act by inhibiting the transport of these ions, which results in loss of sodium and water in the urine. Drugs that block channels of the thick ascending limb of the loop of Henle are known as loop diuretics (e.g., furosemide). Drugs such as hydrochlorothiazide inhibit channels of the distal convoluted tubule.

35.4.3 Connecting Tubules and Collecting Ducts

For most purposes, it is not necessary to distinguish **connecting tubules** and **collecting ducts**; therefore, the focus will be on collecting ducts. **Fig. 35.14** is an electron micrograph of a collecting duct.

Characteristics of collecting ducts include:
• Small cells
• Few microvilli (in most cells)
• Few mitochondria (in most cells)
• Few basolateral infoldings

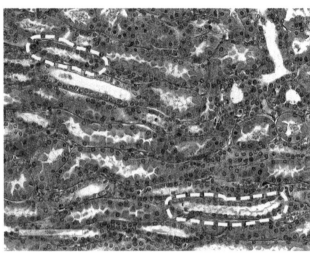

Fig. 35.13 **Ascending thick limbs of loops of Henle.**

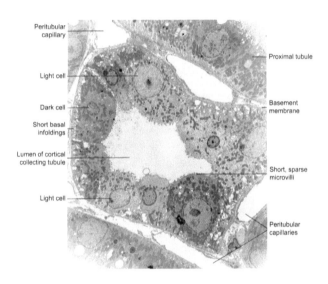

Fig. 35.14 **Electron micrograph of a collecting duct (connecting tubule). Image courtesy of Michael Hortsch, University of Michigan. © 2005 The Regents of the University of Michigan.**

Helpful Hint

Close examination of the collecting duct in **Fig. 35.14** reveals different cell types. Some have numerous mitochondria; however, overall, the collecting duct has fewer mitochondria than the other tubule segments in the kidney. The different cell types here have different functions physiologically, especially with regard to acid-base balance in the plasma. However, it is usually not necessary to distinguish these cell types.

The cellular features of collecting ducts in electron micrographs translate into characteristics in light micrographs, as indicated in **Table 35.4**.

Fig. 35.15 is a light micrograph of a medullary ray, showing a collecting duct (outlined). Note that these tubules have numerous nuclei that are close together, a sharp apical surface with a wide lumen, pale cytoplasm, and borders between the cells visible in several locations.

Table 35.4 Histologic features of collecting ducts

Electron microscopic features	Light microscopic characteristics
Small cells	Nuclei close together, more numerous
Few microvilli	Sharp apical surface, wide lumen
Few mitochondria	Pale cytoplasm
Few basolateral infoldings	Borders between cells visible

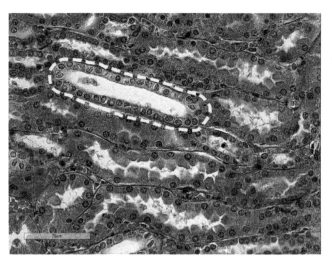

Fig. 35.15 **Collecting duct (outlined).**

Helpful Hint

Although collecting ducts have small cells (so numerous nuclei) and lack microvilli (so a sharp apical border), the most striking features that distinguish these tubules from any other tubules in the kidney are the pale cytoplasm of these cells (less eosinophilic than in the descending and ascending limbs) and the presence of clear borders between adjacent cells.

- Collecting ducts (outlined in red): small, cuboidal cells, pale cytoplasm, borders between cells visible
- Thin limbs of loops of Henle (outlined in yellow): cells categorized as squamous but a little thicker than endothelial cells; no red blood cells (RBCs) in the lumen
- Vasa recta (outlined in black): flat endothelial cells, possible RBCs in the lumen

Video 35.3   Collecting duct

Be able to identify:
— Collecting duct
— Peritubular capillaries
https://www.thieme.de/de/q.htm?p=opn/
tp/308390101/978-1-62623-414-7_c035_v003&t=video

Video 35.4   All ducts and tubule segments

Be able to identify:
— Proximal convoluted tubule
— Distal convoluted tubule
— Descending thick limb
— Ascending thick limb
— Collecting duct
— Peritubular capillaries
https://www.thieme.de/de/q.htm?p=opn/tp/308390101/978-1-
62623-414-7_c035_v004&t=video

35.5   Renal Tubules in the Deep Medulla

Recall that the nephrons in the kidney are oriented such that the loops of Henle are located in the medulla and medullary rays (**Fig. 36.16**), and the turns of the loops are closest to the pelvis. The portion of the medulla closest to the papilla that contains the **thin limbs of the loops of Henle** is a region that can be called the "deep" medulla. The deep medulla also has collecting ducts that will ultimately drain into the minor calyx. In addition, because the loops and collecting ducts in the deep medulla are straight, the capillaries in this region are also straight and are referred to as vasa recta (straight vessels).

The black rectangle in **Fig. 35.1** shows the structures of the nephron that can be found in the deep medulla.

Fig. 35.17 is an image of the deep medulla, showing:

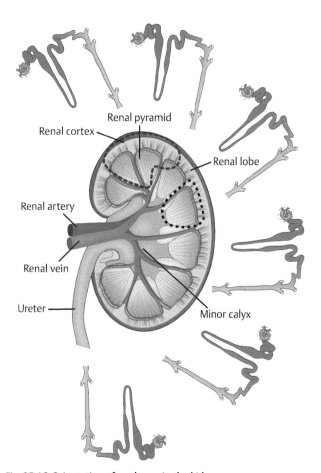

Fig. 35.16 **Orientation of nephrons in the kidney.**

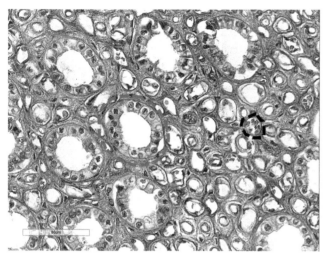

Fig. 35.17 **Deep medulla of the kidney, medium magnification, showing collecting duct (red outline), thin limb of the loop of Henle (yellow outline), and vas rectum (black outline).**

The descending and ascending thin limbs of the loop of Henle are indistinguishable.

Fig. 35.18 is a higher-magnification image of the deep medulla, focusing on the thin limbs of the loop of Henle (yellow outlines) and the vasa recta (outlined in black). Note that the squamous cells are thicker in the thin limbs than in vasa recta; in fact, in the lower of the two outlined vasa recta, which contains RBCs, the endothelial cells are barely seen (one nucleus is at the 9 o'clock position). In the upper vas rectum outlined, no RBCs are present, but the thinness of the endothelial cells strongly suggests that this is a vas rectum and not a thin limb.

Video 35.5 Deep medulla

Be able to identify:
— Collecting duct
— Thin limb of the loop of Henle
— Vas rectum
https://www.thieme.de/de/q.htm?p=opn/tp/308390101/978-1-62623-414-7_c035_v005&t=video

In the renal papilla, the collecting ducts merge into larger collecting ducts called **papillary ducts**. Histologically, papillary ducts have the same appearance as smaller collecting ducts, so identifying them as collecting ducts is sufficient.

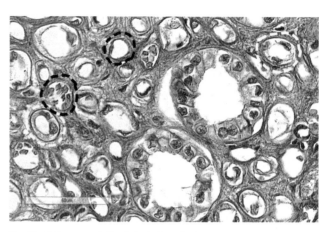

Fig. 35.18 **Deep medulla of the kidney, high magnification. Thin limb of the loop of Henle (yellow outlines) and two vasa recta (black outlines) are indicated.**

Collecting ducts have water transport channels (**aquaporins**) that allow water to move from the urine back into the bloodstream. When these channels are active, water is retained, and the urine is concentrated. The activity of these channels is increased by **antidiuretic hormone** released by the pituitary gland. Drugs such as alcohol inhibit the production or action of antidiuretic hormone and so have a diuretic effect.

35.6 Chapter Review

In addition to removal of waste products, the nephrons in the kidney are responsible for maintaining ideal levels of water, ions, and buffers in the plasma. The nephrons achieve this by first producing an ultrafiltrate (provisional urine) in the renal corpuscle. This ultrafiltrate flows through the lumen of the tubular system; it is in these tubules that the ultrafiltrate is modified according to the body's needs, including selective reabsorption of filtered molecules and active secretion of waste or excess molecules. The cells in the different segments of a tubule have distinct features that can be recognized in electron micrographs and impart characteristics in light micrographs. In addition, the position of these tubule segments in either the medullary rays (and outer medulla) or the pars convoluta allows conclusive identification.

The proximal convoluted tubule is in the pars convoluta, and its wall consists of large cells with numerous microvilli, numerous mitochondria, and basolateral infoldings. In light micrographs, this translates into few nuclei, a fuzzy apical border and narrow lumen, cytoplasmic eosinophilia, and indistinct cell borders. The descending thick limb of the loop of Henle has similar features to the proximal convoluted tubule but is located in medullary rays or the outer cortex.

The distal convoluted tubule has smaller cells and fewer microvilli than the proximal convoluted tubule. In light micrographs, the wall of the distal convoluted tubule has more nuclei and a sharper apical border and wider lumen than the proximal convoluted tubule. The ascending thick limb of the loop of Henle has similar features to the distal convoluted tubule but is located in medullary rays or the outer cortex.

Collecting ducts have few mitochondria, few basolateral infoldings, few microvilli, and small cells. In light micrographs, cells of collecting ducts have a distinctively pale cytoplasm, sharp apical border, and visible borders between the cells.

Collecting ducts are also present in the deep medulla, where they combine to form larger papillary ducts. Also in the deep medulla are thin limbs of the loop of Henle and the vasa recta. Although thin limbs and vasa recta are both lined by simple squamous epithelial cells, cells of the thin limbs are usually slightly thicker, and blood cells are often visible in the vasa recta.

Questions and Answers

An online-only section of questions and answers accompanying this chapter is hosted on Thieme's MedOne Education site: https://medone-education.thieme.com. Use the code on the media page at the front of this book to gain access. An institutional license to the site is required to access these questions in an interactive format, and individual users are required to register for an individual account to track results.

36   Corpuscle of the Kidney

After completing this chapter, you should be able to:
— Identify, at the light microscope level, each of the following:
  - Renal corpuscle
  - Afferent arteriole
  - Efferent arteriole
  - Macula densa
  - Juxtaglomerular cells
— Identify, at the electron microscope level, each of the following:
  - Renal corpuscle
    - Glomerulus
      - Endothelial cells
    - Bowman's capsule
      - Podocytes
        - Primary pedicels (primary foot processes)
        - Secondary pedicels (secondary foot processes)
        - Filtration slits
      - Parietal epithelium
    - Lamina densa
    - Mesangial cells
    - Blood space
    - Urinary space
— Outline the function of each structure and vessel type listed
— Evaluate the process of production of ultrafiltrate (provisional urine)
— Predict the result of damage to the renal corpuscle

36.1   Overview of the Renal Corpuscle

The previous chapters provided an overview of the kidney and the structure and function of the renal tubules. This chapter focuses on the detailed structure of the **renal corpuscle** (**Fig. 36.1**), which filters blood plasma to produce **provisional urine** (**ultrafiltrate**). This provisional urine passes through the lumen of the tubules described in the previous chapter, which modify the urine by recapturing molecules that were filtered as well as adding molecules to the provisional urine that need to be removed from the blood.

36.2   Development of the Renal Corpuscle

To understand the final structure of the renal corpuscle, it is useful to think about the part of the nephron that will form the corpuscle. **Fig. 36.2a** shows that the nephron in this region is a blind-ending tube lined by epithelial cells, with a basement membrane that separates the tubule from the surrounding connective tissue (white background). Blood vessels in the connective tissue form a tuft of capillaries, the **glomerulus**. The glomerulus is flanked by two arterioles (the afferent and efferent arterioles), which bring blood to and from the glomerulus (black arrows in **Fig. 36.2a** indicate direction of blood flow). The **afferent arteriole** is a branch of an **interlobular artery**, while the **efferent arteriole** feeds into the **peritubular capillary plexus** or **vasa recta**.

The renal tubule invaginates, forming a **visceral** and a **parietal layer of Bowman's capsule** (**Fig. 36.2b, c**); the space between these two layers is the **capsular space** (**Bowman's space**). Cells of the visceral layer, called **podocytes**, cover the endothelial cells of the glomerulus. In many places, the connective tissue between the endothelial cells and podocytes is squeezed out, and the two basement membranes fuse to form a single, thick basal lamina, called the **lamina densa**.

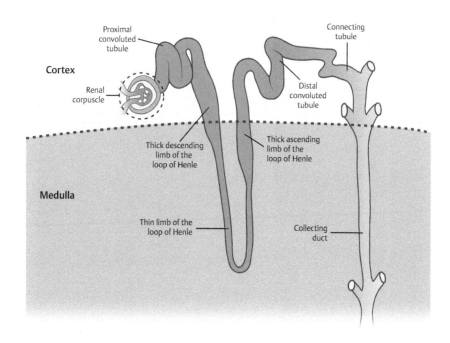

Fig. 36.1 **Nephron.**

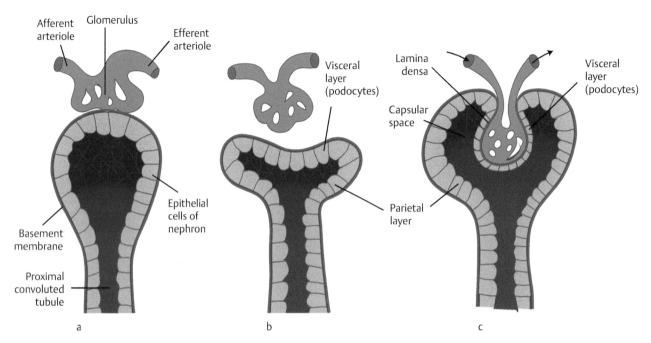

Fig. 36.2   (a–c) Development of the renal corpuscle.

Just to be clear on terminology, the glomerulus is the tuft of capillaries. The visceral layer (podocytes) and the parietal layer together constitute Bowman's capsule. The renal corpuscle is the glomerulus plus the Bowman's capsule. The terms "glomerulus" and "renal corpuscle" are often used interchangeably, but they are not exactly the same.

36.3   Structure of the Renal Corpuscle

Fig. 36.3 is a three-dimensional drawing of a renal corpuscle, which may help visualize its structure. In this image, the glomerular tuft of capillaries is surrounded by the visceral epithelium (podocytes), represented by the brown outer coat (resembling plastic wrap) in this drawing. In this regard, note that the wrapping (podocytes) covers only the outer portions of the glomerular capillaries, moving toward the center of the tuft in some places. However, bridges of connective tissue persist between the capillaries in the central areas not covered by podocytes.

Fig. 36.4 is another three-dimensional drawing of the glomerular capillaries covered by podocytes. Again, the podocytes are represented by the structure resembling plastic wrap, here in green. In locations where the capillaries of the glomerulus are covered tightly by the podocytes, the connective tissue between

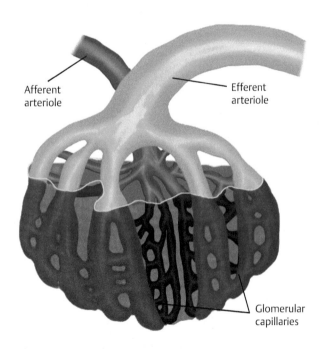

Fig. 36.3   **Three dimensional view of the renal corpuscle. The brown wrapping covering the glomerular capillaries represents the podocytes of the visceral layer of Bowman's capsule.**

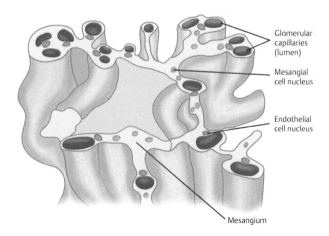

Fig. 36.4   **Three dimensional view of the renal corpuscle. The green wrapping covering the glomerular capillaries represents the podocytes of the visceral layer of Bowman's capsule.**

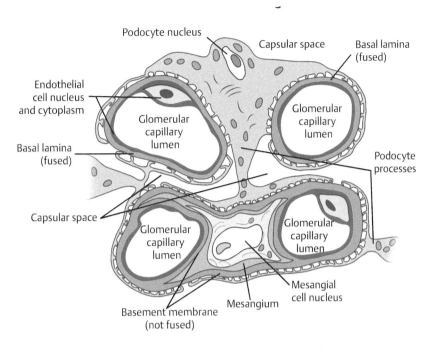

Podocyte nucleus

Capsular space

Basal lamina (fused)

Endothelial cell nucleus and cytoplasm

Glomerular capillary lumen

Glomerular capillary lumen

Basal lamina (fused)

Podocyte processes

Capsular space

Glomerular capillary lumen

Glomerular capillary lumen

Mesangial cell nucleus

Basement membrane (not fused)

Mesangium

Fig. 36.5 Drawing of a section through the corpuscle showing four capillaries, covered by podocyte processes.

the podocytes and endothelial cells of the capillaries is extruded, and their basal laminae fuse (lamina densa). In other areas, the capillaries are connected by stalks of connective tissue, referred to as **mesangium**. Note that endothelial cells, **mesangial cells**, and mesangium are not distinguished in this drawing.

Fig. 36.5 is a more detailed look at four capillaries from the glomerulus. In many areas, podocytes cover the capillaries with extensive processes (described in detail later). In these locations, the connective tissue is extruded, so the basal laminae of the podocytes and endothelial cells fuse. Filtration of blood occurs in these regions, with the ultrafiltrate (provisional urine) accumulating in the capsular space (Bowman's space). In other areas, capillaries are connected by mesangium.

Fig. 36.6 is a light micrograph of a renal corpuscle. The tuft in the center contains the glomerulus, podocytes, and mesangial cells; nuclei in this region are indistinguishable but belong to one of those three cell types. The outer layer consists of **parietal cells**, which are simple squamous. The space between the tuft and parietal cells is the capsular space.

> **Basic Science Correlate: Physiology**
>
> Blood flows through the glomerular capillaries at relatively high pressure, forcing fluid into the capsular space. This fluid is provisional urine (ultrafiltrate) that flows into the proximal convoluted tubule.

The renal corpuscle is polar, because the arterioles are on one side, and the proximal convoluted tubule is attached to the other (**Fig. 36.1**). Some fortuitous sections of renal corpuscles demonstrate these features:

- At the **urinary pole** (**Fig. 36.7a**, blue arrow), the proximal convoluted tubule (dotted blue line) is connected to Bowman's capsule and drains the capsular space.
- At the **vascular pole** (**Fig. 36.7b**, orange arrow), the afferent and efferent arterioles enter and exit the corpuscle (vessels identified by black arrows).

Parietal cells

podocytes/endothelial cells/mesangial cells (cannot distinguish between these three at light micrograph)

Capsular space

Fig. 36.6 Renal corpuscle showing nuclei in the glomerular tuft, nuclei of parietal cells, and the capsular space.

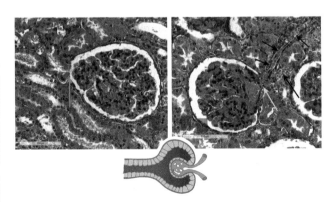

Fig. 36.7 Renal corpuscles showing poles. (a) Urinary pole (blue arrow; blue dotted line indicates the lumen of the proximal convoluted tubule); (b) Vascular pole (orange arrow; black arrows indicate arterioles).

These poles are not necessarily on exact opposite sides of the corpuscle, and sections through corpuscles are at different angles. Therefore, most corpuscles on tissue sections contain neither of these features, while some contain only one. It is rare for one corpuscle to show both.

Video 36.1   Renal corpuscles

Be able to identify:
— Parietal cells
— Capsular space
— Vascular pole
— Urinary pole

https://www.thieme.de/de/q.htm?p=opn/tp/308390101/978-1-62623-414-7_c036_v001&t=video

36.4   Ultrastructure of the Renal Corpuscle in Scanning Electron Micrographs

Although the structure of a corpuscle in light micrographs is fairly straightforward, important details are revealed in electron micrographs. **Fig. 36.8** is a drawing of the corpuscle with part of the parietal epithelium removed, reinforcing key features of the corpuscle:
• Endothelium of glomerulus (not visible, covered by podocytes)
• Podocytes of visceral layer covering glomerulus
• Parietal layer
• Capsular space (Bowman's space)

The red arrows in **Fig. 36.8** indicate the direction of blood flow through the renal vessels (afferent arteriole → glomerulus → efferent arteriole). The yellow arrows indicate filtrate passing from the blood into the capsular space and flowing into the proximal convoluted tubule.

Fig. 36.9 is a scanning electron micrograph of a section of the cortex. Two corpuscles are shown, surrounded by renal tubules (4). In the corpuscle on the left, the central tuft (glomerulus and podocytes) is absent, showing the capsular space (1). The inner aspect of the parietal epithelium can be seen (5 indicates the cut edge of the parietal layer), as well as the vascular pole (2). In the corpuscle to the right, the right half of the tuft is intact, showing the surface (podocytes), while the left half is sectioned, showing the lumen of the glomerular capillaries. (3 marks the macula densa, discussed subsequently).

36.4.1   Glomerulus

The glomerulus is essentially a tuft of fenestrated capillaries. **Fig. 36.10** shows a cast of the glomerular capillaries. At the vascular pole of the glomerulus (1), the afferent (2) and efferent (3) arterioles enter and leave the tuft of capillaries, respectively.

Fig. 36.11 is an image of the wall of a glomerular capillary, showing fenestrations (holes) in the endothelial cells. In contrast to other fenestrated capillaries, the fenestrations in the glomerular capillaries do not have a diaphragm, so they are very porous.

36.4.2   Podocytes

Fig. 36.12 is a detailed drawing of a glomerular capillary covered by podocytes, viewed from within the capsular space. Note:
• The capillary endothelium is fenestrated (without diaphragms).
• Podocytes are elaborate cells, with numerous extensions called **pedicels** (or **foot processes**); larger initial processes are called **primary pedicels**, which have numerous smaller extensions called **secondary pedicels**.
• The pedicels of adjacent podocytes interdigitate, and the spaces between the pedicels are called **filtration slits**.

Fig. 36.13 is a scanning electron micrograph of glomerular capillaries covered by podocytes, viewed from within the capsular space (similar to **Fig. 36.12**). Podocyte cell bodies (1) and primary (2) and secondary (4) pedicels (foot processes)

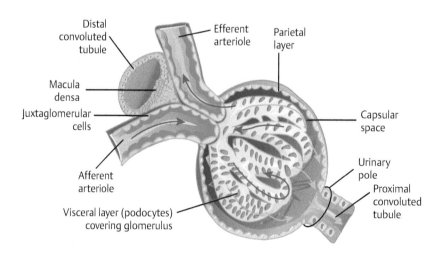

Fig. 36.8   Detailed drawing of an opened renal corpuscle (part of the parietal epithelium removed) showing blood flow though the glomerular capillaries (red arrows) and the flow of ultrafiltrate (yellow arrows).

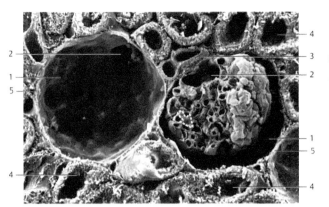

Fig. 36.9   **Two renal corpuscles in scanning electron micrograph. The glomerulus and podocytes were lost during tissue preparation in the left corpuscle, showing the inner wall of the parietal layer. The right corpuscle includes the glomerular tuft, part of which is sectioned to show the lumen of the glomerular capillaries; the part of the tuft not sectioned reveals a surface view of podocytes. Features include (1) capsular space; (2) vascular pole; (3) macula densa; (4) renal tubules; (5) parietal epithelium. Yellow outline marks mesangium (discussed later).**

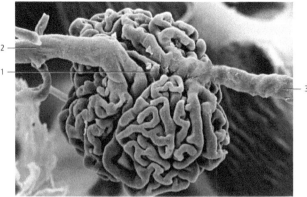

Fig. 36.10 **Cast of the glomerulus. Latex was injected into the glomerular vessels and allowed to harden. The tissue was subsequently removed, leaving behind the latex cast. Note (1) the vascular pole; (2) the afferent arteriole; (3) the efferent arteriole.**

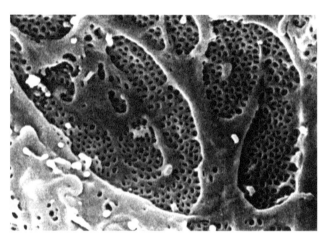

Fig. 36.11 **Wall of the glomerular capillaries.**

are readily seen. The gaps between the secondary pedicels are filtration slits. The large dark spaces between the capillaries (3) are the capsular space.

Fig. 36.14 is a medium-magnification view of the filtration apparatus, as seen from the capsular space. A podocyte cell body (1) and primary (2) and secondary (3) pedicels are shown. The gaps between the secondary pedicels are filtration slits (5). To produce the ultrafiltrate, components of plasma pass from the glomerular capillaries through these slits and into the capsular space (4).

Fig. 36.15 is a high-magnification scanning electron micrograph of the filtration apparatus, as seen from the capsular space, showing primary pedicels (1), secondary pedicels (2), and filtration slits (3).

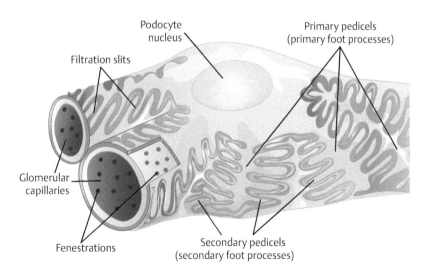

Fig. 36.12 **Podocytes covering glomerular capillaries.**

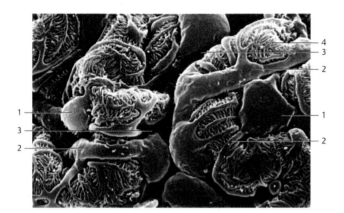

Fig. 36.13 Podocytes covering glomerular capillaries in scanning electron micrograph, low magnification. Note (1) podocyte cell body; (2) primary pedicels; (3) capsular space; (4) secondary pedicel.

Fig. 36.14 Podocytes covering glomerular capillaries in scanning electron micrograph, medium magnification. Note (1) podocyte cell body; (2) primary pedicels; (3) secondary pedicel; (4) capsular space; (5) filtration slits.

36.5   Ultrastructure of the Renal Corpuscle in Transmission Electron Micrographs

Now that the main components of the corpuscle have been examined in scanning electron micrographs, a more detailed look can be made using transmission electron micrographs. **Fig. 36.16** is an electron micrograph similar to a section through the corpuscle represented by the black line in the drawing. The majority of this image shows the tuft of capillaries covered by podocytes. The large empty circular structures are capillaries of the glomerulus (1). Endothelial cell nuclei (4) bulge into the lumen of the capillaries. Some capillaries contain red blood cells (middle right, not labeled). Podocyte nuclei (5) are seen outside the capillaries, and their foot processes (pedicels) can be seen covering the outer surface of each capillary, with a basement membrane (lamina

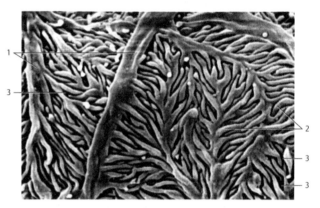

Fig. 36.15 Podocytes covering glomerular capillaries in scanning electron micrograph, high magnification. Note (1) primary pedicels; (2) secondary pedicels; (3) filtration slits.

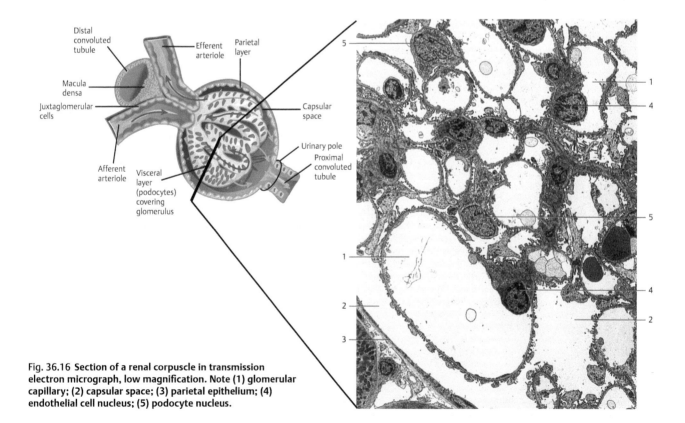

Fig. 36.16 Section of a renal corpuscle in transmission electron micrograph, low magnification. Note (1) glomerular capillary; (2) capsular space; (3) parietal epithelium; (4) endothelial cell nucleus; (5) podocyte nucleus.

densa, not labeled) between the endothelial cells and pedicels. An endothelial cell of the parietal layer of the corpuscle is indicated in the bottom left of this image (3). The capsular space is indicated just inside this layer as well as between the capillaries (2). In living tissue, provisional urine produced by the filtration apparatus fills the capsular space; that is, podocytes are bathed in provisional urine.

Fig. 36.17 is an electron micrograph of a section through the renal corpuscle taken at somewhat higher magnification, similar to a section represented by the black line. This image shows a single capillary (1 is the lumen, 11 is a red blood cell in the lumen, 3 is part of an endothelial cell), with fenestrations indicated by the arrows. Neighboring capillaries can be seen in the upper and lower right. The large nucleated cell is a podocyte (5), including primary (7) and secondary (8) pedicels. The fused basement membrane, the lamina densa, between the endothelial cell and podocyte is more readily recognized at this magnification (4). The capsular space is indicated at (2), as well as the parietal epithelium (9) and supporting connective tissue (10) of the Bowman's capsule.

Fig. 36.18 is a high-magnification micrograph of one wall of a glomerular capillary covered with podocytes, showing the filtration barrier. The capillary lumen is indicated at 8; 1 is the capsular space containing provisional urine. The endothelial cell (7) is clearly fenestrated. Secondary pedicels (2) of podocytes are shown. Adjacent podocytes interdigitate their secondary pedicels (see **Fig. 36.15**), so that, most likely, every other pedicel here belongs to one podocyte, while the remainder belong to another. Filtration slits are indicated by the black arrows. Spanning each filtration slit is a proteinaceous **diaphragm** (3; red arrows are more accurately placed), which is involved in filtration. The basement membrane of the filtration barrier, the lamina densa (4–6), lies between the endothelial cells and podocyte pedicels.

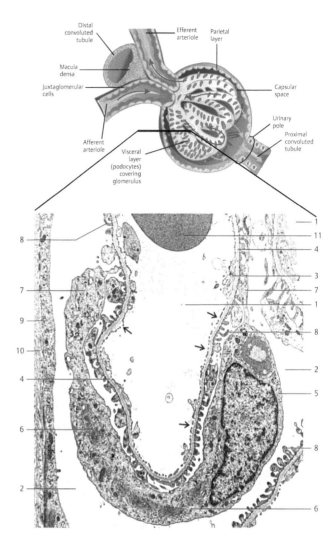

Fig. 36.17 **Section of a renal corpuscle in transmission electron micrograph, low to medium magnification. Note (1) glomerular capillary lumen; (2) capsular space; (3) endothelial cell; (4) lamina densa; (5) podocyte; (6) Golgi apparatus of podocyte; (7) primary pedicel; (8) secondary pedicel; (9) parietal epithelium; (10) supporting connective tissue of Bowman capsule; (11) red blood cell. Arrows indicate fenestrations.**

Basic Science Correlate: Physiology

Because the vessel draining the glomerular capillaries is an arteriole and not a venule, blood flows through the glomerular capillaries at a relatively high pressure. This forces plasma from the blood into the capsular space, passing through the fenestrations in the endothelium, lamina densa, and filtration slits, in that order. This filtration allows most small molecules through (less than around 50 kilodaltons) but keeps larger proteins and formed elements in the blood. There is some selection based on charge, but that is beyond the scope of this book.

Clinical Correlate

Dysfunction of the filtration apparatus occurs when there is inflammation or other pathology that affects renal corpuscles. These **glomerular diseases** can be caused by genetic conditions (e.g., lupus) or metabolic disorders (diabetes). In addition, because this structure is a filter, some malfunctions are caused by antibody deposition in the filtration apparatus during or after an infection or in autoimmune disorders such as lupus. The resulting inflammatory response to the presence of these antibodies damages the filtration apparatus. Proper filtration is disrupted, so larger plasma components, such as proteins or even red blood cells, pass through the filter inappropriately and are lost in the urine.

36.6   Mesangium of the Renal Corpuscle

One other tissue type of the glomerular tuft that needs consideration is the connective tissue of the corpuscle, the **mesangium**. As shown in **Fig. 36.2**, during glomerular formation, the glomerular capillaries become surrounded by the visceral layer of Bowman's capsule (i.e., the podocytes). In most places, the connective tissue between the endothelial cells and podocytes is squeezed out, and their basement membranes fuse to form the lamina densa (see **Fig. 36.3**, **Fig. 36.4**, and **Fig. 36.5**). However, in some locations, the connective tissue remains, forming the mesangium (see **Fig. 36.5**). Cells of the mesangium are called **mesangial cells**. The fused basal lamina between endothelial cells and the podocytes splits on either side of the mesangium, so that there is a basement membrane between the endothelial cells and the mesangium and another between the podocytes and the mesangium (see **Fig. 36.5**).

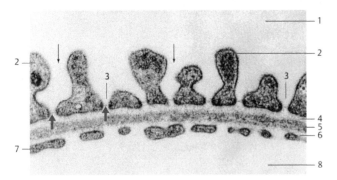

Fig. 36.18 **Filtration barrier in transmission electron micrograph, high magnification. Note (1) capsular space; (2) podocyte secondary pedicels; (3) filtration slit diaphragm; (4–6) lamina densa (light-dark-light regions); (7) endothelial cell (fenestrated); (8) lumen of capillary. Black arrows mark filtration slits; red arrows indicate diaphragm in filtration slit.**

Returning to **Fig. 36.9**, a scanning electron micrograph of a section through two corpuscles, the region outlined in yellow represents the location of the mesangium within the glomerular tuft between capillaries. **Fig. 36.19** shows the transmission electron micrograph from **Fig. 36.16**, with outlines added to show thicker regions that are mesangium and mesangial cells.

Clinical Correlate

Some glomerular pathologies involve the mesangium. For example, one of the features of diabetic glomerular nephropathy is an expansion of the mesangium.

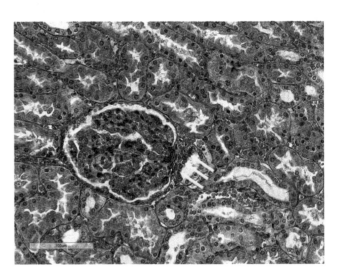

Fig. 36.19 **Section of a renal corpuscle in transmission electron micrograph, low magnification (the same image as Fig. 36.16), with mesangium outlined. Note (1) glomerular capillary; (2) capsular space; (3) parietal epithelium; endothelial cell; (4) endothelial cell nuclei; (5) podocyte nucleus.**

36.7   Juxtaglomerular Apparatus

As shown in **Fig. 36.8**, the distal convoluted tubule of a nephron loops back toward the corpuscle and lies adjacent to the afferent arteriole at the vascular pole of the corpuscle. Cells of the distal convoluted tubule adjacent to the afferent arteriole are specialized cells called the **macula densa**. Cells of the afferent arteriole adjacent to the distal convoluted tubule are **juxtaglomerular cells**. Together, the macula densa and juxtaglomerular cells are called the **juxtaglomerular apparatus**, which is involved in regulating blood volume by releasing hormones such as **renin** and **erythropoietin**.

Fig. 36.20 is a light micrograph showing macula densa cells (yellow arrows) of a distal convoluted tubule. The macula densa can be identified as a flattened part of the distal convoluted tubule, adjacent to the vascular pole of the corpuscle. The nuclei of the cells of the macula densa are close together in almost a straight line, adjacent to the corpuscle. The smaller nuclei just to the left of the macula densa are likely to be either mesangial cells or juxtaglomerular cells (it is difficult to identify with certainty which type).

Video 36.2   Macula densa

Be able to identify:

— Macula densa

https://www.thieme.de/de/q.htm?p=opn/
tp/308390101/978-1-62623-414-7_c036_
v002&t=video

Fig. 36.20 **Macula densa (yellow arrows).**

36.8   Chapter Review

The renal corpuscle produces the initial urine product (the ultrafiltrate or provisional urine) by forcing plasma through a filtration barrier under high pressure. These renal corpuscles are readily identified on light micrographs as tufts of cells surrounded by a capsular space that receives the ultrafiltrate. In some cases, afferent or efferent vessels can be seen associated with the glomerulus (vascular pole). In others, the proximal convoluted tubule can be seen (urinary pole). Important details of the corpuscle are revealed through electron micrographs. The corpuscle consists of a tuft of fenestrated capillaries, without diaphragms across the fenestrations, called the glomerulus, covered by a layer of cells called podocytes, which make up the visceral epithelium of Bowman's capsule. The endothelial cells of the capillaries and the podocytes share a basement membrane: the lamina densa. The podocytes contain elaborate extensions called pedicels, which interdigitate with pedicels from neighboring podocytes. The spaces between the pedicels, the filtration slits, are spanned by a proteinaceous diaphragm. The filtration apparatus thus consists of the fenestrated endothelium (without diaphragms), the lamina densa, and the filtration slits between podocyte pedicels (with diaphragms). Most molecules smaller than 50 kDa pass readily through this barrier; proteins and cells larger than this remain in the plasma. The result is an ultrafiltrate (provisional urine) that passes into the capsular space, which is contained by a parietal epithelium of Bowman's capsule

that forms the outer wall of the corpuscle. This ultrafiltrate flows into the proximal convoluted tubule, where it is modified extensively before release as urine. Mesangium is connective tissue within the tuft of a glomerular capillary. A portion of the distal convoluted tubule of the nephron lies adjacent to the afferent arteriole. In this region, cells of the distal convoluted tubule (the macula densa) and the afferent arteriole (the juxtaglomerular cells) form the juxtaglomerular apparatus, which assesses plasma volume and releases renin and erythropoietin in response to low blood pressure.

Questions and Answers

For further study on this chapter, please see the accompanying Question and Answer material found at http://medone.thieme.com. Code redemption (see inside front cover) required, for personal use only.

37   Extrarenal Excretory Passages

After completing this chapter, you should be able to:
— Identify, at the light microscope level, each of the following:
  • Calyces
  • Ureter
  • Urinary bladder
  • Urethra (female)
— Outline the function of each structure listed
— Correlate the main function of these structures with their histologic features

37.1   Overview of the Extrarenal Excretory Passages

The previous three chapters focused on the kidney and its role in the production of urine. This urine is carried out of the body by structures and organs specialized for urine transport (**Fig. 37.1**).

The major functions of these structures and organs (calyces, ureters, bladder, urethra) are:
• Transport and storage of urine
• Maintaining the composition of urine produced by the kidneys

To achieve these goals, these structures have the following common features (**Fig. 37.2**):
• A **mucosa** (black bracket) which consists of
  • **Transitional epithelium**
  • **Lamina propria**, an irregular connective tissue
• A **muscularis** (yellow bracket), composed mostly of smooth muscle
• An **adventitia** (blue bracket), composed of irregular connective tissue

The qualities of each layer in different structures will vary somewhat depending on function. For example, the bladder, shown in **Fig. 37.2**, has a thick muscularis to provide propulsive force for urination (micturition).

37.1.1   Transitional Epithelium

Transitional epithelium merits special attention because it imparts many of the characteristics of the extrarenal excretory passages:
• It can stretch to allow filling (bladder).
• It is resistant to osmotic movement of ions and water, thus maintaining the composition of urine produced by the kidneys and keeping toxins and wastes from returning to the bloodstream.

Basic Science Correlate: Physiology

The first feature of transitional epithelium (stretching) is fairly obvious in terms of its importance for the bladder. The importance of the second feature (resistance to water and ion movement) cannot be understated. A lot of energy is expended by the kidneys to condition plasma, and the resulting urine reflects the body's current physiologic status. For example, in cases of dehydration, properly functioning kidneys produce a concentrated urine to minimize water loss. During storage, osmotic forces would draw water into the urine if unresisted. The transitional epithelial lining resists these forces and keeps the urine hypertonic.

Recall the histologic features of transitional epithelium (**Fig. 37.3**):
• Basal cells smaller than apical cells
• Surface cells bulging into the lumen
• Dense band (cytoplasmic band, plaques) just under the apical plasma membrane of surface cells (small bracket), which represents folded plasma membrane in the nondistended state
• Occasional binucleate cell (black arrow)

Helpful Hint

Because transitional epithelium is found only in the excretory passages of the urinary system, it is often called **urothelium**, especially by physicians. Also, the apical cells that bulge into the lumen are often called **umbrella cells**.

37.1.2   Muscularis

The smooth muscle in the muscularis is loosely organized into three layers in the bladder: an inner longitudinal layer, an outer circular layer, and an oblique layer. However, in most cases, this organization is not as obvious as that seen in the gastrointestinal tract. In most of the ureter, only the inner longitudinal and outer circular layers are present. The smooth muscle in the muscularis

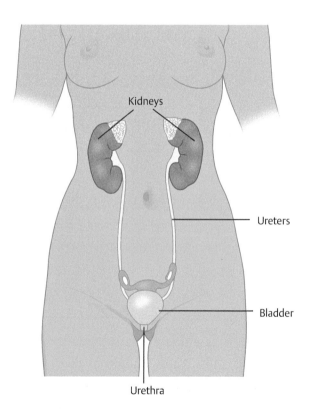

Fig. 37.1   **Urinary system in the female human.**

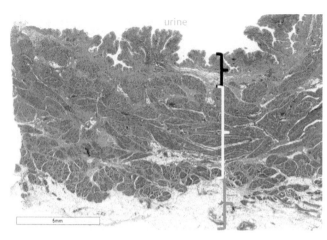

Fig. 37.2 **Histologic structure of urine transport passages (bladder). The wall of these passages is composed of a mucosa (black bracket), muscularis (yellow bracket), and adventitia (blue bracket). The lumen contains urine.**

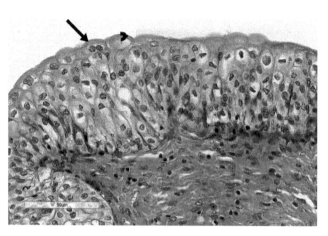

Fig. 37.3 **Transitional epithelium of the bladder. The cytoplasmic band (plaque) is indicated by the bracket. Arrow shows a binucleate cell.**

of the extrarenal passages, especially in the bladder, is mixed with a substantial amount of dense irregular connective tissue, which provides support (**Fig. 37.4**).

37.2 Calyces and Pelvis

Recall that urine passes out of the collecting ducts (papillary ducts) of the kidney and into the **minor calyces**. From there, urine flows through the **major calyces** into the **renal pelvis** (**Fig. 37.5**). Note that the minor calyx surrounds the renal papilla of the pyramid (**Fig. 37.6**). Closer examination of the wall of the minor calyx (**Fig. 37.7**) shows that the epithelium is transitional (note cytoplasmic band in the apical cells). The surface cells do not bulge because this region does not stretch. Scattered smooth muscle cells are seen as elongated nuclei among the connective tissue in the wall of the calyx (bottom right), but they are not organized. The major calyces and renal pelvis have histologic features similar to the minor calyx.

Video 37.1 Minor calyx

Be able to identify:
— Minor calyx
— Transitional epithelium
https://www.thieme.de/de/q.htm?p=opn/
tp/308390101/978-1-62623-414-7_c037_v001&t=video

The histologic features of the calyces are not that striking because these regions do not stretch or contract to a significant extent; they are simply passages to the ureter. In most cases, proper identification is based on the entire histology of the kidney.

37.3 Ureter

The three-layered histology of the extrarenal excretory passages (mucosa, muscularis, adventitia) is more apparent in the ureter and bladder. **Fig. 37.8** is a scanning image of the **ureter**, showing that the mucosa is thrown into folds, which are often described as a star-shaped pattern (with more than five or six points in this case).

Fig. 37.9 shows a closer view of the main histologic features of the ureter. The mucosa consists of transitional epithelium that forms the inner lining of the ureter (A in **Fig. 37.9**). In the upper ureter, the muscularis is only two layers thick: an inner longitudinal layer and an outer circular layer (B in **Fig. 37.9**), though these layers are not always distinct. Lower portions of the ureter, closer to the bladder, add a third oblique layer.

Video 37.2 Ureter

Be able to identify:
— Ureter
https://www.thieme.de/de/q.htm?p=opn/
tp/308390101/978-1-62623-414-7_c037_v002&t=video

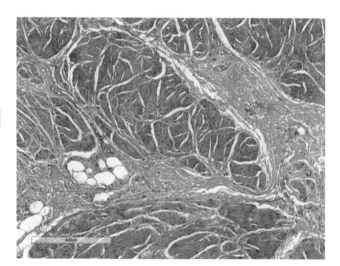

Fig. 37.4 **Smooth muscle of the bladder.**

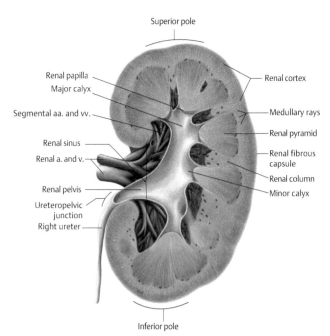

Fig. 37.5   **Kidney, coronal section. From Schuenke M, Schulte E, Schumacher U. *THIEME Atlas of Anatomy. Internal Organs.* Illustrations by Voll M and Wesker K. Second Edition. New York: Thieme Medical Publishers; 2016.**

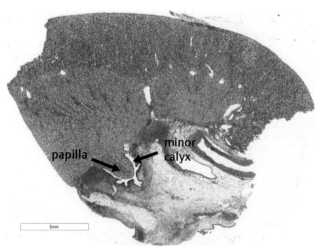

Fig. 37.6   **Scanning light micrograph of the kidney, showing an entire lobe, including the renal papilla, and parts of two adjacent lobes. The space surrounding the papilla is the lumen of the minor calyx.**

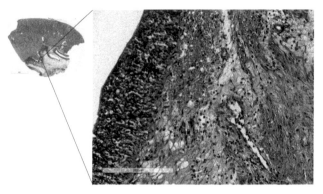

Fig. 37.7   **Light micrograph of the wall of a minor calyx.**

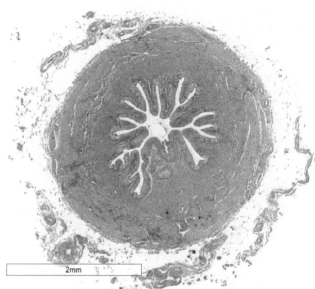

Fig. 37.8   **Scanning light micrograph of the ureter.**

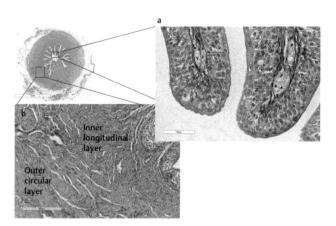

Fig. 37.9   **Histology of the ureter, (a) including transitional epithelium lining the lumen and (b) smooth muscle with the wall.**

Clinical Correlate

Kidney stones (renal calculi) can form within the kidney or calyces and move into the ureter. These stones can become lodged within the ureter, causing excruciating pain. Small stones may eventually pass, whereas larger stones may require surgical intervention.

37.4 Urinary Bladder

As shown in **Fig. 37.2**, the **urinary bladder** has the characteristic three-layered histology of the extrarenal excretory passages (mucosa, muscularis, adventitia). Here, the muscularis (yellow bracket) is quite thick and is called the **detrusor muscle**. This muscle propels urine during **micturition**. The muscularis of the bladder has three layers of smooth muscle: an inner longitudinal layer, a middle circular layer, and an outer longitudinal layer.

Video 37.3   Urinary bladder (adult)

https://www.thieme.de/de/q.htm?p=opn/
tp/308390101/978-1-62623-414-7_c037_
v003&t=video

Video 37.4   Urinary bladder (baby)

Be able to identify:
— Urinary bladder

https://www.thieme.de/de/q.htm?p=opn/
tp/308390101/978-1-62623-414-7_c037_
v004&t=video

Basic Science Correlate: Gross Anatomy

As discussed in the chapters on the gastrointestinal tract, the abdominal cavity is lined with an epithelium called **peritoneum** (**Fig. 37.10**). The **visceral peritoneum** lines the outer surface of the abdominal organs (red arrow), and the **parietal peritoneum** lines the inner surface of the abdominal wall (green arrow). Because of its position in the pelvic cavity, only a portion of the bladder is covered by peritoneum. Sections through most of the bladder (e.g., black line) do not include this epithelial covering. In those locations, the outer layer of the bladder is simply connective tissue and is called an adventitia. However, a section near the apex of the bladder (**Fig. 37.10**, dark blue line) will have an outer layer composed of connective tissue covered with parietal epithelium. This layer is similar to the serosa of the gastrointestinal tract.

Clinical Correlate

Bladder cancer most often originates from the transitional epithelium of the mucosa. These tumors grow into the lumen and can also grow outward to invade surrounding tissues. Certain exposures (e.g., smoking, working in a chemical factory such as a rubber plant) increase the risk of bladder cancer. A typical presentation includes bright red blood in the urine.

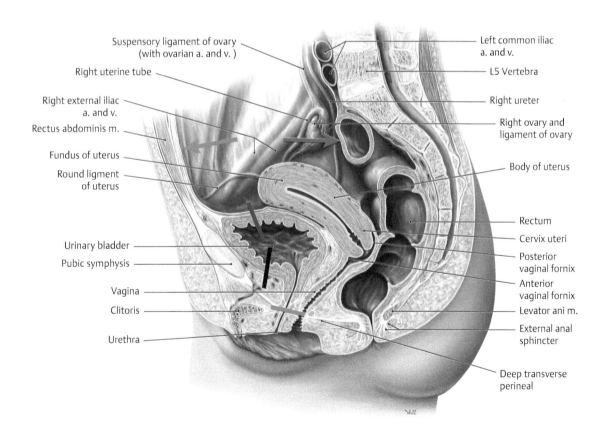

Fig. 37.10 Sagittal view of the female lower abdomen and pelvis. The peritoneum that lines the abdomen includes the outer lining of the visceral organs (visceral peritoneum, red arrow) and the inner lining of the abdominal wall (parietal peritoneum, green arrow). The parietal peritoneum covers the superior aspect of the bladder. Therefore, in sections of the bladder wall in this region (dark blue line), the outer layer is an adventitia covered with parietal peritoneum (similar to a serosa of the gastrointestinal tract). In sections in the inferior aspect of the bladder (black line), the outer layer is simply adventitia. The light blue line indicates a section through the urethra and anterior wall of the vagina (discussed later). Based on the work of Schünke M, Schulte E, Schumacher U. *THIEME Atlas of Anatomy. Internal Organs.* Illustrations by M. Voll and K. Wesker. Second Edition. New York: Thieme Medical Publishers; 2016.

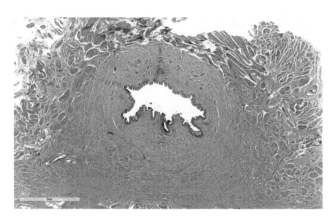

Fig. 37.11 **Scanning light micrograph of the female urethra.**

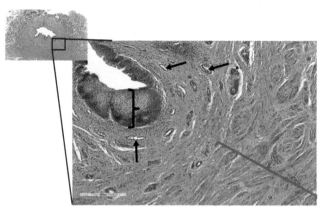

Fig. 37.12 **Histology of the urethra, including stratified squamous nonkeratinized epithelium (black bracket), venous plexus (arrows), and muscularis (green bracket).**

37.5   Urethra

Because passage of urine through the **urethra** is rapid, and the force generated for urination comes from the bladder, the histologic features of the urethra are different from those of other extrarenal excretory structures:

- The epithelium of the urethra near the bladder is transitional, but most of the urethra is lined by stratified squamous nonkeratinized epithelium. This is because the urethra is not required to stretch, and quick urinary passage does not require a barrier that is impermeable to ions and water. On the contrary, an epithelium designed for moist friction is most suitable here. The lumen of the urethra is often crescent-shaped.
- Small mucus glands may be present for lubrication, but they are not obvious on many images.
- The lamina propria has an abundant venous plexus, possibly for heat retention, but it is unlikely that this function is relevant in humans.
- The smooth muscle is less developed and may be interspersed with skeletal muscle of the pelvic floor (e.g., urogenital diaphragm); the muscle here is supportive and not for generating force for urination.

Fig. 37.11 is a scanning image of the female urethra, showing that the lumen is crescent-shaped. (The male urethra will be discussed in the chapters dealing with the male reproductive system.) Even at this low magnification, the thickness of the epithelium and the bundles of smooth muscle in the muscularis can be seen. **Fig. 37.12** is an image of the urethra taken at low to medium magnification, showing that the epithelium is stratified squamous (black bracket), the lamina propria has an elaborate venous plexus (arrows), and the muscularis (green bracket) is a mixture of smooth muscle and connective tissue.

Basic Science Correlate: Gross Anatomy

Due to the proximity of the female urethra and vagina, many histologic slides of the urethra include the anterior wall of the vagina, similar to the section indicated by the blue line in **Fig. 37.10**.

Video 37.5   Urethra

Be able to identify:
— Urethra
https://www.thieme.de/de/q.htm?p=opn/tp/308390101/978-1-62623-414-7_c037_v005&t=video

37.6   Chapter Review

The extrarenal excretory passages are responsible for transport, storage, and elimination of urine. The main features of these structures or organs include a transitional epithelium, which imparts the ability to stretch and provides resistance to the movement of water, ions, and wastes through the walls. The other major feature of these structures and organs is smooth muscle, which moves urine. These features are part of a three-layered structure: mucosa, muscularis, and adventitia. In the calyces, these features are less well developed. The ureter, and especially the bladder, has well-developed smooth muscle. In contrast, the urethra is lined by stratified squamous epithelium rather than transitional, and it has a muscularis that contains much more connective tissue.

Questions and Answers

An online-only section of questions and answers accompanying this chapter is hosted on Thieme's MedOne Education site: https://medone-education.thieme.com. Use the code on the media page at the front of this book to gain access. An institutional license to the site is required to access these questions in an interactive format, and individual users are required to register for an individual account to track results.

38 Upper Respiratory System

After completing this chapter, you should be able to:
- Identify, at the light microscope level, each of the following:
  - General features of structures in the upper respiratory tract:
    - Respiratory epithelium (pseudostratified ciliated columnar with goblet cells)
    - Basement membrane
    - Lamina propria with glands, vessels, nerves, diffuse lymphoid tissue
    - Supporting elements (bone, cartilage, smooth and/or skeletal muscle)
  - Organs and structures
    - Nasal cavity and concha
    - Epiglottis
    - Larynx
      - Vestibular (ventricular, false) vocal fold
      - True vocal fold (vocal fold)
      - Laryngeal ventricle
      - Hyoid bone
      - Epiglottis
      - Thyroid cartilage
      - Cricoid cartilage
    - Trachea
    - Bronchus
- Outline the function of each structure and vessel type listed
- Evaluate the function of the airways in conditioning inspired air
- Correlate the main function of upper respiratory structures with histologic features

38.1 Overview of the Respiratory System

The main functions of the respiratory system (**Fig. 38.1**) are to obtain oxygen from the environment and to eliminate carbon dioxide. The respiratory system is also involved in the production of sound (speech) and the sense of smell.

The respiratory system can be divided into two parts: the upper respiratory system and the lower respiratory system. The transition between upper and lower respiratory systems is the larynx, at the level of the vocal folds. For convenience, everything down to and including the bronchi will be discussed in this chapter on the upper respiratory system. The next chapter will focus on structures within the lungs.

The major structures of the upper respiratory tract covered in this chapter include (**Fig. 38.1**):
- Nasal cavity
- Pharynx (covered in **Chapter 31**)
- Larynx
- Trachea
- Bronchi

Before these structures are considered individually, epithelial features common to all of them will be described.

Clinical Correlate

Physicians broadly divide respiratory tract infections into two categories: upper respiratory tract infections, such as a cold, and lower respiratory tract infections, such as pneumonia.

38.2 Epithelia of the Respiratory Tract

The major function of the respiratory system is gas exchange. To accomplish this, the lungs contain numerous air-filled sacs called **alveoli**, whose walls are composed of a thin layer of well-vascularized connective tissue (**Fig. 38.2**).

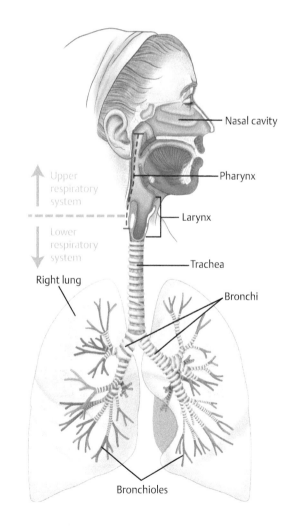

Fig. 38.1 **Respiratory system.**

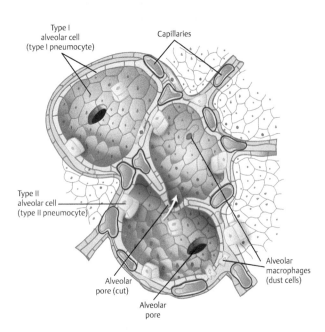

Fig. 38.2   **Alveoli of the lungs.**

Because O_2 and CO_2 are small and hydrophobic, movement of these gas molecules across the alveolar barrier into the bloodstream is accomplished by diffusion. Diffusion is maximized when the distance traveled by the diffusing molecules is small. To achieve this goal, the inner lining of the alveoli is simple squamous epithelium (**Fig. 38.2**, type I pneumocyte). Alveoli will be discussed in detail in the next chapter.

The downside to a simple squamous epithelium is that it is thin and fragile, making it susceptible to infectious agents, dry conditions, and changes in temperature. One major function of the airways (everything in the respiratory tract except alveoli) is to filter, moisturize, and warm the incoming air to reduce damage to the delicate lining of the alveoli. This is largely achieved by a specialized inner lining of the airways, referred to as **respiratory mucosa**. The respiratory mucosa treats the incoming air before it reaches the lungs. The components of the respiratory mucosa include:

- Pseudostratified ciliated columnar epithelium with goblet cells
- Thick basement membrane
- **Lamina propria**: irregular connective tissue with glands and diffuse lymphoid tissue

Because pseudostratified ciliated columnar epithelium with goblet cells is found in only this one location in humans, it is often called simply **respiratory epithelium**.

Fig. 38.3 is an image from the trachea taken at medium magnification. The pseudostratified ciliated columnar epithelium (respiratory epithelium, black bracket) is shown. Below this is the connective tissue of the lamina propria. Numerous serous and mucous glands in that layer are outlined, which excrete their product onto the surface through a duct (arrow).

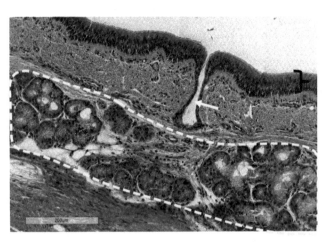

Fig. 38.3   **Respiratory mucosa at medium magnification. The bracket indicates the respiratory epithelium; serous and mucous glands are outlined, with a duct (arrow) connecting to the surface.**

Fig. 38.4 is an image from the trachea taken at high magnification, focusing on the respiratory epithelium. The thick basement membrane of the respiratory epithelium is indicated by the green bracket in the lower right of the image. Above the basement membrane is a pseudostratified columnar epithelium, with cilia and goblet cells (respiratory epithelium, goblet cells indicated by the arrows). Basal cell nuclei of the respiratory epithelium are adjacent to the basement membrane. The respiratory epithelium also has sensory cells called **brush cells** and neuroendocrine cells called **granule cells** (**Kulchitsky cells**); neither of these cells are evident on routinely stained slides.

Basic Science Correlate: Physiology

The epithelial goblet cells and glands in the lamina propria secrete mucus, which coats the inner surface of the respiratory tract and prepares the incoming air (filtering, moisturizing) before exposure to the delicate alveoli. This mucus is produced continuously; cilia sweep this mucus toward the pharynx, where it is swallowed. Because the general direction of movement of most of the mucus is upward (an exception is the nasal cavity), this process is commonly referred to as the **mucociliary escalator**.

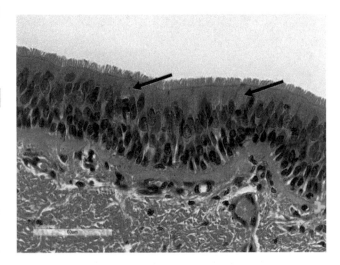

Fig. 38.4   **Respiratory mucosa at high magnification focusing on the respiratory epithelium. The thick basement membrane (green bracket) and goblet cells (black arrows) are indicated.**

Video 38.1   Respiratory mucosa

Be able to identify:
— Respiratory mucosa
  • Respiratory epithelium (pseudostratified ciliated columnar with goblet cells)
  • Thick basement membrane
  • Lamina propria
https://www.thieme.de/de/q.htm?p=opn/tp/308390101/978-1-62623-414-7_c038_v001&t=video

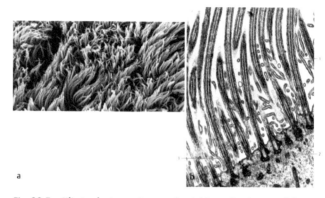

Fig. 38.5   **Cilia in electron micrographs. (a) Scanning image of the inner surface of the trachea. (b) Transmission electron micrograph showing numerous cilia in longitudinal section, each with a core of microtubules.**

Clinical Correlation

There are several conditions that result from an inability to move mucus in the respiratory system. For example, in **cystic fibrosis**, a defective chloride channel results in thick mucus that is difficult for cilia to move properly. Mechanical disruption and drugs that break down the mucus are part of the treatment regimen for these patients. Because mucus movement is not optimal, patients with cystic fibrosis have lifelong complications caused by repeated respiratory infections. These patients also have complications involving the pancreas and other organs.

Fig. 38.5 is a reminder of the basic ultrastructural features of cilia, which were covered in the chapter on epithelial specializations (**Chapter 5**). **Fig. 38.5a** demonstrates nicely the cilia on the inner surface of the trachea. **Fig. 38.5b** is a transmission micrograph (from the female reproductive tract), showing that microtubules are the core protein of cilia. Microtubules are responsible for the active movement characteristic of these surface modifications.

Clinical Correlate

Ciliary motility disorders such as **primary ciliary dyskinesia (Kartagener syndrome)** also cause difficulty with mucus clearance. These patients are often infertile (especially males, due to lack of sperm motility), and half have a condition called **situs inversus**, in which the body's organs are reversed in position (mirror-image reversal).

Now that the features of respiratory mucosa have been discussed, the histologic features of each structure of the upper respiratory system can be considered.

38.3   Nasal Cavity

As mentioned, the airways are designed to filter, warm, and moisturize incoming air.

The **nasal cavity** is well suited for this function because it contains:
• Respiratory epithelium
• An extensive venous plexus

The lateral wall of the nasal cavity has projections called **conchae** (**Fig. 38.6**). These structures increase turbulence of incoming air within the nasal cavity, maximizing the efficiency of conditioning the air. Conchae are supported by cancellous bone; other parts of the respiratory tract are supported by cartilage and smooth muscle.

Fig. 38.7 shows images from a concha, which will serve as a model for the histology of the nasal cavity. These images were taken from a tissue that is overstained. Nevertheless, this figure shows that the lining of the concha is a respiratory mucosa, which includes the respiratory epithelium and a lamina propria that has numerous glands (G) and veins (V), which are part of the venous plexus. As already mentioned, unlike the rest of the

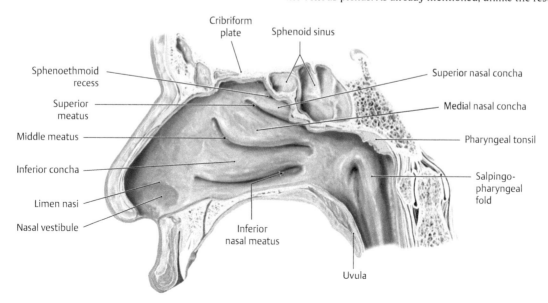

Fig. 38.6   **Lateral wall of the nasal cavity showing conchae. From Schuenke M, Schulte E, Schumacher U.** *THIEME Atlas of Anatomy. Head, Neck, and Neuroanatomy.* **Illustrations by Voll M and Wesker K. Second Edition. New York: Thieme Medical Publishers; 2016.**

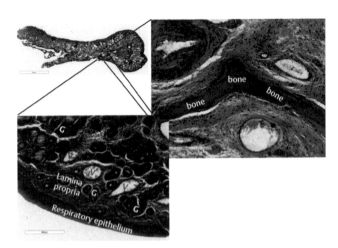

Fig. 38.7   Concha. Bone, respiratory epithelium, and lamina propria are indicated, as well as (G) glands and (V) venous plexus.

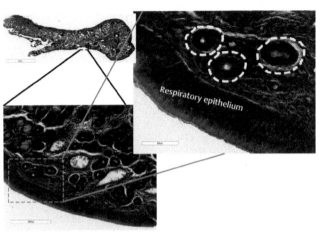

Fig. 38.8   Mucosa of concha showing respiratory epithelium and serous glands (outlined).

respiratory tract, conchae are supported by cancellous bone. **Fig. 38.8** is an image of the mucosa taken at high magnification, showing the respiratory epithelium and three serous glands (outlined).

Video 38.2   Concha

Be able to identify:
— Concha
  • Venous plexus
  • Bone

https://www.thieme.de/de/q.htm?p=opn/tp/308390101/978-1-62623-414-7_c038_v002&t=video

---

Basic Science Correlate: Neuroscience

The roof of the nasal cavity is lined by an **olfactory epithelium**, which is continuous with the respiratory epithelium that lines the rest of the nasal cavity. The olfactory epithelium is similar to respiratory epithelium but has specialized **olfactory receptor cells** that detect chemical odorants and transmit information to the brain via the **olfactory nerve (cranial nerve I)**.

Clinical Correlate

Allergic reactions and infections cause the plexus of vessels in the nasal cavity to dilate and become leaky. The resulting edema in the lamina propria results in the characteristic congestion associated with these conditions. Medications such as oxymetazoline cause vasoconstriction, reducing the edema.

38.4   Pharynx

The pharynx is the common pathway for the digestive and respiratory systems (see **Fig. 38.1** and **Fig. 31.3**). The pharynx is mostly lined by stratified squamous epithelium and was discussed in detail in **Chapter 31**.

Clinical Correlate

Because the pharynx is the common pathway for both ingested food and air, it is not uncommon for food or liquid to be accidentally introduced into the respiratory system, causing irritation of the inner lining of the respiratory tract or, worse, choking.

38.5   Epiglottis

The **epiglottis** helps guide swallowed food toward the esophagus by covering the opening into the **larynx**. **Fig. 38.9** shows the process. In the left image, the bolus of food is in the oral cavity, and the epiglottis is vertical (black arrows), such that the laryngeal inlet (opening into the larynx) is open (**Fig. 38.9**, left). As the bolus of food moves through the pharynx, muscles involved in swallowing reposition the epiglottis so it covers the opening into the larynx (**Fig. 38.9**, right).

The supporting element of the epiglottis is elastic cartilage, which is firm but flexible. Most of the remaining elements of the epiglottis are typical: connective tissue, glands, and so forth. The exception to this is the surface epithelium (see next several slides).

Before discussing the histology of the epiglottis, it helps to describe its orientation. In the open position (**Fig. 38.9**, left), the "top" of the epiglottis faces anteriorly, toward the oral cavity, and is called the anterior surface. The bottom faces posteriorly, so is the posterior surface.

Helpful Hint

In the closed position (**Fig. 38.9**, right) this orientation changes. The names for these surfaces refer to the epiglottis in the open position.

Fig. 38.10a is a scanning view of the epiglottis in longitudinal section; the anterior and posterior surfaces of the epiglottis are indicated. The supporting element of the epiglottis is elastic cartilage. **Fig. 38.10b** is a medium-power image showing elastic cartilage and numerous glands in the core of the epiglottis.

During swallowing, the anterior side of the epiglottis comes to face the pharynx and is exposed to food sliding down toward the

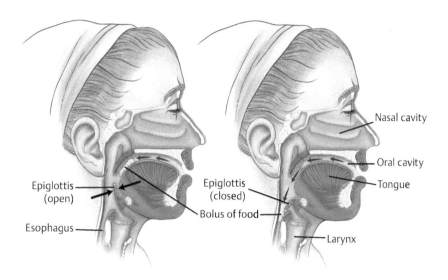

Fig. 38.9   **Role of the epiglottis during swallowing. In the image to the left, food is in the oral cavity, and the epiglottis (black arrows) is in the vertical position such that the opening into the larynx is open. As the bolus of food passes the epiglottis, muscles involved in swallowing result in movement of the epiglottis to cover the opening to the larynx (right image).**

esophagus (**Fig. 38.9**, right). Because of this, the anterior surface of the epiglottis is covered by a stratified squamous nonkeratinized epithelium (similar to the pharynx in this region). The posterior side of the epiglottis faces the lumen of the larynx during swallowing and, therefore, is covered mostly by respiratory epithelium.

Fig. 38.11 shows two drawings and the longitudinal section of the larynx outlining the epithelium covering the epiglottis. In these drawings and image, anterior is to the left. As shown in the schematic in **Fig. 38.11a**, during swallowing, the tip of the epiglottis extends beyond the posterior wall of the larynx. Because of this, both sides of the tip of the epiglottis are exposed to food (see **Fig. 38.11b** and imagine the epiglottis in the closed position). Therefore, the anterior surface and entire tip of the epiglottis is covered by stratified squamous nonkeratinized epithelium (**Fig. 38.11b**, **c**, red arrows). The blue arrows indicate the portion lined by respiratory epithelium.

Fig. 38.12 shows higher-magnification images of the epithelium covering different regions of the epiglottis. In the scanning view in the center, the anterior side is down and the

posterior side is up (the tip is to the left). **Fig. 38.12** shows that the anterior side (a) and the tip of the posterior side (b) are lined by stratified squamous nonkeratinized epithelium, while the inferior portion of the posterior side (c) is lined by respiratory epithelium.

Helpful Hint

The preceding discussion was a little long-winded, however, putting the epiglottis in the context of swallowing and considering the function of these epithelia will aid in remembering which epithelium is covering which aspects of the epiglottis.

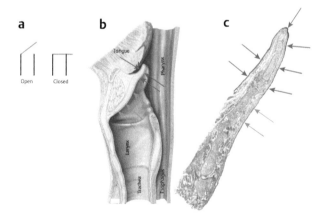

Fig. 38.11 **Epiglottis outlining the epithelium of the epiglottis. In these images, anterior is to the left. (a) Schematic view of the epiglottis (blue line) in the open and closed positions; note that in the closed position, the epiglottis extends past the posterior wall of the larynx. (b) Anatomic drawing of the larynx. Red arrows represent areas covered by stratified squamous epithelium; blue arrows indicate regions covered by respiratory epithelium. From Schuenke M, Schulte E, Schumacher U.** *THIEME Atlas of Anatomy. Head, Neck, and Neuroanatomy.* **Illustrations by Voll M and Wesker K. Second Edition. New York: Thieme Medical Publishers; 2016. (c) Longitudinal section through the epiglottis with arrows similar to those in (b).**

Fig. 38.10   **Epiglottis in longitudinal section (the tip to the left). (a) Scanning view, with the anterior and posterior surfaces indicated, as well as the core of elastic cartilage. (b) Elastic cartilage and glands in the core.**

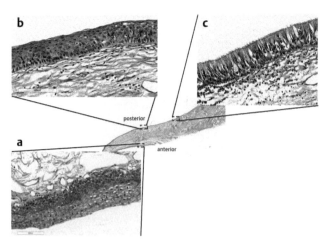

Fig. 38.12 **Epithelium from different regions of the epiglottis.**

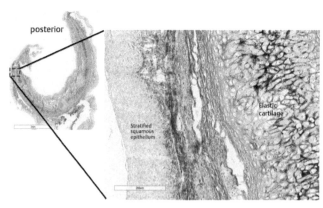

Fig. 38.13 **Epiglottis, tip, cross section, stained for elastic fibers.**

Video 38.3   Epiglottis (longitudinal section)

Be able to identify:
— Epiglottis
  • Epithelium
    ◦ Stratified squamous
    ◦ Respiratory
  • Elastic cartilage
https://www.thieme.de/de/q.htm?p=opn/tp/308390101/978-1-62623-414-7_c038_v003&t=video

Fig. 38.13 is a cross section of the tip of the epiglottis stained for elastic fibers. The elastic cartilage contains numerous elastic fibers, which stain purple/black. The epithelium has fewer elastic fibers, so is poorly stained. Note that the epiglottis is curved posteriorly. Since this is a cross section through the tip of the epiglottis, both sides are lined by stratified squamous epithelium (only one side is shown).

Video 38.4   Epiglottis (tip in cross section) stained for elastic fibers

Be able to identify:
— Epiglottis
  • Elastic cartilage
https://www.thieme.de/de/q.htm?p=opn/tp/308390101/978-1-62623-414-7_c038_v004&t=video

38.6   Larynx

The **larynx** is positioned anterior to the esophagus and is the gateway for inspired air to enter the trachea and the rest of the respiratory tract (see **Fig. 38.1**). As mentioned, the opening to the larynx is covered by the epiglottis during swallowing.

The larynx is supported by the hyoid bone, laryngeal cartilages (thyroid and cricoid cartilages and the epiglottis), and supporting ligaments. **Fig. 38.14a** is a sagittal section through the larynx with the mucosa intact. **Fig. 38.14b** shows the supporting elements of the larynx from the lateral aspect. **Fig. 38.15a, b** are

similar drawings, showing the larynx from the posterior aspect. The **hyoid bone** is U-shaped, open posteriorly, located at the base of the tongue. The **thyroid cartilage** is shaped like a visor and also open posteriorly. The **cricoid cartilage** is a complete ring, thicker in the back than in the front. The epiglottis forms the superior boundary of the larynx. As in the rest of the respiratory system, the inner lining of the larynx is a mucosa. There are two elevations (folds) of the mucosa that project medially (**Fig. 38.14a**); the superior fold is the **vestibular fold** (**ventricular fold**, **false vocal fold**), and the inferior fold is the **vocal fold** (**true vocal fold**). The **laryngeal ventricle** is the space (recess) between the vestibular and vocal folds (not labeled here, see subsequent images).

The vocal and vestibular folds are bulges created by ligaments of the same name that lie just underneath the mucosa (i.e., **vestibular ligament** and **vocal ligament**). The vocal and vestibular ligaments are ligaments, but when they are covered with mucosa, the entire structure (ligament + mucosa) is referred to as a fold (e.g., vocal fold). These terms (vocal ligament vs. vocal fold), although different, are often used interchangeably.

> **Helpful Hint**
>
> The basic histologic features of the larynx are not too tricky, but getting oriented to these images is a little challenging, especially without the benefit of gross anatomy. It may be useful to take a moment and think about these drawings before proceeding.

Fig. 38.16 is a drawing of a coronal section of the larynx, in which the plane of section is similar to that marked by the dotted line in **Fig. 38.14a**. This section passes through the epiglottis and the thyroid and cricoid cartilages (although the cricoid cartilage is not in this drawing). The vestibular and vocal folds are in an anterior-posterior orientation, so in **Fig. 38.16** these structures are in cross section. The vocal fold contains the vocal ligament, and an adjacent **vocalis muscle**, also cut in cross section. The vocalis muscle and other skeletal muscles seen within the larynx are involved in speech.

> **Helpful Hint**
>
> As with the vessels in the kidney, proper identification of structures of the larynx depends largely on position. Reviewing **Fig. 38.14**, **Fig. 38.15**, and **Fig. 38.16** may be beneficial if you are in doubt.

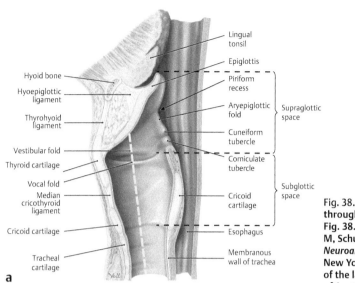

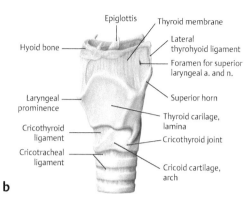

Fig. 38.14 Anatomy of the larynx, lateral views. (a) Sagittal section through the larynx. The dotted line indicates the plane of section for Fig. 38.16, Fig. 38.17, and Fig. 38.18. Based on the work of Schünke M, Schulte E, Schumacher U. *THIEME Atlas of Anatomy. Head, Neck and Neuroanatomy*. Illustrations by M. Voll and K. Wesker. Second Edition. New York: Thieme Medical Publishers; 2016. (b) Supporting elements of the larynx. From Schünke M, Schulte E, Schumacher U. *THIEME Atlas of Anatomy. Head, Neck and Neuroanatomy*. Illustrations by M. Voll and K. Wesker. Second Edition. New York: Thieme Medical Publishers; 2016.

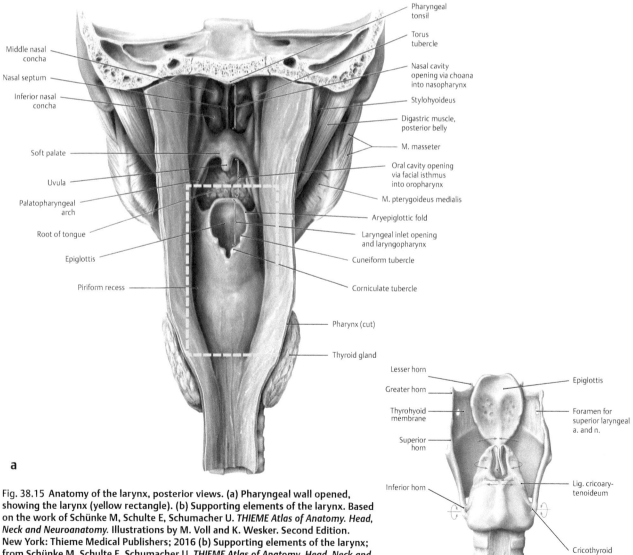

Fig. 38.15 Anatomy of the larynx, posterior views. (a) Pharyngeal wall opened, showing the larynx (yellow rectangle). (b) Supporting elements of the larynx. Based on the work of Schünke M, Schulte E, Schumacher U. *THIEME Atlas of Anatomy. Head, Neck and Neuroanatomy*. Illustrations by M. Voll and K. Wesker. Second Edition. New York: Thieme Medical Publishers; 2016 (b) Supporting elements of the larynx; from Schünke M, Schulte E, Schumacher U. *THIEME Atlas of Anatomy. Head, Neck and Neuroanatomy*. Illustrations by M. Voll and K. Wesker. Second Edition. New York: Thieme Medical Publishers; 2016.

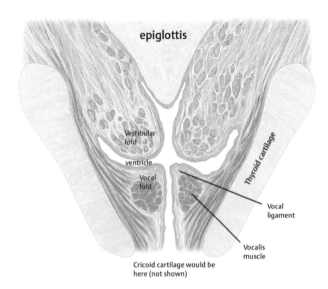

Fig. 38.16 **Drawing of a coronal section through the larynx.**

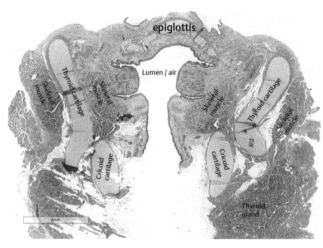

Fig. 38.17 **Coronal section through the larynx, scanning magnification.**

Fig. 38.17 is a scanning image of a coronal section through the larynx, similar to the yellow line in **Fig. 38.14** and similar to the drawing in **Fig. 38.16**. All relevant structures previously discussed are labeled. The thyroid gland is included in this image, but it will be discussed along with the endocrine system (**Chapter 42**). This specimen was taken from an infant, so the cartilage and other tissues are not very well developed.

Fig. 38.18 is a slightly magnified view showing the vestibular (ventricular, false) vocal folds and (true) vocal folds. The laryngeal ventricle is the space between the two folds (arrows).

Video 38.5   Overview of the larynx

Be able to identify:
— Epiglottis
— Larynx
   • Thyroid cartilage
   • Cricoid cartilage
   • Skeletal muscle
   • Vestibular (ventricular, false) fold
   • Vocal fold (true vocal fold)
   • Laryngeal ventricle

https://www.thieme.de/de/q.htm?p=opn/tp/308390101/978-1-62623-414-7_c038_v005&t=video

Helpful Hint

Remember this is a coronal section, so the folds are cut in cross section. Also, remember that the vocal folds include the epithelium and underlying connective tissue, including the vocal ligament.

Fig. 39.19 is a low-magnification image of the laryngeal folds. Note that the vestibular fold contains numerous glands, while the true vocal fold is devoid of glands.

Helpful Hint

Don't forget this fact; it's a quick and easy way to differentiate the false and true vocal folds in images at this magnification when the scanning view is not available.

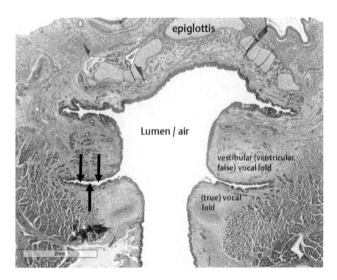

Fig. 38.18 **Coronal section through the larynx, scanning to low magnification. The arrows indicate the laryngeal ventricle.**

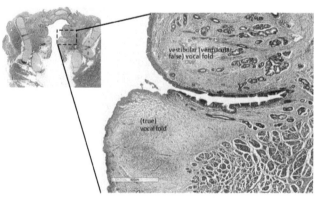

Fig. 38.19 **Coronal section through the larynx, low magnification, showing the vestibular and true vocal folds.**

Another way to differentiate the false from the true vocal folds is by characterizing the epithelium covering the surface. As indicated in **Fig. 38.20**, most of the larynx is lined by respiratory epithelium (green arrows), including the false vocal fold and the laryngeal ventricle. The tip of the true vocal fold, however, is covered by non-keratinized stratified squamous epithelium (black arrows).

This makes sense, because the true vocal folds are exposed to frictional forces as they move against each other during "enthusiastic" speech (yelling) and other activities, such as bearing down, which requires one to close the larynx.

Fig. 38.21 is a closer view of the vocal folds. The epithelium lining each surface is indicated (green arrows point to respiratory epithelium; black arrows indicate stratified squamous nonkeratinized). The vocal ligament cut in cross section is outlined in blue, and the vocalis muscle, also cut in cross section, is outlined in green.

Video 38.6   Vestibular and vocal folds

Be able to identify:
— Larynx
  • Vestibular fold
  • Vocal fold
  • Vocal ligament
  • Vocalis muscle
— Laryngeal ventricle
https://www.thieme.de/de/q.htm?p=opn/tp/308390101/978-1-62623-414-7_c038_v006&t=video

Fig. 38.22 shows images of the larynx taken from a different slide, in which the specimen is turned 90° from the previous images; it shows the respiratory epithelium covering the vestibular fold (A) and the stratified squamous nonkeratinized epithelium covering the true vocal fold (B).

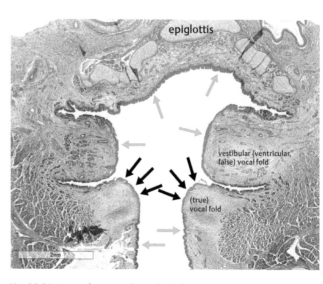

Fig. 38.20 **Coronal section through the larynx, scanning to low magnification, indicating the epithelium lining the larynx. Green arrows indicate respiratory epithelium; black arrows mark stratified squamous nonkeratinized epithelium.**

Video 38.7   Oblique cut through the larynx

Be able to identify:
— Larynx
  • Vestibular fold
  • Vocal fold
  • Vocal ligament
  • Vocalis muscle
  • Laryngeal ventricle
https://www.thieme.de/de/q.htm?p=opn/tp/308390101/978-1-62623-414-7_c038_v007&t=video

38.7   Trachea

Fig. 38.23 is an anatomic drawing of the larynx, trachea, and bronchi. The **trachea** is a single tube passing inferiorly from the larynx until it bifurcates into the **main (primary) bronchi**.

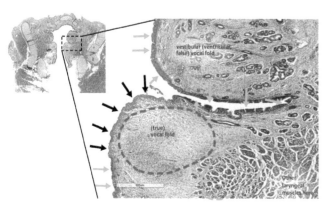

Fig. 38.21 **Coronal section through the larynx, low magnification, showing details of the vestibular and true vocal folds. The epithelium lining the larynx is indicated: Green arrows indicate respiratory epithelium; black arrows mark stratified squamous nonkeratinized epithelium. The vocal ligament (blue outline) and vocalis muscle (green outline) are shown.**

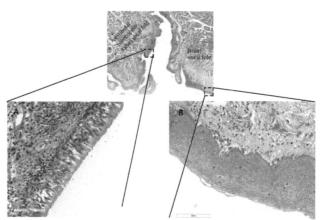

Fig. 38.22 **Oblique section through the larynx, showing the epithelium covering the vestibular fold (A) and true vocal fold (B).**

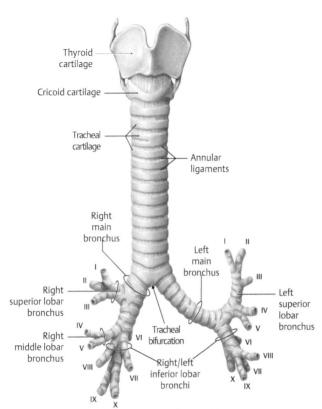

Fig. 38.23 Anatomy of the larynx, trachea, and bronchi. From Schuenke M, Schulte E, Schumacher U. *THIEME Atlas of Anatomy. Internal Organs.* Illustrations by Voll M and Wesker K. Second Edition. New York: Thieme Medical Publishers; 2016.

The trachea is supported by about a dozen C-shaped pieces of cartilage, incomplete posteriorly to allow a bolus of food to pass through the esophagus, which lies posterior to the trachea. The **trachealis muscle** (smooth muscle) spans the open, posterior end of the cartilages and contracts under parasympathetic stimulus during actions such as coughing.

Fig. 38.24 is a scanning image of a cross section of the trachea with the esophagus, a lymph node, and an elastic artery. At this low magnification, you can see the cartilage that supports the trachea (arrows) is C shaped. The open end of the cartilage is on the posterior side, toward the esophagus. There is a separation of the cartilage anteriorly, likely due to sectioning.

Fig. 38.25 is a low-power view of the tracheal wall. The wall of the trachea can be divided into a **mucosa** (blue bracket), a **submucosa** (yellow bracket), **cartilage** (white bracket), and **adventitia** (black bracket). The mucosa includes the previously discussed respiratory epithelium and a lamina propria. Note the numerous glands in the submucosa, and that the cartilage is hyaline cartilage.

Helpful Hint

Unlike the gastrointestinal system, there is no muscularis mucosa in the trachea to provide a distinct border between the mucosa and submucosa. The distinction here is somewhat arbitrary, but is based on the fact that the submucosa is composed of denser connective tissue than the mucosa, and has numerous glands.

Fig. 38.26 is an image showing the posterior wall of the trachea, and it shows the trachealis muscle (arrows), which spans the open ends of the C-shaped cartilage. Contraction of this smooth muscle narrows the lumen slightly, to assist in activities such as coughing.

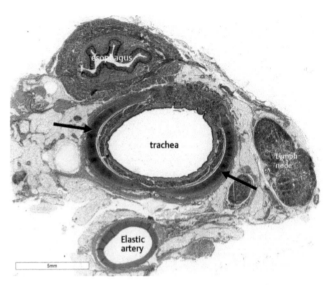

Fig. 38.24 Scanning image of the esophagus and trachea, also showing an elastic artery and lymph node. The cartilage in the trachea is indicated by the arrows.

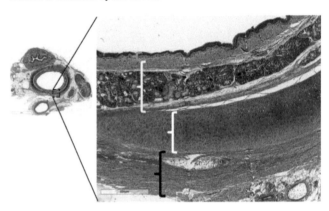

Fig. 38.25 Anterior wall of the trachea, low magnification. The four layers of the wall of the trachea are indicated by the brackets: blue bracket, mucosa; yellow bracket, submucosa; white bracket, cartilage; black bracket, adventitia.

Video 38.8   Trachea

Be able to identify:
— Trachea
  • Mucosa
  • Submucosa
  • Trachealis muscle
  • Cartilage
  • Adventitia
https://www.thieme.de/de/q.htm?p=opn/tp/308390101/978-1-62623-414-7_c038_v008&t=video

38.8   Bronchus

The trachea divides to form the right and left primary (main) **bronchi**, which further divide into secondary (lobar) and then tertiary (lobular) bronchi (see **Fig. 38.23**). As these divisions occur, the cartilage breaks up into smaller pieces, and the smooth muscle component becomes interspersed between the cartilage pieces. Apart from the fact that the cartilage and smooth muscle are interspersed in bronchi, the histology of bronchi is the same as just outlined for the trachea.

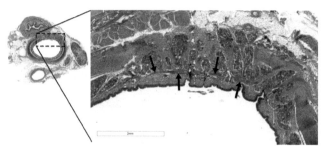

Fig. 38.26 **Posterior wall of the trachea, low magnification, showing the trachealis muscle (arrows).**

Fig. 38.27 is a scanning view of a larger bronchus near the trachea. This specimen has three smaller pieces of cartilage that have the same overall appearance as the trachea. In fact, the transition from the trachea to the bronchi is gradual, so sections of the bronchi near the trachea will look very similar to the trachea. Most or all of the smooth muscle is located posteriorly (arrows), similar to the trachealis.

Video 38.9   Proximal primary bronchus

Be able to identify:
— Bronchus
https://www.thieme.de/de/q.htm?p=opn/
tp/308390101/978-1-62623-414-7_c038_v009&t=video

Fig. 38.28 is a section from the **hilus** of the lung, showing the appearance of a bronchus (outlined) as it is entering the lung. The cartilage here is now separated into several pieces, and the smooth muscle (not readily visible at this magnification) is interspersed between cartilage pieces.

Video 38.10   Hilar bronchus

Be able to identify:
— Bronchus
https://www.thieme.de/de/q.htm?p=opn/
tp/308390101/978-1-62623-414-7_c038_v010&t=video

38.9   Chapter Review

The main functions of the respiratory system are to obtain oxygen and eliminate carbon dioxide. Since these molecules are small and hydrophobic, movement of these molecules into the blood occurs through diffusion. The lung is filled with specialized structures called alveoli that are lined by a simple squamous epithelium that maximizes diffusion efficiency. These alveoli are fragile, and the air that enters them must be moisturized, filtered, and warmed. This occurs during inspiration by the airways, which have an inner lining called the respiratory mucosa specialized for this function. This mucosa consists of a respiratory epithelium (pseudostratified columnar) with numerous glands that secrete mucus, which is moved toward the pharynx by cilia. The nasal cavity is supported by bone and has an elaborate venous plexus that helps to humidify incoming air. The epiglottis is supported by elastic cartilage; it is covered on its anterior side and tip by a stratified squamous

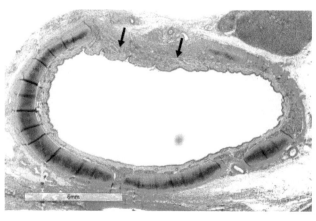

Fig. 38.27   **Upper bronchus, scanning image; arrows show smooth muscle.**

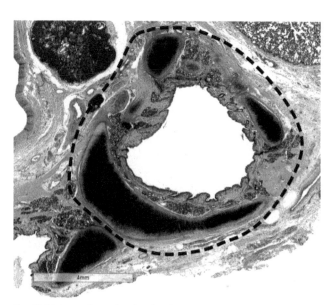

Fig. 38.28   **Lower bronchus (outlined) near hilus of lung, scanning.**

epithelium and on its lower posterior side by a respiratory epithelium. The larynx (voice box) is supported by specialized cartilages and houses the vestibular and true vocal folds. The vestibular fold contains numerous glands, while the true vocal fold lacks glands, contains the vocal ligament and vocalis muscle, and is covered by a stratified squamous epithelium. The trachea is supported by a series of C-shaped cartilages that are open posteriorly; the gap is spanned by the trachealis muscle, which is smooth muscle. The walls of the trachea and bronchi have a four-layered structure: mucosa, submucosa, cartilage, and adventitia. As the trachea branches to form bronchi, and the bronchi branch, the cartilage breaks up into smaller pieces, and the smooth muscle becomes interspersed between the cartilage pieces.

Questions and Answers

An online-only section of questions and answers accompanying this chapter is hosted on Thieme's MedOne Education site: https://medone-education.thieme.com. Use the code on the media page at the front of this book to gain access. An institutional license to the site is required to access these questions in an interactive format, and individual users are required to register for an individual account to track results.

39   Lungs

After completing this chapter, you should be able to:
— Identify, at the light microscope level, each of the following:
  • Bronchus
  • Bronchiole
    ○ (Regular) bronchiole
    ○ Terminal bronchiole
    ○ Respiratory bronchiole
  • Alveolar ducts
  • Alveolar sacs
  • Alveoli
  • Alveolar cells
    ○ Type I alveolar cells (type I pneumocytes)
    ○ Type II alveolar cells (type II pneumocytes
    ○ Alveolar macrophages (dust cells)
  • Pulmonary artery
  • Bronchial artery
  • Pulmonary vein
  • Visceral pleura
— Identify, at the electron microscope level, each of the following:
  • Type I alveolar cells (type I pneumocytes)
  • Type II alveolar cells (type II pneumocytes)
    ○ Lamellar bodies
  • Basal lamina
  • Endothelial cells
  • Components of connective tissue
  • Alveolar macrophage (dust cell)
— Outline the function of each structure and vessel type listed
— Correlate the main function of structures in the lung with histologic features
— Outline the production, function, and recycling of surfactant
— Explain the vasculature of the lungs

39.1   Overview of the Lungs and Airways (Respiratory Passages)

The previous chapter described structures of the upper respiratory system, including the trachea and bronchi (**Fig. 39.1**). The bronchi enter the substance of the lungs, which are the focus of this chapter. Examination of the lungs will include the terminal branches of the bronchi and bronchioles, as well as the site of gas exchange: the alveoli. In addition, the vasculature of the lungs, which includes both the pulmonary and systemic circuits, will be described.

Recall from the previous chapter that the trachea extends inferiorly from the larynx, dividing into right and left **primary (main) bronchi** (**Fig. 39.2**) Subsequent branches of the bronchi include the **secondary (lobar)** and **tertiary (lobular, segmental) bronchi** (tertiary bronchi are assigned Roman numerals in **Fig. 39.2**). The trachea and bronchi are supported by hyaline cartilage and smooth muscle. Sections of the trachea typically include a single, C-shaped cartilage. As the bronchi progress toward and into the lungs, the single cartilage becomes several pieces, and the smooth muscle is interspersed between these pieces.

Within the lung, the bronchi give way to branches that lack cartilage, called **bronchioles**, which lead to the **alveoli**

(**Fig. 39.3a**, **b**). There are several subcategories of each of these, as follows (and discussed subsequently):
• Bronchi
• Bronchioles
  • (Regular) bronchioles
  • Terminal bronchioles
  • Respiratory bronchioles
• Alveoli
  • Alveolar ducts
  • Alveolar sacs

Bronchioles narrow in diameter as they get closer to the alveoli. The smallest bronchioles have some alveoli associated with them and are called **respiratory bronchioles** (**Fig. 39.3a**). The bronchioles immediately proximal to respiratory bronchioles are called **terminal bronchioles**. **Alveolar ducts** are long passages with alveoli; **alveolar sacs** are circular spaces leading to alveoli (**Fig. 39.3b**).

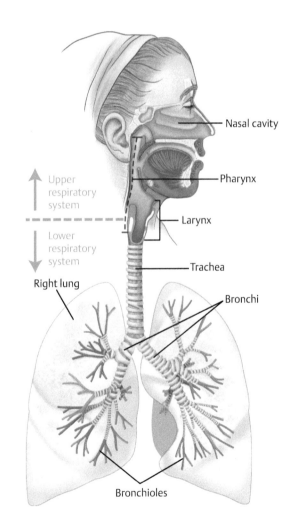

Fig. 39.1   **Respiratory system.**

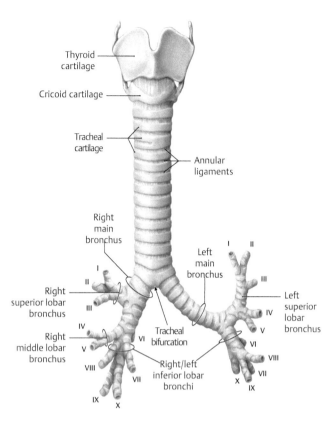

Fig. 39.2 **Anatomy of the larynx, trachea, and bronchi.**

Thyroid cartilage

Cricoid cartilage

Tracheal cartilage

Annular ligaments

Right main bronchus

Left main bronchus

Right superior lobar bronchus

Left superior lobar bronchus

Right middle lobar bronchus

Tracheal bifurcation

Right/left inferior lobar bronchi

As the respiratory passages divide and decrease in diameter, the histologic features of these passages change, including:

- Breakup and then loss of cartilage (bronchi have cartilage, bronchioles lack cartilage)
- Decrease in number of glands
- Relative increase in smooth muscle
- Decrease in height of the epithelium

Helpful Hint

Many sources have tables indicating exactly when the glands disappear, when the epithelium transitions from pseudostratified to simple columnar, and so forth. The exact locations of these transition points are not crucial, and, in many cases, the change is gradual anyway. It is absolutely useful to know that bronchi have cartilage and bronchioles do not. Apart from that specific detail, just knowing the general schema suffices in most cases.

39.2 Recognition of Lung Tissues

The next sections will examine structures of the airways, starting with bronchi and bronchioles, and progressing into the lungs. To start, it is useful to describe lung tissue briefly. Fortunately, lungs are easy to recognize because they have alveoli, which are air sacs with thin walls designed to maximize surface area and minimize diffusion distance between the air and blood. On sections of lung (**Fig. 39.4**), alveoli come in various sizes, and some are open, some collapsed. All are

connected to bronchioles, but because of sectioning, some appear as individual structures (double arrows), while others are connected to a cluster of other alveoli (lines). The details of alveoli will be examined shortly.

39.2.1 Distinguishing Airway from Blood Vessels

In a section of lung, many structures with thick walls and a lumen are present (**Fig. 39.5**). As an initial assessment, it is important to differentiate between components of the airways (bronchi, bronchioles) and blood vessels (arteries and veins).

With the exception of the alveoli, the airways are lined with a respiratory epithelium, either pseudostratified or simple columnar (**Fig. 39.5**, black bracket). The taller, thinner cells in these epithelia result in nuclei that are close together, creating a basophilic inner lining (**Fig. 39.5**, bronchiole). Contrast this with blood vessels, which are lined by a simple squamous epithelium. This inner simple squamous epithelial lining has nuclei that are spread out because the cells are flat; therefore, blood vessels are less basophilic near the lumen.

The structure of the airways will be discussed next, including a detailed look at the alveoli. This will be followed by a consideration of the vasculature supplying the lungs.

39.2.2 Bronchi and Bronchioles

As mentioned, **bronchi** have cartilage, whereas **bronchioles** do not. Bronchioles also lack glands, but it is sometimes difficult to determine whether glands are present. Therefore, the presence or absence of cartilage is a more reliable way to differentiate bronchi from bronchioles. **Fig. 39.6a**, **b** shows an image of two bronchi and a bronchiole, respectively. Note the presence of cartilage in the bronchi and absence of cartilage in the bronchiole.

Fig. 39.7a, **b** is another set of images from a different preparation, showing a much smaller bronchus with a few small pieces of cartilage and a slightly smaller bronchiole lacking cartilage.

Helpful Hint

Size is not a useful indicator to differentiate bronchi from bronchioles, because small bronchi and large bronchioles are approximately the same size. The clincher should always be whether or not cartilage is present. Most sources indicate that the transition from bronchi to bronchioles occurs when the tube is ~ 1 mm in diameter, but the bronchus in **Fig. 39.7a** is smaller than 1 mm. This may be due to slight errors in the scale bars generated by the digital-side software, but it is more likely that the 1-mm cutoff is a little loose.

Video 39.1 Bronchi and bronchioles

Be able to identify:
— Bronchus
— Bronchioles

https://www.thieme.de/de/q.htm?p=opn/tp/308390101/978-1-62623-414-7_c039_v001&t=video

a

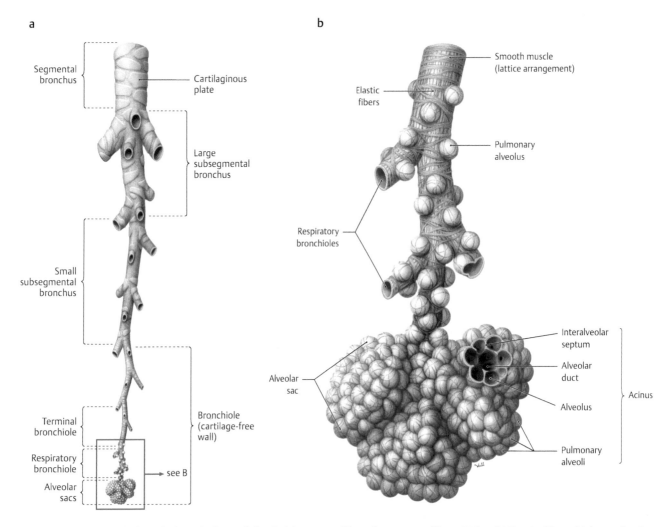

Segmental
bronchus

Cartilaginous
plate

Large
subsegmental
bronchus

Small
subsegmental
bronchus

Terminal
bronchiole

Respiratory
bronchiole

Alveolar
sacs

Bronchiole
(cartilage-free
wall)

see B

b

Smooth muscle
(lattice arrangement)

Elastic
fibers

Pulmonary
alveolus

Respiratory
bronchioles

Interalveolar
septum

Alveolar
duct

Alveolus

Alveolar
sac

Pulmonary
alveoli

Acinus

Fig. 39.3   Anatomy of the bronchi, bronchioles, and alveoli. (a) Segmental bronchi to terminal bronchioles. (b) Terminal bronchioles to alveoli.
From Schuenke M, Schulte E, Schumacher U. *THIEME Atlas of Anatomy. Internal Organs.* Illustrations by Voll M and Wesker K. Second
Edition. New York: Thieme Medical Publishers; 2016.

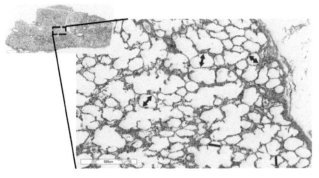

Fig. 39.4   Overview of lungs showing alveoli (double arrows and lines).

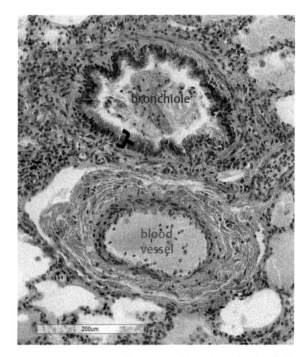

bronchiole

blood
vessel

200um

Fig. 39.5   Comparison of airways and blood vessels. The black
bracket indicates the respiratory epithelium.

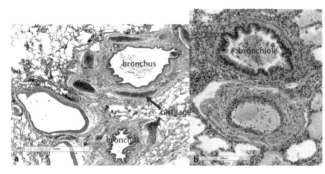

Fig. 39.6 Comparison of (a) bronchi and (b) a bronchiole. Cartilage in the bronchi is indicated.

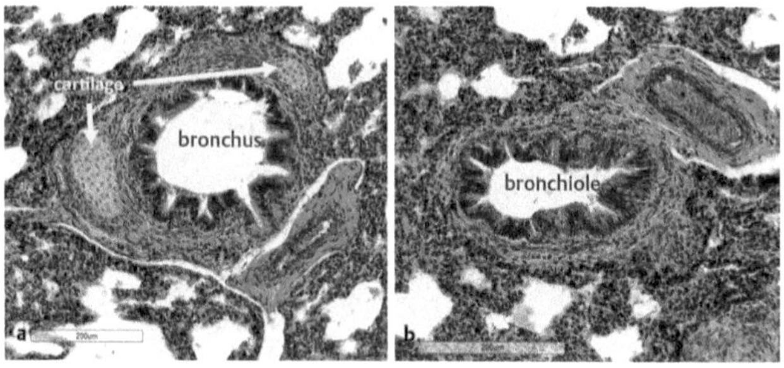

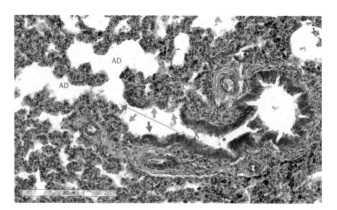

Fig. 39.7 Comparison of (a) a small bronchus and (b) bronchiole. Cartilage in the bronchus is indicated.

39.2.3 Terminal and Respiratory Bronchioles

At the termini of bronchioles, the transition to alveoli is gradual (see **Fig. 39.3**). The smallest bronchioles have some alveoli associated with them and are called **respiratory bronchioles**. The bronchioles immediately proximal to respiratory bronchioles are called **terminal bronchioles**. Terminal bronchioles are important because they include **club cells**, which produce a proteinaceous surfactant. However, club cells are not seen in routine histologic sections.

Recall that bronchioles are relatively thick-walled and lined with respiratory epithelium (though the epithelium in small bronchioles may be simple columnar or even simple cuboidal instead of pseudostratified). Alveoli are thin-walled and lined with a simple squamous epithelium. Therefore, respiratory bronchioles have an epithelial lining that alternates from respiratory epithelium to simple squamous. Terminal bronchioles are lined entirely by respiratory epithelium.

Fig. 39.8 shows a terminal bronchiole (X) giving rise to a respiratory bronchiole (green line). The respiratory bronchiole is partially lined with respiratory epithelium (red arrows) and partially lined with alveolar epithelium (simple squamous, blue arrows). The respiratory bronchiole leads to alveolar ducts (AD, described in the next subsection).

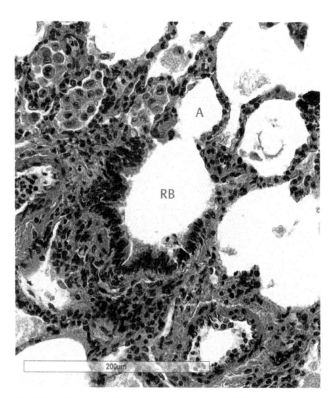

Fig. 39.8 Terminal bronchiole (X) and respiratory bronchiole (green line). The lining of the respiratory bronchiole alternates between respiratory (red arrows) and alveolar (simple squamous, blue arrows). Alveolar ducts (AD) branch from the respiratory bronchiole.

> **Helpful Hint**
>
> Even though the alveoli along this respiratory bronchiole are collapsed, they still demonstrate a simple squamous lining, not respiratory epithelium.

Fig. 39.9 is a cross section through a respiratory bronchiole (RB). The respiratory epithelium lines the duct in the lower and left portions, while the upper right portion of this duct is lined by a simple squamous epithelium and includes at least one alveolus (A).

Video 39.2 Terminal and respiratory bronchioles

Be able to identify:
— Terminal bronchioles
— Respiratory bronchioles

https://www.thieme.de/de/q.htm?p=opn/tp/308390101/978-1-62623-414-7_c039_v002&t=video

Fig. 39.9 Respiratory bronchiole in cross section (RB). A indicates an alveolus.

Terminal and respiratory bronchioles are often challenging to find. Also, note that a terminal bronchiole in cross section will appear similar histologically to any other larger bronchiole. What makes definitive identification of the terminal bronchiole possible in **Fig. 39.8** is the fact that it is continuous with the respiratory bronchiole.

39.2.4   Alveoli, Alveolar Ducts, and Alveolar Sacs

Alveoli are the terminal structures of the respiratory tract (**Fig. 39.10**). They are lined with a simple squamous epithelium, with connective tissue, including an extensive capillary network, within their septa (walls).

Alveoli are lined by a simple squamous epithelium, so the nuclei on the inner surface are spread out. Therefore, alveoli do not have a basophilic inner lining as the airways do.

Fig. 39.11 shows the organization of alveoli in the lung. The terminal portions of airways that lead into individual alveoli can be classified based on shape as either elongated **alveolar ducts** (**Fig. 39.11a**, blue lines) or "rounder" **alveolar sacs** (**Fig. 39.11b**, AS). In **Fig. 39.11a**, alveolar ducts are shown extending from the respiratory bronchiole (RB). The alveolar sac in **Fig. 39.11b** is a central chamber from which alveoli that surround this central chamber arise.

By definition, neither alveolar sacs nor alveolar ducts have respiratory epithelium. Differentiating between alveolar ducts and alveolar sacs on tissue sections is usually not high yield. Although there is indeed a structural difference, there is no functional significance.

Video 39.3   Alveolar ducts and sacs

Be able to identify:
— Alveoli
— Alveolar ducts
— Alveolar sacs
https://www.thieme.de/de/q.htm?p=opn/tp/308390101/978-1-62623-414-7_c039_v003&t=video

Fig. 39.12 is a scanning electron micrograph of a section of a rat lung, showing a bronchiole (1) leading to terminal bronchioles (2), which ultimately lead to alveolar ducts (3) and then alveoli (4).

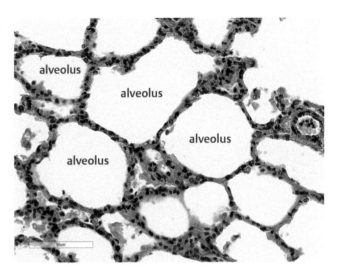

Fig. 39.10 **Alveoli, light micrograph, medium magnification.**

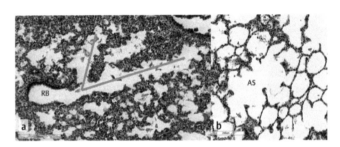

Fig. 39.11 **Organization of alveoli, light micrograph, low-medium magnification. (a) Respiratory bronchiole (RB) leading to two alveolar ducts (blue lines). (b) Alveolar sac (AS).**

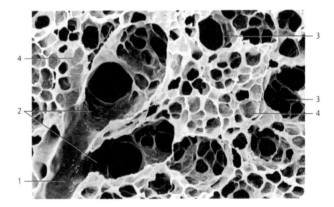

Fig. 39.12 **Scanning electron micrograph from the lung showing a bronchiole (1) leading to terminal bronchioles (2), which lead to alveolar ducts (3) and then alveoli (4).**

39.3 Cells of Alveoli

Fig. 39.13 is a drawing of alveoli, showing that there are three types of cells present in the inner lining of alveoli:

- **Type I alveolar cells (type I pneumocytes)** are simple squamous cells, part of the blood-air barrier.
- **Type II alveolar cells (type II pneumocytes, septal cells)** are cuboidal and produce surfactant.
- **Alveolar macrophages (dust cells)** are often in the lumen of the alveoli.

The walls of the alveoli contain loose connective tissue with many elastic fibers and capillaries.

39.3.1 Pneumocytes and Alveolar Macrophages

Routine preparations of lung tissue are relatively thick sections of the lung (**Fig. 39.14**). Therefore, differentiating the three alveolar cell types with certainty can be challenging. Note that type I and type II alveolar cells are part of the epithelial lining of alveoli. Cells with flattened nuclei are type I alveolar cells (**Fig. 39.14**, black arrow), while cells with round, euchromatic nuclei and eosinophilic cytoplasm are type II alveolar cells (blue arrow). Alveolar macrophages, or dust cells (green arrows), have a much larger nucleus and more extensive cytoplasm than either of these two cells and are more often than not seen within the lumen of the alveoli as opposed to being part of the lining of the alveoli.

Fig. 39.15 shows another image of the alveoli of the lung. This image shows two type II alveolar cells (blue arrows) in a "corner" of adjacent alveoli. Again, note the round, euchromatic nuclei and eosinophilic cytoplasm, suggesting that these cells are quite active in production of surfactant. Still, their nuclei are not as large or irregular as the macrophage has (green arrow); the macrophage has more extensive cytoplasm and is free within an alveolus. Type I alveolar cells are also shown (black arrows, top one a little separated from the wall).

Video 39.4   Alveolar cells

Be able to identify:
- Type I alveolar cells (type I pneumocytes)
- Type II alveolar cells (type II pneumocytes)
- Alveolar macrophages (dust cells)

https://www.thieme.de/de/q.htm?p=opn/tp/308390101/978-1-62623-414-7_c039_v004&t=video

Note that **Fig. 39.14** and **Fig. 39.15** were taken from a specimen of the lungs of a child, in whom the alveolar macrophages did not demonstrate significant accumulation of phagocytosed material. Over time, these resident macrophages accumulate inhaled material not filtered by the mucociliary escalator of the upper respiratory system, so in specimens from older individuals they more often exhibit brown/black cytoplasmic particles (**Fig. 39.16**). This color is not due to staining; it is the natural color of these cells, which appears "dusty"; thus they are also called **dust cells**.

Video 39.5   Alveolar macrophages (dust cells)

Be able to identify:
- Alveolar macrophages (dust cells)

https://www.thieme.de/de/q.htm?p=opn/tp/308390101/978-1-62623-414-7_c039_v005&t=video

39.3.2 Ultrastructure of Alveoli

Fig. 39.17 is a scanning electron micrograph from a section of the lung, showing about a dozen alveoli (the lumina of three alveoli are indicated). The connective tissue in the septa contains numerous capillaries (marked with yellow arrows), underscoring the robust vasculature associated with the alveoli. Note that the alveoli are much larger than the capillaries and that the air-blood barrier is thin (discussed in a later subsection).

The transmission electron micrograph in **Fig. 39.18** shows a detailed view of an alveolar septum. Two complete

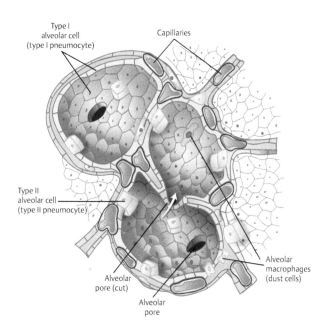

Fig. 39.13 **Alveoli.**

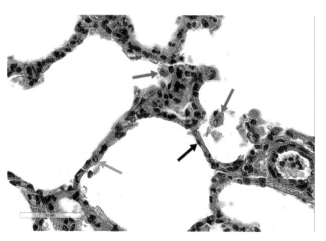

Fig. 39.14 **Alveoli, light micrograph, high magnification, showing type I alveolar cell (black arrow), type II alveolar cell (blue arrow), and alveolar macrophages (green arrows).**

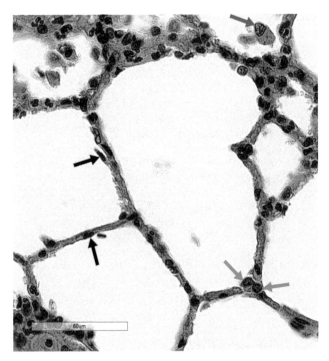

Fig. 39.15 Alveoli, light micrograph, high magnification, showing type I alveolar cells (black arrows), type II alveolar cells (blue arrows), and alveolar macrophage (green arrow).

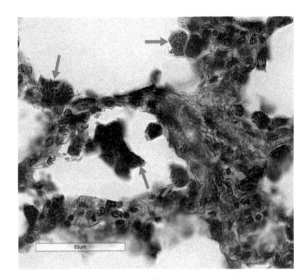

Fig. 39.16 Alveolar macrophages (blue arrows) showing phagocytosed cytoplasmic particles.

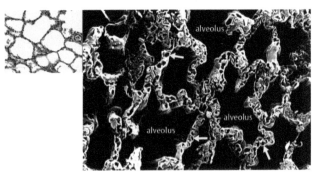

Fig. 39.17 Scanning electron micrograph of a section of lung, showing alveoli and the extensive capillary network (arrows) in the walls of the alveoli. The light micrograph is of approximately the same field for comparison.

capillaries and parts of three others are shown, each with at least one red blood cell in the lumen. The two alveolar lumina containing air are pale. At this magnification only a small portion of each alveolus is seen; the capillaries are much smaller than the alveoli. The nucleus of an endothelial cell can be seen bulging into the lumen of a capillary. Most of the inner lining of the alveoli in contact with air is the thin portions of type I alveolar cells, barely visible at this magnification. The air-blood barrier (between arrows) is very thin in most places and is composed of a type I alveolar cell, a fused basal lamina, and the capillary endothelial cell. The type II alveolar cell is also in contact with air, and small inclusions in the cytoplasm of this cell can be seen.

Clinical Correlate

Chronic obstructive pulmonary disorder (COPD) is a progressive disease in which patients have **emphysema**, chronic bronchitis, or both. Emphysema is characterized by destruction of alveolar walls and results in enlarged alveoli with a decrease in surface area for gas exchange. **Chronic bronchitis** is irritation and inflammation of the bronchi and bronchioles, reducing the luminal diameter. Smoking and other exposures are common causes of COPD.

Fig. 39.19 is a higher-magnification electron micrograph showing a single alveolar capillary, with a red blood cell in the lumen. The alveolar lumen containing air is pale. As in **Fig. 39.18**, the air-blood barrier in **Fig. 39.19** is very thin in most places and is composed of a type I alveolar cell (green arrow), a fused basal lamina (orange arrow), and a capillary endothelial cell (black arrow). To the lower right of these arrows, the fused basal lamina splits; the material between the basement membranes below the split is connective tissue.

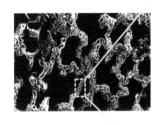

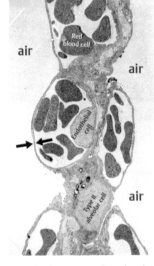

Fig. 39.18 Transmission electron micrograph of a section of an alveolar septum corresponding to the boxed area of the scanning electron micrograph of Fig. 39.17, showing alveoli (marked as "air") and the capillaries with red blood cells. Nuclei belonging to an endothelial cell and a type II alveolar cell are indicated. The arrows show the thin air-blood barrier. Image courtesy of Michael Hortsch, University of Michigan. © 2005 The Regents of the University of Michigan.

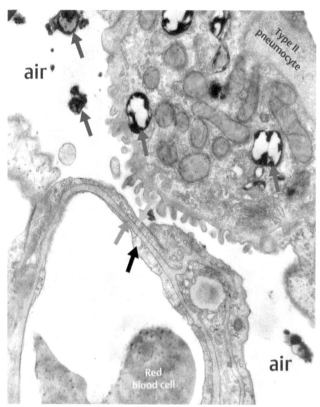

Fig. 39.19 **Transmission electron micrograph of a section of lung, showing alveoli (labeled "air") and a capillary. A type II alveolar cell is at upper right, demonstrating lamellar bodies containing surfactant (red arrows). Surfactant in the alveolar lumen (purple arrow) is also shown. The air-blood barrier includes a type I alveolar cell (type I pneumocyte, green arrow), a fused basal lamina (orange arrow), and an endothelial cell (black arrow). Image courtesy of Michael Hortsch, University of Michigan. © 2005 The Regents of the University of Michigan.**

39.3.3 Surfactant

A type II pneumocyte is shown in the upper right of **Fig. 39.19**. **Surfactant** produced by these cells is stored in large vesicles usually demonstrating a lamellar structure (red arrows); these structures are often called **lamellar bodies**. In many images of these cells, the lamellar structure washes away during tissue preparation, as is seen here. Newly released surfactant can also be seen (purple arrow); the lamella will unravel, and the surfactant will cover the inner surface of the alveoli, reducing surface tension to prevent alveolar collapse. Though not shown here, type II alveolar cells form tight junctions with their type I neighbors and are therefore part of the alveolar epithelium and air-blood barrier.

Helpful Hint

Surfactant is recycled by alveolar macrophages, so the lysosomal compartment in these cells can have a lamellar appearance similar to the lamellar bodies in type II alveolar cells. When in doubt, identifying tight junctions between type II alveolar cells and type I alveolar cells will help distinguish type II cells from alveolar macrophages, which do not have tight junctions.

Clinical Correlate

In a fetus, surfactant production occurs during the last months of pregnancy. Therefore, babies born prematurely often have insufficient surfactant, with reduced activity. Since surfactant reduces surface tension, these infants have difficulty with respiration as they struggle to inflate their lungs with each breath. This condition is called **neonatal respiratory distress syndrome**. Treatment options include supportive care, such as positive pressure ventilation, and exogenous (animal) surfactant. If a mother is at risk for premature delivery, she may receive corticosteroids, which stimulate the fetal lungs to increase surfactant production.

39.3.4 Air-Blood Barrier

Fig. 39.20 is an electron micrograph focusing on the air-blood barrier. The lumen of the alveolus (air) is at the bottom of the image (4), while the capillary lumen is the clear space at the top (5). The molecules exchanged here—oxygen and carbon dioxide—are small, hydrophobic molecules that readily diffuse from air to blood or vice versa. To maximize this diffusion-driven process, the air-blood barrier is very thin. Therefore, the type I pneumocyte of the alveolar wall (1) and capillary endothelial cell (2) are simple squamous and share a fused basal lamina (3) without intervening connective tissue.

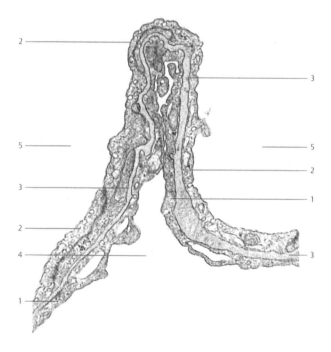

Fig. 39.20 **Transmission electron micrograph showing details of the air-blood barrier: (1) type I alveolar cell (type I pneumocyte); (2) endothelial cell; (3) fused basal lamina; (4) alveolar lumen; (5) lumen of capillary.**

In an image such as this, the large spaces separated by a thin barrier readily identify this as a relatively high-magnification image of the lung. To differentiate between type I alveolar cells and endothelial cells at this high magnification without red blood cells as an aid, recall that endothelial cells are one of the two cell types that have numerous **pinocytotic vesicles**, or **caveolae** (the other is smooth muscle cells). The endothelial cell in **Fig. 39.20** (2) has more caveolae and vesicles than the type I alveolar cell (1).

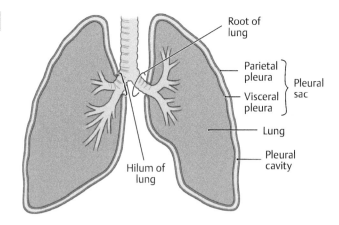

Fig. 39.21 **Pleura of the lungs.**

39.4   Visceral Pleura

Fig. 39.21 shows the **pleura** of the lungs: the lining that encases the lungs and contains pleural fluid. The outer surface of the lungs is covered by the **visceral pleura**, an epithelium, usually simple squamous or low cuboidal. The **parietal pleura** lines the inner aspect of the thorax, the superior part of the diaphragm, and the lateral aspect of the pericardial sac. **Fig. 39.22** is an image showing the visceral pleura as an epithelium on the outer surface of the lung (blue arrows; here it appears low cuboidal).

The outer surface of the lung shows much variation in prepared specimens. In many cases, cells of the visceral pleura are visible, as shown here. In other samples, the outer layer of the lung will appear smooth but with no visible cells, suggesting a simple squamous epithelium. In other cases the epithelium was lost during tissue preparation.

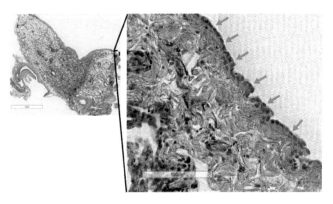

Fig. 39.22 **Visceral pleura (blue arrows).**

Video 39.6   Visceral pleura

Be able to identify:
— Visceral pleura

https://www.thieme.de/de/q.htm?p=opn/
tp/308390101/978-1-62623-414-7_c039_v006&t=video

39.5   Vasculature of the Lung

The lungs are relatively unique in that they have a dual blood supply (**Fig. 39.23**).
1. Most of the blood going to the lungs is deoxygenated, delivered from the right side of the heart through the **pulmonary arteries** (**Fig. 39.23a**). This blood is destined to become oxygenated in the alveoli, so these arteries do not give rise to capillaries until that point.
2. A small amount of blood is carried to the lungs by the **bronchial arteries**, branches of the aorta (**Fig. 39.23b**). Because this oxygenated blood is necessary to supply the cells of the trachea, bronchi, and bronchioles, these vessels branch into arterioles and capillaries within the walls of these structures.

Each lung is composed of about 10 **bronchopulmonary segments**. **Fig. 39.24** is a drawing of a segment of lung supplied by a terminal bronchiole. Things to note:
1. Both arteries (pulmonary and bronchial) and branches of the airways are positioned in the center of the segment, while the **pulmonary veins** return along the partitions between adjacent segments.
2. The pulmonary artery is approximately the same size as the airways (this image shows it smaller, but, as you will see, the pulmonary arteries are indeed close to the size of the associated airway). The bronchial artery is much smaller and within the wall of the airways.

The pulmonary arteries are under lower pressure than arteries of the systemic circuit, so they have thinner walls. Therefore, it is difficult to distinguish pulmonary arteries from veins based on wall thickness. As will be described below, the position and size of these vessels is the best way to distinguish them.

a

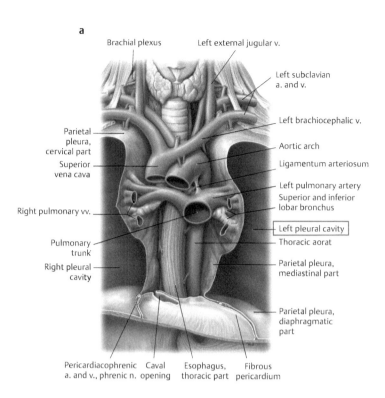

Brachial plexus

Left external jugular v.

Left subclavian
a. and v.

Left brachiocephalic v.

Parietal
pleura,
cervical part

Aortic arch

Ligamentum arteriosum

Superior
vena cava

Left pulmonary artery

Superior and inferior
lobar bronchus

Right pulmonary vv.

Left pleural cavity

Pulmonary
trunk

Thoracic aorat

Right pleural
cavity

Parietal pleura,
mediastinal part

Parietal pleura,
diaphragmatic
part

Pericardiacophrenic   Caval   Esophagus,   Fibrous
a. and v., phrenic n. opening   thoracic part pericardium

Fig. 39.23 Vasculature of the lung. The lung receives a dual blood supply. (a) The entire cardiac output from the right ventricle, consisting of deoxygenated blood, reaches the lungs via the pulmonary arteries. Based on the work of Schuenke M, Schulte E, Schumacher U. *THIEME Atlas of Anatomy. Internal Organs.* Illustrations by Voll M and Wesker K. Second Edition. New York: Thieme Medical Publishers; 2016. (b) The lungs receive a small amount of oxygenated blood from the systemic circuit from bronchial arteries, which supply oxygen to the bronchi and bronchioles. From Schuenke M, Schulte E, Schumacher U. *THIEME Atlas of Anatomy. Internal Organs.* Illustrations by Voll M and Wesker K. Second Edition. New York: Thieme Medical Publishers; 2016.

b

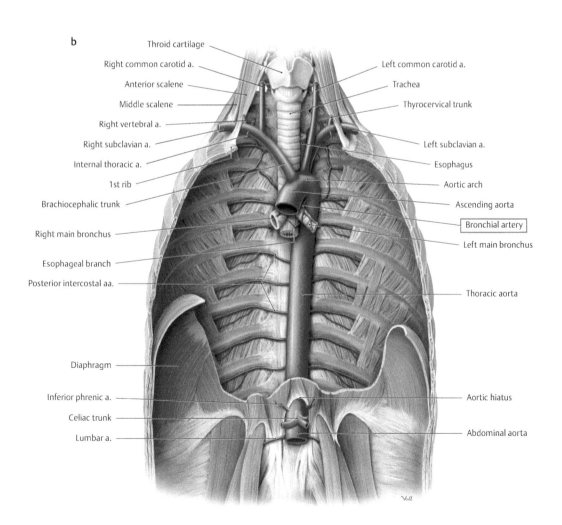

Throid cartilage

Right common carotid a.

Left common carotid a.

Anterior scalene

Trachea

Middle scalene

Thyrocervical trunk

Right vertebral a.

Right subclavian a.

Left subclavian a.

Internal thoracic a.

Esophagus

1st rib

Aortic arch

Brachiocephalic trunk

Ascending aorta

Bronchial artery

Right main bronchus

Left main bronchus

Esophageal branch

Posterior intercostal aa.

Thoracic aorta

Diaphragm

Inferior phrenic a.

Aortic hiatus

Celiac trunk

Lumbar a.

Abdominal aorta

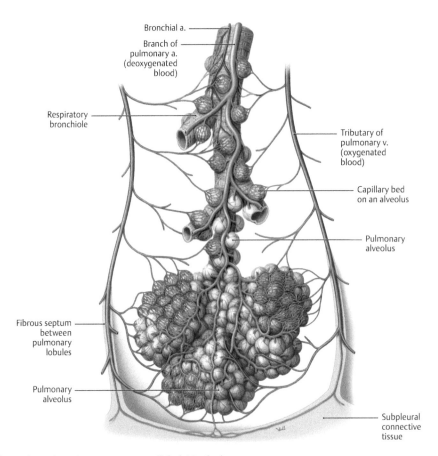

Fig. 39.24 **Blood supply to a bronchopulmonary segment (lobule) in the lung.**

Basic Science Correlate: Physiology

It may be useful to think about the function of these vessels to understand their anatomy and histology. The pulmonary arteries are bringing deoxygenated blood to the alveoli, the purpose of this is to pick up oxygen. Therefore, they will not branch into capillaries until they get to the alveoli. This is why they are approximately the same size as the airways (bronchi, bronchioles), because their target is the same: namely the alveoli.

The bronchial arteries, on the other hand, are designed to *deliver* oxygen to cells within the walls of the bronchi and bronchioles. Therefore, they branch into capillaries within the walls of the airways. They are located within the walls of the airways and are much smaller vessels. Functionally, the bronchial arteries are not intended to reach the alveoli at all (even though some blood from these vessels does reach the alveolar capillaries). Blood from all capillaries in the lungs, including alveolar capillaries and capillaries in the bronchi and bronchioles, flows into the pulmonary veins.

Because of these properties of the lung vasculature, when looking at histologic sections, note that (**Fig. 39.24**):

1. The airways, pulmonary artery, and bronchial artery are together in the same bundle, while the pulmonary veins are isolated.
2. The pulmonary artery is approximately the same size as the associated airway, while the bronchial arteries are much smaller and within the wall of the bronchus/bronchiole.

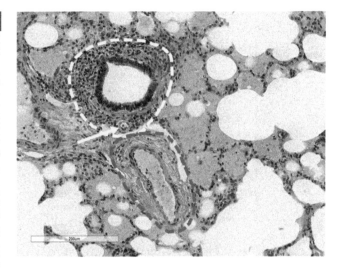

Fig. 39.25 **Center of a pulmonary segment showing a bronchiole (yellow outline), pulmonary artery (blue outline), and bronchial artery (yellow arrow).**

Fig. 39.25 is an image showing a region in the center of a pulmonary segment. The bronchiole (yellow outline) is recognized by its respiratory epithelium and lack of cartilage. The pulmonary artery (blue outline) has approximately the same diameter as the bronchiole that it accompanies. The bronchial artery (arrow) is within the wall of, and much smaller in diameter than, the bronchiole it supplies.

Fig. 39.26 is an image taken at lower magnification to include the center and edge of a pulmonary segment. Note that branches of the airways are each paired with a pulmonary artery of the same size (blue outlines). The pulmonary veins are found in the partitions between the lobules and are isolated structures (green outline). There are small lymphatic vessels associated with the airways, as well as in the partitions between lobules; these are small at this level, so they are difficult to identify definitively.

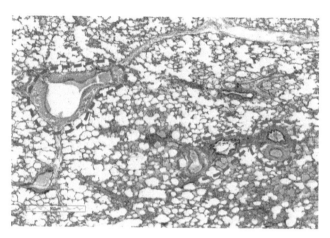

Fig. 39.26 **Lung segment showing the airways and pulmonary arteries in the center of the segments (blue outlines) and the pulmonary vein in the septa between segments (green outline).**

Video 39.7 Pulmonary vasculature, part 1

https://www.thieme.de/de/q.htm?p=opn/
tp/308390101/978-1-62623-414-7_c039_
v007&t=video

Video 39.8 Pulmonary vasculature, part 2

https://www.thieme.de/de/q.htm?p=opn/
tp/308390101/978-1-62623-414-7_c039_
v008&t=video

Be able to identify:
— Pulmonary arteries
— Bronchial arteries
— Pulmonary veins

Clinical Correlate

Each bronchopulmonary segment in the lungs functions independently, supplied by a tertiary (segmental) bronchus and its branches and the accompanying branch of the pulmonary artery. In patients with tumors or other pathology restricted to one or a few bronchopulmonary segments, the affected segments can be removed without disrupting the architecture of the remaining segments.

39.6 Chapter Review

The lungs contain the lower portion of the airways, including bronchi, bronchioles (including terminal and respiratory bronchioles), and alveoli (including alveolar ducts and sacs). The airways, except for the alveoli, are lined by respiratory epithelium (pseudostratified columnar, with cilia and goblet cells). The bronchi are characterized by the presence of cartilage and glands in the wall; bronchioles lack these structures. Terminal bronchioles are the smallest bronchioles that do not have associated alveoli. Respiratory bronchioles are bronchioles that have some alveoli, and they eventually lead to alveolar ducts and sacs.

Cell types in the alveoli include type I alveolar cells (type I pneumocytes), which are simple squamous, minimizing the diffusion distance between air and blood. In the thinnest portions of the alveoli, type I alveolar cells share a basal lamina with endothelial cells of capillary walls, so the air–blood barrier consists of a type I alveolar cell, basal lamina, and endothelial cell. Type II alveolar cells (type II pneumocytes) are cuboidal, with a euchromatic nucleus and eosinophilic cytoplasm, and they secrete surfactant, which reduces surface tension. In electron micrographs, these cells contain surfactant in the form of lamellar bodies and are joined to type I alveolar cells by tight junctions. Alveolar macrophages (dust cells) are found in many locations in the alveoli, including the lumen. They are large cells, with a frothy eosinophilic cytoplasm, and often contain accumulated inhaled particulate material.

The outer lining of the lungs is the visceral pleura, seen as a simple cuboidal or simple squamous epithelium.

The lungs receive a dual blood supply. Deoxygenated blood is delivered via pulmonary arteries, and oxygenated blood is supplied by the bronchial arteries. The airways, pulmonary arteries, and bronchial arteries branch together in the lung, in the center of a pulmonary segment. The pulmonary arteries are thin-walled but can be recognized because they are approximately the same diameter as the airways with which they are associated. Bronchial arteries are small and in the wall of the airways. Pulmonary veins are located in the connective tissue septa between segments and are not associated with any of these other structures.

Questions and Answers

An online-only section of questions and answers accompanying this chapter is hosted on Thieme's MedOne Education site: https://medone-education.thieme.com. Use the code on the media page at the front of this book to gain access. An institutional license to the site is required to access these questions in an interactive format, and individual users are required to register for an individual account to track results.

40   Pituitary Gland

After completing this chapter, you should be able to:
— Identify, at the light microscope level, each of the following:
  • Pituitary gland
    ◦ Adenohypophysis/pars distalis/anterior pituitary
      ▪ Acidophils
      ▪ Basophils
      ▪ Chromophobes
      ▪ Sinusoids
    ◦ Neurohypophysis/pars nervosa/posterior pituitary
      ▪ Pituicytes
      ▪ Herring bodies (best seen with PAS stain)
    ◦ Pars intermedia
      ▪ Colloid
— Outline the function of each cell and structure listed, including the specific types of cells of the pituitary gland
— Illustrate the development of the pituitary gland
— Correlate the appearance of each cell type or structure with its function
— Describe the principles of immunocytochemistry and the use of this procedure

40.1   Overview of Endocrine Organs

Recall that glandular formation begins with proliferation of an epithelium, creating a growth of epithelial cells into the underlying connective tissue (**Fig. 40.1a–c**). The basement membrane remains between the glandular epithelial cells and connective tissue, so the epithelial cells maintain apical-basal polarity. During **exocrine gland** formation (**Fig. 40.1e**), the glandular cells retain a connection to the surface epithelium through a duct and secrete product apically. Examples of exocrine glands include sweat and salivary glands as well as the liver and exocrine pancreas.

Endocrine gland formation occurs through a similar process, except that the epithelial cells separate from the originating epithelium to form a cluster of cells that secrete product basally into the connective tissue and bloodstream (**Fig. 40.1d**). Note that the basement membrane persists, surrounding the cluster of endocrine cells.

This series of chapters presents the pituitary, adrenal, thyroid, and parathyroid glands. These organs are considered endocrine glands because their main (or only) function is to secrete hormones. Most organs are now known to have an endocrine function; for example, adipose tissue secretes leptin, the heart releases atrial natriuretic peptide, and the kidneys produce renin. However, these other organs do not develop in the manner just described—that is, they are not derived from epithelia—and they have multiple functions, only one of which is secretion of hormone. Therefore, "the endocrine system" as a unit includes only organs that function primarily as endocrine glands.

40.2   Development of the Pituitary Gland

The **pituitary gland** develops from neural tissue and oral ectoderm, both of which are epithelial. **Fig. 40.2** is a drawing of the early embryo in sagittal section. The ventricle (space with

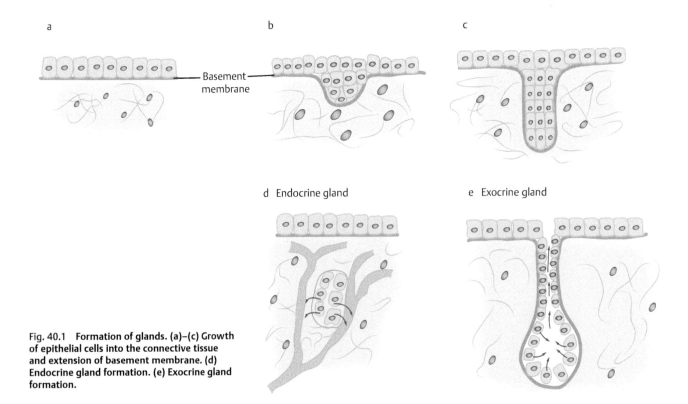

a

b

c

Basement membrane

d Endocrine gland

e Exocrine gland

Fig. 40.1   **Formation of glands. (a)–(c) Growth of epithelial cells into the connective tissue and extension of basement membrane. (d) Endocrine gland formation. (e) Exocrine gland formation.**

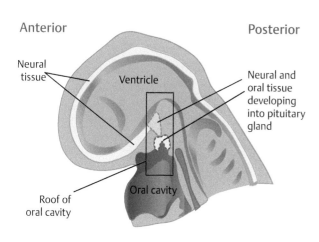

Anterior   Posterior

Neural tissue

Ventricle

Neural and oral tissue developing into pituitary gland

Oral cavity

Roof of oral cavity

Fig. 40.2 **Origin of the pituitary gland.**

Fig. 40.3 shows details of the development of the pituitary gland. The floor of the brain, specifically the diencephalon in the area of the future **hypothalamus**, grows inferiorly (**Figure 40.3b, c**). This **neurohypophyseal diverticulum** forms the **posterior lobe of the pituitary gland** (**neurohypophysis, pars nervosa**), which remains connected to the hypothalamus via the **infundibulum** (**Fig. 40.3e, f**). At the same time, the **hypophyseal diverticulum** from the oral ectoderm migrates superiorly, separating from the oral cavity to form a fluid-filled vesicle that becomes situated anterior to the infundibulum and posterior lobe (**Fig. 40.3b–d**). The anterior wall of this vesicle develops robustly, forming the **anterior lobe of the pituitary gland** (**adenohypophysis, pars distalis**), while the posterior wall of this vesicle is fairly vestigial, forming a thin **intermediate lobe of the pituitary gland** (**pars intermedia**) (**Fig. 40.3e, f**). The lumen of this vesicle is called **Rathke's pouch**, which fills with **colloid** (**Fig. 40.3d–f**). The mesenchyme surrounding these structures forms bones of the floor of the skull (sphenoid bone) (**Fig. 40.3f**).

cerebrospinal fluid) is exaggerated in this drawing. The wall of the developing brain (i.e., the neural tissue) is indicated by the pale blue and dark blue border. Specialized cells on the floor of the brain (gray-blue) in the area of the developing hypothalamus form the neural contribution to the pituitary gland. As this is happening, a specialized portion of the oral epithelium grows superiorly from the roof of the oral cavity to form the oral contribution to the pituitary gland.

Clinical Correlate

Occasionally, **Rathke's pouch** can form an abnormal fluid-filled cyst, called a **Rathke's cleft cyst.** Although often asymptomatic, these cysts can enlarge enough to cause complications, such as loss of peripheral vision. In other cases, epithelial cells along the path of the hypophyseal diverticulum can form an abnormal growth called a **craniopharyngioma.** Although these tumors are usually benign, they can cause a variety of endocrine disorders associated with abnormal function of the pituitary gland.

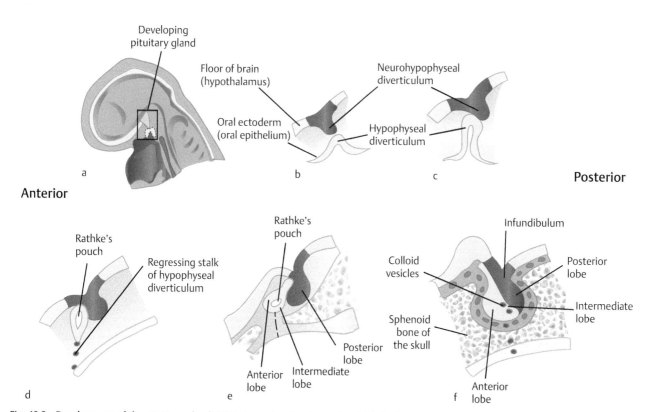

Fig. 40.3 **Development of the pituitary gland. (a)** Embryo showing tissues in which the lobes originate. **(b)** About 25 days, neurohypophyseal and hypophyseal diverticula begin to form. **(c)** About 29 days, diverticula come into contact. **(d)** About 36 days, stalk of hypophyseal diverticulum degenerates. **(e)** Anterior and intermediate lobes develop from the hypophyseal diverticulum of the oral cavity; posterior lobe and infundibulum develop from the neurohypophyseal diverticulum from the hypothalamus. **(f)** Mature pituitary.

40.3 Overview of the Pituitary Gland

Fig. 40.4 is a drawing showing the developed pituitary gland and associated hypothalamus. Note the anterior-posterior orientation is opposite to that in **Fig. 40.2** and **Fig. 40.3**. The optic chiasm and mammillary body of the brain are indicated for orientation. The posterior lobe does not separate from the floor of the brain (see **Fig. 40.3f**), so it is really an extension of the hypothalamus; neurons from hypothalamic nuclei send axons into the posterior lobe. As will be seen, the posterior lobe has a similar histologic appearance to neural tissue. The anterior lobe (and intermediate lobe) is derived from oral ectoderm, has a glandular appearance, and stains more darkly than the posterior lobe. The **median eminence** is a well-vascularized region of the floor of the hypothalamus that picks up stimulating hormones secreted by cells in the floor of the hypothalamus, which are carried to the anterior lobe (more on this later).

As shown in **Fig. 40.5**, a horizontal section through the pituitary gland (blue line) passes through the anterior and posterior lobes, but not through the infundibulum. At scanning magnification, the pituitary gland can be recognized by the juxtapositioning of the neural-like posterior lobe and the more glandular-appearing anterior lobe, often with colloid between them in the area of the intermediate lobe.

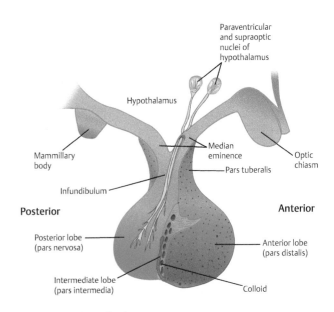

Fig. 40.4 **Pituitary gland.**

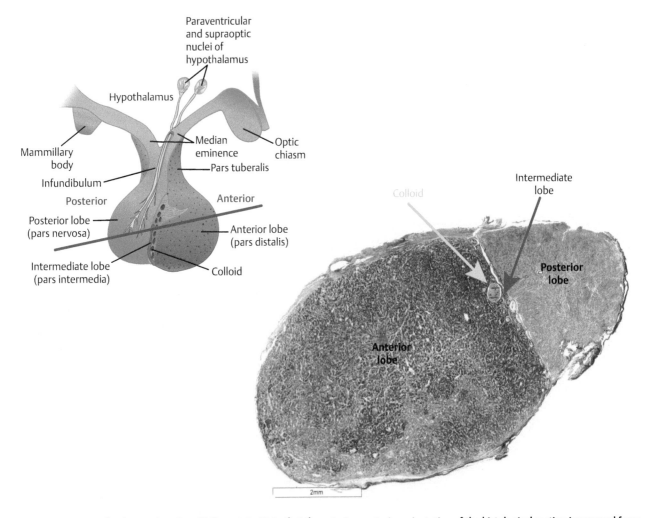

Fig. 40.5 **Pituitary gland, scanning view, Mallory stain. Note that the anterior-posterior orientation of the histological section is reversed from the drawing.**

Video 40.1   Pituitary gland overview

Be able to identify:
— Pituitary gland
  • Anterior lobe (adenohypophysis, pars distalis)
  • Posterior lobe (neurohypophysis, pars nervosa)
  • Intermediate lobe
  • Colloid

https://www.thieme.de/de/q.htm?p=opn/tp/308390101/978-1-62623-414-7_c040_v001&t=video

40.4   Anterior Lobe of the Pituitary Gland

The pituitary gland is often called the "master gland" because it secretes a large number of hormones, many of which are involved in regulating the function of other endocrine organs (e.g., the adrenal gland). The pituitary gland is largely under the influence of the hypothalamus.

40.4.1   Cell Types in the Anterior Lobe

There are several cell types in the **anterior pituitary**, which are listed here with the hormones they secrete:

1. **Somatotrophs** secrete **growth hormone** (*somatotropin*), which stimulates cell and tissue growth.
2. **Mammotrophs** (**lactotrophs**) secrete *prolactin*, which stimulates milk production in the breast.
3. **Corticotrophs** secrete *adrenocorticotropic hormone* (ACTH), which stimulates the adrenal cortex.
4. **Gonadotrophs** secrete *luteinizing hormone* (LH) and *follicle-stimulating hormone* (FSH), involved in reproduction.
5. **Thyrotrophs** secrete *thyroid-stimulating hormone*, which stimulates the thyroid gland.

These cell types can be specifically identified using antibodies to cell-type specific markers. In routine histologic stains, including H & E, PAS, and trichrome (Mallory) stains, the cell types in the anterior lobe of the pituitary can be classified into one of three categories:

• **Acidophils** (include somatotrophs and mammotrophs)
• **Basophils** (include corticotrophs, gonadotrophs, and thyrotrophs)
• **Chromophobes** (pale cytoplasm, may be cells that have recently released granule content)

Helpful Hint

One mnemonic used here is "SAM" (Somatotrophs are Acidophils and so are Mammotrophs); the rest of the cells are basophils.

Fig. 40.6 is an image of the anterior pituitary stained with a trichrome stain (called Mallory stain). With this stain, basophils (yellow arrows) are seen as large cells with a purple cytoplasm, and acidophils (blue arrows) are slightly smaller and have a cytoplasm that is orange to red. Chromophobes (green arrows) have a pale cytoplasm.

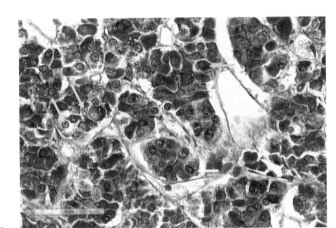

Fig. 40.6   Anterior lobe of the pituitary gland, high magnification, Mallory stain showing basophils (yellow arrows), acidophils (blue arrows), and chromophobes (green arrows).

Video 40.2   Pituitary gland showing cells of anterior lobe stained with Mallory trichrome

Be able to identify:
— Acidophils
— Basophils
— Chromophobes

https://www.thieme.de/de/q.htm?p=opn/tp/308390101/978-1-62623-414-7_c040_v002&t=video

Fig. 40.7 is an image of the anterior pituitary stained with PAS and counterstained with orange G. Hormones secreted by basophils are glycoproteins, so the granules in these cells are PAS+ (yellow arrows). Orange G is used as a counterstain that highlights acidophils (blue arrows). Chromophobes are identified by lack of cytoplasmic staining (green arrow; a cluster of chromophobes is outlined).

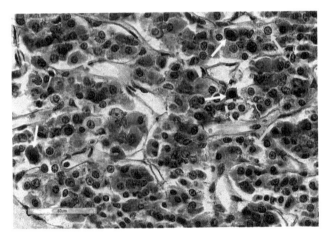

Fig. 40.7   Anterior lobe of the pituitary gland, high magnification, PAS and orange G stain, showing basophils (yellow arrows), acidophils (blue arrows), and chromophobes (green arrow and outline).

Video 40.3   Pituitary gland showing cells of anterior lobe stained with PAS

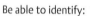

Be able to identify:
— Acidophils
— Basophils
— Chromophobes

https://www.thieme.de/de/q.htm?p=opn/tp/308390101/978-1-62623-414-7_c040_v003&t=video

Fig. **40.8** is an image of the anterior pituitary stained with H & E; red is eosinophilic and blue is basophilic. In this image, the staining is more subtle, so there are more cells that are difficult to identify with confidence. Nevertheless, a few good examples of basophils (yellow arrows), acidophils (blue arrows), and chromophobes (green arrow) can be identified.

Video 40.4   Pituitary gland showing cells of anterior lobe stained with H & E

Be able to identify:
— Acidophils
— Basophils
— Chromophobes

https://www.thieme.de/de/q.htm?p=opn/tp/308390101/978-1-62623-414-7_c040_v004&t=video

Helpful Hint

Different stains are used for the anterior pituitary because the difference between acidophils and basophils is sometimes subtle in H & E-stained images. However, note that, regardless of the stain, basophils are on the blue/purple side and acidophils are red/pink/orange.

As mentioned, routine histologic stains such as H & E can distinguish between acidophils and basophils, but they cannot identify specific cell types. Individual cell types can be differentiated using antibodies to the hormones secreted by each cell type. As an example, **Fig. 40.9** shows such a slide. Using immunocytochemical techniques, a brown reaction product is precipitated over somatotrophs, which secrete growth hormone, and a pink reaction product is produced near thyrotrophs, which secrete thyroid-stimulating hormone. This image as well as the

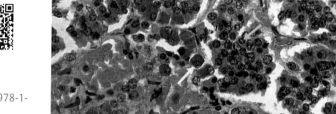

Fig. 40.8   Anterior lobe of the pituitary gland, high magnification, H & E stain, showing basophils (yellow arrows), acidophils (blue arrows), and chromophobes (green arrow).

preceding figures show that cell types in the anterior pituitary are not evenly distributed. This is particularly obvious in the scanning view in **Fig. 40.9**, which shows pink reaction product in the left and lower left regions and more brown precipitate in the right upper regions.

Video 40.5   Pituitary gland showing immunocytochemistry

https://www.thieme.de/de/q.htm?p=opn/tp/308390101/978-1-62623-414-7_c040_v005&t=video

Be able to:
— Describe the use of immunocytochemistry to identify specific cell types in the anterior pituitary

Helpful Hint

Abnormal growths of the pituitary gland, **pituitary adenomas**, are not uncommon. The abnormally growing cells may release excessive hormone, or they may impinge on other cells, reducing their activity. This results in a wide variety of hormonal disorders affecting growth, reproductive function, weight, and metabolism. In addition, the increased mass of the pituitary gland can compress the optic chiasm, resulting in peripheral visual loss. In addition, headaches are a common symptom.

40.4.2   Blood Supply to the Anterior Lobe

The anterior pituitary utilizes a *portal circulatory system*. In a portal system, such as that of the liver, there are two capillary beds in the systemic circuit to maximize delivery of specific substances from one organ to the other. In the **hypophyseal portal system**, shown in **Fig. 40.10**, the superior hypophyseal artery feeds blood to the first capillary bed in the median eminence and infundibulum, where it picks up releasing and inhibiting factors secreted by hypothalamic cells. These capillaries merge inferiorly to form the **hypophyseal portal veins**, which carry blood to the anterior lobe, where they branch into a second capillary

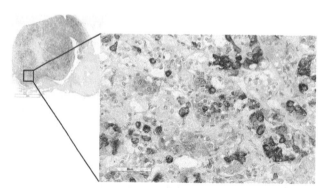

Fig. 40.9   Immunocytochemistry of the anterior lobe of the pituitary gland, labeling somatotrophs (brown) and thyrotrophs (pink).

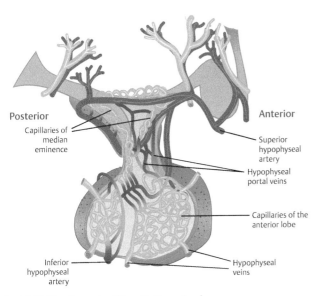

Posterior

Capillaries of
median
eminence

Anterior

Superior
hypophyseal
artery

Hypophyseal
portal veins

Capillaries of the
anterior lobe

Inferior
hypophyseal
artery

Hypophyseal
veins

Fig. 40.10 **Blood supply of the pituitary gland.**

bed. In this way, hypothalamic factors have a direct influence on secretory activity of cells in the anterior pituitary. For example, dopamine released by the hypothalamus inhibits the release of prolactin from mammotrophs in the anterior pituitary.

The capillaries in the anterior pituitary are **fenestrated sinusoids** (fenestrated sinuses):

- Fenestrated means that the endothelial cells have fenestrations.
- Sinusoids means the vessels have a wider diameter than most capillaries.

Fig. 40.11 is two images from the anterior pituitary, showing numerous sinusoids (one in each image is outlined) among the cells of the anterior pituitary. **Fig. 40.11a** is stained with H & E, showing red blood cells within the lumen of the sinusoid. In **Fig. 40.11b** stained with Mallory trichrome, red blood cells are not visible, but the trichrome stain highlights the vessel walls nicely, which are lined by simple squamous endothelial cells.

Light micrographs clearly demonstrate that these capillaries have a wide diameter and are thin-walled. However, fenestrations are not visible in light micrographs. For review, **Fig. 40.12** shows a comparison of types of capillaries (**Fig. 40.12a**) and an electron micrograph of a fenestrated capillary (**Fig. 40.12b**). Although the electron micrograph is from the pancreatic islet of

Langerhans, the endothelial cells of the sinusoids in the pituitary gland have a similar fenestrated structure.

Video 40.6   Pituitary gland showing fenestrated sinusoids (H & E)

https://www.thieme.de/de/q.htm?p=opn/tp/308390101/978-1-62623-414-7_c040_v006&t=video

Video 40.7   Pituitary gland showing fenestrated sinusoids (Mallory's trichrome)

Be able to identify:
— Sinusoids

https://www.thieme.de/de/q.htm?p=opn/tp/308390101/978-1-62623-414-7_c040_v007&t=video

40.5   Intermediate Lobe of the Pituitary Gland

As the name implies, the **intermediate lobe** (**pars intermedia**) is situated between the anterior and posterior lobes (see **Fig. 40.5**). **Fig. 40.13** is an image of the boundary between the anterior and posterior lobes, showing detail of the **colloid** and intermediate lobe (portion of this lobe is outlined). The cells of the intermediate lobe are, for the most part, similar to the cells in the anterior lobe. In humans, the intermediate lobe is not prominent, and the function of this region, if any, is not known.

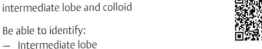

Video 40.8   Pituitary gland showing intermediate lobe and colloid

Be able to identify:
— Intermediate lobe
— Colloid

https://www.thieme.de/de/q.htm?p=opn/tp/308390101/978-1-62623-414-7_c040_v008&t=video

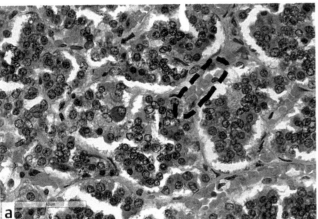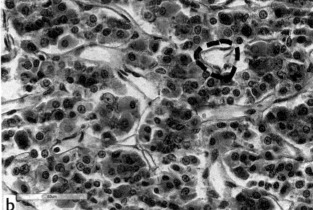

Fig. 40.11 **Fenestrated sinusoids in the anterior pituitary (outlined). (a) H & E stain. (b) Trichrome stain.**

a

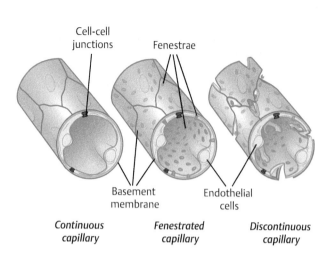

Continuous capillary   *Fenestrated capillary*   *Discontinuous capillary*

b

Fig. 40.12 Fenestrated capillaries. (a) Drawing showing the three types of capillaries. (b) Electron micrograph of a fenestrated capillary (from the endocrine pancreas), showing (1) fenestrated membrane with diaphragm; (2) Golgi apparatus; (3) endothelial cell nucleus; (4) mitochondrion; (5) endocrine cells (of the islets of Langerhans).

40.6   Posterior Lobe of the Pituitary Gland

There are two hormones produced by the **posterior pituitary**:

- *Antidiuretic hormone* (*ADH, vasopressin*) increases the permeability of the collecting ducts of the kidney, resulting in water retention, and also causes vasoconstriction; both effects raise blood pressure.

- **Oxytocin** stimulates smooth muscle contraction in the uterus during childbirth and the milk letdown reflex in the mammary glands.

These hormones are synthesized in neuronal cell bodies located in the hypothalamus (paraventricular and supraoptic hypothalamic nuclei, see **Fig. 40.4**). These cells of the hypothalamus send axons down through the infundibulum and into the posterior pituitary. Once synthesized, antidiuretic hormone and oxytocin are transported in vesicles down the axons of these cells, to be stored in synaptic termini (called **Herring bodies**). Signals received by the cell bodies in the hypothalamic nuclei result in action potentials that travel down the axons to trigger the release of ADH or oxytocin from the posterior pituitary.

> **Helpful Hint**
>
> No hormones are synthesized in the posterior pituitary; hormones released from the posterior pituitary are synthesized in the hypothalamus.

Fig. 40.14 is an image of the posterior pituitary stained with H & E. Because the posterior pituitary consists largely of unmyelinated axons, its appearance is quite similar to a peripheral nerve, with numerous pale eosinophilic threads. The neuronal cell bodies that belong to these axons are in the hypothalamus. The synaptic terminals (Herring bodies) of the neurons are not readily visible on this H & E-stained tissue. Most of the nuclei in this section belong to specialized glial cells called **pituicytes**.

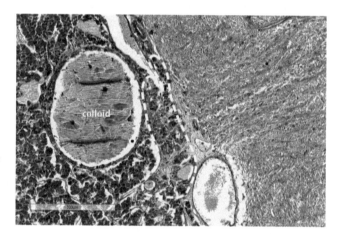

Fig. 40.13 Intermediate lobe of the pituitary gland (a portion is outlined) and colloid.

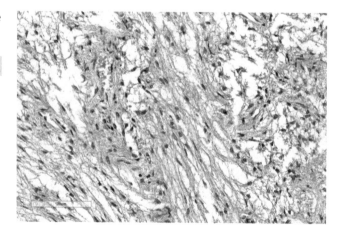

Fig. 40.14 Posterior lobe of the pituitary gland, H & E stain.

Video 40.9 Pituitary gland showing the posterior lobe (H & E)

Be able to identify:
— Posterior pituitary
— Pituicytes

https://www.thieme.de/de/q.htm?p=opn/tp/308390101/978-1-62623-414-7_c040_v009&t=video

Fig. 40.15 is an image of the posterior pituitary stained with PAS and counterstained with orange G. The synaptic accumulations within the posterior pituitary (Herring bodies) are PAS+ (outlined). Note that most are adjacent to blood vessels (blue arrows), where their contents can be released immediately into the bloodstream. The counterstain with orange G stains the red blood cells.

Video 40.10 Pituitary gland showing the posterior lobe (PAS)

Be able to identify:
— Posterior pituitary
— Herring bodies

https://www.thieme.de/de/q.htm?p=opn/tp/308390101/978-1-62623-414-7_c040_v010&t=video

40.7 Chapter Review

The pituitary gland is also called the "master gland" because it releases a large number of hormones, many of which regulate the function of other endocrine glands. The pituitary gland develops from the floor of the hypothalamus and the roof of the oral cavity, forming a glandular structure attached to the hypothalamus by the infundibulum. The pituitary gland consists of three parts: the anterior, intermediate, and posterior lobes. The anterior pituitary is the most diverse, consisting of at least five different cell types. Based on staining characteristics, these can be classified as either acidophils (mammotrophs and somatotrophs), basophils (corticotrophs, gonadotrophs, and thyrotrophs), or chromophobes (cells of the other types that have released their hormones). Immunocytochemical techniques can be used to

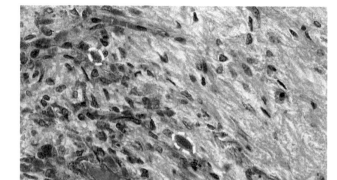

Fig. 40.15 **Posterior lobe of the pituitary gland, PAS and orange G stain, showing synaptic termini (Herring bodies, outlined) and blood vessels (blue arrows).**

stain cells according to their specific products. The blood supply to the anterior pituitary is a portal system. Hormones from the median eminence of the hypothalamus are delivered directly to the anterior pituitary through this portal system. The capillaries in the anterior pituitary are fenestrated sinusoids. The intermediate lobe is relatively inactive in humans and has histologic features of the anterior pituitary. Colloid is also present in the intermediate lobe in spaces that are remnants of Rathke's pouch. The hormones released by the posterior pituitary are synthesized by neurons whose cell bodies are in the hypothalamus. These hormones are transported down axons and stored in synaptic termini called Herring bodies, from which they are released. Glial cells in the posterior pituitary are called pituicytes. Because the posterior pituitary consists of axons and glial cells, it has the appearance of neural tissue.

Questions and Answers

An online-only section of questions and answers accompanying this chapter is hosted on Thieme's MedOne Education site: https://medone-education.thieme.com. Use the code on the media page at the front of this book to gain access. An institutional license to the site is required to access these questions in an interactive format, and individual users are required to register for an individual account to track results.

41   Adrenal Gland

After completing this chapter, you should be able to:
— Identify, at the light microscope level, each of the following:
- Adrenal gland (suprarenal glands)
    ◦ Cortex
        ▪ Zona glomerulosa
        ▪ Zona fasciculata
        ▪ Zona reticularis
    ◦ Medulla
        ▪ Medullary cells (chromaffin cells)
        ▪ Central vein
— Outline the function of each cell and structure listed
— Correlate the appearance of each cell type or structure with its function
— Describe the vasculature of the adrenal gland

41.1   Overview of the Adrenal Glands

As shown in **Fig. 41.1**, the **adrenal glands** (**suprarenal glands**) are situated above the kidneys in the posterior abdominal wall, surrounded by a connective tissue capsule and adipose tissue. Each adrenal gland is organized into an outer **cortex** and an inner **medulla**. These regions are distinct embryologically, histologically, and in terms of function:

1. The **adrenal cortex** is derived from **intermediate mesoderm** and secretes steroid hormones.
2. The **adrenal medulla** is derived from **neural crest cells** and secretes epinephrine and norepinephrine.

Fig. 41.2 shows two scanning images of adrenal glands. The border between the cortex and medulla is indicated by the series of arrows in both images.

Helpful Hint

Staining of adrenal glands varies, as shown by the two images in **Fig. 41.2** (both are H & E). The adrenal gland in **Fig. 41.2a** is more intensely basophilic overall, while the staining in **Fig. 41.2b** tends toward the eosinophilic side. Images from both preparations will be shown in the upcoming discussions.

Video 41.1   Adrenal gland overview–1

https://www.thieme.de/de/q.htm?p=opn/
tp/308390101/978-1-62623-414-7_c041_
v001&t=video

Video 41.2   Adrenal gland overview–2

https://www.thieme.de/de/q.htm?p=opn/
tp/308390101/978-1-62623-414-7_c041_
v002&t=video

Be able to identify:
— Adrenal gland
— Cortex
— Medulla

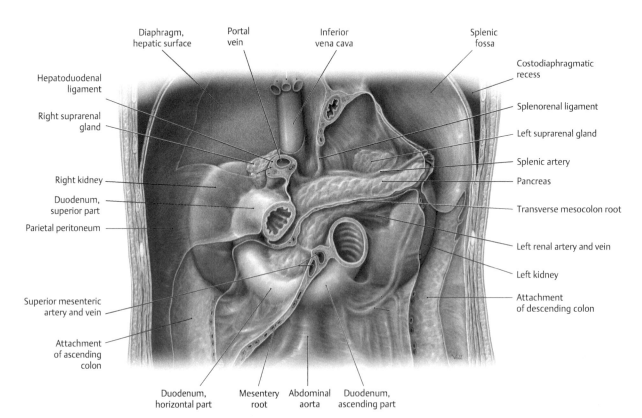

Fig. 41.1   Adrenal (suprarenal) glands. From Schuenke M, Schulte E, Schumacher U. *THIEME Atlas of Anatomy. Internal Organs.* Illustrations by Voll M and Wesker K. Second Edition. New York: Thieme Medical Publishers; 2016.

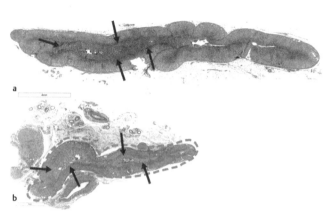

Fig. 41.2 (a, b) Adrenal glands, scanning magnification image. b includes surrounding connective tissue and other structures; the adrenal gland is outlined. In both a and b, the tips of the arrows indicate the border between the outer cortex and inner medulla.

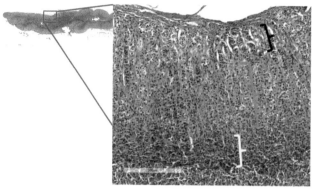

Fig. 41.3 Adrenal cortex. The three zones are indicated: zona glomerulosa (black bracket); zona fasciculata (blue bracket); zona reticularis (yellow bracket).

41.2 Adrenal Cortex

The adrenal cortex consists of three zones (**Fig. 41.3**):

1. The **zona glomerulosa** (black bracket) secretes **mineralocorticoids**, mainly **aldosterone**, which are involved in ion regulation (salt and water retention)
2. The **zona fasciculata** (blue bracket) secretes **glucocorticoids**, mainly **cortisol**, which increases blood sugar and suppresses the immune system.
3. The **zona reticularis** (yellow bracket) secretes weak androgens (male sex hormones).

The steroid-secreting cells in all three regions contain lipid droplets, so the cells are pale in H & E-stained sections (lipid is extracted away during tissue preparation). The zona fasciculata is often the palest, and the zona reticularis is more eosinophilic. Cells in the glomerulosa and, to a lesser extent, the reticularis tend to organize into round clusters, while cells in the fasciculata organize into columns.

Fig. 41.4 shows two high-magnification images of the zona fasciculata. The cells in this region are large (two are outlined) and are organized into columns oriented toward the adrenal medulla (more obvious in **Fig. 41.4a**). These cells contain numerous small lipid droplets (yellow arrows; individual droplets are better seen in **Fig. 41.4b**). The lipid droplets provide substrate for steroid hormone production. The lipid droplets wash away during tissue preparation, so all that

remains in the cytoplasm are threads of eosinophilia staining the remaining cytoplasmic components. The black arrows indicated fenestrated capillaries.

> **Helpful Hint**
>
> Cells of the zona fasciculata typically have more lipid droplets than cells of the zona glomerulosa or zona reticularis. Therefore, in low-magnification images (see **Fig. 41.3**, blue bracket), the zona fasciculata is typically paler than the other two regions. This is subtle, especially since the zona glomerulosa has clear spaces belonging to blood vessels. In addition, note the columnar organization of the cells in the zona fasciculata in **Fig. 41.3**, compared to the clusters of cells in the other regions.

Fig. 41.5 shows two images: one from the zona glomerulosa (**Fig. 41.5a**) and the other from the zona reticularis (**Fig. 41.5b**). Like the cells in the zona fasciculata, the cells in these regions also have lipid droplets that wash away on tissue preparation. However, in contrast to the zona fasciculata, cells of the zona glomerulosa and zona reticularis are smaller and form clusters instead of columns (the zona reticularis has some columnar organization). The cells of the zona glomerulosa (**Fig. 41.5a**) form more distinct clusters and tend to be the smallest cells of the three regions. The cells of the zona reticularis have few lipid droplets (**Fig. 41.5b**), so they exhibit more cytoplasmic eosinophilia than cells from the other two regions.

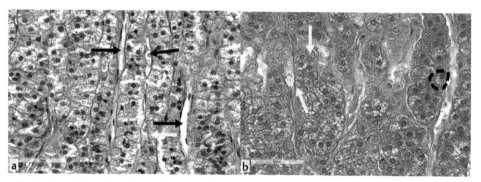

Fig. 41.4 (a, b) Zona fasciculata of the adrenal cortex from two different preparations. Individual cells (outlined) and lipid droplets (yellow arrows) are indicated. Fenestrated sinusoids are indicated by the black arrows.

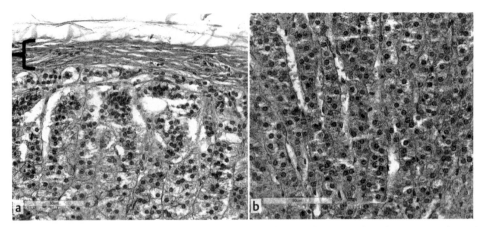

Fig. 41.5   (a) Zona glomerulosa and (b) zona reticularis of the adrenal cortex. The capsule surrounding the organ is indicated (bracket).

In the adrenal cortex, it is always useful to return to low-magnification images (**Fig. 41.3**). The small cells in the zona glomerulosa create a high nuclear density, giving that region an overall basophilic appearance (black bracket) with clusters. The zona reticularis has more cytoplasmic eosinophilia than the other two regions (yellow bracket) and forms less distinct clusters than the zona glomerulosa does. Nonetheless, in both of these regions, the cells form clusters, contrasting with the columns seen in the zona fasciculata (blue bracket).

Video 41.3   Adrenal cortex–1

https://www.thieme.de/de/q.htm?p=opn/
tp/308390101/978-1-62623-414-7_c041_
v003&t=video

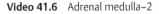

Video 41.4   Adrenal cortex–2

https://www.thieme.de/de/q.htm?p=opn/
tp/308390101/978-1-62623-414-7_c041_
v004&t=video

Be able to identify:
— Adrenal cortex
  • Zona glomerulosa
  • Zona fasciculata
  • Zona reticularis

Adrenal insufficiency, also known as **Addison disease**, is a disorder caused by destruction of the adrenal cortex. Although this primarily affects cortisol production, a decrease in mineralocorticoids can also occur. Decreased cortisol causes muscle weakness, fatigue, and weight loss. If aldosterone is involved, salt and water loss may result in hypotension.

41.3   Adrenal Medulla

The **adrenal medulla** (**Fig. 41.6**, bracket) is populated by cells of neural crest origin, called **chromaffin cells**, which secrete the catecholamines **epinephrine** and **norepinephrine**. In this image with more intense basophilic staining, the basophilia in these cells

is in contrast to the cells of the zona reticularis that flank it (above and below). The cells often appear disorganized and indistinct.

Fig. 41.7 shows high-magnification images of the adrenal medulla. The cells of the adrenal medulla are less organized than in the cortex. Although the cells vary in size, most cells have nuclei that are large and euchromatic (yellow arrows), while a few have nuclei that are smaller and heterochromatic (blue arrows). The staining in the cytoplasm can vary in different preparations; in **Fig. 41.7a** the cytoplasm is basophilic, while in **Fig. 41.7b** the cytoplasm is eosinophilic. In both preparations, areas of the cytoplasm are washed away (more obvious in **Fig. 41.7b**).

By itself, the adrenal medulla is not very distinct. In most cases, identification is made based on its location in the center of the adrenal gland.

Video 41.5   Adrenal medulla–1

https://www.thieme.de/de/q.htm?p=opn/
tp/308390101/978-1-62623-414-7_c041_
v005&t=video

Video 41.6   Adrenal medulla–2

https://www.thieme.de/de/q.htm?p=opn/
tp/308390101/978-1-62623-414-7_c041_
v006&t=video

Be able to identify:
— Adrenal medulla
— Medullary (chromaffin) cells

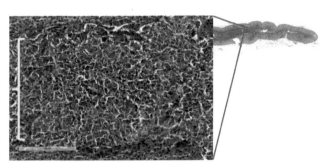

Fig. 41.6   Adrenal medulla (bracket), medium magnification.

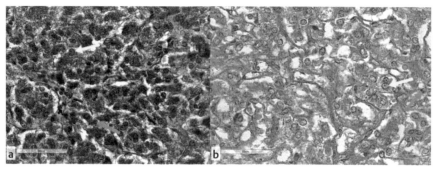

Fig. 41.7   **Adrenal medulla, high magnification, from two different preparations. (a) More basophilic stain. (b) More eosinophilia. Some cells exhibit large euchromatic nuclei (yellow arrows), while other cells have smaller nuclei (blue arrows).**

Basic Science Correlate: Gross Anatomy

The autonomic nervous system is a motor system that innervates visceral structures, namely cardiac muscle, smooth muscle, and glands. This system is a two-neuron chain. The first neuron, called the **preganglionic (presynaptic) neuron**, has a cell body in the brain or spinal cord and extends its axon to a ganglion, where it synapses with a **postganglionic (postsynaptic) neuron**. In most cases, the postganglionic neuron extends an axon to target cells. The cells of the adrenal medulla are equivalent to postganglionic sympathetic neurons, but they do not extend axons. Instead, these cells release their neurotransmitters into the bloodstream for a more widespread sympathetic response (the so-called "adrenalin rush" felt during heightened emotional responses).

The adrenal medulla receives both direct arterial blood (medullary arteriole) as well as blood that has percolated through the cortex, picking up steroid hormones (vessels on the left side of the drawing). Because of this circulatory arrangement, although the cortex and medulla are derived from different tissues embryologically and release distinct hormones, the secretions from the cortex have an influence on activity in the medulla.

The capillaries in the cortex match the organization of the surrounding cells, so there are convoluted vessels in the glomerulosa and parts of the reticularis and longitudinal vessels in the fasciculata. In **Fig. 41.4**, an image from the zona fasciculata of the adrenal cortex, several sinusoids are shown (black arrows) in longitudinal section, oriented in the same direction as the columns of cells in this region.

41.4   Blood Supply to the Adrenal Gland

Like all endocrine organs, the adrenal gland has a rich blood supply, highlighted by capillaries that are fenestrated (**Fig. 41.8**). In the adrenal cortex, as in the anterior pituitary, the capillaries have a wider diameter than other capillaries, so they are referred to as sinusoids.

Video 41.7   Adrenal gland showing sinusoids–1

https://www.thieme.de/de/q.htm?p=opn/tp/308390101/978-1-62623-414-7_c041_v007&t=video

Video 41.8   Adrenal gland showing sinusoids–2

Be able to identify:
— Fenestrated sinusoids

https://www.thieme.de/de/q.htm?p=opn/tp/308390101/978-1-62623-414-7_c041_v008&t=video

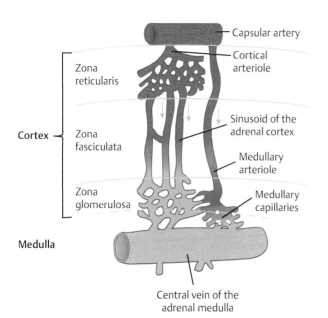

- Capsular artery
- Cortical arteriole
- Zona reticularis
- Cortex
- Zona fasciculata
- Sinusoid of the adrenal cortex
- Medullary arteriole
- Zona glomerulosa
- Medullary capillaries
- Medulla
- Central vein of the adrenal medulla

Fig. 41.8   **Blood supply of the adrenal gland.**

Another unusual feature of adrenal circulation is the **central vein** of the adrenal medulla (**central medullary vein**), which drains blood from the adrenal gland (see **Fig. 41.8**). Veins typically have very little smooth muscle. The central medullary vein, however, has thick bundles of smooth muscle oriented longitudinally (**Fig. 41.9**, outlined). Contraction of these muscles reduces the size of the adrenal gland; it is thought that this action enhances the release of adrenal hormones.

Video 41.9   Adrenal gland showing central medullary vein–1

https://www.thieme.de/de/q.htm?p=opn/tp/308390101/978-1-62623-414-7_c041_v009&t=video

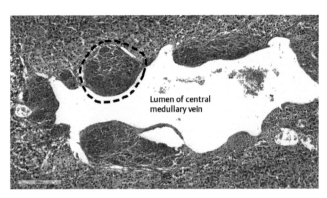

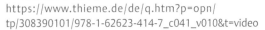

Fig. 41.9   **Central vein of the adrenal medulla. The lumen is indicated, and the thick, longitudinally oriented smooth muscle is outlined.**

Video 41.10 Adrenal gland showing central medullary vein–2

Be able to identify:
— Central medullary vein
https://www.thieme.de/de/q.htm?p=opn/
tp/308390101/978-1-62623-414-7_c041_v010&t=video

41.5   Chapter Review

The adrenal glands are located in the posterior abdominal wall, superior to the kidneys, so they are also called suprarenal glands. They are composed of an outer cortex, derived from intermediate mesoderm, and an inner medulla that develops from neural crest cells. The cortex synthesizes steroid hormones; therefore, the cells in the cortex contain lipid droplets, which are substrates for synthesis of these hormones. The cortex consists of three zones. The zona glomerulosa is composed of small cells that form clusters, so it is more basophilic than other regions of the adrenal cortex due to the relative abundance of nuclei.. Cells of the zona fasciculata are organized into columns, and the cells are paler because they contain abundant lipid droplets. Cells of the zona reticularis also form clusters and contain fewer lipid droplets than the other regions of the cortex, so they are more eosinophilic. The adrenal medulla, which secretes epinephrine and norepinephrine (which are not steroids), is less organized, and the cells are more variably stained. The blood supply to the cortex consists of fenestrated sinusoids. Blood flow to the medulla is either indirect from the capsular artery, percolating through these fenestrated sinusoids, or direct from the medullary arteriole, bypassing the cortex. The central vein of the adrenal medulla has large bundles of smooth muscle that contract to assist in squeezing hormone-laden blood from the gland into the circulation.

Questions and Answers

An online-only section of questions and answers accompanying this chapter is hosted on Thieme's MedOne Education site: https://medone-education.thieme.com. Use the code on the media page at the front of this book to gain access. An institutional license to the site is required to access these questions in an interactive format, and individual users are required to register for an individual account to track results.

42 Thyroid and Parathyroid Glands

After completing this chapter, you should be able to:
— Identify, at the light microscope level, each of the following:
  • Thyroid gland
    ◦ Follicle
      ▪ Colloid
      ▪ Follicular cells
      ▪ Parafollicular cells (C cells)
  • Parathyroid gland
    ◦ Chief cells
    ◦ Oxyphil cells
— Identify, at the electron microscope level, each of the following:
  • Thyroid gland
    ◦ Follicular cell
    ◦ Colloid
    ◦ Parafollicular cells (C cells)
— Outline the function of each cell and structure listed
— Correlate the appearance of each cell type or structure with its function
— Describe the synthesis, storage, and secretion of thyroid hormone

42.1 Overview of the Thyroid and Parathyroid Glands

The final endocrine organs to be discussed are the **thyroid** and **parathyroid glands**. The thyroid gland releases **thyroid hormones**, which are primarily involved in regulation of metabolism. The thyroid gland also contains specialized cells that release **calcitonin**, which decreases serum calcium. There are usually four parathyroid glands that release **parathyroid hormone**, which increase blood calcium.

Both organs are located in the neck but develop from the oral cavity. **Fig. 42.1a** shows an anterior view of the thyroid gland, situated anterior to the cricoid cartilage and upper trachea. **Fig. 42.1b** is a posterior view of the pharynx, showing the thyroid gland as it wraps around the trachea and pharynx. Embedded in the posterior aspect of the thyroid gland are the parathyroid glands.

42.2 Development of the Thyroid Gland

The thyroid gland develops from the **foramen cecum** of the tongue, a small depression located on the midline about two-thirds of the way back (**Fig. 42.2**). **Fig. 42.3** shows sagittal views of the developing embryo (**Fig. 42.3a–Fig. 4.23c**) and of the adult (**Fig. 42.3d**). The cranial end of the embryo is to the left (neck is flexed). Yellow is the lumen of the digestive tract: in this image, the future oral cavity and pharynx are shown. Epithelial cells migrate from the foramen cecum of the developing tongue to their final position anterior to the trachea. As they migrate, they remain temporarily connected to the foramen cecum by a **thyroglossal duct**, which normally degenerates. The migrating cells that become the thyroid gland come to lie anterior to the larynx and trachea.

Clinical Correlate

Cells of the thyroglossal duct may persist and form a **thyroglossal duct cyst**. These cysts present as a swelling on the midline of the neck, often associated with the hyoid bone. Treatment is by surgical removal of the cyst and middle portion of the hyoid bone (Sistrunk procedure).

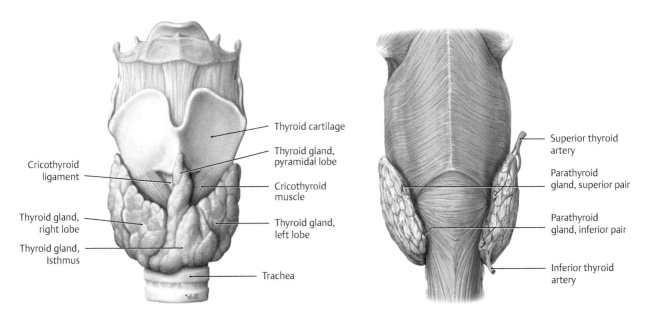

Fig. 42.1 **Thyroid and parathyroid glands in the neck. (a) Anterior view. (b) Posterior view. From Schuenke M, Schulte E, Schumacher U.** *THIEME Atlas of Anatomy. Head, Neck, and Neuroanatomy.* **Illustrations by Voll M and Wesker K. Second Edition. New York: Thieme Medical Publishers; 2016.**

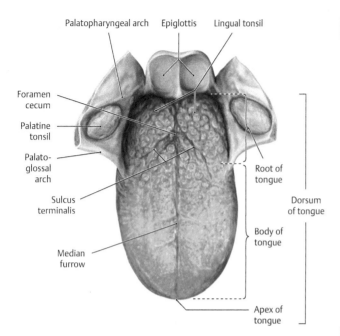

Fig. 42.2   **Dorsal surface of the tongue showing the foramen cecum.** From Schuenke M, Schulte E, Schumacher U. *THIEME Atlas of Anatomy. Head, Neck, and Neuroanatomy.* **Illustrations by Voll M and Wesker K. Second Edition. New York: Thieme Medical Publishers; 2016.**

42.3   Thyroid Gland

The epithelial cells of the thyroid gland organize into hundreds of **thyroid follicles** (**Fig. 42.4**, one follicle is outlined). Loose connective tissue between the follicles contains numerous blood vessels. The follicles are lined by epithelial **follicular cells** (or **principal cells**) and filled with **colloid**, which contains a precursor to mature **thyroid hormone** called **thyroglobulin**. Although many follicular cells are cuboidal (blue arrows), some are squamous (green arrows). The height of the cells is related to physiologic activity; in very active glands, follicular cells may be columnar. Cells with pale cytoplasm (black arrow) may be **clear cells** (**C cells**, **parafollicular cells**), which secrete **calcitonin**, though it is difficult to identify them definitively in routine H & E-stained tissues.

Follicular cells are epithelial, with their apical side facing the colloid and their basal side facing the connective tissue surrounding the follicles.

Video 42.1   Thyroid gland

Be able to identify:
— Thyroid gland
  • Colloid
  • Follicular cells
  • Clear cells (C cells or parafollicular cells, not definitively identified)
https://www.thieme.de/de/q.htm?p=opn/tp/308390101/978-1-62623-414-7_c042_v001&t=video

The main product of the thyroid gland, thyroid hormone, is produced by the follicular cells. In **Fig. 42.5** two follicular cells are shown. The cell to the left shows the exocytic pathway, while the cell on the right shows the endocytic pathway. Note that all follicular cells use both pathways; the division here is just for clarity.

Thyroid hormone synthesis begins with the production of thyroglobulin, a glycoprotein synthesized in the rough endoplasmic reticulum (RER), processed by the Golgi apparatus, and released into the colloid by exocytosis. Iodide is transported from the blood to the colloid using transport proteins (sodium/iodide symporter [NIS], pendrin) on the basal and apical membranes of the follicular cells. Enzymes on the microvilli convert iodide to iodine and enzymatically add it to tyrosine residues of thyroglobulin.

Upon stimulation by thyroid-stimulating hormone (TSH), thyroglobulin is brought back into follicular cell by endocytosis. Endocytic vesicles fuse with lysosomes, where thyroglobulin is degraded and the resulting iodinated tyrosine is released as thyroid hormones T_3 and T_4 into the bloodstream.

Fig. 42.6 is an electron micrograph of a portion of a thyroid follicle. The follicular cells are the three cells across the top (the left of the three indicated at 1 lacks a visible nucleus). Even at

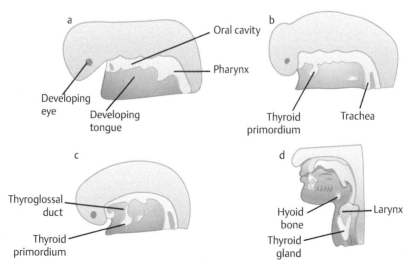

Fig. 42.3   **Development of the thyroid gland. A is a drawing of an early embryo showing the developing tongue in the oral cavity. The epithelium of the tongue near the foramen cecum proliferates, and migrates inferiorly (thyroid primordium, b and c). This primordium migrates to a final position anterior to the larynx to form the thyroid gland (d). The thyroglossal duct connecting the thyroid primordium to the tongue (c) normally degenerates.**

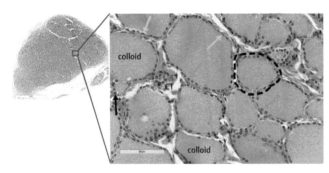

Fig. 42.4 The thyroid gland is composed of hundreds of follicles (one is outlined), each filled with colloid. Loose connective tissue (CT) is between each follicle. The epithelial cells (follicular cells) that line the follicles may be cuboidal (blue arrows) or squamous (green arrows). Clear cells may also be present (black arrow).

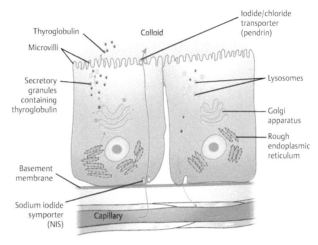

Fig. 42.5 Production of thyroid hormone. Thyroglobin is produced by the follicular cells, and exocytosed into the lumen (colloid), where it is iodinated and stored. Thyroid stimulating hormone stimulates endocytosis of iodinated thyroglobin, whch is degraded by lysosomes, and released as thyroid hormone (iodinated tyrosines).

this low magnification, the follicular cells demonstrate abundant RER (3) and prominent Golgi apparatuses (4). Colloid (2) containing thyroglobulin is in the lumen of the follicle, opposite the underlying connective tissue (6).

A clear cell (C cell, 5) can be seen in the basal aspect of this follicle. These cells secrete calcitonin and typically demonstrate numerous secretory vesicles in their basal aspect. Although the basal secretory vesicles are not abundant in this micrograph, this C cell can be recognized because it has significantly less RER than the follicular cells do.

42.4 Development of the Parathyroid Glands

Fig. 42.7 shows a posterior view of the oral-pharyngeal region of a developing embryo, with the posterior wall opened to show the floor of the oral cavity, including the developing tongue and pharynx. By way of review, the foramen cecum on the midline of the developing tongue is shown (**Fig. 42.7b**); **Fig. 42.7c** shows the migration of this thyroid tissue into the neck to form the thyroid gland (straight black arrow).

In the embryo there are grooves on the inside of the oral-pharyngeal cavity, called **pharyngeal pouches** (**Fig. 42.7a**). These are lined by endoderm, with underlying mesoderm. The parathyroid glands are derived from the third and fourth pharyngeal pouches. Cells from these regions migrate into the neck (curved black arrows)

and become embedded in the posterior aspect of the thyroid gland to form the parathyroid glands. This is similar to formation of the thymus, which is derived from the third pharyngeal pouches.

Usually, there are four parathyroid glands: a superior and an inferior gland on each side of the body (see **Fig. 42.1b**). In most cases, they are embedded in the posterior aspect of the thyroid gland. All are histologically similar.

Fig. 42.8 is a medium-power image of the parathyroid gland, which reveals that the parathyroid gland consists of two major cell types:

- **Chief (principal) cells** (not outlined) are more numerous, smaller, with a slightly eosinophilic cytoplasm and possibly some cytoplasmic basophilia. These cells release parathyroid hormone.

- **Oxyphil cells** (**outlined**) are less numerous, larger, and have a very eosinophilic cytoplasm because they have numerous mitochondria. They are found individually or clustered in groups as seen here. The function of these cells is unknown, yet their presence assists in identifying this organ.

The parathyroid gland typically has adipose tissue interspersed throughout; a few unilocular adipose cells are seen here.

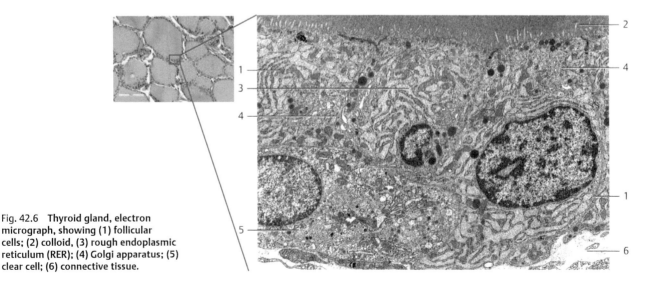

Fig. 42.6 Thyroid gland, electron micrograph, showing (1) follicular cells; (2) colloid, (3) rough endoplasmic reticulum (RER); (4) Golgi apparatus; (5) clear cell; (6) connective tissue.

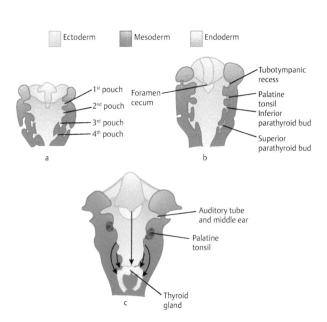

Fig. 42.7   **Development of structures derived from the pharyngeal pouches. The pharyngeal pouches line the oral and pharyngeal cavity in the developing embryo, and are numbered cranially to caudally (a). Cells lining the 3rd and 4th pharygeal pouches migrate into the neck (b,c) and become embedded in the thyroid gland to form the inferior and superior parathyroid glands, respectively.**

Helpful Hint

The overall basophilia of a region on a slide under low to medium power is often due to nuclear density. This is particularly useful in the parathyroid gland. In the regions where the smaller chief (principal) cells are located, the nuclei are closer together, giving an overall basophilic appearance. In regions of larger oxyphil cells, nuclei are further apart. This, in combination with the highly eosinophilic cytoplasm, gives those regions of the parathyroid gland intense eosinophilia.

Fig. 42.9 is a high-power image of the parathyroid gland; note that the nuclear density is highest in areas of smaller chief cells (left half of the image). Also, note the eosinophilia in the cytoplasm of oxyphil cells (right half of the image).

Video 42.2   Parathyroid gland

Be able to identify:
– Parathyroid gland
– Chief (principal) cells
– Oxyphil cells
https://www.thieme.de/de/q.htm?p=opn/tp/308390101/978-1-62623-414-7_c042_v002&t=video

42.5   Chapter Review

Both the thyroid and parathyroid glands are located in the neck but develop from the epithelium of the oral cavity. The thyroid gland is derived from the foramen cecum of the tongue. The thyroid gland is composed of thyroid follicles, lined by follicular cells and filled with colloid. The follicular cells synthesize the precursor to thyroid

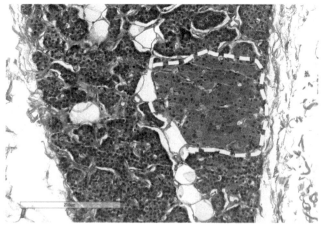

Fig. 42.8   **Parathyroid gland, medium magnification. Oxyphil cells are outlined.**

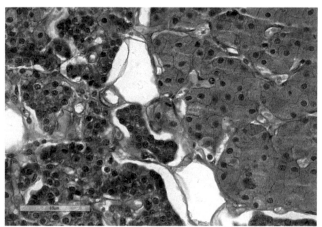

Fig. 42.9   **Parathyroid gland, high magnification.**

hormone, called thyroglobulin, and secrete it into the lumen of the follicles to be stored as colloid. Thyroglobulin is iodinated in the lumen of the follicle. Upon stimulation by thyroid-stimulating hormone, the cells take up thyroglobulin and degrade it in their lysosomes, releasing thyroid hormone. The thyroid gland also contains C cells (clear cells, parafollicular cells), recognized by their pale cytoplasm. C cells release calcitonin, which lowers blood calcium.

The parathyroid glands are derived from the third and fourth pharyngeal pouches. These glands (usually four of them) are embedded in the posterior aspect of the thyroid gland. The principal (or chief) cells of the parathyroid gland release parathyroid hormone, which raises blood calcium. Oxyphil cells in the parathyroid gland are large and have intense cytoplasmic eosinophilia due to numerous mitochondria. Although the function of oxyphil cells is unknown, they are distinct cells that aid in identifying the parathyroid gland.

Questions and Answers

An online-only section of questions and answers accompanying this chapter is hosted on Thieme's MedOne Education site: https://medone-education.thieme.com. Use the code on the media page at the front of this book to gain access. An institutional license to the site is required to access these questions in an interactive format, and individual users are required to register for an individual account to track results.

43   Testes and Genital Ducts

After completing this chapter, you should be able to:
— Identify, at the light microscope level, each of the following:
   • Testis
      ○ Regions
         ▪ Tunica albuginea
         ▪ Mediastinum testis
         ▪ Seminiferous tubules
      ○ Cell types
         ▪ Germ cells
            – Spermatogonia
            – Primary spermatocytes
            – Secondary spermatocytes (not seen on most images)
            – Spermatids
            – Spermatozoa
         ▪ Sertoli cells
         ▪ Leydig cells
         ▪ Myoid cells
      ○ Ducts associated with testis
         ▪ Rete testis
         ▪ Efferent ductules
         ▪ Epididymis
         ▪ Vas deferens (ductus deferens)
            – Spermatic cord
            – Cremaster muscle
            – Testicular artery
            – Pampiniform plexus of veins
— Identify, at the electron microscope level, each of the following:
   • Spermatid
      ○ Nucleus
      ○ Acrosome
      ○ Flagella
      ○ Mitochondria
— Outline the function of each cell and structure listed
— Correlate the appearance of each cell type or structure with its function
— Describe gametogenesis in the male
— Describe the structure and role of the blood-testis barrier

43.1   Overview of the Reproductive Systems

The overall goal of the male and female reproductive systems is to make more humans. This is carried out by organs specialized to produce cells called **gametes** (sperm and egg), which are products of a type of cell division called **meiosis**. The reproductive systems are also designed to facilitate the coming together and fusion of gametes, a process called **fertilization**. In addition, the female reproductive system provides a supportive environment for the development of the resulting fertilized product.

This next series of chapters will describe the male and female reproductive systems. The first two chapters in this series describe the male reproductive system; the final four address the female reproductive system. Before beginning a discussion of these reproductive systems, it is useful to provide an overview of mitosis and meiosis.

43.2   Overview of Mitosis and Meiosis

A **genome** is a complete set of an individual's **genes**. Human cells carry two copies of the genome; one copy inherited from the mother and the other inherited from the father (**Fig. 43.1**). These genes are located on **chromosomes**, which are composed of DNA and protein and contain a central **centromere** and a **chromatid** that has two arms. Each cell contains two copies of each chromosome; again, one from the mother, one from the father. Pairs of chromosomes are referred to as **homologous chromosomes**. In **Fig. 43.1**, the two blue chromosomes are homologous because their chromatids are the same size, and they have similar genes along the length of these chromatids. By the same token, the two green chromosomes are also a homologous pair.

Human cells have 23 pairs of chromosomes, for a total of 46. However, for simplicity, **Fig. 43.1** and subsequent drawings show a cell with only two pairs of chromosomes (four chromosomes total). Also, only the nucleus of each cell is shown.

43.2.1   Mitosis

Cell division in most tissues occurs through **mitosis** (**Fig. 43.2**). During the **S phase** of the cell cycle (see **Chapter 2**), the genome is duplicated. When this occurs, each **chromatid** is duplicated, but the centromeres are not, and the duplicated chromatids remain attached at the centromere. Division through mitosis involves duplication of the centromere and separation of the chromatids on each chromosome, one going to each cell. After mitosis, the two resulting cells have the same genetic complement as the original cell.

Mitosis is used for growth of tissues, cell turnover, and tissue regeneration.

43.2.2   Meiosis

Meiosis is used for sexual reproduction. Meiosis begins in the same way as mitosis, with the S phase duplicating the genome (**Fig. 43.3**). However, meiosis has two cell divisions: **meiosis I** and **meiosis II**. In meiosis I, homologous chromosomes separate,

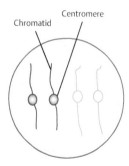

Fig. 43.1   **Schematic drawing of the nucleus of a theoretical human cell. For simplicity, only four chromosomes are shown. Homologous chromosomes are shown in the same color; for each pair, one of these chromosomes came from the mother, the other from the father. Humans have a total of 46 chromosomes (23 pairs).**

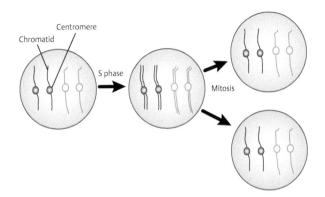

Fig. 43.2   Mitosis. Cells prepare for division by duplicating the genome during the S phase of the cell cycle. During mitosis, the centromere is duplicated so that chromatid copies can move into separate cells. The resulting progeny contain the same genetic complement as the original cell.

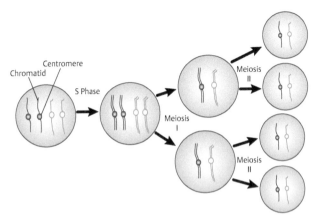

Fig. 43.3   Meiosis. Like mitosis, preparation for meiosis includes duplication of the genome during S phase. There are two divisions in meiosis. In meiosis I, homologous chromosomes move to different cells. Meiosis II is similar to mitosis; duplication of centromeres allows the chromatids to move to different cells.

so that the resulting cells have half the number of chromosomes; each chromosome is composed of two chromatids attached at the centromere. Meiosis II is similar to mitosis because the centromeres duplicate and the two chromatids on a chromosome separate into different cells. The end result of meiosis is that each cell has only one copy of the genome. These cells will fuse with a similar cell from the opposite sex to create a new cell that has two copies of the genome and will grow into a new individual.

Basic Science Correlate: Genetics

Due to independent assortment and crossing over, the products of meiosis produced by an individual are genetically different. The details of independent assortment and crossing over are beyond the scope of this publication, but, in essence, they involve shuffling of an individual's genome during meiosis.

43.3   Spermatogenesis

Spermatogenesis—that is, the production of spermatozoa—begins at puberty and, in most cases, continues throughout the lifetime of the individual (**Fig. 43.4**). Because meiosis is a terminal division (that is, a cell that proceeds through meiosis cannot divide again), a stem cell population of cells, called **spermatogonia**, divide mitotically to generate progeny that can then enter meiosis. Cells that enter meiosis in the male go through the following stages:

1. **Primary spermatocyte**: a cell that has gone through S phase and has begun meiosis (i.e., is in **meiosis I**)
2. **Secondary spermatocyte**: a cell that has completed the first meiotic division (i.e., is in **meiosis II**)
3. **Spermatid**: a cell that has completed meiosis but has not transformed into a mature spermatozoon
4. **Spermatozoon**: a cell that is genetically identical to a spermatid but has undergone physical transformations, including nuclear condensation, loss of excess cytoplasm, and generation of a flagellum and acrosome

---

Helpful Hint

Note that when a spermatogonium divides to produce two cells, one of the cells "stays behind"; it does not enter meiosis but divides again by mitosis. Since meiosis is a terminal division, this is necessary to ensure continued production of spermatozoa.

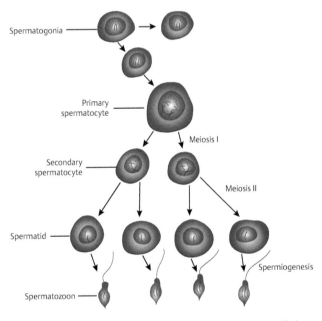

Fig. 43.4   Spermatogenesis. Cells that divide mitotically are called spermatogonia; these divisions continually produce cells that enter meiosis. Cells in meiosis I are called primary spermatocytes; cells in meiosis II are called secondary spermatocytes. The final products of meiosis in the male are called spermatids, which remodel to form spermatozoa.

As shown in **Fig. 43.4**, the final products of meiosis in males, the spermatids, are round cells. These cells undergo a transformation called **spermiogenesis** to produce **spermatozoa**, cells that are streamlined for movement through the female reproductive tract and able to fuse with the ovulated oocyte. The main features of the resulting spermatozoa include (**Fig. 43.5**):

- An **acrosome** (2), a large organelle adjacent to the nucleus, filled with digestive enzymes, similar to a lysosome; the acrosome enzymes break apart the corona radiata and zona pellucida of the egg during fertilization
- A condensed nucleus (3)
- Numerous mitochondria within a sheath (7)
- Axoneme (microtubules) of a **flagellum** (10)

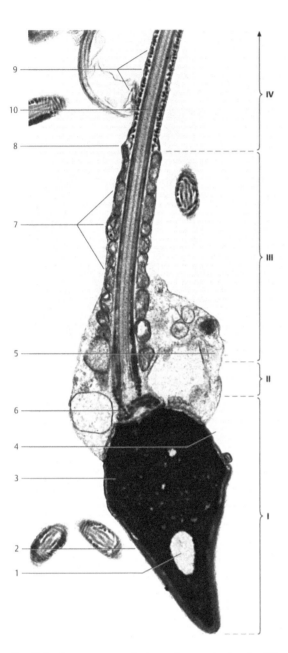

Fig. 43.5 **Spermatozoon, electron micrograph, showing (1) nuclear vesicle; (2) acrosome; (3) condensed nucleus; (4) postacrosomal region; (5) cytoplasmic droplet; (6) connecting piece; (7) numerous mitochondria within sheath; (8) annulus; (9) fibrous sheath; (10) axoneme (microtubules) of flagellum**

43.4 Overview of the Male Reproductive System

Major structures of the male reproductive system that serve in production and transmission of spermatozoa include (**Fig. 43.6**):

- The **testis** or **testicle** produces spermatozoa; it is housed in the **scrotum**.
- The **epididymis** provides for storage and maturation of spermatozoa.
- The **ductus deferens** or **vas deferens** transports spermatozoa to the prostatic urethra during arousal.
- The male **urethra** has three parts—prostatic, membranous, and penile—named for the structures surrounding the urethra.

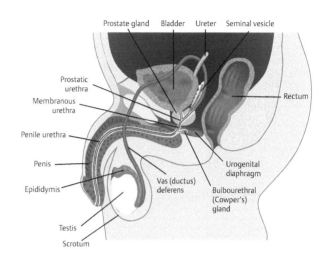

Fig. 43.6 **Male reproductive system.**

The **urogenital diaphragm** is a thin sheet of mostly skeletal muscle that includes the external urethral sphincter. "Membranous" refers to the part of the urethra that passes through the urogenital diaphragm. The membranous urethra is about 1 cm in length.

The male reproductive system also includes accessory glands that are adjacent to the main pathway for spermatozoa. These accessory glands secrete fluids (**Fig. 43.6**):

- The **seminal vesicles** (or **seminal glands**, one on each side) produce 65% of **semen**; the duct of each seminal vesicle joins with the vas deferens to become the **ejaculatory duct**, which passes through the prostate to drain into the prostatic urethra.
- The **prostate gland** produces 30% of semen and surrounds the prostatic urethra.
- The **bulbourethral (Cowper's) gland** secretes mucus during arousal for lubrication of the urethra.

The accessory glands and the penis will be covered in the next chapter. This chapter will begin with the testes, the organs that produce spermatozoa. This will be followed by a discussion of the ducts that carry mature spermatozoa toward the urethra: rete testis, efferent ductules, epididymis, and vas (ductus) deferens.

43.5 Overview of the Testes

The testes are housed in a pouch of skin called the scrotum. Each testis (**Fig. 43.7**) is bounded by an outer dense irregular connective tissue called the **tunica albuginea**. The posterior aspect of the tunica albuginea is thickened and is referred to as the **mediastinum testis (testicular mediastinum)** because it projects toward the middle of the testis.

Each testis contains hundreds of **seminiferous tubules**; the inner lining of these tubules is an epithelium containing **spermatogenic cells** and supportive **Sertoli cells**. The spermatogenic cells are the aforementioned cells undergoing mitosis and meiosis to produce mature spermatozoa. The seminiferous tubules are surrounded by loose connective tissue containing blood vessels and testosterone-secreting **Leydig cells**.

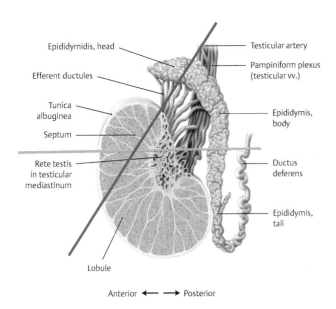

Fig. 43.7   **Testis and associated structures. The two colored lines indicate the planes of the sections through the testis and associated structures that will be seen in the following figures. Based on the work of Schuenke M, Schulte E, Schumacher U.** *THIEME Atlas of Anatomy. Head, Neck, and Neuroanatomy.* **Illustrations by Voll M and Wesker K. Second Edition. New York: Thieme Medical Publishers; 2016.**

Fig. 43.8 shows a scanning view of a horizontal section through the testis (yellow line in **Fig. 43.7**). This section includes the testis and surrounding tunica albuginea and passes through the mediastinum testis (yellow outline), epididymis (blue outline), and vas deferens (green outline). Surrounding the epididymis and vas deferens is connective tissue.

Video 43.1   Testis overview (horizontal section)

Be able to identify:
— Testis
— Tunica albuginea
— Mediastinum testis
— Other structures (epididymis, vas deferens) generally, just to get oriented

https://www.thieme.de/de/q.htm?p=opn/tp/308390101/978-1-62623-414-7_c043_v001&t=video

Fig. 43.9 is a scanning view of an oblique section through the testis (red line in **Fig. 43.7**). This section includes the testis, efferent ductules (black outline), and epididymis (blue outline). The tunica albuginea (arrows) encapsulates the testis; the mediastinum testis is not in this plane of section.

Video 43.2   Testis overview (oblique section)

Be able to identify:
— Testis
— Tunica albuginea
— Other structures (efferent ductules, vas deferens) generally, just to get oriented

https://www.thieme.de/de/q.htm?p=opn/tp/308390101/978-1-62623-414-7_c043_v002&t=video

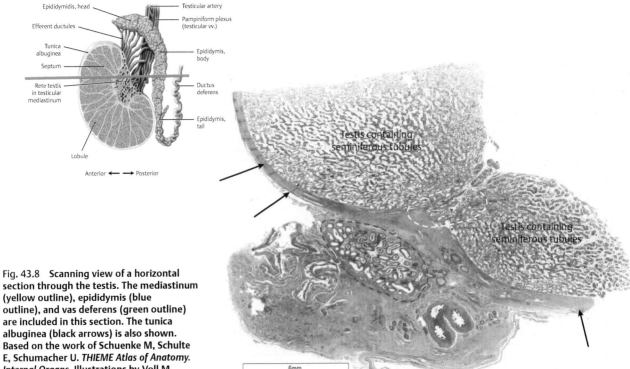

Fig. 43.8   **Scanning view of a horizontal section through the testis. The mediastinum (yellow outline), epididymis (blue outline), and vas deferens (green outline) are included in this section. The tunica albuginea (black arrows) is also shown. Based on the work of Schuenke M, Schulte E, Schumacher U.** *THIEME Atlas of Anatomy. Internal Organs.* **Illustrations by Voll M and Wesker K. Second Edition. New York: Thieme Medical Publishers; 2016.**

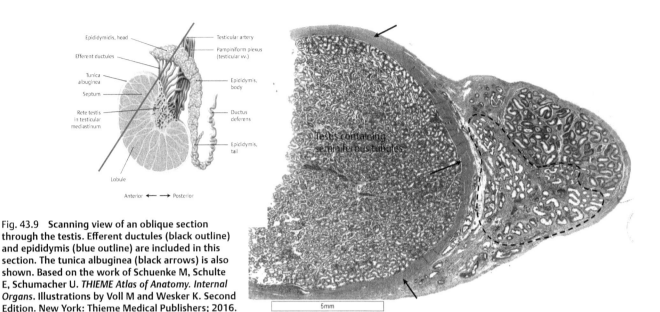

Fig. 43.9   **Scanning view of an oblique section through the testis. Efferent ductules (black outline) and epididymis (blue outline) are included in this section. The tunica albuginea (black arrows) is also shown.** Based on the work of Schuenke M, Schulte E, Schumacher U. *THIEME Atlas of Anatomy. Internal Organs.* Illustrations by Voll M and Wesker K. Second Edition. New York: Thieme Medical Publishers; 2016.

The previous images and associated videos were presented simply for orientation to the specific slides that were used to generate future images and videos. They also provide a sense of the gross anatomy of structures in the scrotum. Sections of these tissues from other sources may be in different orientations.

43.6   Seminiferous Tubules

As mentioned, each testis contains hundreds of **seminiferous tubules**, which produce spermatozoa. **Fig. 43.10** is an image of a testis taken at medium magnification, showing about six seminiferous tubules (one indicated by the double arrow). Seminiferous tubules consist of an epithelium; the basement membrane of two of these tubules is indicated by the arrows. The connective tissue between the tubules contains steroid-secreting Leydig cells (described subsequently; one cluster of Leydig cells is outlined).

Fig. 43.11 highlights a single seminiferous tubule, which consists of an epithelium, with the basement membrane (arrows) and lumen indicated. Between tubules is connective tissue containing Leydig cells.

Fig. 43.12 is a drawing of a region of the seminiferous tubule (within the rectangle), showing the cells of the testes. By way of overview, note the following:

- Spermatogonia (cells in mitosis) remain close to the basement membrane. Developing spermatozoa, including primary spermatocytes and spermatids, move toward the lumen as they progress through meiosis. Meiosis II progresses rapidly, so secondary spermatocytes are rarely seen.

- Supportive Sertoli cells surround the spermatogenic cells; the cytoplasm of Sertoli cells is extensive. Sertoli cells form tight junctions with neighboring Sertoli cells, just above the spermatogonia, creating a **blood-testis barrier**. Before spermatogenic cells begin meiosis, they pass between the Sertoli cells to the apical side of this barrier, where they are protected from cells of the immune system.

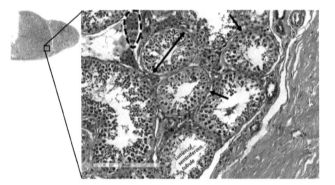

Fig. 43.10 **Testis, medium magnification, showing seminiferous tubules (one indicated by the double arrow), basement membrane (arrows), and a cluster of Leydig cells (outlined) in the surrounding connective tissue.**

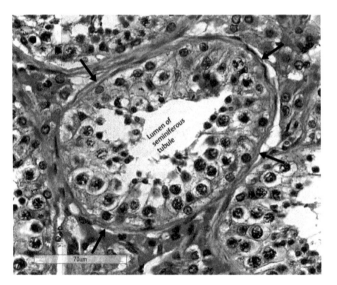

Fig. 43.11 **Seminiferous tubule, medium-high magnification. The lumen and basement membrane (arrows) of the epithelium of the seminiferous tubule are indicated.**

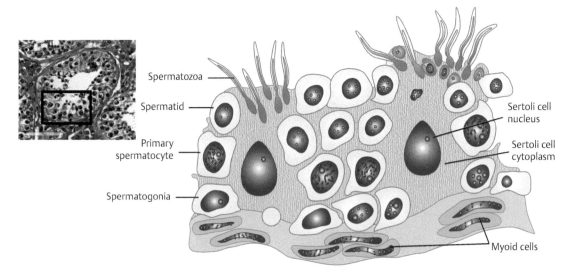

Spermatozoa

Spermatid

Primary spermatocyte

Spermatogonia

Sertoli cell nucleus

Sertoli cell cytoplasm

Myoid cells

Fig. 43.12 Drawing of a portion of the wall of a seminiferous tubule. Each seminiferous tubule is an epithelium. Spermatogonia are basal cells, and as cells progress through meiosis, they move toward the lumen, and are ultimately released. Sertoli cells support the developing spermatogenic cells. Myoid cells in the connective tissue have a contractile function.

- **Myoid cells** are connective tissue cells that have some contractile function; they are found adjacent to or within the thick basement membrane.

The following discussion provides details of the specific cell types in the testes.

43.6.1   Sertoli Cells

Sertoli cells are supporting cells for the developing spermatogenic cells. As mentioned, they create the blood-testis barrier, protecting developing spermatozoa from the immune system. As shown in **Fig. 43.13**, Sertoli cells are characterized by a large euchromatic nucleus, with a prominent nucleolus, and extensive cytoplasm that spans from the basement membrane all the way to the lumen of the tubule. Their nuclei are usually positioned in the "second" row from the basement membrane (staggering of nuclei results in indistinct and uneven rows).

   Fig. 43.14 shows two images that are enlargements of **Fig. 43.13**, focusing on a single Sertoli cell. The nuclear envelope (**Fig. 43.14a**, yellow arrows) and nucleolus (blue arrow) of the Sertoli cell are indicated. **Fig. 43.14b** shows at least part of the cytoplasm of this Sertoli cell (labeled between the dotted lines).

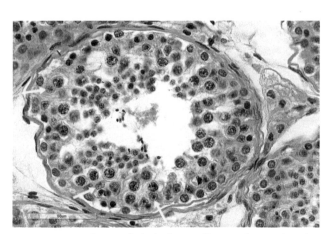

Fig. 43.13 Seminiferous tubule, high magnification, showing Sertoli cells (arrows).

The outer outline in **Fig. 43.14b** is an approximation based on the location of neighboring cells and provides an indication of the extent of the cytoplasm of Sertoli cells. The exact boundary of this cell is not critical to identify. However, it is important to understand that Sertoli cell cytoplasm is extensive and that neighboring Sertoli cells make contact with each other and form the tight junctions responsible for the blood-testis barrier. In addition, Sertoli cells surround spermatogenic cells throughout and play a role in degradation of excess cytoplasm shed during the process of spermiogenesis (see **Fig. 43.4**).

Video 43.3   Sertoli cells (horizontal section through the testes)

https://www.thieme.de/de/q.htm?p=opn/tp/308390101/978-1-62623-414-7_c043_v003&t=video

Video 43.4   Sertoli cells (oblique section through the testes)

https://www.thieme.de/de/q.htm?p=opn/tp/308390101/978-1-62623-414-7_c043_v004&t=video

Be able to identify:
— Sertoli cells

Basic Science Correlate: Embryology

Sertoli cells also play a role in development by secreting a hormone called *antiMüllerian hormone*. All male and female embryos develop primordial structures for both sexes. In males, *antiMüllerian hormone*, produced by Sertoli cells, inhibits further development of the female reproductive tract (oviducts, uterus).

Fig. 43.14 **Seminiferous tubule, high magnification, pseudomagnification to highlight a Sertoli cell. (a) Nuclear envelope (yellow arrows) and nucleolus of a Sertoli cell. (b) Two outlines indicate the nuclear envelope and approximate location of the plasma membrane, showing the extent of the cytoplasm of this Sertoli cell.**

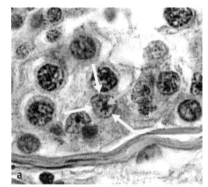
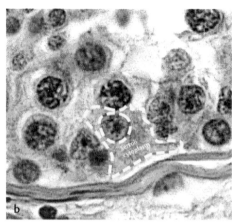

43.6.2 Developing Spermatozoa

Recall that developing spermatozoa (spermatogenic cells) are part of the epithelium of the seminiferous tubules. Mitotically active cells (spermatogonia) are located at the basal aspect of the epithelium, close to the basement membrane. As the progeny of these cells enter meiosis, they progress toward the lumen, so that the mature spermatozoa are closest to the lumen. Before spermatogenic cells begin meiosis, they pass between Sertoli cells to the apical side of the blood-testis barrier.

In a sense, this apical progression is not much different from the development of cells in other epithelia (e.g., skin, sebaceous glands). The only difference here is that cells progress through meiosis as they progress toward the surface.

- Spermatogonia (**Fig. 43.15**, black arrows) are adjacent to the basement membrane. Although the density of their nuclei varies somewhat, they often lack an easily recognizable nucleolus and do not have "clumpy" chromatin as primary spermatocytes do.
- Primary spermatocytes (**Fig. 43.15**, red arrows) are on the luminal (apical) side of Sertoli cells and have a larger nucleus than those of spermatogonia that contains "clumpy" chromatin. A thin rim of cytoplasm may be evident but is often not seen.
- Because meiosis II proceeds quickly, secondary spermatocytes are not typically seen.
- The products of meiosis, spermatids, are small cells with small, round nuclei (**Fig. 43.15**, blue arrows). As they mature into spermatozoa, the nucleus condenses, becoming smaller and narrower (green arrows). Note that throughout this condensation, they are still called spermatids; mature spermatozoa are released into the lumen.

Spermatozoa are released into the lumen immediately upon maturation; therefore, they will be seen free within the lumen, and not part of the epithelium as are the spermatids in **Fig. 43.15**. It is likely that even the ones that appear in the lumen in this image are still part of the epithelium, having been separated from the epithelium during tissue preparation.

Fig. 43.16 is another image showing all these cell types for reinforcement. Notice the large number of spermatids in this seminiferous tubule (green outline). Complete spermatogenesis (from spermatogonia to mature spermatozoa) takes approximately 74 days in humans and occurs in "waves" in different regions of the tubules. Therefore, it is not unusual to see a seminiferous tubule with a large number of one cell type, and not all sections will demonstrate all cell types.

Video 43.5 Developing spermatozoa (oblique section)

https://www.thieme.de/de/q.htm?p=opn/
tp/308390101/978-1-62623-414-7_c043_
v005&t=video

Video 43.6 Developing spermatozoa (horizontal section)

https://www.thieme.de/de/q.htm?p=opn/
tp/308390101/978-1-62623-414-7_c043_
v006&t=video

Be able to identify:
- Spermatogonia
- Primary spermatocytes
- Spermatids

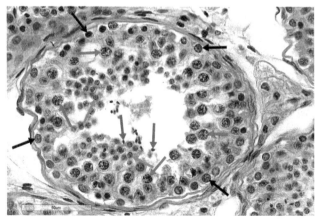

Fig. 43.15 **Seminiferous tubule, high magnification, showing spermatogenic cells: spermatogonia (black arrows), primary spermatocytes (red arrows), spermatids (blue arrows), and spermatids that are nearly spermatozoa (green arrows).**

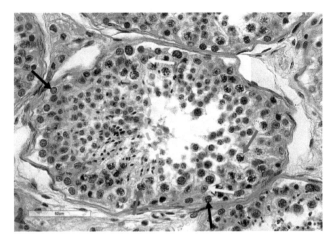

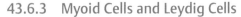

Fig. 43.16 **Seminiferous tubule, high magnification, showing Sertoli cells (yellow arrows) and spermatogenic cells: spermatogonia (black arrows), primary spermatocytes (red arrows), and spermatids in various stages (green outline).**

43.6.3   Myoid Cells and Leydig Cells

The interstitial connective tissue of the testis contains myoid cells and Leydig cells. Myoid cells are specialized connective tissue cells that are similar to smooth muscle cells. They synthesize some of the extracellular components (e.g., collagen) of connective tissue, but they also produce mild peristaltic contractions that move mature spermatozoa toward the ducts. Myoid cells are recognized by their flattened nuclei on the connective tissue side of the basement membrane of seminiferous tubules (**Fig. 43.17**, arrows).

> **Helpful Hint**
>
> **Myoepithelial cells** (e.g., in the sweat glands, mammary glands) are also contractile and have a flattened nucleus. However, myoepithelial cells arise from the epithelium and, therefore, are on the epithelial side of the basement membrane.

Leydig (interstitial) cells (**Fig. 43.18**, outlined) secrete testosterone, a steroid hormone. Although steroid-secreting cells are typically pale in H & E sections due to removal of lipid precursors on tissue preparation, Leydig cells are a notable exception. Although many are indeed pale, most exhibit a fairly intense cytoplasmic eosinophilia. Leydig cells have extensive smooth endoplasmic reticulum, which is involved in testosterone synthesis.

> **Helpful Hint**
>
> Recall that cytoplasmic eosinophilia is also a feature of androgen-secreting cells of the zona reticularis of the adrenal gland.

Video 43.7   Myoid cells and Leydig cells (oblique section)

https://www.thieme.de/de/q.htm?p=opn/ tp/308390101/978-1-62623-414-7_c043_ v007&t=video

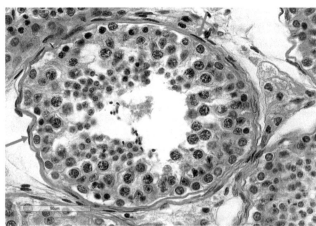

Fig. 43.17 **Seminiferous tubule, high magnification, showing myoid cells (arrows).**

Video 43.8   Myoid cells and Leydig cells (horizontal section)

Be able to identify:
— Myoid cells
— Leydig cells

https://www.thieme.de/de/q.htm?p=opn/tp/308390101/978-1-62623-414-7_c043_v008&t=video

> **Clinical Correlate**
>
> Testicular cancers typically present as a nodular mass within the testes. Malignancy may bring about other symptoms including back pain, gastrointestinal distress, and dyspnea. It most commonly occurs in men between the ages of 20 and 39, and it has a high cure rate. Testicular self-exam is an important screening tool.

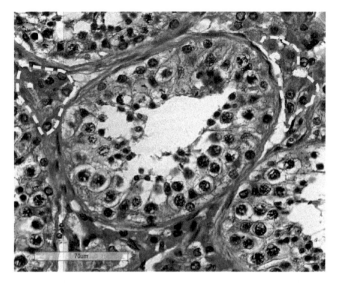

Fig. 43.18 **Seminiferous tubule, medium-high magnification, showing Leydig cells (outlined).**

43.7   Ducts Exiting the Testes

Once spermatozoa are produced by the seminiferous tubules, they are moved along the remainder of the male reproductive tract toward the penile urethra.

The remainder of this chapter will discuss the initial portion of this pathway:

Seminiferous tubules → rete testis → efferent ductules →
epididymis → vas (ductus) deferens

43.7.1   Rete Testis

The **rete testis** is an anastomosing network of wide-diameter tubes, lined by cuboidal epithelium (**Fig. 43.19**). Because these tubes are in the mediastinum testis, which is part of the tunica albuginea, the rete testis is embedded in a dense connective tissue (see **Fig. 43.7**). The lumen of the rete testis is often filled with cells from the seminiferous tubules; many are spermatozoa, but some likely sloughed during tissue preparation.

Video 43.9   Rete testis

Be able to identify:
— Rete testis
https://www.thieme.de/de/q.htm?p=opn/
tp/308390101/978-1-62623-414-7_c043_
v009&t=video

43.7.2   Efferent Ductules and Epididymis

The **efferent ductules** connect the rete testis to the **epididymis** (see **Fig. 43.7**). Because both of these tubules are outside the mediastinum testis, they are surrounded by a dense connective tissue that is not as compact as the tissue that surrounds the rete testis.

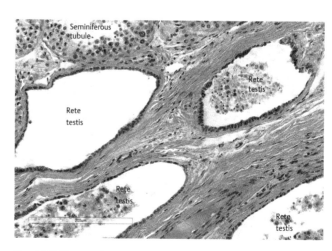

Fig. 43.19 **Rete testis.**

Fig. 43.20 is an image of an efferent ductule. The efferent ductules are lined by a pseudostratified epithelium. However, the cells here alternate between tall ciliated cells and shorter cells with microvilli, giving the epithelium a characteristic undulating appearance. Each tubule is supported by dense irregular connective tissue that may contain scattered smooth muscle cells. Efferent ductules reabsorb most of the fluid produced by the seminiferous tubules. Movement of spermatozoa is assisted by both the cilia and peristaltic movements generated by the smooth muscle cells.

The **epididymis** receives spermatozoa from the efferent ductules and is the major site for storage of sperm. Final maturation of the spermatozoa, notably development of motility, occurs in the epididymis. The regions of the epididymis (head, body, tail; see **Fig. 43.7**) are similar in histologic sections. **Fig. 43.21** is an image of the epididymis, showing that these tubes are lined by a very tall, pseudostratified epithelium with an even luminal border and long stereocilia. The surrounding connective tissue is dense irregular, with sparse smooth muscle.

Video 43.10 Efferent ductules and epididymis

Be able to identify:
— Efferent ductules
— Epididymis
https://www.thieme.de/de/q.htm?p=opn/tp/308390101/978-1-
62623-414-7_c043_v010&t=video

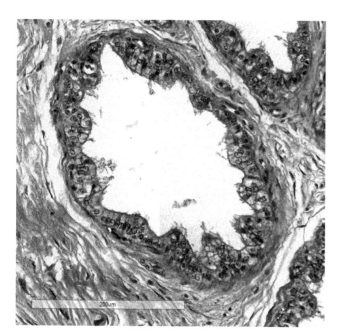

Fig. 43.20 **Efferent ductule.**

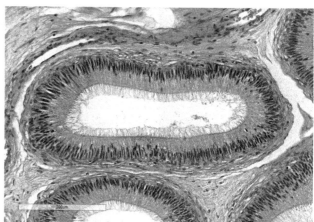

Fig. 43.21 **Epididymis.**

43.7.3   Vas Deferens and the Spermatic Cord

The vas (ductus) deferens is a continuation of the epididymis (see **Fig. 43.6** and **Fig. 43.7**). During arousal, the vas deferens propels spermatozoa from the epididymis to the prostatic urethra.

Much of the vas (ductus) deferens is within the **spermatic cord**, which contains a **testicular artery**, numerous veins called the **pampiniform plexus of veins**, nerves, skeletal muscle called the **cremaster muscle**, and supporting connective tissue and coverings (**Fig. 43.22**). The spermatic cord passes through the inguinal canal of the abdominal wall.

Fig. 43.23 is a scanning image from the spermatic cord, showing:

1. The vas (ductus) deferens (outlined)
2. The cremaster muscle (CM), a skeletal muscle derived from the abdominal wall
3. The testicular artery (TA), surrounded by numerous veins of the pampiniform plexus, which have walls that are thicker than those of typical veins

---

Clinical Correlate

The cremaster muscle is the motor component of the **cremasteric** reflex. This reflex is elicited by scratching the inner thigh, which causes the testicles on the same side to be raised slightly. This reflex can be used to test for spinal injury at the L1/L2 level or for other conditions such as **testicular torsion**, in which the spermatic cord is twisted, compressing blood supply to the testicle.

Fig. 43.24 is an image of the vas (ductus) deferens. The epithelium of the vas (ductus) deferens is similar to that of the epididymis: pseudostratified, with cuboidal basal cells and tall principal cells with stereocilia. There are three features that differentiate the vas deferens from the epididymis and efferent ductules:

1. The stereocilia are typically shorter, and the cells are not as tall as those found in the epididymis.
2. The epithelium contains a few longitudinal ridges (arrows). Note that these are fewer, larger folds, as opposed to the numerous smaller undulations created by the different-sized epithelial cells of the efferent ductules.
3. The wall is composed of three layers of thick smooth muscle (brackets), responsible for the peristaltic action that propels sperm toward the prostatic urethra during arousal. These muscle layers are oriented as inner and outer longitudinal (L) layers, with a middle circular (C) layer.

Video 43.11 Vas deferens (H & E)

https://www.thieme.de/de/q.htm?p=opn/
tp/308390101/978-1-62623-414-7_c043_
v011&t=video

Video 43.12 Vas deferens (trichrome)

https://www.thieme.de/de/q.htm?p=opn/
tp/308390101/978-1-62623-414-7_c043_
v012&t=video

Be able to identify:

— Vas (ductus) deferens
— Other structures of the spermatic cord: cremaster muscle, testicular artery, pampiniform plexus of veins

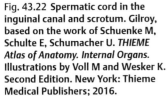

Fig. 43.22 Spermatic cord in the inguinal canal and scrotum. Gilroy, based on the work of Schuenke M, Schulte E, Schumacher U. *THIEME Atlas of Anatomy. Internal Organs.* Illustrations by Voll M and Wesker K. Second Edition. New York: Thieme Medical Publishers; 2016.

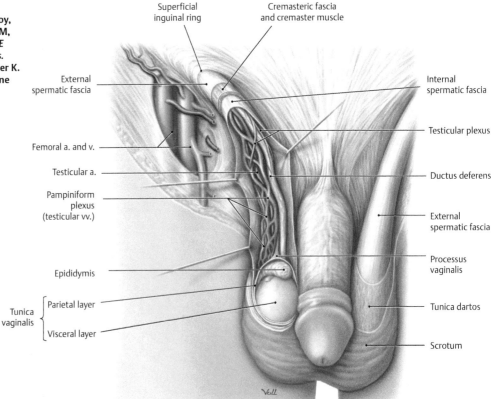

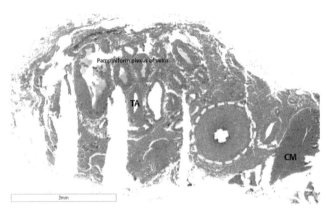

Fig. 43.23 **Spermatic cord, scanning image. The vas deferens (yellow outline), cremaster muscle (CM), and testicular artery (TA) are indicated. The other structures with lumina surrounding the testicular artery are the veins of the pampiniform plexus.**

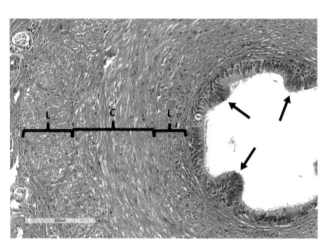

Fig. 43.24 **Vas deferens, showing the inner pseudostratified epithelium with ridges (arrows), and three layers of muscle in the muscularis (L = longitudinal, C = circular).**

43.8 Chapter Review

The male and female reproductive systems are designed to produce more humans. Because normal human cells contain two copies of the genome, the first step in reproduction is to produce cells with only one copy of the genome. This is accomplished through a cell division called meiosis, which, in males, occurs in the testes. The testes are housed in the scrotum and have an outer connective tissue called the tunica albuginea, which extends into the center of the testis as the mediastinum testis. Each testis contains hundreds of seminiferous tubules, epithelial-lined tubes that produce spermatozoa. Supportive cells in the seminiferous tubules are Sertoli cells, large cells with euchromatic nuclei and abundant cytoplasm. Sertoli cells nourish spermatogenic cells and form tight junctions with neighboring Sertoli cells to form the blood-testis barrier, which protects developing spermatozoa from rejection by the immune system. Spermatozoa production is initiated by mitotically active spermatogonia, which are located in the basal aspect of seminiferous tubules. The progeny of these mitotic divisions cross the blood-testis barrier and enter meiosis, becoming primary spermatocytes. Primary spermatocytes are characterized by large nuclei with clumpy cytoplasm. Primary spermatocytes complete meiosis I and enter meiosis II as secondary spermatocytes, which quickly finish meiosis II and, therefore, are not readily seen. The final product of meiosis is spermatids, small round cells with round nuclei. Spermiogenesis involves maturation of spermatids to spermatozoa, which includes condensation of the nucleus, loss of cytoplasm, and generation

of a single flagellum. Cells of the connective tissue of the testis includes flattened myoid cells, which have a contractile function, and large eosinophilic Leydig cells, which secrete testosterone. The spermatozoa are moved through the duct system, which includes the rete testis within the dense connective tissue of the mediastinum testis. From there they are passed to the efferent ductules, characterized by a pseudostratified epithelium that alternates between tall and short cells. The efferent ductules connect to the epididymis, which stores spermatozoa and is characterized by a pseudostratified epithelium with an even apical surface and abundant long stereocilia. The vas deferens carries spermatozoa from the epididymis to the penile urethra during arousal. The vas deferens is lined by a pseudostratified epithelium that has ridges, and it has three layers of thick smooth muscle in its wall. The vas deferens is located, in part, within the spermatic cord, which also contains the testicular artery, pampiniform plexus of veins, cremaster muscle, and connective tissue coverings.

Questions and Answers

An online-only section of questions and answers accompanying this chapter is hosted on Thieme's MedOne Education site: https://medone-education.thieme.com. Use the code on the media page at the front of this book to gain access. An institutional license to the site is required to access these questions in an interactive format, and individual users are required to register for an individual account to track results.

44   Male Accessory Glands and the Penis

After completing this chapter, you should be able to:
— Identify, at the light microscope level, each of the following:
  • Seminal vesicle
  • Prostate gland
    ○ Concretions
    ○ Urethral crest (colliculus seminalis)
    ○ Utricle
    ○ Ejaculatory ducts
  • Bulbourethral gland
  • Membranous urethra
  • Penis
    ○ Penile (spongy) urethra
    ○ Corpus spongiosum
    ○ Corpus cavernosum
— Outline the function of each cell and structure listed
— Correlate the appearance of each cell type or structure with its function
— Describe the process of erection

44.1   Overview of Male Accessory Structures and the Penis

The previous chapter discussed meiosis and production of spermatozoa, as well as the testes that produce these gametes. It also covered the initial portion of the male reproductive tract, including rete testis, efferent ductules, epididymis, and vas deferens.

This chapter will focus on the remainder of the male reproductive system: the accessory glands, urethra, and penis (**Fig. 44.1**). There are three accessory glands: **seminal vesicles**, **prostate gland**, and **bulbourethral glands**. The **urethra** can be divided into three parts based on the structures surrounding that portion of the urethra: **prostatic urethra**, **membranous urethra**, and **penile (spongy) urethra**. The membranous urethra is about 1 cm in length and is the part that passes through the **urogenital diaphragm**, a sheet of skeletal muscle in the floor of the pelvic cavity, which includes the **external urethral sphincter**.

44.2   Male Accessory Organs

Fig. 44.2 is a posterior view of the bladder showing the accessory glands of the male reproductive system. These glands include:
• **Seminal vesicles** (**seminal glands**) produce 65% of semen.
• **Prostate gland** produces 30% of semen, surrounds prostatic urethra.
• **Bulbourethral (Cowper's) gland** secretes mucus during arousal for lubrication of the urethra.

44.2.1   Seminal Vesicles

Each seminal vesicle (seminal gland) develops as an evagination from the vas (ductus) deferens, forming a highly folded tubular structure (**Fig. 44.3**). As shown below, sections of the seminal vesicle reveal several apparently distinct lumina; however, note

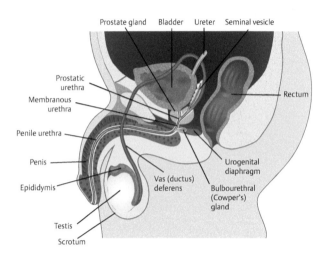

Fig. 44.1   **Male reproductive system.**

that these are all part of an interconnected lumen. The duct of each seminal vesicle joins with the vas (ductus) deferens on the same side to form the **ejaculatory duct**, which passes through the prostate to drain into the **prostatic urethra**.

Fig. 44.4 is a scanning light micrograph showing several profiles of a seminal vesicle. The wall of the seminal vesicle has three regions (from inside to outside):
1. **Mucosa**: epithelium plus loose connective tissue
2. **Muscularis**: thick, fibrous smooth muscle layer that is highly eosinophilic
3. **Adventitia**: outer connective tissue

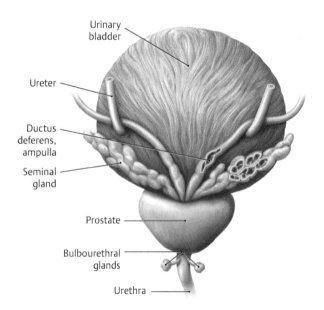

Fig. 44.2   **Male accessory glands, posterior view. From Schuenke M, Schulte E, Schumacher U. THIEME Atlas of Anatomy. Internal Organs. Illustrations by Voll M and Wesker K. Second Edition. New York: Thieme Medical Publishers; 2016,**

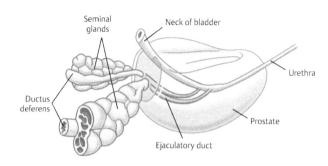

Fig. 44.3 **Seminal vesicles (seminal glands), vas (ductus) deferens, prostate gland, and urethra, lateral view.**

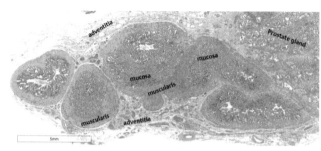

Fig. 44.4 **Seminal vesicle, scanning magnification. Mucosa, muscularis, and adventitia of the seminal vesicle are indicated, as well as a portion of the prostate.**

Helpful Hint

These features have been seen before in several other organs. Tubes or organs with lumina that are continuous with the outside world are lined by a mucosa. The muscularis region is for contraction, and the adventitia is connective tissue surrounding the organ, adhering it to adjacent structures.

Fig. 44.5 is an image taken at low to medium magnification. Each region of the seminal vesicle contains numerous folds of mucosa, which is often described as "lacy." The muscularis consists of brightly eosinophilic bundles of a fibrous smooth muscle. Dashed lines mark the borders between the muscularis and mucosa. Note that this is not the location of the basement membrane; the basement membrane is between the epithelium and connective tissue within the mucosa. The elaborate mucosal folds create numerous "pockets" that seem to be cut off from the main lumen (e.g., black arrows indicate several of these); actually, each pocket is connected to the main lumen in a different plane of section.

Fig. 44.6 is taken at medium magnification, focusing on the mucosa. Although the epithelium of the seminal vesicle is officially pseudostratified, the basal cells are less numerous, so the epithelium appears to be simple columnar. There is some variation in cell height, from cuboidal to columnar, but this is not as prominent as was seen in, for example, the efferent ductules. The epithelium is supported by loose connective tissue (black arrows), which forms the core of the folds, and it contains little, if any, smooth muscle. The muscularis that surrounds each region of the seminal vesicle has thin projections (green arrows) that subdivide each segment to some extent; these contain some smooth muscle cells but are mostly dense irregular connective tissue.

Video 44.1 Seminal vesicle overview

https://www.thieme.de/de/q.htm?p=opn/ tp/308390101/978-1-62623-414-7_c044_ v001&t=video

Video 44.2 Seminal vesicle (with prostate)

https://www.thieme.de/de/q.htm?p=opn/ tp/308390101/978-1-62623-414-7_c044_ v002&t=video

Video 44.3 Seminal vesicle (isolated)

https://www.thieme.de/de/q.htm?p=opn/ tp/308390101/978-1-62623-414-7_c044_ v003&t=video

Be able to identify:
- Seminal vesicle
  - Mucosa
  - Muscularis
  - Adventitia

44.2.2 Prostate Gland

The prostate gland (**Fig. 44.7**) has the same general features as the seminal vesicle: mucosa with pseudostratified epithelium, muscularis, adventitia. However, there are notable differences:

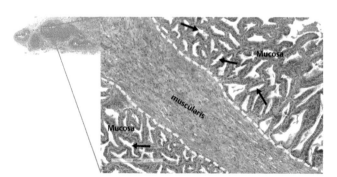

Fig. 44.5 **Seminal vesicle, low-medium magnification. Mucosa and muscularis are indicated; the borders between them are indicated by the dashed lines. Arrows represent the lumen.**

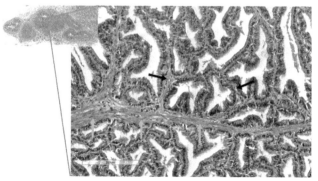

Fig. 44.6 **Seminal vesicle, medium magnification. Thin projections of the muscularis (green arrows) and loose connective tissue of the mucosa (black arrows) are shown.**

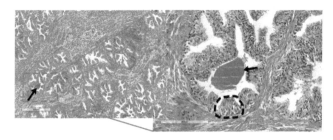

Fig. 44.7 Prostate gland, low-medium magnification. The epithelium is pseudostratified, with taller regions that appear stratified (outlined). A concretion (arrow) is evident.

1. The lumen contains brightly eosinophilic **concretions** (black arrows), which are formed from precipitated secretions.
2. The "lobules" of the prostate are much smaller than the segments of the seminal vesicle, with noticeable smooth muscle interspersed between them.
3. The folds of mucosa are much less elaborate.
4. The epithelium undulates; the taller regions appear to be stratified (outlined), even though the epithelium, like the seminal vesicle, is classified as pseudostratified.

Video 44.4 Prostate (with seminal vesicle)

https://www.thieme.de/de/q.htm?p=opn/
tp/308390101/978-1-62623-414-7_c044_
v004&t=video

Video 44.5 Prostate (isolated)

https://www.thieme.de/de/q.htm?p=opn/
tp/308390101/978-1-62623-414-7_c044_
v005&t=video

Be able to identify:
— Prostate gland
  • Concretions

The duct of each seminal vesicle is very short and joins with the vas (ductus) deferens to become the **ejaculatory duct**, which runs anteriorly and inferiorly within the substance of the prostate gland to join with the prostatic urethra (see **Fig. 44.3**). Not shown in **Fig. 44.3** is the **prostatic utricle**, a blind-ending remnant of what would have developed into the female reproductive tract (essentially the uterus) that is connected to the **prostatic urethra** at the same location as the ejaculatory ducts, but on the midline. These structures run through the substance of the prostate gland, so they are seen in some sections of this gland.

Fig. 44.8 is an anterior view of the urethra, showing its three parts: **prostatic**, **membranous**, and **spongy (penile)**. To get this view, imagine the anterior half of the prostate has been cut away, including the anterior wall of the urethra, to show the posterior wall of the urethra. There is an elevation on the posterior wall of the prostatic urethra, called the **seminal colliculus (urethral crest)**. In this location, the two ejaculatory ducts drain into the urethra (green arrows). On the midline is the opening to the prostatic utricle (red arrow).

Fig. 44.9 shows a horizontal section through the prostate in the region where the ejaculatory ducts and utricle connect to the prostatic urethra. Note that the lumen of the urethra is U-shaped due to the presence of the seminal colliculus (not labeled, the bulge into the urethra). The ejaculatory ducts are shown in cross section just before they join with the urethra. The midline invagination of the urethra is the prostatic utricle (arrow).

Fig. 44.10 is a scanning image of the prostate gland. In this image, the anterior wall of the prostatic urethra and some of the

Fig. 44.8 Parts of the urethra: prostatic, membranous, spongy (penile). The green arrows indicate the openings of the ejaculatory ducts; the red arrow indicates the opening of the prostatic utricle. Based on the work of Schuenke M, Schulte E, Schumacher U. *THIEME Atlas of Anatomy. Internal Organs.* Illustrations by Voll M and Wesker K. Second Edition. New York: Thieme Medical Publishers; 2016.

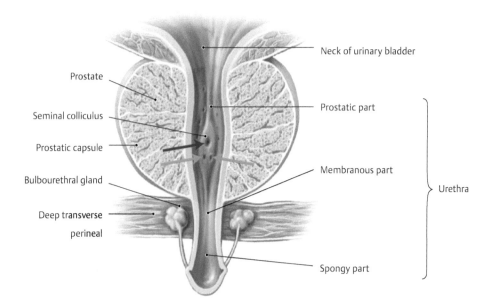

Neck of urinary bladder

Prostate

Seminal colliculus

Prostatic capsule

Bulbourethral gland

Deep transverse

perineal

Prostatic part

Membranous part

Urethra

Spongy part

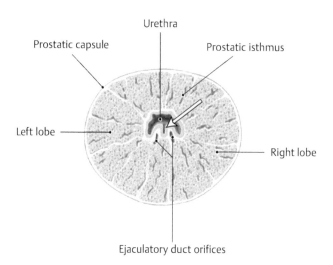

Urethra
Prostatic capsule
Prostatic isthmus
Left lobe
Right lobe
Ejaculatory duct orifices

Fig. 44.9 Prostatic urethra in horizontal section; arrow indicates the prostatic utricle. Based on the work of Schuenke M, Schulte E, Schumacher U. *THIEME Atlas of Anatomy. Internal Organs.* Illustrations by Voll M and Wesker K. Second Edition. New York: Thieme Medical Publishers; 2016.

anterior portion of the prostate are torn away, so only the posterior portion of the prostate gland is present (region within the red rectangle in drawing). In addition, this section is cut slightly superior to the drawing, so the ejaculatory ducts are farther from the prostatic urethra, and the utricle is seen as a separate structure.

The urethral crest is indicated; the U-shaped lumen of the prostatic urethra is marked by the dashed line. Even at low power, the three structures indicated by the arrows exhibit a more stratified-appearing epithelium than the surrounding glandular units. These structures are the utricle (green arrow) and ejaculatory ducts (black arrows).

Video 44.6 Prostatic ducts

Be able to identify:
— Prostate gland
  • Prostatic urethra
  • Urethral crest (colliculus seminalis)
  • Utricle
  • Ejaculatory ducts
https://www.thieme.de/de/q.htm?p=opn/tp/308390101/978-1-62623-414-7_c044_v007&t=video

Clinical Correlate

The prostate grows throughout the lifespan of an individual, mostly in response to **dihydrotestosterone**, a derivative of testosterone. Excessive growth of prostatic tissue is referred to as **benign prostatic hyperplasia**, which is more common as men age. Because this results in the formation of nodules of prostatic tissue around the urethra, benign prostatic hyperplasia results in obstruction of urinary outflow. This causes incomplete voiding, increasing urinary frequency and nocturia.

44.2.3 Bulbourethral Gland

The urogenital diaphragm is a thin sheet of skeletal muscle that includes the external urethral sphincter (see **Fig. 44.1**). The bulbourethral gland (**Cowper's gland**) is a mucous gland that is embedded within the urogenital diaphragm. The mucus secreted by the bulbourethral gland lines the urethra just before ejaculation. As shown in **Fig. 44.11**, the bulbourethral gland has skeletal muscle fibers of the urogenital diaphragm interspersed among the mucous acini.

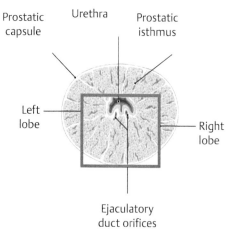
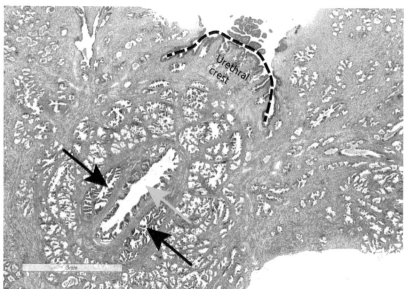

Prostatic capsule
Urethra
Prostatic isthmus
Left lobe
Right lobe
Ejaculatory duct orifices
Urethral crest

Fig. 44.10 Prostate gland including posterior wall of prostatic urethra, showing the urethral crest. The dotted line represents the lumen of the prostatic urethra. The ejaculatory ducts (black arrows) and prostatic utricle (green arrow) are shown. Based on the work of Schuenke M, Schulte E, Schumacher U. *THIEME Atlas of Anatomy. Internal Organs.* Illustrations by Voll M and Wesker K. Second Edition. New York: Thieme Medical Publishers; 2016.

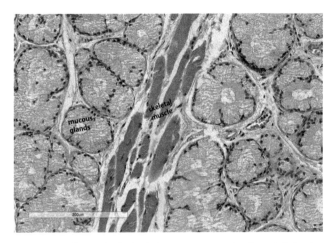

Fig. 44.11 Bulbourethral gland showing mucous glands and skeletal muscle.

Helpful Hint

The combination of all mucous acini and skeletal muscle is unique to the bulbourethral gland.

Video 44.7 Bulbourethral gland

Be able to identify:
— Bulbourethral (Cowper) gland
  • Mucous acini
  • Skeletal muscle
https://www.thieme.de/de/q.htm?p=opn/tp/308390101/978-1-62623-414-7_c044_v008&t=video

44.3 Membranous Urethra

As mentioned above, the urethra in the male has three parts—prostatic, membranous, and penile—named based on the structures that surround it (see **Fig. 44.1**). The prostatic urethra has already been discussed. The membranous urethra, which is about 1 cm in length, is the part of the urethra that passes through the urogenital diaphragm.

Fig. 44.12 shows a cross section through the membranous urethra. Like other organs that line internal spaces, the membranous urethra has three regions:

1. **Mucosa** (orange bracket), consisting of
   a. **Epithelium**; here, the epithelium is stratified or pseudostratified, but varies considerably
   b. **Lamina propria**; contains connective tissue with extensive venous sinuses (V)
2. **Muscularis** (green outlined areas); mostly smooth muscle with some connective tissue
3. **Adventitia** (black arrows); contains some skeletal muscle (area of blue arrow) that is part of the urogenital diaphragm/external urethral sphincter

The urethra also has mucous glands (of Littre) for lubrication, but these are not well demonstrated in this specimen.

Video 44.8 Membranous urethra

Be able to identify:
— Membranous urethra
https://www.thieme.de/de/q.htm?p=opn/tp/308390101/978-1-62623-414-7_c044_v009&t=video

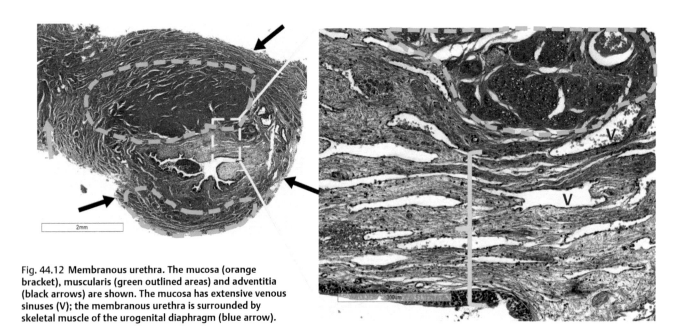

Fig. 44.12 Membranous urethra. The mucosa (orange bracket), muscularis (green outlined areas) and adventitia (black arrows) are shown. The mucosa has extensive venous sinuses (V); the membranous urethra is surrounded by skeletal muscle of the urogenital diaphragm (blue arrow).

44.4 Penis

Fig. 44.13 shows drawings of the penis in longitudinal (**Fig. 44.13**) and cross (**Fig. 44.13**) section. The penis contains three erectile elements: two dorsal **corpora cavernosa** and a single ventral **corpus spongiosum**. All three engorge with blood during erection. Each erectile element is composed of a dense connective tissue capsule (**tunica albuginea**) and **venous sinuses**. The **penile** (**spongy**) **urethra** passes through the corpus spongiosum.

Fig. 44.14 is a scanning image of the penis, showing the corpora cavernosa (black outline) and corpus spongiosum (yellow outline). The lumen of the penile (spongy) urethra is indicated by the arrow.

The corpora cavernosa tend to fuse toward the distal end of the shaft of the penis, as in this specimen.

Fig. 44.15 shows a closer view of the spongy urethra and corpus spongiosum. Like the membranous urethra, the penile (spongy) urethra (U) is lined by a stratified/pseudostratified epithelium. Each corpus contains connective tissue and numerous venous sinuses (V). The outer tunica albuginea of each is typically dense irregular connective tissue, with some scattered smooth muscle in the outer layer of the corpus spongiosum (arrows). The corpora cavernosa have a similar appearance as the corpus spongiosum.

Basic Science Correlate: Physiology

In a flaccid state, blood flow to the tissues of the penis is minimal—just enough to supply the cells with nutrients. Upon arousal, activation of the parasympathetic nervous system results in vasodilation of the arterioles in the penis, and the increased blood flow pools in the venous sinuses. Because the erectile tissues are bounded by the dense connective tissue of the tunica albuginea, the increase in blood pressure results in stiffness of the penis (erection).

Video 44.10 Penis

Be able to identify:
— Penis
  • Corpus spongiosum
    ◦ Penile (spongy) urethra
  • Corpora cavernosa

https://www.thieme.de/de/q.htm?p=opn/tp/308390101/978-1-62623-414-7_c044_v010&t=video

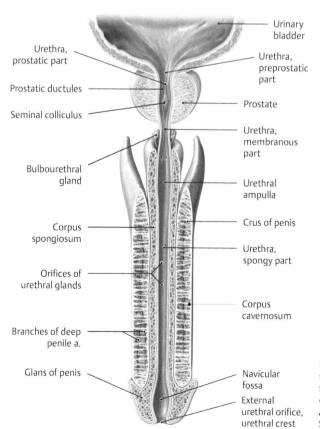

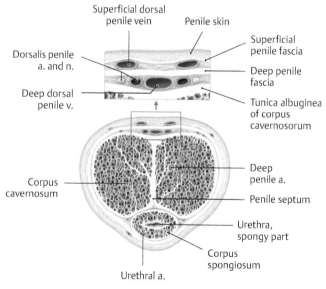

Fig. 44.13 Drawings of the penis. (a) Longitudinal view. (b) Cross-sectional view. The penis contains erectile tissue, including the corpus spongiosum which surrounds the penile urethra, and two corpora cavernosa dorsally. From Schuenke M, Schulte E, Schumacher U. *THIEME Atlas of Anatomy. Internal Organs.* Illustrations by Voll M and Wesker K. Second Edition. New York: Thieme Medical Publishers; 2016.

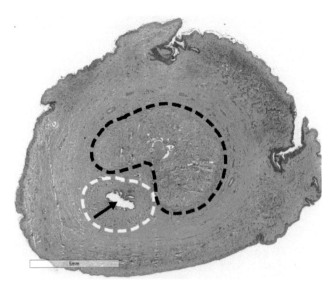

Fig. 44.14 Penis, scanning magnification (cross-section). The corpus cavernosa (black outline), corpus spongiosum (yellow outline), and the penile (spongy) urethra (arrow) are indicated.

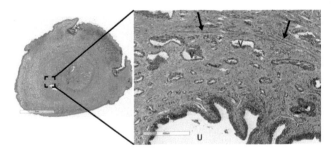

Fig. 44.15 Penis, focusing on the spongy urethra (U) and corpus spongiosum. The corpus spongiosum has extensive venous sinuses (V); the outer tunica albuginea is dense connective tissue with scattered smooth muscle (arrows).

44.5   Chapter Review

The male accessory structures produce secretions that contribute to semen and lubricate the urethra before ejaculation. The two seminal vesicles have a three-layered structure: mucosa, muscularis, adventitia. The mucosa is thrown up into elaborate folds lined by a pseudostratified epithelium. The muscularis is fibromuscular, so it exhibits intense eosinophilia, and it surrounds each profile of the seminal vesicle on section. The prostate gland has a similar structure but is composed of more numerous, smaller glandular units, with the fibromuscular muscularis extending between these glandular units. The pseudostratified epithelium in the prostate undulates due to regions of the epithelium that appear stratified. The lumen of the prostate often has characteristic concretions. The prostatic urethra passes through the prostate gland and has a characteristic U shape in cross section, due to the presence of the urethral crest. Some sections of the prostate in this region demonstrate the ejaculatory ducts and prostatic utricle. The bulbourethral gland is unique because it consists of all mucous glands and skeletal muscle. The membranous urethra is short, contains a venous plexus and smooth muscle, and is surrounded by skeletal muscle of the urogenital diaphragm. The spongy (penile) urethra is within the penis, which consists of erectile tissues including the corpus spongiosum and two corpora cavernosa. The erectile tissues fill with blood during erection.

Questions and Answers

An online-only section of questions and answers accompanying this chapter is hosted on Thieme's MedOne Education site: https://medone-education.thieme.com. Use the code on the media page at the front of this book to gain access. An institutional license to the site is required to access these questions in an interactive format, and individual users are required to register for an individual account to track results.

45 Ovary

After completing this chapter, you should be able to:
— Identify, at the light microscope level, each of the following:
  • Ovary
    ◦ Regions and structures
      ▪ Cortex
      ▪ Medulla
      ▪ Germinal epithelium
      ▪ Tunica albuginea
      ▪ Mesovarium
    ◦ Cell types and extracellular structures
      ▪ Oocyte
      ▪ Zona pellucida
      ▪ Follicular cells
      ▪ Granulosa cells
        – Cumulus oophorus
        – Corona radiata
      ▪ Theca interna
      ▪ Theca externa
    ◦ Follicles
      ▪ Primordial follicle
      ▪ Primary follicle
      ▪ Secondary follicle
        – Antrum
      ▪ Tertiary (Graafian) follicle
    ◦ Corpora
      ▪ Corpus luteum
        – Granulosa luteal cells
        – Theca luteal cells
      ▪ Corpus albicans
    ◦ Interstitial glands
    ◦ Atretic follicles
      ▪ Eosinophilic bands
      ▪ Glassy membranes
      ▪ Corpora fibrosa
— Identify, at the electron microscope level, each of the following:
  • Oocyte
  • Zona pellucida
  • Granulosa cells
— Outline the function of each cell and structure listed
— Correlate the appearance of each cell type or structure with its function
— Describe gametogenesis in the female (oogenesis)
— Describe the female reproductive cycle, including the hormones that drive this process

45.1 Overview of the Female Reproductive System

The female reproductive system is designed to produce **oocytes** (eggs) and to provide a site for fertilization and growth of the developing organism. In addition, the mammary glands produce milk for the newborn. This chapter will begin with an overview of the structures of the female reproductive system, including a description of the peritoneal coverings of these structures. This will be followed by a description of the female reproductive cycle and female gametogenesis (oogenesis), followed by an in-depth

look at the ovary. Subsequent chapters will discuss the remaining structures of the female reproductive system, the mammary glands, and placenta and umbilical cord.

Major structures of the female reproductive system that contribute to the production and transmission of the oocyte include (**Fig. 45.1**):
• **Ovary**: produces oocytes
• **Oviduct (uterine tube, fallopian tube)**: transport of oocyte, usual site of fertilization, transport of zygote
• **Uterus**: site of implantation and development of the embryo/fetus, contracts during childbirth
• **Vagina**: organ of copulation and birth canal

These structures are located in the pelvic cavity; most are covered by a layer of **peritoneum**.

45.2 Peritoneal Coverings of the Female Reproductive System

Fig. 45.2 is a drawing of a posterior view of the female reproductive structures and their peritoneal coverings. Note that as the sheet of peritoneum drapes over the oviducts, lateral to the uterus, there is a double layer of peritoneum with connective tissues, vessels, and nerves between these two layers. This is called the **broad ligament**. Because the ovary is posterior to the oviducts, a portion of the broad ligament extends posteriorly from the main sheet; this portion is called the **mesovarium**. The point where the horizontal mesovarium is attached to the vertical portion of the broad ligament separates this vertical portion into two parts: the **mesosalpinx** (above the mesovarium) and **mesometrium** (below the mesovarium).

Helpful Hint

Because this concept is challenging to grasp, an analogy may be useful (**Fig. 45.3**). The standing person represents the female reproductive structures. The legs, trunk, and head are the uterus, and the arms are the oviducts. This person is standing in a giant salad bowl (not sure why), which represents the floor of the pelvis (brown curve; **Fig. 45.3a**). Now think about draping a bed sheet over this person, creating something similar to a ghost costume (**Fig. 45.3b**). Note that below the arms (oviducts) and to the side of the trunk (uterus) are two layers of the bed sheet with a space between the two layers of the sheet (for connective tissue, vessels, nerves, etc.). This double-layered sheet to the sides of the uterus represents the vertical portion of the broad ligament.

In **Fig. 45.3c**, add two beach balls (to represent the ovaries) to the side of the trunk (uterus), between the two layers of the sheet (i.e., within the vertical broad ligament). If the balls are then moved toward you, they will pull out the posterior side of the bed sheet and create a new double-layered sheet oriented horizontally, connecting the vertical portion of the bed sheet to the beach balls. This horizontal double layer is the mesovarium, and where it joins the vertical part, it divides this vertical part into two (above the junction is mesosalpinx, below is mesometrium).

It may be useful to go back to the anatomic drawing and confirm understanding.

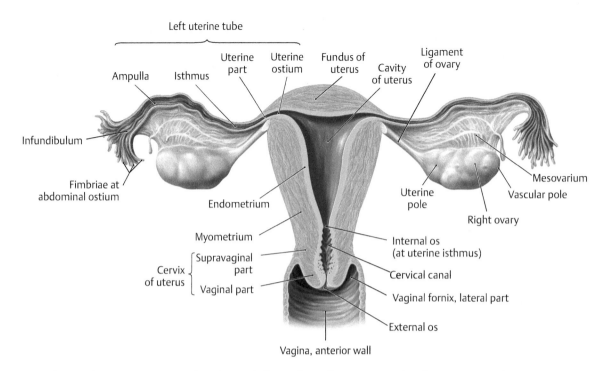

Fig. 45.1 Female reproductive system. From Schuenke M, Schulte E, Schumacher U. *THIEME Atlas of Anatomy. Internal Organs.* Illustrations by Voll M and Wesker K. Second Edition. New York: Thieme Medical Publishers; 2016.

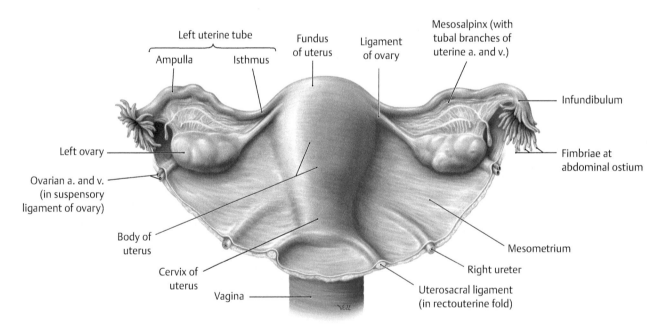

Fig. 45.2 Female reproductive system, posterior view, showing the peritoneal coverings of these structures and organs. The mesovarium is the peritoneal covering that comes off of the ovary and projects anteriorly (just above the ovary in this drawing). The mesovarium, mesosalpinx, and mesometrium together form the broad ligament. From Schuenke M, Schulte E, Schumacher U. *THIEME Atlas of Anatomy. Internal Organs.* Illustrations by Voll M and Wesker K. Second Edition. New York: Thieme Medical Publishers; 2016.

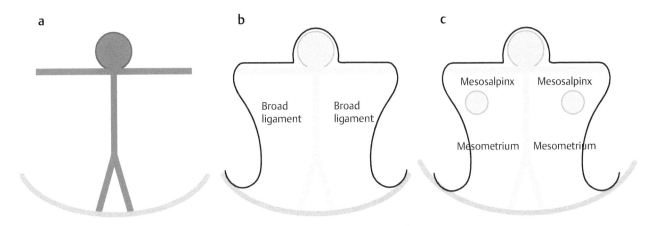

Fig. 45.3   (a)–(c) An analogy to represent the peritoneal coverings of the female reproductive system.

In **Fig. 45.4**, the upper left drawing is a posterior view of the female reproductive system, similar to **Fig. 45.2**. The larger drawing shows a parasagittal section through the female reproductive structures, as indicated by the red line (view indicated by the arrow) to show the broad ligament in more detail. Note that:

- The floor of the pelvic cavity is the bottom of the drawing, and the peritoneum comes off the floor of the pelvic cavity to sweep over the reproductive structures.
- The mesometrium, mesosalpinx, and mesovarium are double-layered sheets of peritoneum, with connective tissue forming the core of these structures.
- The **germinal epithelium** is the outer surface of the ovary; the peritoneal covering and germinal epithelium are a continuous epithelium.

Fig. 45.5 is a scanning view of the female reproductive structures from a fetus, showing the ovary, oviduct (uterine tube), and broad ligament (similar to **Fig. 45.4**). The floor of the pelvis is at the bottom of the image; anterior is to the left.

Fig. 45.6 is an image showing two close-up views of the epithelium covering the female reproductive structures. The peritoneal layer covering the mesometrium is a simple squamous epithelium (black arrows). The core of the broad ligament is connective tissue with vessels and nerves that supply the visceral structures. The outer layer of the ovary, the germinal epithelium, is a cuboidal epithelium (green arrows).

Video 45.1   Overview of broad ligament

Be able to identify:

— Mesovarium
— Mesometrium
— Mesosalpinx

https://www.thieme.de/de/q.htm?p=opn/tp/308390101/978-1-62623-414-7_c045_v001&t=video

Helpful Hint

This is not much different from the peritoneum and mesentery of the intestinal tract.

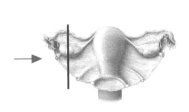

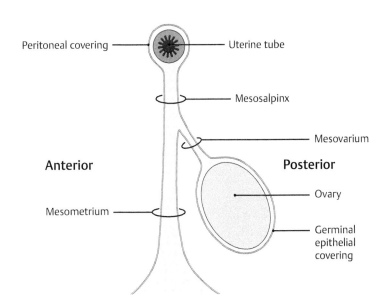

Fig. 45.4   **Parasagittal section through the female reproductive system, showing the peritoneal coverings. From Schuenke M, Schulte E, Schumacher U.** *THIEME Atlas of Anatomy. Internal Organs.* **Illustrations by Voll M and Wesker K. Second Edition. New York: Thieme Medical Publishers; 2016.**

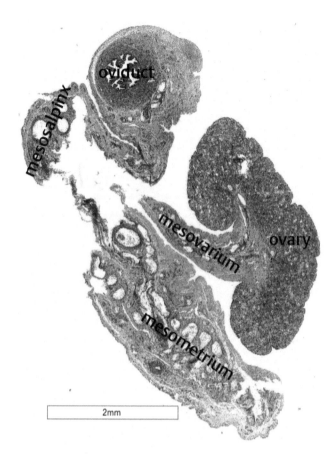

Fig. 45.5   **Female reproductive structures similar to Fig. 45.4, scanning magnification.**

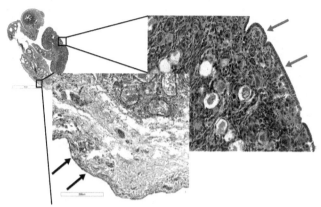

Fig. 45.6   **Epithelium covering the mesometrium (black arrows) and the germinal epithelium covering the ovary (green arrows).**

45.3   Female Reproductive Cycle

Before presenting the histology of the organs of the female reproductive tract, it is useful to consider the female reproductive cycle, which is designed to coordinate the function of the ovaries and uterus to maximize the chances of successful reproduction (**Fig. 45.7**).

This discussion will assume a cycle that is 28 days long (indicated at the bottom of **Fig. 45.7**). Ovulation occurs on day 14. The day after day 28 of any given cycle is day 1 of the next cycle. The second half of the cycle is pretty consistent in length: 14 days. In women who have reproductive cycles that are shorter or longer than 28 days, it is usually the first half of the cycle that reflects this variation.

The process of oocyte maturation is driven by two hormones, **follicle-stimulating hormone** (FSH) and **luteinizing hormone** (LH), both secreted by **gonadotrophs** (one of the basophil cell types) of the **anterior pituitary gland**. FSH predominates during the first half of the menstrual cycle (days 1–14) and stimulates maturation of **follicles** in the ovary. These follicles release mainly **estrogen**. This period in the ovary is referred to as the **follicular phase of the ovarian cycle** and ultimately results in one large **Graafian (tertiary) follicle**. At mid-cycle, day 14, a surge of LH induces **ovulation** of the oocyte in the Graafian follicle. The cells of the follicle that remain in the ovary (not ovulated) form a structure called the **corpus luteum**, which releases mostly **progesterone** (and some estrogen). Because the corpus luteum is

the dominant structure of the ovary after ovulation, the second half of the cycle is referred to as the **luteal phase of the ovarian cycle**. In the absence of fertilization and implantation, the corpus luteum degenerates around day 26, becoming an inactive **corpus albicans**, and a new cycle begins two days later.

The hormones that are released by the ovary—estrogen and progesterone—drive changes in the uterus. The uterine cycle begins with the **menstrual phase of the uterine cycle**, in which the endodermal lining of the uterus is sloughed off. This occurs because at day 28 of the previous cycle, the ovaries are no longer releasing either progesterone or estrogen. Around day 5, the growing follicles in the ovary begin to secrete enough estrogen to stimulate the endometrial lining to regenerate. Because this regeneration requires cell division, this phase of the uterine cycle is called the **proliferative phase of the uterine cycle**. After ovulation, progesterone from the corpus luteum induces the endometrial lining to enter the **secretory phase of the uterine cycle**. In this phase, glandular secretion increases (thus the name), and the tissue becomes edematous and more vascular. Around day 26, the corpus luteum degenerates, and when circulating progesterone and estrogen levels drop back to baseline 2 days later, the menstrual phase of the next uterine cycle begins.

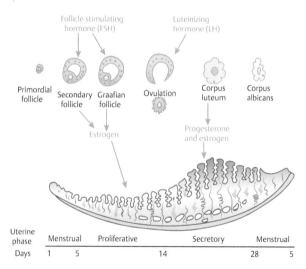

Fig. 45.7   **Female reproductive cycle.**

This is a lot of information, especially on first exposure, and is meant as an overview. Follicular development in the ovary and changes in the uterus will be discussed in this and the subsequent chapter, respectively. It may be useful to return to this chart during those discussions to solidify understanding once mental pictures of these structures are established.

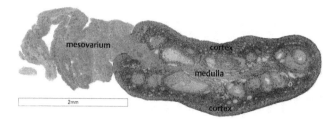

Fig. 45.8 Ovary with attached mesovarium. Cortex and medulla are indicated.

45.4 Overview of the Ovary

Fig. 45.8 is a scanning image from a monkey ovary with the mesovarium attached. The ovary consists of an outer **cortex**, which contains most of the early-stage follicles, and an inner **medulla** that contains more mature follicles and most of the larger vessels supplying the ovary. As with the testis, the outermost portion of the ovary (i.e., the outer region of the cortex) is composed of thick connective tissue called the **tunica albuginea** (not labeled), but this is not as distinct as in the testis because much of the ovary is dense irregular connective tissue. The ovary is covered by the germinal epithelium.

Video 45.2 Overview of ovary

Be able to identify:
— Ovary
— Cortex
— Medulla
— Germinal epithelium
— Tunica albuginea
— Mesovarium

https://www.thieme.de/de/q.htm?p=opn/tp/308390101/978-1-62623-414-7_c045_v002&t=video

The term "germinal epithelium" came about because it was once thought that these cells were the source of the germ cells (i.e., oocytes). It is now known that this is not the case and that the germinal epithelium is simply a peritoneal covering of the ovary, but the name has stuck. Remember that this layer is continuous with the epithelial coverings of the mesovarium and rest of the broad ligament.

45.5 Oogenesis

The process of gamete production in the female, **oogenesis** (**Fig. 45.9**), is similar to spermatogenesis in the male (compare to **Fig. 43.4**). The cells of oogenesis include:

- **Oogonium**: a cell that divides mitotically, produces progeny that enter meiosis
- **Primary oocyte**: a cell that has begun meiosis (i.e., is in meiosis I)
- **Secondary oocyte**: a cell that has completed the first meiotic division (i.e., is in meiosis II)
- **Ovum** (haploid, N): a cell that has completed meiosis

Despite the similarities between male and female gamete production, there are some very distinct differences. In the female:

- During fetal development, *all* oogonia divide by mitosis and all enter meiosis I, becoming primary oocytes. These are arrested in meiosis I at birth and remain in this state until ovulation.
- At puberty (and every month thereafter), just before ovulation, (usually) one primary oocyte finishes meiosis I, becoming a secondary oocyte, where it arrests in meiosis II and is ovulated.
- At fertilization, the secondary oocyte finishes meiosis II. If unfertilized, the secondary oocyte does not divide.
- Also note that division of the cytoplasm is unequal, so that only one cell, the ovum, receives most of the cytoplasm. Smaller cells, called **polar bodies**, ultimately degenerate.

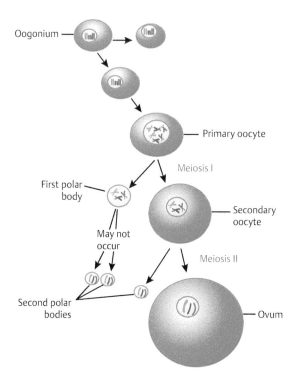

Fig. 45.9 **Oogenesis. Germ cells undergoing mitosis are called oogonia, which divide to produce the population of cells that will enter meiosis, which is two cell divisions. In females, these divisions are unequal, so that most of the cytoplasm is retained in one of the resulting cells, the ovum, while the other three products of mitosis, called polar bodies, contain little cytoplasm and degenerate.**

Although polar bodies are not used during natural reproduction, they can be biopsied during *in vitro* **fertilization**. Because they are products of meiosis complementary to the ovum, analysis of the genes in polar bodies can indicate which genes are in the oocyte. This information is used to select oocytes for *in vitro* fertilization and implantation that do not carry a disease gene. These **polar body biopsies** are one of the strategies used in **preimplantation genetic diagnosis** to assist couples who carry disease genes but do not want to pass them down to their offspring.

45.6   Basic Structure of Ovarian Follicles

Oocytes develop within the ovary as part of follicles, which include the oocyte, supportive cells (**follicular cells** or **granulosa cells**, and **thecal cells**), and extracellular components, notably the **zona pellucida** (**Fig. 45.10**).

Before describing the details of the histology of the different types of follicles, it is useful to describe the most mature follicle, the Graafian follicle, because it demonstrates all the structures within a follicle clearly.

Fig. 45.11 is a drawing of a graafian follicle (or a follicle close to this stage). The oocyte is the largest cell shown and contains a large, euchromatic nucleus and extensive eosinophilic cytoplasm. The smaller cells surrounding the oocyte are called granulosa cells. The collection of granulosa cells immediately surrounding the oocyte are referred to as the **corona radiata**. Granulosa cells that surround the corona radiata and attach it to the remainder of the follicle make up the **cumulus oophorus** (corona radiata and cumulus oophorus are not labeled in **Fig. 45.11**). Between the oocyte and granulosa cells of the corona radiata is an extracellular glycoprotein layer, the zona pellucida. Fluid has accumulated within this follicle, in a space called the **antrum**. Surrounding the outer layer of granulosa cells are **theca interna** (producing steroids, mostly estrogen) and **theca externa** (fibroblastlike) cells. The granulosa cells are epithelial, so there is a basement membrane between the granulosa cells and theca interna cells.

Fig. 45.12 is a low- to medium-magnification image of a Graafian follicle. The nucleus of the oocyte is out of the plane of section, but it is still apparent that the oocyte is a large cell, with abundant eosinophilic cytoplasm. At this late stage, there are hundreds of granulosa cells surrounding the ovary and fluid-filled antrum. The granulosa cells are much smaller than the oocyte, and they surround the oocyte and line the antrum. Between the granulosa cells and the oocyte is the highly eosinophilic zona pellucida (purple arrow), a glycoprotein structure produced by the combined actions of the oocyte and granulosa cells. The granulosa cells immediately adjacent to the zona pellucida are collectively the corona radiata (yellow arrows), which are ejected at ovulation along with the oocyte and zona pellucida. The granulosa cells that connect the oocyte/zona pellucida/corona radiata to the granulosa cells surrounding the antrum are called the cumulus oophorus (green arrows). Immediately outside the granulosa cells that line the antrum is the thecal region,

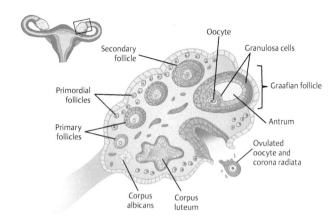

Fig. 45.10 **Ovarian follicles.**

which includes the steroid-secreting theca interna cells (blue arrow) and fibroblastlike theca externa (orange arrow). There is a basement membrane between the granulosa and thecal cells (at location of the black arrows).

Fig. 45.13 is a higher-magnification image of the oocyte and surrounding structures within the Graafian follicle. Again, the nucleus of the oocyte is not in the plane of section; the oocyte cytoplasm is eosinophilic. The eosinophilic region surrounding the oocyte is the zona pellucida (purple arrows). The corona radiata consists of the granulosa cells nearest the zona pellucida (yellow brackets). The remainder of the granulosa cells surrounding the oocyte, and attaching this complex to the granulosa cells surrounding the antrum, form the cumulus oophorus (green brackets). The pale region between the zona pellucida and corona radiata is artifact.

Basic Science Correlate: Physiology

Just before ovulation, the cumulus oophorus disperses, and the cumulus mass (oocyte, zona pellucida, corona radiata, and some of the cumulus) floats free in the antrum for a short time before it is ovulated.

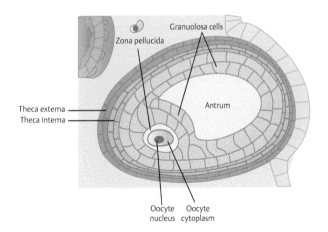

Fig. 45.11 **Graafian follicle.**

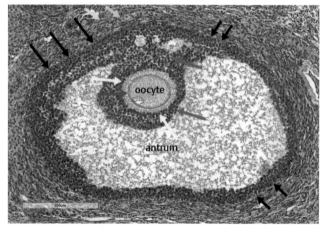

Fig. 45.12 **Graafian follicle, low to medium magnification. The oocyte and antrum are labeled. The zona pellucida (purple arrow), corona radiata (yellow arrows), cumulus oophorus (green arrows), basement membrane (black arrows), theca interna cells (blue arrow), and theca external cells (orange arrow) are indicated.**

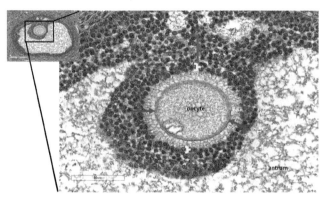

Fig. 45.13 Graafian follicle, medium magnification showing oocyte and surrounding structures. The oocyte and antrum are labeled. The zona pellucida (purple arrows), corona radiata (yellow brackets), and cumulus oophorus (green brackets) are indicated.

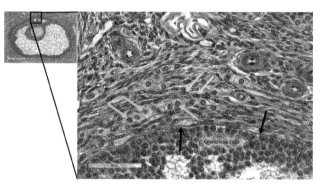

Fig. 45.14 Graafian follicle, high magnification showing outer region of Graafian follicle. The outer granulosa cells are labeled. The basement membrane (black arrows), theca interna cells (blue arrows), and theca externa cells (orange arrows) are indicated.

Fig. 45.14 is a high-magnification image of the outer region of the follicle. The theca interna cells (blue arrows) have an abundant cytoplasm that is palely eosinophilic, underscoring the fact that these are steroid-secreting cells (mostly estrogen). The theca externa cells are more fibroblastlike (orange arrows). The granulosa cells are epithelial-like and are separated from the connective tissue (thecal cells and surrounding interstitial tissue) by a basement membrane (black arrows).

Helpful Hint

There are some fibroblastlike cells between the theca interna and the basement membrane, as if the theca externa were inside the theca interna. This is not unusual on many slides, and it may represent less active cells of the theca interna. Identification of thecal cells is based on cellular morphology, not position.

Fig. 45.15 is an image of an earlier stage of follicular development (a primary follicle), indicating the large, euchromatic nucleus within the oocyte (nuclear envelope at the tips of the black arrows). The cytoplasm demonstrates pale, almost watery eosinophilia.

Video 45.3 Overview of follicular structure

Be able to identify:
— • Follicle
  • Oocyte
    ◦ Nucleus and cytoplasm
  • Zona pellucida
  • Granulosa cells
    ◦ Cumulus oophorus
    ◦ Corona radiata
  • Theca interna
  • Theca externa
https://www.thieme.de/de/q.htm?p=opn/tp/308390101/978-1-62623-414-7_c045_v003&t=video

Fig. 45.16 is an electron micrograph showing the outer portion of the oocyte cytoplasm (1), the zona pellucida (2), and surrounding granulosa cells (3). The granulosa cells have processes that project into the zona pellucida (4) to make contact with microvilli from the oocyte plasma membrane, enabling cell-cell signaling.

45.7 Development of Ovarian Follicles

Now that the cellular and extracellular features of follicles have been described, the different stages of follicular development can be discussed.

As shown in **Fig. 45.10**, follicle maturation occurs largely through proliferation and organization of the cells and extracellular structures surrounding the oocyte. All the oocytes in the ovary, with the exception of the oocyte in a Graafian follicle just before ovulation, are arrested in meiosis I and are, therefore, primary oocytes. Therefore, the oocyte itself undergoes very little change during follicular maturation.

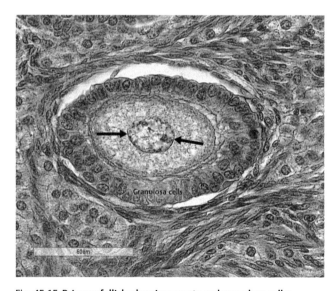

Fig. 45.15 Primary follicle showing oocyte and granulosa cells; nuclear envelope is indicated (arrows).

Fig. 45.16 Electron micrograph showing outer cytoplasm of oocyte (1), zona pellucida (2), granulosa cells (3), and granulosa cell processes (4).

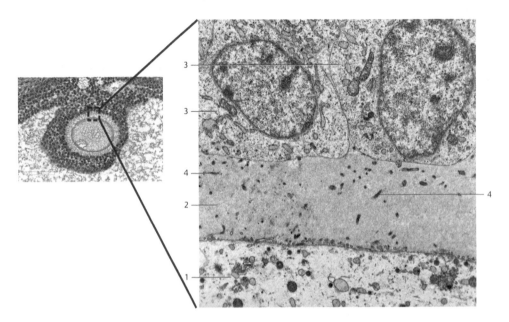

The stages of follicular development are as follows (see also **Fig. 45.10**):

1. A **primordial follicle** consists of an oocyte surrounded by a single layer of squamous cells, called **follicular cells**.
2. In the **primary follicle**, the follicular cells become cuboidal. With the change in shape, the follicular cells are typically referred to as granulosa cells. Initially, these remain a single layer of cells, but later they become stratified. Connective tissue cells organize around the basement membrane of the granulosa cells to become thecal cells (interna and externa). Synthesis of the zona pellucida is evident.
3. In a **secondary follicle**, a fluid-filled antrum forms among the granulosa cells.
4. In a **Graafian (tertiary) follicle**, the antrum enlarges, surrounding the oocyte and corona radiata on all sides except where cells of the cumulus oophorus connect the corona radiata to the outer granulosa cells.

Helpful Hint

Do not confuse primary and secondary *follicles* with primary and secondary *oocytes*. The oocyte is a single cell, while the follicles include the oocyte, granulosa and thecal cells, and zona pellucida.

Remember that all oocytes become arrested in meiosis I during fetal development and, therefore, are primary oocytes within primordial follicles. Completion of meiosis I and arrest in meiosis II do not occur until just before ovulation. Therefore, all the follicles—primordial, primary, secondary—include a primary oocyte. The exception to this is the very mature Graafian follicle just before ovulation.

45.7.1   Primordial Follicles

Primordial follicles (**Fig. 45.17**) consist of an oocyte surrounded by a single layer of squamous cells, called follicular cells (black and yellow arrows). Note the large, euchromatic nucleus and abundant eosinophilic cytoplasm of the oocyte. A basement membrane separates the follicular cells from the surrounding connective tissue, seen as a prominent eosinophilic band in some follicles (red arrow). The theca is not developed at this stage.

Helpful Hint

Primordial follicles are typically found in the periphery (cortex) of the ovary. Primordial follicles are formed during fetal development and then become arrested, most remaining in this stage until puberty.

Video 45.4   Primordial follicles

Be able to identify:
— Primordial follicle
  • Oocyte
  • Follicular cells
https://www.thieme.de/de/q.htm?p=opn/tp/308390101/978-1-62623-414-7_c045_v004&t=video

45.7.2   Primary Follicles

In primary follicles (**Fig. 45.18**) the squamous follicular cells have become cuboidal (black and yellow arrows). The zona pellucida and thecal cells begin to develop at this stage but may not be well developed. In **Fig. 45.18a**, the zona pellucida is more evident (blue arrow), as this is a later stage of development than the follicle in **Fig. 45.18b**.

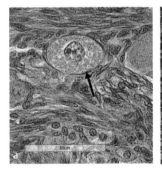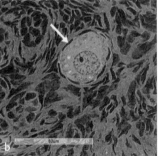

Fig. 45.17 Primordial follicles from (a) a cat and (b) a monkey. The squamous follicular cells (black and yellow arrows) and basement membrane (red arrow) are indicated.

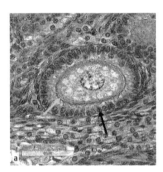
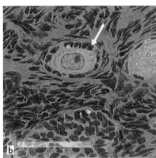

Fig. 45.18 **Primary follicles from (a) a cat and (b) a monkey. Granulosa cells (black and yellow arrows) and zona pellucida (blue arrow) are indicated.**

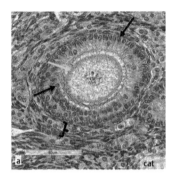
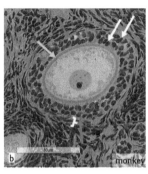

Fig. 45.19 **Late primary follicles from (a) a cat and (b) a monkey. Granulosa cells (black and yellow arrows), zona pellucida (blue arrows), theca (black and yellow brackets), and basement membrane (red arrows) are indicated.**

In late primary follicles (**Fig. 45.19**), the granulosa cells have proliferated and become a stratified layer (black and yellow arrows). By this stage, the zona pellucida (blue arrows) is more easily seen, especially in **Fig. 45.19b**. Thecal cells (black and yellow brackets) have begun to organize against the basement membrane (red arrows).

Video 45.6   Secondary follicles

Be able to identify:
— Secondary follicle
   • Oocyte
   • Granulosa cells
   • Zona pellucida
   • Antrum
   • Theca interna
   • Theca externa
https://www.thieme.de/de/q.htm?p=opn/tp/308390101/978-1-62623-414-7_c045_v006&t=video

45.7.4   Graafian (Tertiary) Follicles

The Graafian follicle (or tertiary follicle, **Fig. 45.22**) is characterized by a very large antrum, surrounding the oocyte nearly completely, with the exception of a thinning region of granulosa cells of the cumulus oophorus that form a "stalk" (arrow). Just before ovulation, the granulosa cells in this stalk will disperse, and the oocyte/zona pellucida/corona radiata with some cumulus cells will float freely in the antral fluid. The thecal cells are fully developed (bracket). In humans, the final Graafian follicle just before ovulation is approximately 1 cm in diameter, extending from one end of the ovary to the other. This growing follicle enlarges the overall size of the ovary.

Video 45.5   Primary follicles

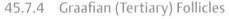

Be able to identify:
— Primary follicle
   • Oocyte
   • Follicular cells/granulosa cells
   • Zona pellucida
https://www.thieme.de/de/q.htm?p=opn/tp/308390101/978-1-62623-414-7_c045_v005&t=video

45.7.3   Secondary Follicles

Secondary follicles (also known as antral follicles; **Fig. 45.20**) are characterized by the appearance of a fluid-filled space, the antrum, between the granulosa cells. The zona pellucida is usually more pronounced (not in this image), and the thecal cells have become more organized, forming distinct theca interna (black bracket, steroid secreting) and theca externa layers (blue bracket, fibroblastlike).

As the antrum continues to enlarge, the oocyte is moved to one side of the follicle (**Fig. 45.21**). The mound of granulosa cells surrounding the oocyte is referred to as the cumulus oophorus (labeled "CO" and marked with arrow).

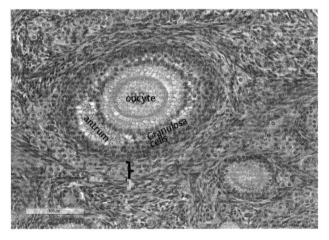

Fig. 45.20 **Secondary follicle from a cat. The oocyte, granulosa cells, and antrum are labeled. Theca interna (black bracket) and theca externa (blue bracket) are indicated.**

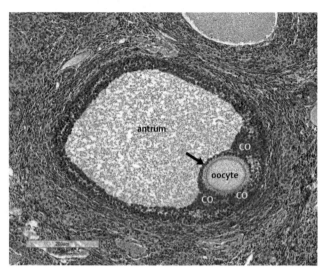

Fig. 45.21 **Late secondary follicle from a cat. The oocyte, antrum, and cumulus oophorus (CO and arrow) are labeled.**

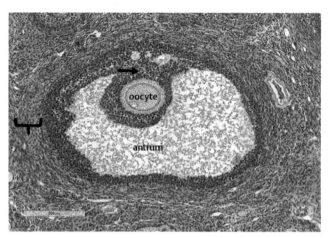

Fig. 45.22 **Graafian follicle from a cat. The oocyte and antrum are labeled. The theca (bracket) and narrowing stalk of the cumulus oophorus (arrow) are indicated.**

Video 45.7   Graafian (tertiary) follicles

Be able to identify:
— Graafian (tertiary) follicle
  • Oocyte
  • Follicular cells / Granulosa cells
  • Corona radiata
  • Cumulus oophorus
  • Zona pellucida
  • Antrum
  • Theca interna
  • Theca externa
https://www.thieme.de/de/q.htm?p=opn/tp/308390101/978-1-62623-414-7_c045_v007&t=video

Helpful Hint

The types of follicles present in the ovary change throughout the lifespan of an individual. A fetal ovary consists of mostly primordial follicles, with a few primary follicles. An active ovary contains all types of follicles, while the ovary of a postmenopausal woman contains no active follicles.

Clinical Correlate

Follicular cysts are very common and are derived from Graafian follicles that either fail to rupture, or rupture and reseal. Polycystic ovaries (ovaries with multiple cysts) are associated with **polycystic ovary syndrome**, an endocrine disorder that presents with menstrual irregularity, male-pattern hair distribution, acne, and metabolic disorders (metabolic syndrome, diabetes). **Ovarian tumors** are neoplasms derived from the ovary, and they can be benign or malignant. Although not the most frequent type of female reproductive cancer, they are commonly fatal because they are not diagnosed until later stages.

45.8   Corpus Luteum and Corpus Albicans

Ovulation occurs on day 14 of the female reproductive cycle (see **Fig. 45.7** and **Fig. 45.10**) During this process, the oocyte, zona pellucida, and corona radiata are released into the peritoneal cavity near the oviduct. The ovulated oocyte will be discussed in **Chapter 48**.

The structures that are left behind in the ovary after ovulation include the outer granulosa cells, the thecal cells, and the basement membrane between them. These structures collapse and reorganize into a **corpus luteum** ("yellow body"); the cells are renamed **granulosa luteal** and **theca luteal cells**, respectively. These cells now produce (mostly) progesterone, which is important for inducing and maintaining the secretory phase of the uterine cycle. Typically, there is a clot where the antrum was located; this breaks down during the luteal phase.

In the absence of fertilization and human chorionic gonadotropin, the corpus luteum will degenerate 12 days after ovulation, forming a connective tissue–like structure called the **corpus albicans** (white body), which does not secrete hormones.

In humans, most cycles result in a single ovulation, so only one corpus luteum (on one side) exists at a time. Corpora albicantia last for several months, so each ovary in a reproductive woman will contain a few of them, representing previous cycles.

45.8.1   Corpus Luteum

The corpus luteum is a very large structure, dominating large regions of the ovary containing it; **Fig. 45.23** shows one that is close to a centimeter in diameter (outlined). Early after it is formed, the central cavity contains clotted blood, which is a remnant of ovulation, while the walls contain granulosa luteal cells and thecal luteal cells. Because the corpus is the collapsed wall of the follicle, the thecal cells are thrown into folds (arrows) that partition the granulosa cells.

Fig. 45.24 is a closer view of the outer wall of the corpus luteum in the area of a fold. The basement membrane between the granulosa luteal cells and theca luteal cells breaks down; its location is indicated by the dashed lines. The granulosa luteal cells are to the upper and lower left, while the theca luteal cells are between the dashed lines and to the right. Although both types of cells appear to be histologically steroid secreting (large

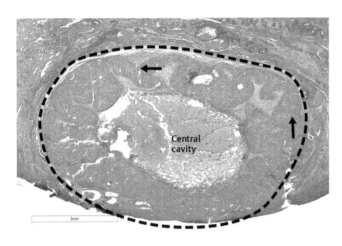

Fig. 45.23 **Corpus luteum (outlined). The central cavity is labeled. Folds of the corpus luteum (arrows) contain thecal cells.**

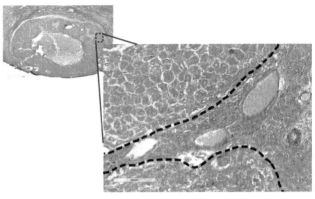

Fig. 45.24 **Wall of the corpus luteum showing the approximate location of the basement membrane (dashed lines). Granulosa luteal cells are above and below the dashed lines and thecal luteal cells are between the dashed lines.**

euchromatic nucleus, eosinophilic or pale eosinophilic cytoplasm), the granulosa cells typically have more cytoplasm, so they are much larger.

Helpful Hint

In fact, the scanning view shows that the wall of the corpus luteum is quite thick, much thicker than the wall of the corresponding graafian follicle from which it was derived (compare to **Fig. 45.22**, which is not at the same magnification). Much of this increased thickness is accounted for by the large size of the granulosa luteal cells.

Fig. 45.25 is another view of the wall of the corpus luteum at a later stage. Again, the location of the basement membrane is indicated by the dashed lines. In this preparation, it is easier to see the difference between the granulosa luteal cells (left and right of the dashed lines) and the theca luteal cells (between the dashed lines). The granulosa luteal cells are steroid secreting, exhibiting a large, euchromatic nucleus with eosinophilic or pale eosinophilic cytoplasm. The theca luteal cells are smaller than the granulosa luteal cells, with a cytoplasm that is more eosinophilic than pale (black arrows). Fibroblastlike cells with flattened nuclei within the thecal region are likely cells of the former theca externa.

Video 45.8   Corpus luteum—1

https://www.thieme.de/de/q.htm?p=opn/tp/308390101/978-1-62623-414-7_c045_v008&t=video

Video 45.9   Corpus luteum—2

https://www.thieme.de/de/q.htm?p=opn/tp/308390101/978-1-62623-414-7_c045_v009&t=video

Be able to identify:
— Corpus luteum
  • Granulosa luteal cells
  • Thecal luteal cells

45.8.2   Corpus Albicans

After about 12 days, the corpus luteum stops secreting progesterone and estrogen. Once steroid production ceases, the remnant of the corpus luteum becomes a fibrous, connective tissue–like "scar" called the **corpus albicans** (**Fig. 45.26**, outlined). This structure consists of extracellular matrix components, with scattered fibroblastlike cells.

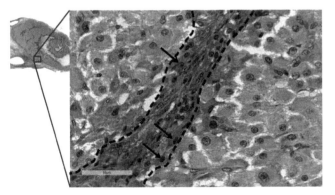

Fig. 45.25 **Wall of the corpus luteum showing the approximate location of the basement membrane (dashed lines). Granulosa luteal cells are to the right and left of the dashed lines, and thecal luteal cells are between the dashed lines indicated by the arrows.**

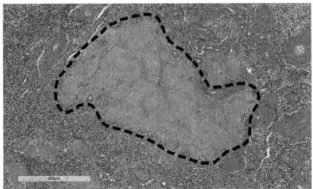

Fig. 45.26 **Corpus albicans (outlined).**

Histologically, the corpus albicans is often described as eosinophilic, and it clearly is in **Fig. 45.26**. However, because much of the surrounding ovarian tissue stains fairly well, the corpus albicans is often pale in comparison to the surrounding tissues. Its name, which means "white body," derives from its appearance on fresh tissue (unstained). The corpus luteum means "yellow body," again as seen in fresh tissues.

Video 45.10 Corpus albicans

Be able to identify:
— Corpus albicans
https://www.thieme.de/de/q.htm?p=opn/
tp/308390101/978-1-62623-414-7_c045_v010&t=video

45.9   Atresia

Progression from a primordial follicle to a Graafian follicle, ovulation, and the resulting corpus luteum and corpus albicans are part of "normal" follicular development (see **Fig. 45.10**).

Fetal ovaries generate millions of primordial follicles, but only several hundred of these reach maturation. The remaining follicles undergo **atresia**, a degenerative process that some believe is the result of selection of the best oocytes. Atresia can occur at any stage of follicular development and gives rise to several structures in the ovary.

Fig. 45.27 is an image of an **atretic follicle**; the dashed line is in the approximate location of the basement membrane (line placed only on the left side of the follicle). The granulosa cells have lost cell-cell adhesion and demonstrate apoptotic features: condensed chromatin and vesicular cytoplasm. The oocyte is not present; it has likely degenerated, but it may be merely out of the plane of section. In this example, thecal cells remain fairly intact, but they will also undergo degeneration.

Apoptotic cells typically demonstrate condensed and broken-down nuclei, a term referred to as **pyknosis**.

Video 45.11 Atretic follicles

Be able to identify:
— Atretic follicle
https://www.thieme.de/de/q.htm?p=opn/
tp/308390101/978-1-62623-414-7_c045_v011&t=video

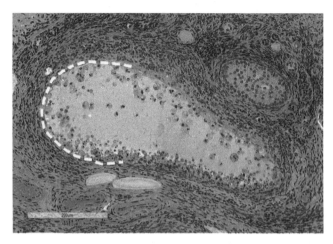

Fig. 45.27 **Follicle undergoing atresia. The dashed yellow line indicates the location of the basement membrane.**

Atresia causes degeneration of the follicle. Remnants of atresia can persist in the ovary, some of them for quite some time. These include:
- Interstitial glands
- Eosinophilic bands
- Glassy membranes
- Corpora fibrosa

45.9.1   Interstitial Glands

The most important remnants of atresia are **interstitial glands** (**Fig. 45.28**, outlined), which are derived from theca interna cells. These cells retain their steroid-secreting function (mostly estrogen) within the interstitial tissue of the ovary.

Because they are steroid secreting, interstitial glands consist of large cells with a pale eosinophilic cytoplasm. They tend to cluster together.

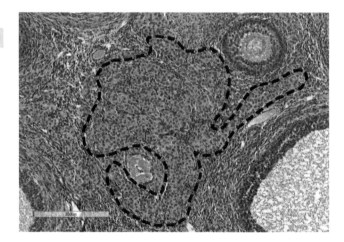

Fig. 45.28 **Interstitial gland of the ovary (outlined).**

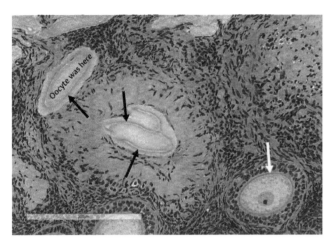

Fig. 45.29 **Eosinophilic bands (black arrows). A normal zona pellucida is shown for comparison (yellow arrow).**

Video 45.12 Interstitial glands

Be able to identify:
— Interstitial glands
https://www.thieme.de/de/q.htm?p=opn/
tp/308390101/978-1-62623-414-7_c045_v012&t=video

45.9.2 Eosinophilic Bands

Eosinophilic bands (**Fig. 45.29**, black arrows) are remnants of the zona pellucida. As the name implies, they are brightly eosinophilic and either oval or wavy. A normal zona pellucida (yellow arrow) is shown for comparison; note that eosinophilic bands are a similar color and brightness.

Helpful Hint

Because slide staining varies, it helps to find a normal zona pellucida for comparison to help distinguish eosinophilic bands from other atretic or connective tissue structures.

Video 45.13 Eosinophilic bands

Be able to identify:
— Eosinophilic bands
https://www.thieme.de/de/q.htm?p=opn/
tp/308390101/978-1-62623-414-7_c045_v013&t=video

45.9.3 Glassy Membranes

Glassy membranes (**Fig. 45.30**, black arrows) are remnants of the basement membrane between the granulosa and thecal

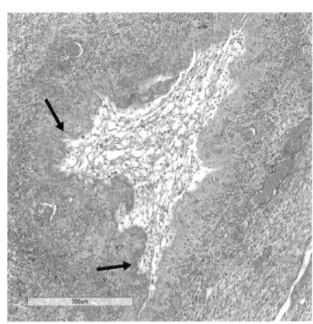

Fig. 45.30 **Glassy membrane (black arrows).**

cells. Note that because most of the granulosa cells have undergone apoptosis, the glassy membrane lines the large space that was once the antrum. As the name implies, it has a "glassy" appearance (though this is not always the case) and is typically wavy.

Helpful Hint

Eosinophilic bands and glassy membranes can be difficult to distinguish. Eosinophilic bands are remnants of the zona pellucida, so they are typically smaller than glassy membranes. In addition, because the oocyte breaks down readily, eosinophilic bands usually have nothing inside them. Glassy membranes are remnants of the basement membrane, so they surround degenerating granulosa cells and antral debris.

Video 45.14 Glassy membrane

Be able to identify:
— Glassy membrane
https://www.thieme.de/de/q.htm?p=opn/
tp/308390101/978-1-62623-414-7_c045_v014&t=video

45.9.4 Corpora Fibrosa

Corpora fibrosa (**Fig. 45.31**, outlined) are large, wavy, eosinophilic bands. These are more commonly seen in senile ovaries and are thought to be remnants of thecal cells that persist for some time after atresia.

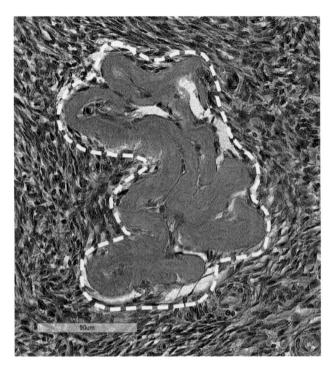

Fig. 45.31 Corpus fibrosum (outlined).

A corpus fibrosum looks similar to an eosinophilic band from a degenerating zona pellucida. However, corpora fibrosa are thicker, wavier, and not as shiny as eosinophilic bands. Corpora fibrosa have the same eosinophilic appearance as a corpus albicans but are much smaller.

Video 45.15 Corpora fibrosa

Be able to identify:
— Corpora fibrosa
https://www.thieme.de/de/q.htm?p=opn/
tp/308390101/978-1-62623-414-7_c045_v015&t=video

Bottom line here: Identifying eosinophilic bands, glassy membranes, and corpora fibrosa is low yield because they are simply remnants of atretic follicles (even though a few may be in the questions for this chapter). The interstitial glands are useful to recognize because they secrete hormones, particularly estrogen, and so have a physiologic function.

45.10   Chapter Review

The female reproductive system generates oocytes (eggs) and provides sites for fertilization and growth of the developing organism. Most structures (except for the mammary glands) reside in the pelvic cavity, covered by peritoneum, which forms ligaments (broad ligament and its parts) that support these structures. The female reproductive cycle is designed to coordinate the function of the ovary and uterus and is directed by the release of FSH and LH from the anterior pituitary gland.

Oogenesis is similar to spermatogenesis, except that all oogonia enter meiosis I before birth and are surrounded by a simple squamous layer of follicular cells. These primordial follicles are in stasis until puberty. FSH drives follicle development in the first half of the female reproductive cycle. Initially, follicular cells become cuboidal, proliferate, and become stratified; follicles in this stage are called primary follicles. A zona pellucida is produced that surrounds the oocyte, and thecal cells organize from the surrounding connective tissue. The granulosa and thecal cells of these follicles release estrogen, which stimulates the proliferative phase of the uterine cycle. Eventually, a fluid-filled space, the antrum, develops among the granulosa cells, and the follicle is called a secondary follicle. The antrum enlarges to surround the oocyte, associated zona pellucida, and granulosa cells, which are now called the corona radiata. The largest follicle, the Graafian follicle, ovulates under the influence of LH, and the oocyte completes meiosis I and becomes arrested in meiosis II. Meiosis II will not be completed until fertilization.

The structures that are released from the ovary at ovulation include the oocyte, zona pellucida, and corona radiata. After ovulation, the remaining granulosa and thecal cells of the Graafian follicle collapse to form a corpus luteum. The cells of the corpus luteum (the granulosa luteal and theca luteal cells) produce progesterone, which induces the uterine endometrial lining to become secretory. If fertilization does not occur, the corpus luteum degenerates after 12 days, forming an inactive corpus albicans.

Millions of follicles are produced during fetal development, the vast majority of which undergo a degenerative process called atresia. Of note, interstitial glands, a remnant of atresia, remain active and synthesize estrogen.

An online-only section of questions and answers accompanying this chapter is hosted on Thieme's MedOne Education site: https://medone-education.thieme.com. Use the code on the media page at the front of this book to gain access. An institutional license to the site is required to access these questions in an interactive format, and individual users are required to register for an individual account to track results.

46   Uterine Tubes, Uterus, and Vagina

After completing this chapter, you should be able to:
— Identify, at the light microscope level, each of the following:
  • Oviduct (uterine tube, fallopian tube)
    ○ Ciliated cells
    ○ Secretory (peg) cells
  • Uterus
    ○ Body
      ▪ Layers
        – Endometrium
          ◊ Functional zone
          ◊ Basal zone
        – Myometrium
        – Perimetrium
      ▪ Stages
        – Proliferative
        – Early secretory
        – Late secretory
        – Menstrual
    ○ Cervix
  • Vagina
— Outline the function of each cell and structure listed
— Correlate the appearance of each cell type or structure with its function
— Describe the female reproductive cycle, including the predominant hormones in each phase, and the effects these hormones have on the stages of the uterine cycle

46.1   Overview of the Female Reproductive System

Recall the major structures of the female reproductive system that contribute to the production and transmission of the oocyte and gestation of the offspring (**Fig. 46.1**):
• **Ovary**: site of production of oocytes
• **Oviduct** (uterine tube, fallopian tube): transport of oocyte, usual site of fertilization, transport of zygote
• **Uterus**: site of implantation and development of the embryo/fetus, contracts during childbirth
• **Vagina**: organ of copulation and birth canal

The ovaries were covered in the previous chapter. This chapter describes the oviducts, uterus, and vagina.

46.2   Oviducts (Uterine Tubes, Fallopian Tubes)

The oviducts (uterine tubes, fallopian tubes, see **Fig. 46.1**) are connected to the uterus, but laterally are open to the peritoneal cavity. Grossly, there are several regions of the oviducts (intramural, isthmus, ampulla, and infundibulum). The mucosa of the oviducts is thrown up into folds that are more prominent in the infundibulum and ampulla and are attenuated in regions closer to the uterus. However, it is usually not necessary to distinguish the different portions of the oviduct in histologic sections.

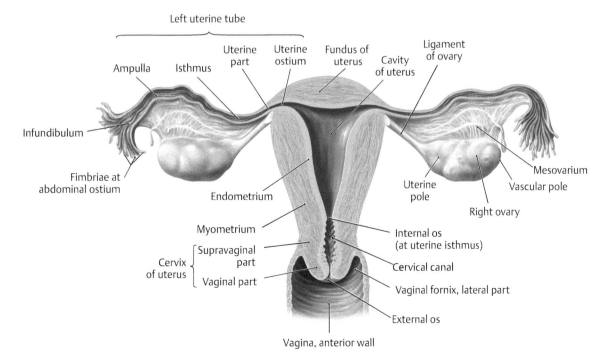

Fig. 46.1   Female reproductive system. From Schuenke M, Schulte E, Schumacher U. *THIEME Atlas of Anatomy. Internal Organs.* Illustrations by Voll M and Wesker K. Second Edition. New York: Thieme Medical Publishers; 2016.

Recall that the oviduct is at the top edge of the broad ligament (**Fig. 46.2**). **Fig. 46.3** is a scanning image of the oviduct and mesosalpinx; both are covered by an epithelium that is part of the peritoneal membrane (see discussion in the previous chapter). Even at this scanning magnification, the inner mucosa of the oviduct can be seen to be thrown up into folds, similar to the seminal vesicles.

The mucosal folds of the oviduct and seminal vesicles look similar. However, note that there is only one profile of the oviduct because it is a relatively straight tube. Recall that the seminal vesicle is lobulated, so it typically shows several profiles on sectioning. Other ways to distinguish the two will be discussed subsequently.

46.2.1   Wall of Oviduct

Fig. 46.4 is a low-magnification image of the wall of the oviduct, showing that the wall of the oviduct has three regions:

- **Mucosa**: epithelium with underlying loose connective tissue; this is thrown up into folds
- **Muscularis**: smooth muscle layer around the periphery of the mucosa
- **Serosa**: connective tissue containing blood vessels, nerves, and so on, covered by an epithelium (peritoneum, so it is a serosa rather than an adventitia)

Fig. 46.5 is a high-magnification image showing that the epithelium lining the oviduct is a simple columnar epithelium containing ciliated cells (black arrows) and nonciliated **secretory (peg) cells** (green arrows). The cilia propel the ovulated oocyte (or developing organism, if fertilized) toward the uterus. The secretory cells release nutritive fluid.

The peg cells are best characterized as lacking cilia, with a nucleus that is located in the apical portion of the cell, typically causing a bulging of the surface. The apical nuclei create the illusion of a pseudostratified epithelium, but it is classified as simple columnar.

Video 46.1   Oviduct

Be able to identify:
— Oviduct
  - Mucosa
    ∘ Ciliated cells
    ∘ Secretory (peg) cells
  - Muscularis
  - Serosa

https://www.thieme.de/de/q.htm?p=opn/tp/308390101/978-1-62623-414-7_c046_v001&t=video

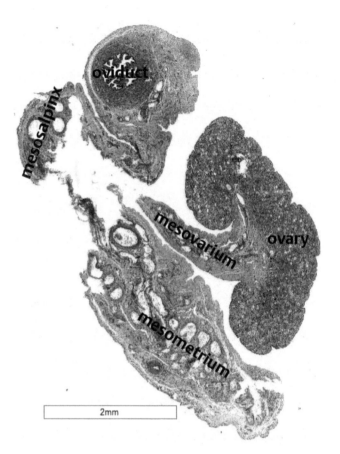

Fig. 46.2   **Female reproductive structures of a fetus. The floor of the pelvis is at the bottom of this slide, ventral is to the left. The mesosalpinx is torn.**

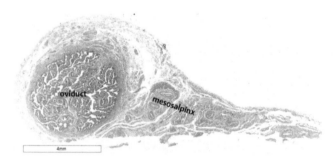

Fig. 46.3   **Oviduct and mesosalpinx, scanning magnification.**

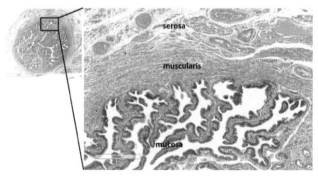

Fig. 46.4   **Oviduct, low magnification, showing mucosa, muscularis, and serosa.**

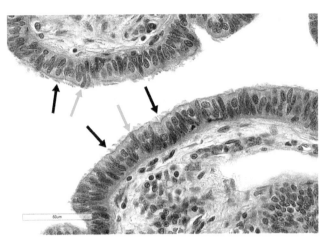

Fig. 46.5 **Epithelium of the oviduct, showing ciliated cells (black arrows) and peg cells (green arrows).**

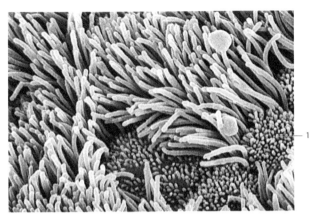

Fig. 46.6 **Scanning electron micrograph of the inner lining of the oviduct. Large projections are cilia; short projections are microvilli of peg cells (1).**

Fig. 46.6 is a scanning electron micrograph of the inner surface of the oviduct. The larger surface modifications are cilia. The shorter projections are microvilli on the surface of secretory (peg) cells (1).

Clinical Correlate

As mentioned, cilia, in combination with peristaltic movements of the muscularis, propel the ovulated oocyte or fertilized developing organism toward the uterus. Any condition that disrupts the action of the oviduct or compromises the luminal diameter (e.g., inflammation or scarring from pelvic inflammatory disease caused by sexually transmitted infections) can result in infertility.

46.2.2 Fimbriae of the Oviducts

The end of the oviduct closest to the ovary is open to the peritoneal cavity. Here, the oviduct extends fingerlike projections called **fimbriae**. **Fig. 46.7** is a scanning image of a section of the oviduct close to the ovary, on a plane similar to that marked by the blue line in the drawing on the left. Note that this cuts the oviduct in cross section, as before, but it also includes the open fingerlike projections of the fimbriae. Histologically, the fimbriae have a structure similar to the oviducts, with the exception that the muscularis layer is not as well developed.

Video 46.2 Oviduct with fimbriae

Be able to identify:
— Oviduct
  • Mucosa
    ◦ Ciliated cells
    ◦ Secretory (peg) cells
  • Muscularis
  • Serosa

https://www.thieme.de/de/q.htm?p=opn/tp/308390101/978-1-62623-414-7_c046_v002&t=video

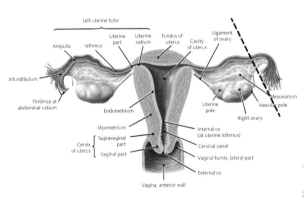

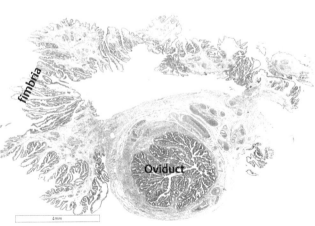

Fig. 46.7 **Oviduct and fimbriae of oviduct, scanning magnification. Based on the work of Schuenke M, Schulte E, Schumacher U. *THIEME Atlas of Anatomy. Internal Organs.* Illustrations by Voll M and Wesker K. Second Edition. New York: Thieme Medical Publishers; 2016.**

46.2.3 Mesonephric (Wolffian) Ducts

During early embryonic development, embryos develop both male and female reproductive structures. Later in development, normally the structures appropriate for the embryo's sex are elaborated, while structures of the other sex regress. In females, remnants of the vestigial male reproductive tract (i.e., the **mesonephric** or **Wolffian ducts**) persist in the broad ligament as structures called the **epoophoron** or **paroophoron**. As shown in **Fig. 46.8**, histologically, these are fairly indistinct tubes lined by simple cuboidal epithelium and surrounded by connective tissue (outlined).

Video 46.3 Oviduct showing remnants of mesonephric ducts

Be able to identify:
— Remnants of mesonephric ducts
https://www.thieme.de/de/q.htm?p=opn/
tp/308390101/978-1-62623-414-7_c046_v003&t=video

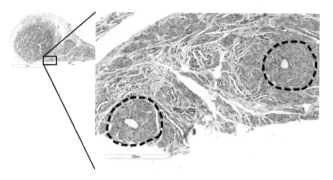

Fig. 46.8 **Oviduct and mesosalpinx showing mesonephric duct remnants (outlined).**

Clinical Correlate

It is usually not critical to identify the epoophoron or paroophoron. They are mentioned here because they can form benign cysts called **Gartner cysts**. These structures are almost always benign, but they can present as a mass lateral to the vagina or uterus that causes discomfort during intercourse or tampon insertion.

46.3 Uterus

The uterus is the site of implantation of the embryo and contains thick smooth muscle that contracts during childbirth (see **Fig. 46.1**). Histologically and anatomically, the uterus can be divided into the **body** (including the **fundus**) and **cervix** (superior and inferior to the **internal os**, respectively). Both regions consist of three layers:

1. **Endometrium**: inner lining, consisting of epithelium and connective tissue, similar to a mucosa
2. **Myometrium**: very thick layer of smooth muscle in the body (and fundus), less muscular in the cervix
3. **Perimetrium**: very thin outer connective tissue layer, covered by an epithelium on most of its surface (similar to a serosa)

This discussion of the uterus will begin by taking a look at the body, including the histologic changes that occur in this region during the female reproductive cycle. This will be followed by a look at the cervix, including the vaginal surface.

Fig. 46.9 is a scanning image showing one wall of the body of the uterus. The lumen of the uterus is indicated, as are the three layers of the wall. Even at this low magnification, it may be evident that the endometrium consists of an epithelium and connective tissue, similar to a mucosal layer in other organs. The myometrium is bright pink/red and contains abundant smooth muscle with interspersed bundles of connective tissue. The perimetrium is very thin, hardly visible at this magnification.

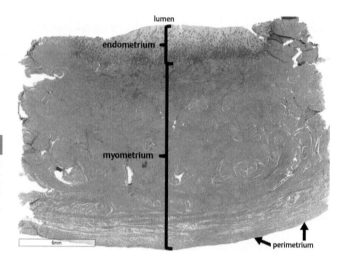

Fig. 46.9 **Uterus, scanning magnification, showing endometrium, myometrium, and perimetrium.**

46.3.1 Myometrium and Perimetrium

The myometrium and perimetrium do not change during the uterine cycle, so they can be discussed briefly (**Fig. 46.10**). **Fig. 46.10a** is an image of the myometrium, which is dominated by bundles of smooth muscle in all orientations, with some connective tissue between the bundles. The myometrium provides protection for the developing embryo/fetus and contracts to expel the fetus during childbirth. **Fig. 46.10b** shows the perimetrium (bracket),

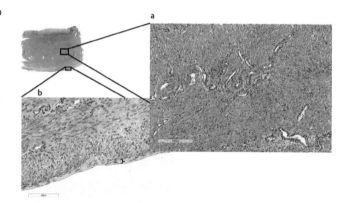

Fig. 46.10 **Uterus, showing closer views of (a) the myometrium and (b) the perimetrium bracket.**

consisting of a thin layer of connective tissue covered by a simple squamous epithelium. The remainder of the lower left image (above the perimetrium) is smooth muscle of the myometrium.

Video 46.4   Overview of uterus layers—1

https://www.thieme.de/de/q.htm?p=opn/
tp/308390101/978-1-62623-414-7_c046_
v004&t=video

Video 46.5   Overview of uterus layers—2

https://www.thieme.de/de/q.htm?p=opn/
tp/308390101/978-1-62623-414-7_c046_
v005&t=video

Be able to identify:
— Uterus
  • Endometrium
  • Myometrium
  • Perimetrium

Fig. 46.11 **Uterus, endometrium, showing functional zone and basal zone.**

> **Helpful Hint**
>
> The term *stroma* refers to the connective tissue of a tissue or structure and usually implies that the cells or tissues are structural, as opposed to performing a specific function such as secretion. It is not specific to the uterus.

46.3.2   Endometrium

Fig. 46.11 is an image focusing on the endometrium. Even at this magnification, it is evident that the endometrium has very deep glands that extend all the way to the myometrium. The basal portion of the endometrium, near the myometrium, stains more darkly. This region is the **basal zone**, while the paler region is the **functional zone**. During menstruation, the functional zone is sloughed off, and the epithelial cells at the base of the glands and surrounding connective tissue of the basal zone regenerate the functional zone during the subsequent menstrual cycle.

Fig. 46.12 is an image of the surface endometrium lining the lumen of the uterus. The epithelium of the endometrium is simple columnar epithelium. Many of the cells are ciliated, though not as prominently as in the oviduct. The lamina propria is very cellular and includes fibroblastlike cells referred to as **stromal cells**. In addition, numerous white blood cells populate the lamina propria. Glands are numerous in the lamina propria, extending all the way to the basal layer, and are lined by columnar cells similar to the cells that line the uterine lumen. The surface and glandular epithelial cells have pale eosinophilia when they are actively secreting, as shown here.

Video 46.6   Overview of the endometrium

Be able to identify:
— Uterus
  • Endometrium
    ◦ Basal zone
    ◦ Functional zone
    ◦ Surface and glandular epithelial cells
    ◦ Stroma

https://www.thieme.de/de/q.htm?p=opn/tp/308390101/978-1-62623-414-7_c046_v006&t=video

46.4   Phases of the Uterine Cycle

The uterus undergoes changes during the menstrual cycle in response to hormones released by the ovary (**Fig. 46.13**). Most or all of these changes occur in the endometrium.

At the end of the female reproductive cycle, the corpus luteum of the ovary degenerates. The resulting decrease in circulating progesterone (and estrogen) levels causes changes in blood flow to the functional zone of the uterus. Ultimately, the functional zone sloughs off; this process, **menstruation**, takes place during approximately the first five days of the subsequent uterine cycle.

Around day 5, developing follicles in the ovary produce enough **estrogen** to induce the **proliferative phase of the uterus**. In this phase, the functional zone is replaced through proliferation of epithelial and connective tissue cells of the remaining basilar zone.

After ovulation, **progesterone** released by the corpus luteum induces the endometrial tissue to enter the **secretory phase of the uterus**; glands become more numerous and secretory, and stromal tissue becomes more vascularized and edematous. The secretory phase lasts approximately 12 days, after which the corpus luteum degenerates and the loss of progesterone results in another menstrual phase, continuing the cycle.

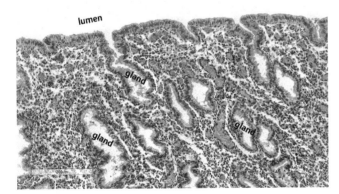

Fig. 46.12 **Surface endometrium of the uterus, showing uterine glands.**

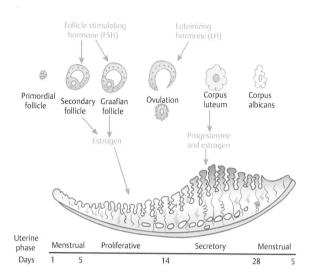

Fig. 46.13 **Female reproductive cycle.**

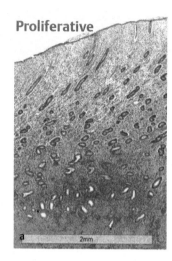

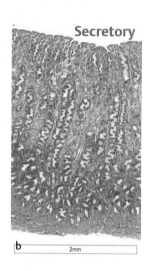

Fig. 46.14 **Uterine endometrium in the (a) proliferative and (b) secretory phases.**

To begin differentiating these states, it is easiest to compare major differences in the endometrium between the proliferative and secretory phases, as shown in low-magnification images in **Fig. 46.14**. Note that the glands in the **proliferative endometrium** are not as numerous, are straighter, and have a narrow lumen. In contrast, the glands in the **secretory endometrium** are more numerous, with dilated lumina that give them a "sawtooth" appearance.

Helpful Hint

The stroma of the endometrium also undergoes changes, such as edema and increased blood supply in the secretory uterus. However, these changes are more subtle; therefore, it is easier to look at the number and features of the glands to differentiate these phases.

46.4.1   Proliferative Phase of the Uterine Cycle

Under the influence of estrogen from developing ovarian follicles, the functional zone of the endometrium is regenerated during the proliferative phase of the uterine cycle. The proliferative endometrium has straight glands, each with a narrow lumen (**Fig. 46.15**). The lamina propria is very cellular, and blood vessels are evident. Regeneration of the epithelial and connective tissue cells from the basal layer of the endometrium requires cell division, so mitotic figures can be seen in the proliferative endometrium (**Fig. 46.15**, arrow).

Helpful Hint

Even though regeneration of the functional zone requires a lot of cell division, finding mitotic figures is somewhat challenging. Therefore, it is best to utilize the straight, narrow glands as the key to identifying the proliferative phase of the uterus.

Video 46.7   Uterus in the proliferative phase

Be able to identify:
— Uterus, proliferative phase
https://www.thieme.de/de/q.htm?p=opn/
tp/308390101/978-1-62623-414-7_c046_
v007&t=video

46.4.2   Secretory Phase of the Uterine Cycle

After ovulation, the corpus luteum from the ovary releases progesterone (and some estrogen). In response to progesterone, the cells of the endometrial epithelium become highly secretory and release their product into the lumen, causing the glands to dilate and become sacculated (**Fig. 46.16**, "sawtooth" appearance). The lamina propria becomes edematous, and the vasculature becomes much more elaborate.

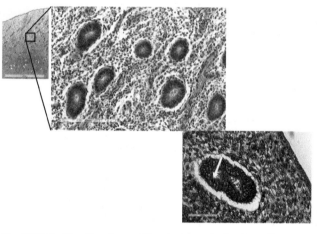

Fig. 46.15 **Proliferative phase of the uterine cycle. A mitotic figure is shown (arrow).**

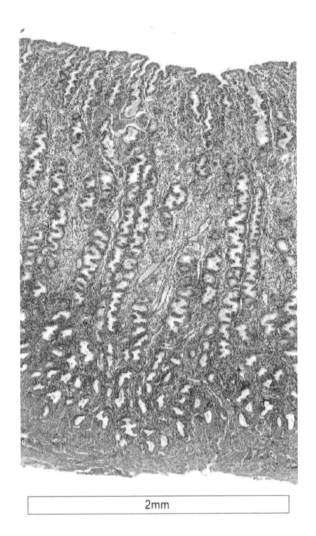

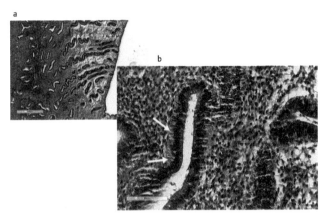

Fig. 46.17 **Early secretory phase of the uterine cycle, shown at (a) low and (b) medium magnification. Arrows indicate glycogen.**

Video 46.8   Uterus in early secretory phase

Be able to identify:
— Uterus, early secretory phase
https://www.thieme.de/de/q.htm?p=opn/
tp/308390101/978-1-62623-414-7_c046_
v008&t=video

During the later part of the secretory phase (**Fig. 46.18**), the secretory product is moved to the apical side of the cell (**Fig. 46.18b**, arrows) and released into the lumen of the gland. The nuclei are repositioned back to the basal aspect of the cells (**Fig. 46.18b**), and the glands become more dilated and tortuous (**Fig. 46.18a**).

Video 46.9   Uterus in late secretory phase

Be able to identify:
— Uterus, late secretory phase
https://www.thieme.de/de/q.htm?p=opn/
tp/308390101/978-1-62623-414-7_c046_
v009&t=video

2mm

Fig. 46.16 **Secretory phase of the uterine cycle.**

Basic Science Correlate: Embryology

Given the presence of spermatozoa, fertilization occurs in the oviducts shortly after ovulation. Through the action of cilia and the muscularis, the embryo will reach the uterus 3–4 days later and begin implanting around day 6 after fertilization. Therefore, the embryo will arrive at the uterus around day 20–22 of the uterine cycle, right in the middle of this secretory phase. This provides an enriched environment for the embryo to implant, full of nutrient-rich secretory product, fluid, and vasculature.

The secretory phase can be roughly divided into early and late secretory phases. In the early portion of the secretory phase, the glands begin to become tortuous, with a wider lumen (**Fig. 46.17a**). This change is due to increased activity of the glandular cells. One of the main products secreted by the endometrium is glycogen, which is initially located in the basal aspect of the glandular cells (**Fig. 46.17b**, arrows), displacing the nucleus toward the apical side of the cell.

Helpful Hint

Recall that glycogen does not stain well in routine H & E preparations.

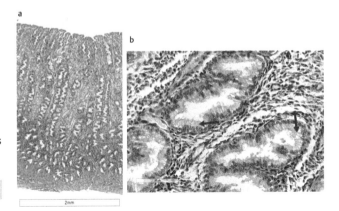

2mm

Fig. 46.18 **Late secretory phase of the uterine cycle, shown at (a) low and (b) medium magnification. Arrows indicate glycogen.**

46.4.3 Menstrual Phase of the Uterine Cycle

During the menstrual phase, the functional zone of the endometrium is sloughed off, leaving only the basal zone. Histologically, this appears as an incomplete surface epithelial layer of the endometrium (**Fig. 46.19**). The increased cellularity in the stroma is due to an increase in the number of white blood cells.

Helpful Hint

The "tears" in the surface epithelium of the menstrual uterus appear similar to artifacts. However, careful tissue preparation, and knowledge of the fact that this is the endometrium, a tissue known to undergo this process, allows definitive identification. Other phases of the endometrium (proliferative, secretory) may have small "tears" as a result of tissue preparation, but not to this extent.

Video 46.10 Uterus in menstrual phase

Be able to identify:
— Uterus, menstrual phase
https://www.thieme.de/de/q.htm?p=opn/
tp/308390101/978-1-62623-414-7_c046_
v010&t=video

Clinical Correlate

There are a variety of pathologies of the uterus. Many involve the endometrium, including malignant cancers and polyps. Furthermore, many women experience irregular or uncomfortable menstrual cycles (**dysmenorrhea**). **Fibroids (leiomyomas)** are usually asymptomatic, noncancerous growths within the myometrium, thought to be present in 75% of the female population.

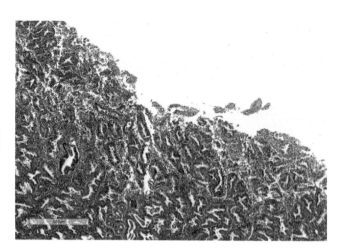

Fig. 46.19 **Menstrual phase of the uterine cycle.**

46.5 Cervix of the Uterus

The cervix of the uterus (**Fig. 46.20**, black box) contains the same three layers as the body of the uterus. However, there are distinctions:

- The endometrium consists of mucous glands and surface epithelial cells that secrete mucus; it does not slough off during the menstrual phase.
- In the myometrium, the smooth muscle in the cervix is much thinner than in the body of the uterus, so this layer is mostly connective tissue.
- The perimetrium in the cervix is covered by little, if any, peritoneum, so it is an adventitia rather than a serosa.

Also note that the inferior surface of the cervix is facing the vagina (**Fig. 46.20**, arrows), and, therefore, is lined by vaginal epithelium, namely, stratified squamous nonkeratinized.

Fig. 46.21 shows the cervix of the uterus. **Fig. 46.21a** is the same drawing as **Fig. 46.20**, turned 90°, with a rectangle indicating one wall of the cervix. **Fig. 46.21b** is a scanning image

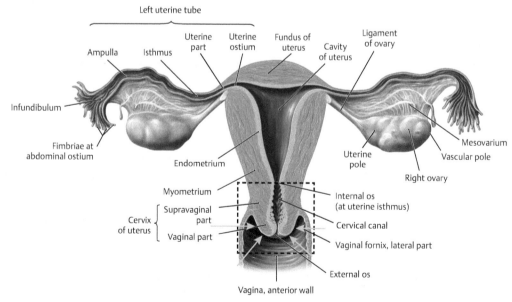

Fig. 46.20 **Female reproductive system focusing on the cervix (black box).** Arrows indicate the vaginal surface of the cervix. Based on the work of Schuenke M, Schulte E, Schumacher U. *THIEME Atlas of Anatomy. Internal Organs.* Illustrations by Voll M and Wesker K. Second Edition. New York: Thieme Medical Publishers; 2016.

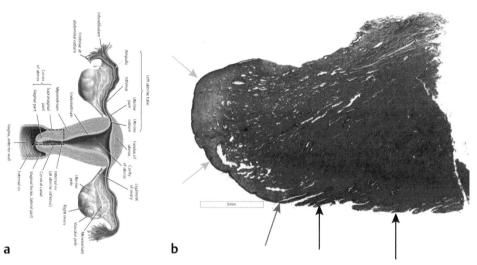

a   **b**

Fig. 46.21 Cervix of the uterus. (a) The drawing from Fig. 46.20. (b) Scanning image of the part of the cervix corresponding to the rectangle in a. The arrows represent the sides of the cervix: blue, vaginal side; black, cervical side; purple, transition point (external os). Fig. 46.21a from Schuenke M, Schulte E, Schumacher U. *THIEME Atlas of Anatomy. Internal Organs.* Illustrations by Voll M and Wesker K. Second Edition. New York: Thieme Medical Publishers; 2016.

showing the wall of the cervix corresponding to the rectangle in **Fig. 46.21a**. The side of the cervix facing the lumen of the cervical uterus (**endocervix**) is indicated by the black arrows, while the side facing the vagina (**ectocervix**) is indicated by the blue arrows. The transition between the uterine and vaginal sides of the cervix (purple arrow) is in the area of the **external os**.

Clinical Correlate

The external os is the opening into the cervix seen in a pelvic examination.

Fig. 46.22 shows images of the side of the cervix that faces the lumen of the uterus, which consists of columnar, mucus-secreting epithelial cells and mucous glands in a very cellular

lamina propria. The myometrium (shown only in the scanning image) has much less smooth muscle than is found in the body of the uterus.

Fig. 46.23 is an image of the vaginal side of the cervix, which is lined by a stratified squamous nonkeratinized epithelium, with a dense irregular connective tissue that contains numerous blood vessels. This is similar to the lining of the rest of the vagina, discussed in the following section.

Video 46.11 Cervix

Be able to identify:
— Cervix of uterus
https://www.thieme.de/de/q.htm?p=opn/tp/308390101/978-1-62623-414-7_c046_v011&t=video

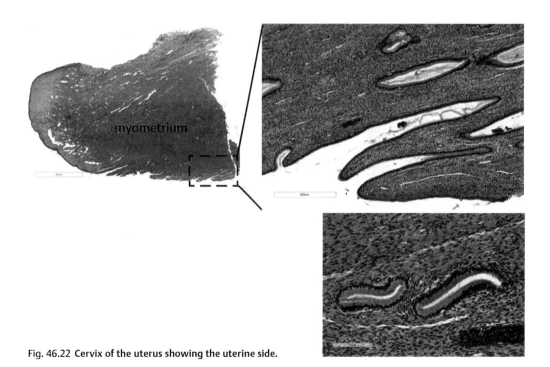

Fig. 46.22 Cervix of the uterus showing the uterine side.

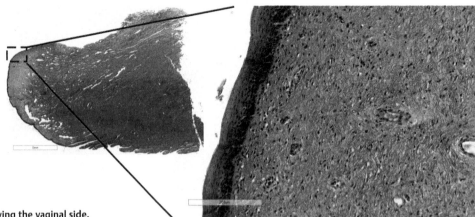

Fig. 46.23 **Cervix of the uterus showing the vaginal side.**

46.6   Vagina

The vagina is a muscular-elastic organ. It is the organ of copulation and the birth canal.

Like the oviduct and uterus, the vagina has three regions (**Fig. 46.24**):

1. Mucosa: epithelium with underlying elastic connective tissue
2. Muscularis: smooth muscle layer
3. Adventitia: connective tissue containing blood vessels, nerves, and other structures

Fig. 46.25 is a low-magnification image focusing on the epithelium of the vagina, which is stratified squamous, nokeratinized, and specialized for moist friction. The mature epithelial cells contain cytoplasmic glycogen; these pale cells are a characteristic feature that distinguishes the vagina from other tissues with a similar epithelium (e.g., esophagus). To assist in withstanding friction, the underlying connective tissue contains papillalike structures (arrow) that project into the epithelium. As might be expected in an organ of copulation and childbirth, the connective tissue is quite dense and contains numerous elastic fibers, but it contains no glands (glandular secretions during arousal come from the cervix and external genitalia). The muscularis is a mixture of smooth muscle and dense irregular connective tissue.

Video 46.12 Vagina

Be able to identify:
— Vagina
https://www.thieme.de/de/q.htm?p=opn/
tp/308390101/978-1-62623-414-7_c046_v012&t=video

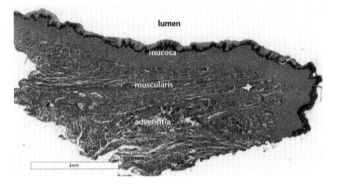

Fig. 46.24 **Vagina, scanning view, showing three regions (mucosa, muscularis, adventitia).**

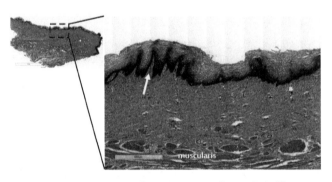

Fig. 46.25 **Vagina, low magnification. Arrow indicates fingerlike projection of the lamina propria.**

The next two images show sections that include portions of the urinary tract (**Fig. 46.26**). These images are useful because they provide review of the urinary system and reinforce anatomic relationships between the urinary and reproductive structures. The yellow line marks the plane of a section through the anterior wall of the vagina and the posterior wall of the bladder. The green line indicates a plane of section through the anterior wall of the vagina and the entire urethra. Where the adventitia of the vagina is adjacent to the adventitia of the bladder or the urethra, these tissues merge.

Fig. 46.27 is a scanning image of a section through the anterior wall of the vagina and the posterior wall of the bladder at the level of the yellow line in **Fig. 46.26**. The dashed line indicates the approximate border between the two, although

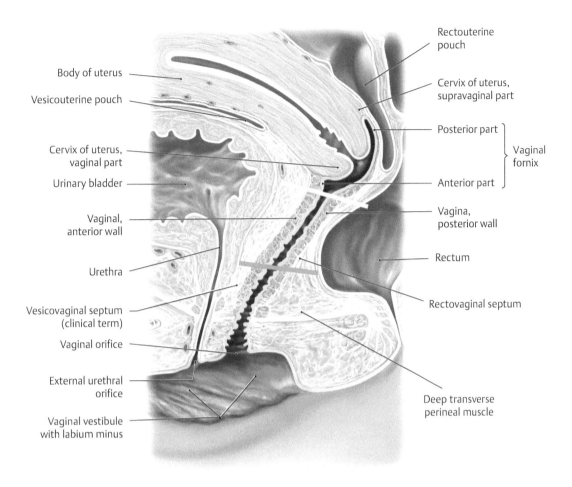

Rectouterine pouch

Body of uterus

Vesicouterine pouch

Cervix of uterus, supravaginal part

Posterior part

Vaginal fornix

Cervix of uterus, vaginal part

Anterior part

Urinary bladder

Vagina, posterior wall

Vaginal, anterior wall

Rectum

Urethra

Rectovaginal septum

Vesicovaginal septum (clinical term)

Vaginal orifice

External urethral orifice

Deep transverse perineal muscle

Vaginal vestibule with labium minus

Fig. 46.26 Female pelvis showing relationship between urinary and reproductive structures. Green and yellow lines indicate tissue sections on subsequent images. Based on the work of Schuenke M, Schulte E, Schumacher U. *THIEME Atlas of Anatomy. Internal Organs.* Illustrations by Voll M and Wesker K. Second Edition. New York: Thieme Medical Publishers; 2016.

the adventitial layers are fused. Recall that the surface of the bladder is a transitional epithelium, with an underlying lamina propria, and that the muscularis of the bladder has substantial smooth muscle.

Video 46.13 Vagina and bladder

Be able to identify:
— Vagina
— Review bladder

https://www.thieme.de/de/q.htm?p=opn/
tp/308390101/978-1-62623-414-7_c046_v013&t=video

Fig. 46.28 is an image of the anterior wall of the vagina and the entire urethra at the level of the green line in **Fig. 46.26**. The border of the urethra is indicated by the dashed line.

The female urethra is essentially the same as the membranous urethra in the male:

1. A mucosa with an ill-defined epithelium and a lamina propria with numerous blood vessels
2. A muscularis containing smooth muscle and connective tissue
3. An adventitia composed of connective tissue, which may contain skeletal muscle from the urogenital diaphragm

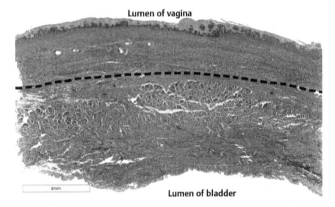

Lumen of vagina

4mm

Lumen of bladder

Fig. 46.27 Vagina and bladder, scanning view at the level of the yellow line in Fig. 46.26. Dashed line indicates the approximate border between these two structures.

Video 46.14 Vagina and urethra

Be able to identify:
— Vagina
— Review urethra

https://www.thieme.de/de/q.htm?p=opn/
tp/308390101/978-1-62623-414-7_c046_v014&t=video

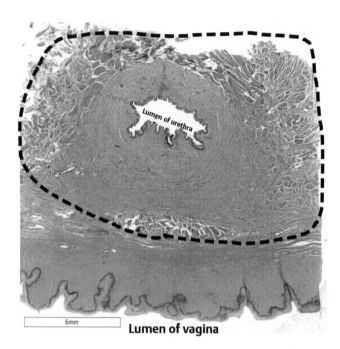

Lumen of urethra

5mm

Lumen of vagina

Fig. 46.28 Vagina and urethra, scanning view at the level of the green line in Fig. 46.26. Dashed line indicates the approximate border of the urethra.

46.7 Chapter Review

The female reproductive structures provide a site for fertilization, growth of the embryo, and the birth canal. The oviduct is the site of fertilization and is composed of three histologic layers; mucosa, submucosa, adventitia. It contains thin wisps of smooth muscle in the muscularis, and has ciliated and secretory (peg) cells in the epithelium. The cilia and muscularis move the ovulated oocyte toward the uterus. The uterus is also composed of three layers, but they are called the endometrium, myometrium,

and perimetrium. The uterus has a thick, very muscular myometrium that provides protection for the developing fetus and contracts during childbirth. The endometrium consists of a simple columnar epithelium and lamina propria composed of a very cellular connective tissue. A portion of the endometrium, called the functional zone, sloughs off during menstruation and is regenerated by the remaining basal zone. This regeneration occurs under the influence of estrogen secreted by ovarian follicles, which induces cell proliferation in the epithelial and connective tissue cells. After ovulation, progesterone from the corpus luteum induces the endometrium to become secretory. Epithelial cells produce and release a secretory product rich in glycogen, and the lamina propria becomes edematous and well vascularized. When the corpus luteum degenerates, and progesterone secretion ceases, menstruation ensues. The cervix is similar to the body of the uterus, but its myometrium is composed of mostly connective tissue. The epithelial cells facing the lumen of the uterus are simple columnar and, along with the extensive glands in this region, secrete mucus. The vaginal surface of the cervix is lined by stratified squamous nonkeratinized epithelium. The vagina consists of three layers: a mucosa, a muscularis, and an adventitia. The epithelium that lines the vagina is stratified squamous nonkeratinized; the cells contain glycogen. The lamina propria of the vagina has abundant elastic fibers, and the muscularis is composed of smooth muscle with interspersed connective tissue.

47 Mammary Glands

After completing this chapter, you should be able to:
— Identify, at the light microscope level, each of the following:
  • Mammary gland
    ○ Lobes and lobules
      ▪ Acini
      ▪ Ducts
      ▪ Stroma
      ▪ Cells and structures
        – Secretory cells
        – Myoepithelial cells
        – Plasma cells and other lymphocytes
    ○ Stages
      ▪ Immature/Inactive
      ▪ Mammary gland of pregnancy
      ▪ Lactating mammary gland
      ▪ Regressing (difficult to distinguish from poorly preserved tissue)
    ○ Nipple
      ▪ Lactiferous ducts / sinuses
— Identify, at the electron microscope level, each of the following:
  • Mammary gland
    ○ Acinar cells
      ▪ Lipid product
      ▪ Protein product
    ○ Myoepithelial cells
— Outline the function of each cell and structure listed
— Correlate the appearance of each cell type or structure with its function
— Describe the development of the mammary gland through life stages

47.1 Overview of the Mammary Gland

Mammary glands are located in the breast, or the skin of the anterior thoracic wall (**Fig. 47.1**). These glands produce milk for sustenance of newborns, a process called **lactation**.

Each breast has a **nipple**, which is a conical elevation containing sebaceous glands and smooth muscle for erection. There are 12 to 15 mammary glands in each breast, each with a separate opening onto the nipple. Like other glands, the mammary glands can be divided into lobes and lobules. Secretory cells of mammary glands are organized into **acini**, which are surrounded by loose connective tissue. **Lactiferous ducts** drain the acini. Near the nipple, a dilation of each duct, called the **lactiferous sinus**, provides a reservoir for milk between feedings.

This chapter will examine four different stages of mammary gland development:
1. Immature/inactive
2. Mammary gland of pregnancy
3. Mammary gland of lactation
4. Regressing
These discussions will be followed by a discussion of the nipple.

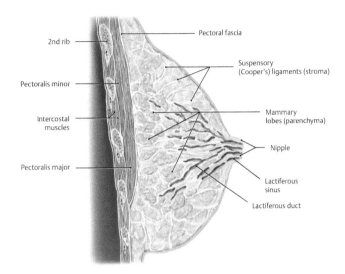

Fig. 47.1 Gross anatomy of the mammary gland. From Schuenke M, Schulte E, Schumacher U. *THIEME Atlas of Anatomy. General Anatomy and Musculoskeletal System*. Illustrations by Voll M and Wesker K. Second Edition. New York: Thieme Medical Publishers; 2016.

47.2 Immature/Inactive Mammary Gland

The **immature (prepubertal) mammary gland** is mostly connective tissue mixed with some adipose tissue (**Fig. 47.2**). There are some rudimentary ducts and secretory units (outlined).

At this stage, the male and immature female mammary glands are indistinguishable. Male breast tissue will remain in this stage.

> **Helpful Hint**
>
> The connective tissue of a structure or organ is sometimes referred to as **stroma**. This is in contrast with **parenchyma**, which consists of the active cells in an organ.

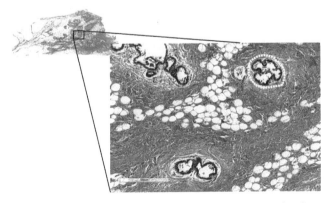

Fig. 47.2 Immature mammary gland. A secretory unit is outlined.

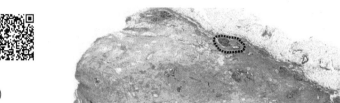

Be able to identify:
— Immature mammary gland
  • Rudimentary ducts and glands
    ○ Stroma
    ○ Connective tissue (dense irregular and loose)
    ○ Adipose

https://www.thieme.de/de/q.htm?p=opn/tp/308390101/978-1-62623-414-7_c047_v001&t=video

Estrogen and **progesterone** drive development of the glandular structures of the female mammary gland tissues and induce growth of the female breasts. However, in the absence of fertilization and implantation, the effect of these hormones on glandular development is minimal. Histologically, the inactive mammary gland in the female, postpuberty, demonstrates some elaboration of the glandular structures (**Fig. 47.3**, outlined). However, because this increase is relatively modest, most regions of the inactive mammary gland are connective and adipose tissue, the expansion of which accounts for the increase in size in the breasts during puberty. Therefore, it is difficult to distinguish immature and inactive mammary glands with certainty.

Fig. 47.4 is a medium magnification image focusing on a region of glandular tissue in an inactive mammary gland, showing minimally developed acinar secretory units (outlined) and an associated duct (arrows). The stroma at this stage is mostly loose or dense irregular connective tissue, with adipose tissue.

Video **47.2**   Inactive mammary gland

Be able to identify:
— Inactive mammary gland (indistinguishable from immature)
  • Ducts and glands
    ○ Stroma
    ○ Connective tissue (dense irregular and loose)
    ○ Adipose

https://www.thieme.de/de/q.htm?p=opn/tp/308390101/978-1-62623-414-7_c047_v002&t=video

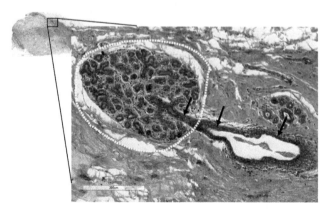

Fig. 47.4   Inactive mammary gland, medium magnification. Secretory units are outlined, and the duct draining these units is indicated by the arrows.

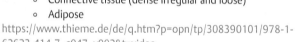

Fig. 47.3   Inactive mammary gland, scanning magnification. Secretory units are outlined.

47.3   Mammary Gland of a Pregnant Woman

During **pregnancy**, estrogen and progesterone levels increase significantly. **Fig. 47.5** is a scanning image of the mammary gland from a woman 7 months pregnant. Even at low magnification, when this image is compared to inactive mammary glands, it is evident that these hormones stimulate extensive elaboration of the ducts and glands, replacing the stromal tissue. Continued proliferation of the glandular units continues throughout pregnancy, so at term (**Fig. 47.6**), most of the breast consists of glandular units.

Like other glandular structures, the secretory units of the mammary gland are organized into **lobes** (**Fig. 47.7**, yellow outline) and **lobules** (green outline). In the upper right portion of the image in **Fig. 47.7**, the structure with the large lumen is the main duct that drains the entire lobe.

Fig. 47.8 is an image showing an enlargement of a portion of a lobule (yellow outline) and an adjacent duct. The lobule is composed of acini (one is outlined in green) consisting of a simple cuboidal epithelium, similar to secretory end pieces in other glands. The cells are mildly active at this stage, producing

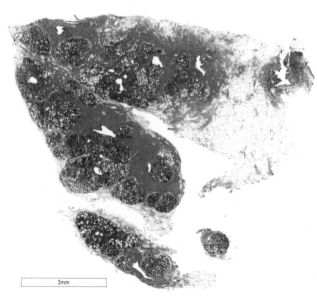

Fig. 47.5   Mammary gland from a woman 7 months pregnant, scanning magnification.

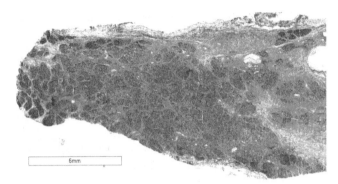

Fig. 47.6   **Mammary gland from a woman at term, scanning magnification.**

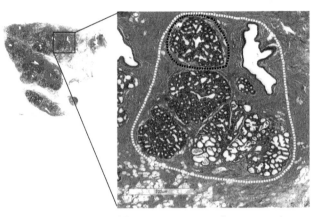

Fig. 47.7   **Mammary gland from a woman 7 months pregnant, low magnification, showing secretory units organized into lobes (yellow outline) and lobules (green outline).**

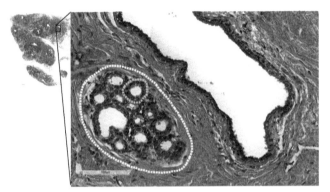

Fig. 47.8   **Mammary gland from a woman 7 months pregnant, medium magnification, showing a lobule (yellow outline) and individual secretory acinus (green outline).**

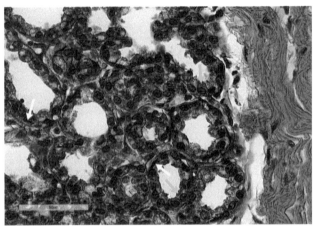

Fig. 47.9   **Mammary gland from a woman 7 months pregnant, high magnification, showing an acinar cells (green arrows) and myoepithelial cells (yellow arrows).**

colostrum. Colostrum is a fluid similar to milk, but it lacks significant fat and contains a laxative and antibodies. The **acinar cells** are fairly nondistinct, with large nuclei and cytoplasmic basophilia. The duct has a much wider lumen and is lined by a stratified epithelium.

Fig. 47.9 is a high-magnification image of a secretory region. The acinar cells (green arrows) are cuboidal/columnar, with round nuclei and cytoplasmic basophilia. The epithelium also includes **myoepithelial cells** (yellow arrows), which have smaller or flattened nuclei on the *epithelial side* of the basement membrane. These myoepithelial cells have contractile proteins that are involved in moving secretory product out of the gland during lactation. Sparse connective tissue stroma is between the acini.

Helpful Hint

Both myoepithelial cells of the mammary gland and myoid cells in the testes are involved in contraction. However, myoepithelial cells (**Fig. 47.10a**, yellow arrow) are derived from the epithelium and, therefore, are located on the epithelial side of the basement membrane (basement membrane indicated by the blue arrows). In contrast, myoid cells (**Fig. 47.10b**, black arrow) are derived from connective tissue and are positioned on the connective tissue side of the basement membrane.

Colostrum and milk produced by the mammary gland contain antibodies, which provide passive immunity. These are produced by plasma cells within the connective tissue of the mammary gland and transported across the epithelium of the acini into the lumen. **Fig. 47.11** shows a plasma cell (arrow) in the connective

tissue of the mammary gland, recognized by its intense cytoplasmic basophilia.

Helpful Hint

Plasma cells can be found in the loose connective tissue between the acini. However, due to the highly cellular nature of these regions where acini are packed together, it is often difficult to identify plasma cells in that location.

Video 47.3   Mammary gland of pregnancy

Be able to identify:
— Mammary gland from a pregnant woman
  • Ducts and glands
  • Acinar cells
  • Myoepithelial cells
  • Connective tissue
  • Plasma cells

https://www.thieme.de/de/q.htm?p=opn/tp/308390101/978-1-62623-414-7_c047_v003&t=video

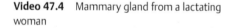

Fig. 47.10 **Comparison of (a) myoepithelial cells (yellow arrow) and (b) myoid cells of the seminiferous tubules (black arrow). The basement membrane is indicated by blue arrows.**

47.4 Mammary Gland of a Lactating Woman

As mentioned, during pregnancy, the mammary glands fill with colostrum, a milklike substance that contains protein, a small amount of fat, a mild laxative, and antibodies produced by plasma cells in the mammary gland. The newborn feeds on colostrum during the first few days after birth; the laxative helps clear the intestinal lumen of cellular debris and bilirubin that accumulates during development.

After birth, the mammary glands begin producing **milk**, which contains fat and protein as well as carbohydrates, minerals, and ions. Histologically, this transition includes some proliferation of the ducts and glands, as shown in **Fig, 47.12**.

Milk contains a substantial amount of fat. Acinar cells from lactating mammary glands demonstrate large lipid droplets (**Fig. 47.13**, black arrows) in their cytoplasm, which washes away on tissue preparation. In addition, the lumen of the acini are dilated because they are filled with milk, and some milk product can be seen precipitated within the lumen (blue arrows).

Video 47.4   Mammary gland from a lactating woman

Be able to identify:
— Mammary gland from a lactating woman
  • Ducts and glands
  • Acinar cells
  • Myoepithelial cells
  • Connective tissue septa
https://www.thieme.de/de/q.htm?p=opn/tp/308390101/978-1-62623-414-7_c047_v004&t=video

Milk contains both fat and protein and is stored in the lumina of the acini and lactiferous ducts and sinuses in between feedings. **Fig. 47.14** is an electron micrograph taken from the mammary gland of a lactating woman, showing about four acinar cells. In the lumen, large lipid droplets (1) and smaller protein precipitates (5) are evident. Secretory vesicles (4) containing protein are in transit to the cell surface. These cells also demonstrate the rough endoplasmic reticulum (RER; 2) and Golgi apparatus (3) necessary for milk production; the RER imparts cytoplasmic basophilia in these cells in light micrographs (see **Fig. 47.13**).

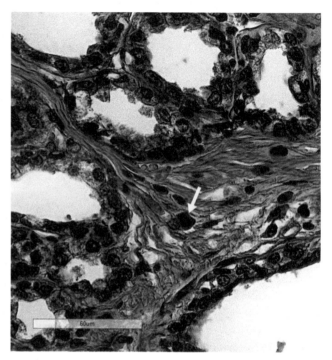

Fig. 47.11 **Mammary gland from a woman 7 months pregnant, high magnification, showing plasma cell (yellow arrow).**

47.5 Regressing Mammary Gland

After lactation, the secretory units regress. **Fig. 47.15a** is a scanning image from a woman shortly after weaning, showing faint outlines of lobules, with sparse secretory tissue within them. **Fig. 47.15b** is taken at higher magnification, showing that the epithelial component within the lobules is being replaced by connective tissue.

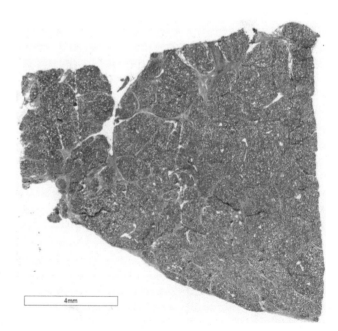

Fig. 47.12 **Mammary gland from a lactating woman, scanning magnification.**

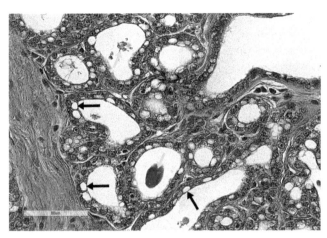

Fig. 47.13 Mammary gland from a lactating woman, medium magnification, showing lipid droplets in acinar cells (black arrows) and precipitated milk in the lumen (blue arrows).

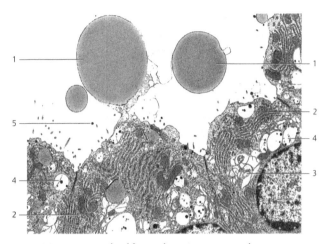

Fig. 47.14 Mammary gland from a lactating woman, electron micrograph, showing (1) lipid droplets; (2) rough endoplasmic reticulum; (3) Golgi apparatus; (4) secretory vesicles; (5) small proteins.

Video 47.5 Regressing mammary gland

Be able to identify:
— Regressing mammary gland
https://www.thieme.de/de/q.htm?p=opn/
tp/308390101/978-1-62623-414-7_c047_
v005&t=video

Clinical Correlate

Breast cancer is one of the most common cancers, affecting about one in eight women in the United States. The incidence is much lower in men (1 in 1,000). Although the mortality rate is still quite high, it has dropped dramatically as a result of early detection through active screening, including self-exams and mammograms. Common presentations include pain, presence of a palpable mass, and discharge from the nipple. Some are asymptomatic, detected by mammograms. There are several forms of breast cancer; most are derived from the epithelial cells of the ducts or acini. Over half of these tumors express receptors to estrogen and respond to therapies that target this hormone or hormone receptors. It should be noted that benign lesions of the breast (e.g., cysts, fibrosis) also present as lumps or densities on mammograms.

47.6 Nipple

The **nipple** is a conical projection on the surface of the breast designed for suckling (see **Fig. 47.1**). Each breast contains 12 to 15 lactiferous ducts, each with a separate opening on the nipple. The **lactiferous ducts** dilate in the area near the nipple, forming a **lactiferous sinus** that is a reservoir for easily accessible milk. The surface of the nipple is a lightly keratinized epidermis. The connective tissue of the nipple is scattered dense irregular connective tissue and smooth muscle, the latter responsible for erection during feeding as well as arousal.

Fig. 47.16 is a scanning image taken from the nipple; note the stratified squamous keratinized epithelium (black arrows) on the surface. Dense irregular connective tissue and smooth muscle are deep to the epithelium; within this region can be seen lactiferous ducts / lactiferous sinuses (yellow arrows).

Fig. 47.17 is an image from the nipple just underneath the surface epithelium, showing smooth muscle wisps (outlined) scattered among dense irregular connective tissue. The lactiferous ducts and sinuses (black arrows) have fairly dense connective tissue surrounding them and are lined by a stratified epithelium.

Helpful Hint

The histology of the lactiferous ducts and sinuses is the same; the difference is in the diameter of the lumen. Therefore, it is difficult to distinguish the lactiferous sinuses definitively from lactiferous ducts.

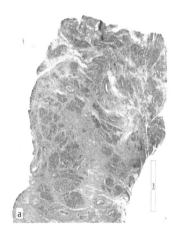
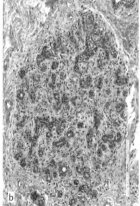

Fig. 47.15 Regressing mammary gland, at (a) scanning magnification and (b) medium magnification.

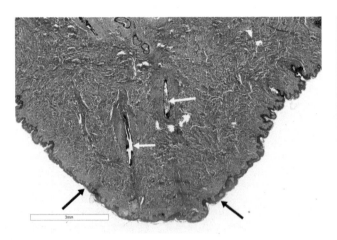

Fig. 47.16 **Nipple of the breast, scanning magnification, showing surface epithelium (black arrows) and lactiferous ducts (yellow arrows).**

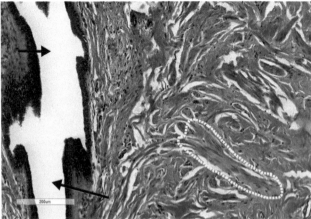

Fig. 47.17 **Nipple of the breast, low to medium magnification, showing lactiferous duct (arrows) and smooth muscle (outlined).**

Video 47.6   Nipple of breast

Be able to identify:
— Nipple
  • Stratified squamous keratinized epithelium
  • Smooth muscle
  • Lactiferous ducts
https://www.thieme.de/de/q.htm?p=opn/tp/308390101/978-1-62623-414-7_c047_v006&t=video

47.7   Chapter Review

The mammary glands are located in the anterior thoracic wall (breast) and are designed to produce milk to provide nutrition for newborns. Before puberty, the breasts are composed of connective tissue and adipose, with rudimentary ducts and secretory acini. Although these secretory units proliferate slightly at puberty, the visible increase in size of the breasts during this period is due to expansion of the connective and adipose tissue. Pregnancy increases circulating estrogen and progesterone significantly, which stimulates extensive proliferation of the epithelial ducts

and secretory acini. During this time, colostrum is produced, a milklike product with less fat than milk but containing laxative and antibodies as well as protein. After birth, the fully lactating breast produces milk, laden with fat and proteins. The acinar cells exhibit lipid droplets in their cytoplasm, and the lumen shows precipitated milk product. In electron micrographs, lipid droplets are readily seen in the cytoplasm and lumen. In addition, the acinar cells have prominent rough endoplasmic reticulum and Golgi apparatus, which produce the protein component of milk. After lactation ends, the secretory structures regress. The lactiferous ducts from the lobes of the mammary gland converge and widen into lactiferous sinuses at the nipple, where they are surrounded with dense irregular connective tissue and smooth muscle. The nipple is covered with a lightly keratinized epithelium.

Questions and Answers

An online-only section of questions and answers accompanying this chapter is hosted on Thieme's MedOne Education site: https://medone-education.thieme.com. Use the code on the media page at the front of this book to gain access. An institutional license to the site is required to access these questions in an interactive format, and individual users are required to register for an individual account to track results.

48 Placenta and Umbilical Cord

After completing this chapter, you should be able to:
— Identify, at the light microscope level, each of the following:
  • Placenta
    ○ Fetal portion
      ▪ Chorion
      ▪ Amnion
      ▪ Stem villi
      ▪ Branch villi
      ▪ Mesenchyme
      ▪ Cytotrophoblast
      ▪ Syncytiotrophoblast
        – Syncytial knots
      ▪ Anchoring villi (same substructures as stem villi)
    ○ Maternal portion
      ▪ Basal plate
        – Fibrinoid
        – Decidual tissue
        – Myometrium
      ▪ Decidua parietalis
        – Decidual cells
  • Umbilical cord
    ○ Amnion
    ○ Mesenchyme
    ○ Umbilical arteries and veins
— Identify, at the electron microscope level, each of the following:
  • Placenta
    ○ Cytotrophoblasts
    ○ Syncytiotrophoblast
— Outline the function of each cell and structure listed
— Correlate the appearance of each cell type or structure with its function
— Describe the development of the placenta and umbilical cord

48.1 Early Embryology

The **placenta** is an elaborate organ designed to exchange nutrients and waste products between the mother and the embryo. It is formed from tissues derived from the developing embryo combined with the maternal endometrial lining into which the embryo implants. Therefore, before examining the structure of the placenta, it is useful to provide a general overview of early embryonic development, with a focus on formation of the tissues that will give rise to the placenta.

48.1.1 First Week of Development

As discussed in **Chapter 46**, the ovulated **oocyte** is surrounded by a **zona pellucida** and **corona radiata** (**Fig. 48.1**). The ovulated oocyte enters the **oviduct**, which, given the presence of spermatozoa, is the site of **fertilization**. The product of fertilization, the single-celled **zygote**, undergoes mitotic divisions. Because there is little cell growth between cell divisions, the organism does not grow significantly during this time. By day 4, the resulting ball of cells is called a **morula**. Fluid accumulates within the morula, and the cells reorganize, forming a structure called the **blastocyst**. During this entire process, the developing organism is moved toward the uterus by ciliary action from the oviduct epithelium, so that the blastocyst arrives in the lumen of the uterus around day 4 or day 5. Around day 6, the zona pellucida breaks apart, and the outer layer of cells of the blastocyst makes contact with the endometrial epithelium to begin implantation.

Clinical Correlate

Early development of the organism is timed appropriately with its movement toward the uterus by ciliary action and muscular contraction of the oviduct, so that when the organism is ready to implant, it is within the lumen of the uterus. Conditions that reduce the ability of the oviducts to move the organism result in an organism ready to implant while still in the oviduct. The result is an **ectopic pregnancy**, also called a **tubal pregnancy**. In almost all cases, the organism cannot be sustained, and the life of the mother is at risk. Therefore, these must be surgically removed. Conditions that increase the risk for tubal pregnancies include a history of pelvic infections (sexually transmitted infections) that scar or disrupt the function of the oviducts.

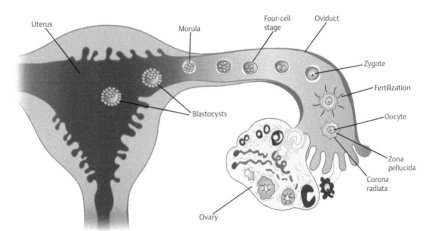

Fig. 48.1 First week of development. The oocyte ovulated from the ovary is surrounded by an extracellular zona pellucida and a collection of granulosa cells called the corona radiata. This ovulated complex is brought into the oviduct, where fertilization takes place. The resulting cell, the zygote, begins to divide rapidly. During this early development, cilia of the oviduct move the newly formed organism toward the uterus. The organism reaches the uterus around day 4 or 5, when it has developed into the blastocyst stage.

The blastocyst consists of a fluid-filled **blastocyst cavity** and two cell types: an outer layer called the **trophoblast (outer cell mass)** and a collection of cells at one end called the **inner cell mass (embryoblast, Fig. 48.2)**. Trophoblast cells adjacent to the inner cell mass make contact with the endometrial epithelium, initiating **implantation**. At this time, the uterine endometrial lining is in the secretory phase (about day 20–22 of the uterine cycle), including well-developed endometrial glands and a vascular and edematous endometrial connective tissue.

48.1.2 Implantation

Contact with the endometrial epithelium stimulates proliferation of the trophoblast cells (**Fig. 48.3**). Progeny from these cell divisions fuse to produce a multinuclear mass, the **syncytiotrophoblast**. Cells of the trophoblast that remain unfused are renamed the **cytotrophoblast**. Cytotrophoblast cells continue to proliferate, and the progeny fuse with the ever-growing syncytiotrophoblast mass.

The syncytiotrophoblast is responsible for implantation, a process by which the growing organism burrows into the endometrial lining. When implantation is complete, the organism is completely surrounded by endometrial connective tissue, and the endometrial epithelium reseals at the site of implantation (B in **Fig. 48.3**). In addition to providing the driving force for implantation, the syncytiotrophoblast is important for preventing immunologic rejection of the invading organism.

48.1.3 Establishing Early Maternal and Fetal Circulations

By the end of the second week, the organism has fully embedded into the endometrial lining of the uterus (**Fig. 48.4**). The syncytiotrophoblast has grown and will continue to grow as cells of the cytotrophoblast divide and fuse with the syncytiotrophoblast. Spaces appear within the syncytiotrophoblast, called **trophoblastic lacunae**. These lacunae connect to maternal blood vessels within the endometrial connective tissue, establishing a maternal circulation, which includes maternal arterial blood flowing into the trophoblastic lacunae and then draining via maternal

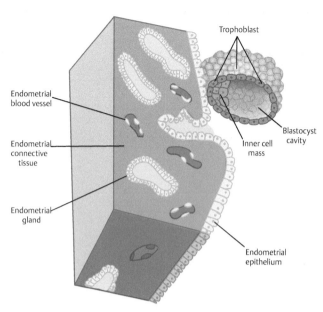

Fig. 48.2 Implantation, initial contact of the blastocyst with the endometrial lining of the uterus.

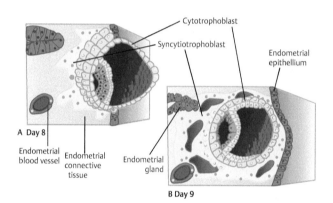

Fig. 48.3 Implantation, second week. Initial contact of the blastocyst with the endometrial epithelium causes proliferation of the trophoblast cells. The progeny of these divisions fuse, forming a multinuclear mass called the syncytiotrophoblast, which breaches the uterine epithelium and burrows into the underlying connective tissue.

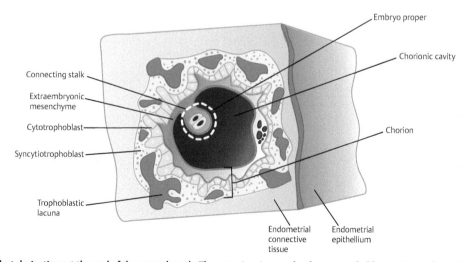

Fig. 48.4 Trophoblast derivatives at the end of the second week. The organism is completely surrounded by uterine endometrial connective tissue. The trophoblast is now two separate layers: a multicellular syncytiotrophoblast, and the cytotrophoblast. A connective tissue called extraembryonic mesenchyme develops inside the cytotrophoblast, and these three layers (syncytiotrophoblast, cytotrophoblast, and extraembronic mesenchyme) collectively form the chorion. Spaces called trophoblastic lacunae form within the syncytiotrophoblast, and fill with maternal blood. The blastocyst cavity is now called the chorionic cavity. The inner cell mass continues to develop, and is labeled embryo proper here.

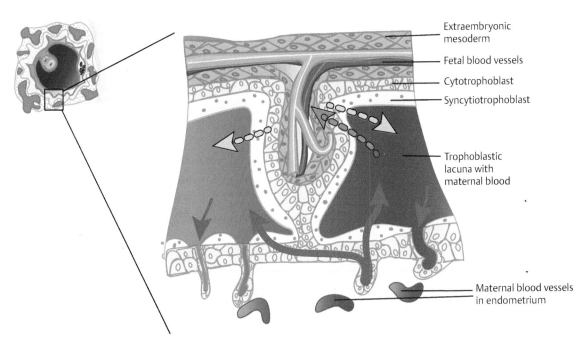

Extraembryonic mesoderm

Fetal blood vessels

Cytotrophoblast

Syncytiotrophoblast

Trophoblastic lacuna with maternal blood

Maternal blood vessels in endometrium

Fig. 48.5 Detailed drawing of the chorion, showing a single chorionic (placental) villus. The villi are projections of the chorion, and, therefore, consist of three layers: extraembryonic mesoderm, cytotrophoblast, syncytiotrophoblast. Embryonic/fetal blood vessels form within the extraembryonic mesoderm of the chorion and villi; fetal blood circulates from the developing embryo in the embryo proper through vessels in the connecting stalk, and into these vessels. Maternal blood flows into and out of the trophoblastic lacuna, which surround the placental villi (solid red arrows). Molecular exchange between maternal and embryonic/fetal blood occurs across the layers of the villi (dashed arrows).

veins. A layer of **extraembryonic mesenchyme** (embryonic connective tissue; see **Chapter 7**) appears deep to the cytotrophoblast, completing formation of the **chorion**, which includes the extraembryonic mesenchyme, cytotrophoblast, and syncytiotrophoblast layers. Within the chorion is a space, the **chorionic cavity**. The "embryo proper," derived from the inner cell mass, is surrounded by the chorionic cavity, connected to the chorion by a **connecting stalk** made from extraembryonic mesoderm.

During subsequent weeks, **chorionic villi** extend from the chorion into the trophoblastic lacunae (**Fig. 48.5**). These finger-like projections contain all three layers of the chorion: a core of extraembryonic mesenchyme, covered by cytotrophoblast and syncytiotrophoblast. These villi branch to increase surface area. Fetal blood vessels develop within the extraembryonic mesenchyme, which connect to blood vessels developing within the connecting stalk and embryo proper. Thus, a fetal circulation is established, whereby fetal blood vessels carry fetal blood into the vessels within the chorionic villi, from which it flows back to the fetus. Maternal blood in the trophoblastic lacunae bathes the chorionic villi. Therefore, nutrients in the maternal circulation can diffuse from maternal blood, through the trophoblast and extra-embryonic mesenchyme, and into the fetal circulation (dashed red arrows), while waste products can move in the opposite direction (dashed blue arrows).

Helpful Hint

Technically, the organism at the end of week two is entering the embryonic stage, and doesn't become a fetus until week nine. The terms "fetal blood" and "fetal blood vessels" are used here for convenience because slides shown later in this chapter are from the fetal stage. However, at this stage, these are more appropriately called "embryonic blood" and "embryonic blood vessels."

48.1.4 The Amnion

As for the structures derived from the inner cell mass, the early embryo at the end of the second week is a **bilaminar germ disk** (**Fig. 48.6**). The bilaminar germ disk will elaborate into a fully developed fetus, a process addressed in an embryology course or text. The **amniotic cavity** is a fluid-filled space bounded by the **amnion** or **amniotic membrane**. The amnion is composed of two layers: an inner layer in contact with amniotic fluid (blue), which is an epithelium referred to as **amnioblasts** or **extraembryonic ectoderm**, and an outer layer of extraembryonic mesenchyme (red). As will be discussed subsequently, the amniotic cavity expands, and the amnion makes contact with the chorion to become part of the fully formed placenta.

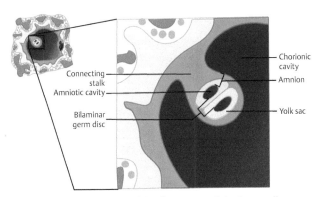

Connecting stalk

Amniotic cavity

Bilaminar germ disc

Chorionic cavity

Amnion

Yolk sac

Fig. 48.6 Detailed drawing of the derivatives of the inner cell mass. The cells of the inner cell mass differentiate, and organize into a bilaminar germ disk, flanked by a yolk sac and amnion. The connecting stalk, composed of extraembryonic mesoderm, connects the entire structure to the chorion.

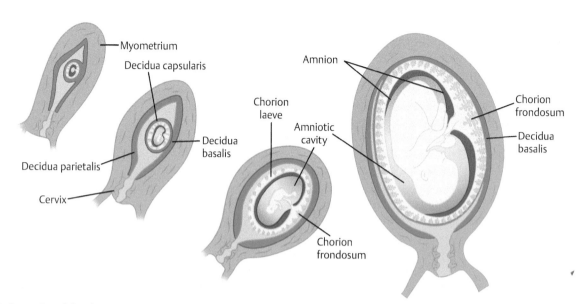

Fig. 48.7 Formation of the placenta. As implantation occurs, the uterine endometrium can be divided into three regions; the decidua basalis is between the organism and myometrium, the decidua capsularis is a thin layer covering the embedded organism, and locations away from the site of implantation are referred to as the decidua parietalis. The chorionic villi adjacent to the decidua basalis elaborate; this portion of the chorion is called the chorion frondosum (villous chorion). Villi adjacent to the decidua capsularis do not grow; this region of the chorion is called the chorion laeve (smooth chorion). The amniotic expands so that the amnion becomes opposed to the chorion.

48.2 Formation of the Placenta

Once implantation occurs, the endometrial lining of the uterus undergoes histologic and physiologic changes (**Fig. 48.7**). Because of this, the endometrial tissue of the uterus is now referred to as the **decidual layer**. This can be divided into three regions based on where the embryo implanted. That portion of the decidua between the implanted embryo and myometrium is called the **decidua basalis**, which will form part of the placenta. The decidua covering the implanted embryo is called the **decidua capsularis**, which thins as the embryo expands, eventually degenerating. Any decidua where implantation did not occur is called the **decidua parietalis**.

In addition, as mentioned, chorionic villi will form from the chorion. Early on, villi are well distributed on the chorion, surrounding the entire embryo. However, as development progresses, the villi closest to the decidua basalis continue to grow, and this region of the chorion is referred to as the **villous chorion** (**chorion frondosum**). Villi adjacent to the decidua capsularis regress; as this region of the chorion thins, it is referred to as the **smooth chorion** (**chorion laeve**).

Finally, the amniotic cavity expands, and the amnion becomes apposed to the chorion.

The final placenta is formed by the union of three structures. In **Fig. 48.8**, the placenta is to the right of the embryo. Starting from the amniotic cavity and moving to the right, the placenta consists of:

1. The amnion (amniotic membrane) contains an inner epithelium, covered by extraembryonic mesenchyme.
2. The chorion frondosum (villous chorion) contains extraembryonic mesenchyme, cytotrophoblast, and syncytiotrophoblast.
3. The maternal decidua basalis that was formerly the endometrium.

The chorion is tightly attached to the maternal decidua when the organism implants into the uterine lining. In contrast, expansion of the amniotic cavity brings the amnion adjacent to the chorion, obliterating the chorionic cavity. However, the amnion is only loosely apposed to the chorion, and these layers will separate during tissue preparation.

The mature placenta is a disk-shaped structure and is ejected as part of the afterbirth. This occurs via separation of the **decidua basalis** from the uterine wall (somewhat similar to menstruation). The ejected placenta has two sides (**Fig. 48.9**):

- A rough **maternal side** is composed of decidual (endometrial) tissue. This region is broken into segments, called **cotyledons**.
- The fetal side is smooth because it is covered by the amniotic membrane.

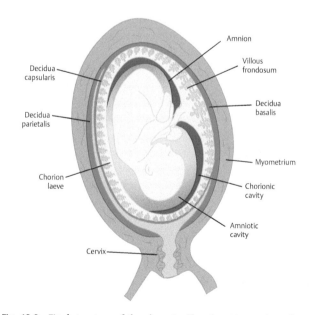

Fig. 48.8 Final structure of the placenta. The placenta consists of three layers (from fetus to myometrium): the amnion, villous chorion, decidua basalis. As the fetus grows, the lumen of the uterus is obliterated, and the smooth chorion and decidua capsularis thins.

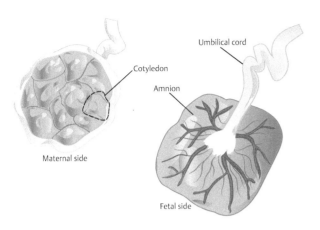

Fig. 48.9   **Gross anatomy of the placenta, showing the maternal and fetal sides.**

48.3   Overview of the Histology of the Placenta

Fig. 48.10 shows a scanning image of a 5-month placenta, similar to the region in the rectangle in the inset. The fetal side is to the right, and the maternal side to the left. At this magnification, the amnion and flat portion of the chorion are not distinguishable (green bracket). The space to the right of this was once occupied by amniotic fluid. The trophoblastic lacunae have merged to form one large space with numerous chorionic villi; this large region is referred to as the villous space (black bracket). The maternal side includes the decidua (blue bracket) and myometrium (red bracket). The myometrium is covered by a very thin perimetrium; the space to the left of the myometrium/perimetrium is the pelvic cavity.

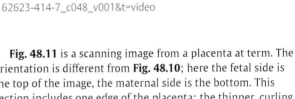

Video 48.1   Overview of placenta at 5 months

Be able to identify:
— Fetal side
— Villous space
— Maternal side
https://www.thieme.de/de/q.htm?p=opn/tp/308390101/978-1-62623-414-7_c048_v001&t=video

Fig. 48.11 is a scanning image from a placenta at term. The orientation is different from **Fig. 48.10**; here the fetal side is the top of the image, the maternal side is the bottom. This section includes one edge of the placenta; the thinner, curling tissue to the left is the tissue adjacent to the placenta (amnion, smooth chorion, and decidua parietalis). Again, note the amnion/chorion (green bracket), villous space (black bracket), and decidua (red bracket). Because this is a placenta at term, sloughed from the uterus as part of the afterbirth, the myometrium is not included.

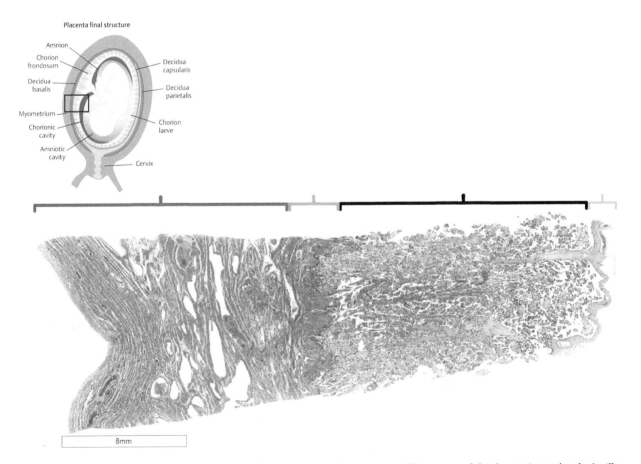

Fig. 48.10 **Placenta, 5 months pregnancy, scanning magnification, showing the amnion and flat portion of the chorion (green bracket), villous space (black bracket), decidua (blue bracket), and myometrium (red bracket).**

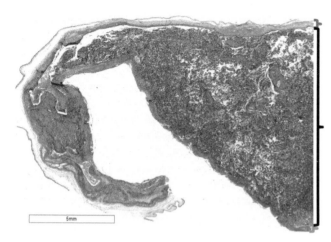

Fig. 48.11 Placenta at term, scanning magnification, showing the amnion and flat portion of the chorion (green bracket), villous space (black bracket), and decidua (blue bracket).

Video 48.2   Overview of placenta at term

Be able to identify:
— Fetal side
— Villous space
— Maternal side

https://www.thieme.de/de/q.htm?p=opn/tp/308390101/978-1-62623-414-7_c048_v002&t=video

48.4   Amnion and Chorion

Fig. 48.12 is taken from the fetal side of the placenta in a region where the amnion is separated from the chorion. The point of separation is indicated by the black arrow; below that point the fetal side includes both amnion and chorion (black bracket), above that point it is simply chorion (green bracket). The separated amnion is seen curving toward the right (green arrows). There is a large fetal blood vessel (X) in the chorion above the separation point.

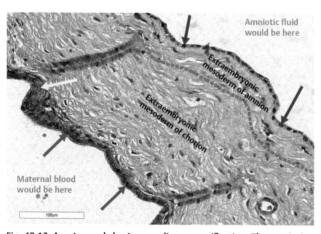

Fig. 48.13 Amnion and chorion, medium magnification. The amniotic fluid on the fetal side and maternal blood in the villous space are indicated. Amniotic epithelium (amnioblasts) are indicated by the blue arrows, as well as cytotrophoblasts (yellow arrow) and syncytiotrophoblast (red arrows). Fused extraembryonic mesenchyme from the amnion and chorion forms the core of this structure; the approximate fusion point is indicated by the green dashed line.

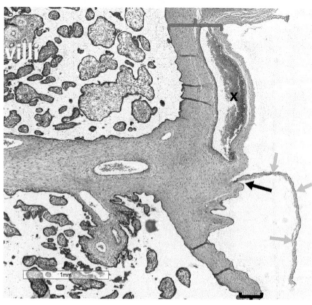

Fig. 48.12 Amnion and chorion, low magnification. The villous space with villi is indicated. The amnion and chorion are fused at the bottom of the slide (black bracket) but have come apart in the middle; the point of separation is indicated by the black arrow. Only the chorion is intact at the top (green bracket), and the torn amnion peels off to the right (green arrows). X marks a fetal blood vessel.

Fig. 48.13 is a medium-magnification image from a region of the fetal side of the placenta in which the amnion has remained attached to the chorion. The green dashed line represents the approximate border between these two layers (i.e., the approximate location of the obliterated chorionic cavity).

Closer examination of the amnion reveals that it consists of two layers:
• Amniotic epithelium (amnioblasts, blue arrows in **Fig. 48.13**)
• Extraembryonic mesenchyme

The chorion is composed of three layers:
• Extraembryonic mesenchyme
• Cytotrophoblasts (yellow arrow)
• Syncytiotrophoblast (red arrows)

The two darker, horizontally oriented double bands in **Fig. 48.13** are artifacts.

Video 48.3   Amnion and chorion in a placenta at 5 months

https://www.thieme.de/de/q.htm?p=opn/tp/308390101/978-1-62623-414-7_c048_v003&t=video

Video 48.4   Amnion and chorion in a placenta at term

https://www.thieme.de/de/q.htm?p=opn/tp/308390101/978-1-62623-414-7_c048_v004&t=video

Be able to identify:
— Amnion
  • Amnioblasts
  • Extraembryonic mesenchyme
— Chorion
  • Extraembryonic mesenchyme
  • Trophoblasts

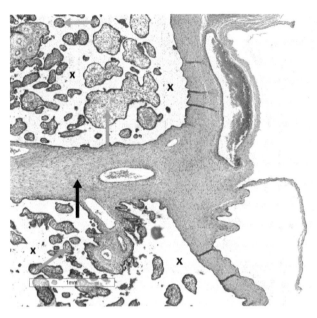

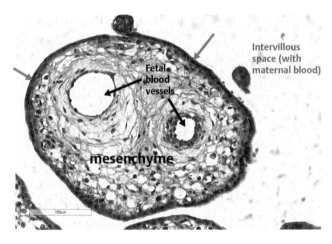

Fig. 48.15 **Villus in the intervillous space, 5 months pregnancy, medium magnification. The intervillous space is indicated. The core of a villus is mesenchyme, with fetal blood vessels. Villi are covered by cytotrophoblasts (blue arrows) and syncytiotrophoblast (red arrows).**

Fig. 48.14 **Villi in the intervillous space, 5 months pregnancy, low magnification. X marks the intervillous space, the location of maternal blood. A stem villus (black arrow) projects directly from the chorion; branch villi (blue arrows) are indicated.**

48.5 Villi and Intervillous Space at 5 Months Pregnancy

Villi are projections of the chorion and are bathed in maternal blood (**Fig. 48.14**). They contain fetal blood vessels and are the site of molecular exchange between maternal and fetal circulations. Villi that project directly from the chorion are called **stem villi** (black arrow). Branches from the stem villi, called **branch villi** (blue arrows), are quite numerous and vary in shape and size. The empty space (Xs) between the villi, normally filled with maternal blood, is the **intervillous space**.

Fig. 48.15 shows a villus at medium magnification. Since villi are projections of the chorion, they are composed of a core of mesenchyme with fetal blood vessels covered by trophoblast. The outermost layer, the syncytiotrophoblast (red arrows), is a complete layer in contact with maternal blood. The nuclei of the

syncytiotrophoblast are typically small and round or oval shaped; the cytoplasm is darkly eosinophilic. Cytotrophoblasts (blue arrows) form an incomplete cell layer underneath the syncytiotrophoblast.

Fig. 48.16 is an image taken at high magnification, showing a portion of a few villi. Maternal blood normally occupies the intervillous space; a few maternal red blood cells can be seen on the outer surface of the villus in the bottom left. Cytotrophoblasts (blue arrows) typically have larger, more euchromatic nuclei and paler cytoplasm than the syncytiotrophoblast layer (red arrows). The cytotrophoblast cells serve as stem cells. The syncytiotrophoblast layer, on the other hand, is very active metabolically, with prominent rough and smooth endoplasmic reticulum, Golgi apparatus, and secretory vesicles, which accounts for its darkly stained cytoplasm. This layer has numerous microvilli, seen as a brush border on the surface in contact with maternal blood (most obvious on the surface of the largest villus).

Video 48.5 Villi at 5 months pregnancy

Be able to identify:
— Villi
  • Stem villi
  • Branch villi
— Mesenchyme
  • Cytotrophoblast
  • Syncytiotrophoblast
  • Intervillous space
— The location of fetal blood
— The location of maternal blood
https://www.thieme.de/de/q.htm?p=opn/tp/308390101/978-1-62623-414-7_c048_v005&t=video

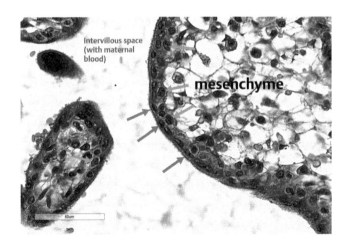

Fig. 48.16 **Villi in the intervillous space, 5 months pregnancy, high magnification. The intervillous space is indicated. Villi are covered by cytotrophoblasts (blue arrows) and syncytiotrophoblast (red arrows); the latter shows a brush border in contact with maternal blood.**

48.6 Villi and Intervillous Space at Term

The placenta at 5 months has a villus network able to provide sufficient exchange of nutrients and waste products between maternal and fetal blood. However, as the embryo grows, the efficiency of this exchange must be improved. The villi undergo morphological changes that increase molecular exchange, including:

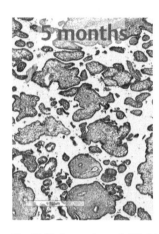
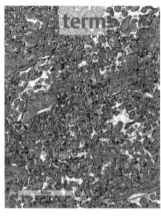

Fig. 48.17 **Comparison of villi at (a) 5 months pregnancy and (b) term.**

- More elaborate branching of the villus network to increase surface area
- A decreased distance between maternal and fetal blood, increasing the efficiency of diffusion. This occurs by a combination of the following:
  - A decrease in the number of cytotrophoblast cells; at term, cytotrophoblast cells are essentially nonexistent
  - Clustering of syncytiotrophoblast nuclei, forming **syncytial knots**, which allowing the remainder of the syncytiotrophoblast to thin
  - Movement of fetal blood vessels to the edge of the villi, where the **basement membrane** of the fetal endothelial cells fuse with the basement membrane of the trophoblast

Fig. 48.17 compares villi at 5 months pregnancy with villi at term. Both images are of the intervillous space, at similar magnification. As the placenta develops during pregnancy, the villi continue to branch, resulting in a larger number of smaller villi that provide more surface area for molecular exchange.

Fig. 48.18 is an image of several villi from a placenta at term. There are few, if any, cytotrophoblasts at this stage. The nuclei at the edge of the villi (blue arrows) likely belong to the syncytiotrophoblast layer. Syncytiotrophoblast nuclei cluster together to form syncytial knots (outlined), allowing the remainder of the syncytiotrophoblast to form a very thin but highly eosinophilic outer layer of the villi (black arrows). Fetal blood vessels (yellow arrows) are close to the edge of the villi, adjacent to the thinner regions of the syncytiotrophoblast. The basement membranes of the fetal endothelial cells and syncytiotrophoblast cell layer fuse. Therefore, the final barrier between maternal and fetal blood is as thin as the air-blood barrier in the lung:

Syncytiotrophoblast → fused basement membrane → fetal endothelial cells

Video 48.6   Villi at term

Be able to identify:
- Villi
  - Stem villi
  - Branch villi
- Mesenchyme
- Syncytiotrophoblast
- Intervillous space
- The location of fetal blood
- The location of maternal blood
- Changes at term relative to 5 months pregnancy
  - Increased number of villi
  - Lack of cytotrophoblasts
  - Syncytial knots
  - Areas of fused basal lamina

https://www.thieme.de/de/q.htm?p=opn/tp/308390101/978-1-62623-414-7_c048_v006&t=video

Helpful Hint

The lack of numerous cytotrophoblast cells should not be surprising. These cells are stem cells, which divide and fuse with the syncytiotrophoblast cell mass. Once enough syncytiotrophoblast is present, cytotrophoblast cells are no longer necessary.

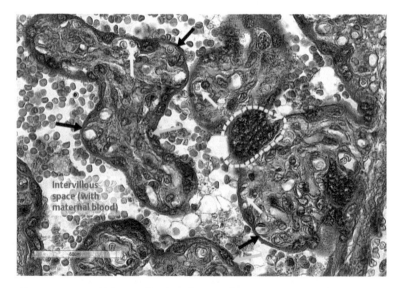

Figure 48.18   Villi in the intervillous space, term, high magnification. The intervillous space is indicated. At term, cytotrophoblasts are essentially absent. The syncytiotrophoblast nuclei are clustered into syncytial knots (outlined), allowing the remainder of the syncytiotrophoblast cytoplasm to thin (black arrows). Single syncytiotrophoblast nuclei can be seen (blue arrows). Fetal blood vessels (yellow arrows) have moved to the edge of villi, and the basement membranes of the endothelial cells have fused with the trophoblast basement membrane.

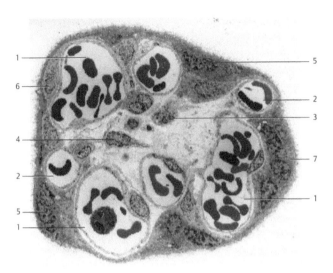

Fig. 48.19 Placental villus, electron micrograph, showing (1, 2) fetal blood vessels (capillaries); (3) fetal macrophage; (4) fibroblast; (5) syncytiotrophoblast nucleus; (6) cytotrophoblast nucleus; (7) syncytial knot.

Clinical Correlate

If a couple has a family history of a genetic condition, or in a mother of advanced maternal age, a **chorionic villus sample** can be obtained. In this procedure, an ultrasound-guided needle is placed into the villous space, and a sample is withdrawn. This sample has fetal cells (the villi are derived from the fetus) and can inform the parents of the genetic makeup of the fetus.

Fig. 48.19 is an electron micrograph of a villus from a mature placenta. The space surrounding the villus is the intervillous space, which contained maternal blood that washed away during tissue preparation. Fetal blood cells can be seen within fetal vessels (1 and 2). The connective tissue core of the villus includes a fetal macrophage (3) and fibroblasts (4). The outermost layer is syncytiotrophoblast, with nuclei that are either singular (5) or in clusters (syncytial knots, 7). The cytotrophoblast cell seen here (6) can be recognized because it is under a thin layer of syncytiotrophoblast and has paler cytoplasm than the syncytiotrophoblast. Note areas where fetal vessels are close to the surface of the villus; in these locations the basement membrane of fetal blood vessels fuses with the basement membrane of the trophoblast layer.

48.7 Maternal Side of the Placenta

Fig. 48.20 is a scanning image showing the maternal side of the placenta, including:
- Villi in the intervillous space
- Decidua, covered on the villous side by syncytiotrophoblast (not visible at this magnification; recall that the trophoblastic lacunae are lined by syncytiotrophoblast)
- Myometrium

Fig. 48.21 is a low-magnification image of the maternal side of the placenta, showing that some villi extend across the intervillus space and make contact with the syncytiotrophoblast that lines the decidual tissue. These villi are called **anchoring villi** (arrows).

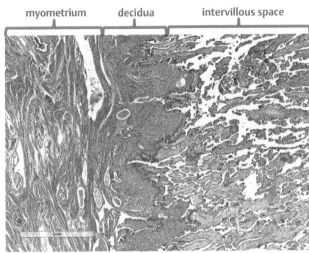

Fig. 48.20 Maternal side of the placenta, 5 months pregnancy, scanning magnification.

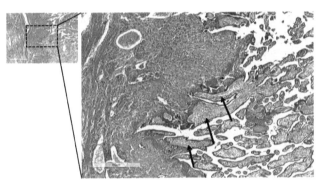

Fig. 48.21 Maternal side of the placenta, 5 months pregnancy, low magnification, showing anchoring villi (arrows).

Fig. 48.22 is a medium-magnification image of the junction between an anchoring villius and the decidua. The anchoring villi have many cytotrophoblasts (yellow outline); these cells migrate between the syncytiotrophoblast and decidual tissue to form a **cytotrophoblastic shell** (not visible on this image). Other cells derived from the cytotrophoblast migrate into the maternal vasculature, replacing maternal endothelial cells. This remodeling also includes loss of the tunica media in endometrial vessels, enabling consistent perfusion of the placenta even in the presence of vasoactive hormones.

Clinical Correlate

Failure of cytotrophoblasts to migrate into the maternal vasculature, or their failure to replace maternal endothelial cells, results in maternal arteries that remain small and constrictive. This reduces flow to the placenta and can lead to a number of pregnancy complications, including intrauterine growth restriction and fetal death. In addition, the resulting inadequate placental flow has detrimental effects on maternal circulation and is a known cause of **preeclampsia**, which is new-onset hypertension and proteinuria in a pregnant woman.

Similar to syncytial knots in villi, clusters of more condensed nuclei within eosinophilic cytoplasm belong to the syncytiotrophoblast (**Fig. 48.22**, green outline). **Decidual cells** in the

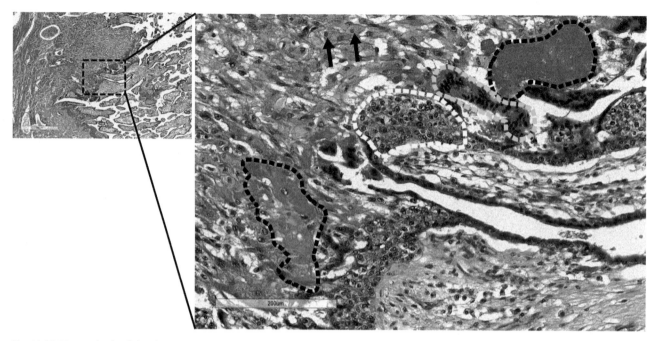

Fig. 48.22 Maternal side of the placenta, 5 months pregnancy, medium magnification. The anchoring villi show cytotrophoblast clusters (yellow outline) and syncytiotrophoblast nuclei (green outline). Decidual cells (black arrows) and fibrinoid (black outlines) are shown.

maternal tissue (arrows) have pale eosinophilia, characteristic of hormone-secreting cells (e.g., relaxin, which plays a role in softening pelvic ligaments and the cervix). The syncytiotrophoblast, cytotrophoblastic shell, and maternal decidual tissue are collectively called the **decidual plate**. Maternal decidual cells and blood form a highly eosinophilic **fibrinoid** (black outlines), which accumulates throughout pregnancy. The function of fibrinoid is not completely understood.

Video 48.7   Maternal side of placenta at 5 months pregnancy

https://www.thieme.de/de/q.htm?p=opn/tp/308390101/978-1-62623-414-7_c048_v007&t=video

Video 48.8   Maternal side of placenta at term

https://www.thieme.de/de/q.htm?p=opn/tp/308390101/978-1-62623-414-7_c048_v008&t=video

Be able to identify:
— Villi
  • Anchoring villi
  • Cytotrophoblasts
— Decidua
  • Fibrinoid
  • Large, eosinophilic cells (decidual or trophoblastic cells)
— Myometrium

48.8   Decidua Parietalis

Recall that the decidua in regions where implantation did not occur is referred to as the decidua parietalis (see **Fig. 48.7**). This region is not inactive. **Fig. 48.23** is a scanning image of the decidua parietalis and associated myometrium. At low magnification, it is evident that the decidual tissue has the appearance of the secretory phase of the endometrium.

Fig. 48.24 is a high-magnification image from the decidua parietalis close to the surface. The surface epithelium is thin (black arrow). **Decidual cells** (blue arrows) in the lamina propria are easily recognized as large cells with a large, euchromatic nucleus and abundant eosinophilic cytoplasm. Like decidual cells of the placenta, the decidual cells here also secrete hormones important for pregnancy.

Video 48.9   Decidua parietalis

Be able to identify:
— Decidua parietalis
  • Endometrial glands
  • Decidual cells
https://www.thieme.de/de/q.htm?p=opn/tp/308390101/978-1-62623-414-7_c048_v009&t=video

48.9   Umbilical Cord

The umbilical cord is largely derived from extraembryonic mesenchyme of the connecting stalk, covered by amnion (see **Fig. 48.6**). **Fig. 48.25** is a scanning image of the umbilical cord at 5 months. Note:
• The outer layer of the umbilical cord is epithelial (amnioblasts, black arrows).
• The core of the umbilical cord is mesenchyme.
• There is a central **umbilical vein** (blue arrow), flanked by two **umbilical arteries** (red arrows).

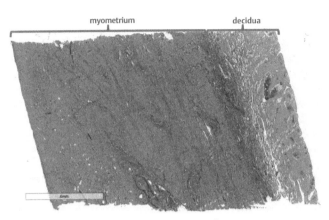

Fig. 48.23 **Decidua parietalis, scanning magnification.**

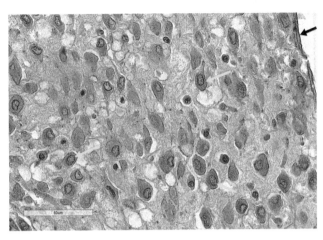

Fig. 48.24 **Decidua parietalis, high magnification, showing decidual cells (blue arrows) and decidual epithelium (black arrow).**

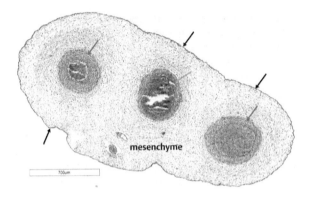

Fig. 48.25 **Umbilical cord at 5 months pregnancy, low magnification. The core of mesenchyme contains the developing umbilical vein (blue arrow) flanked by umbilical arteries (red arrows). The umbilical cord is covered by amnioblasts continuous with the amnioblasts of the amniotic membrane (black arrows).**

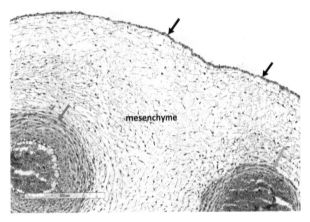

Fig. 48.26 **Umbilical cord at 5 months pregnancy, low-medium magnification. The core of mesenchyme contains the developing umbilical vein (blue arrow) and umbilical arteries (one is shown at red arrow). The umbilical cord is covered by amnioblasts continuous with the amnioblasts of the amniotic membrane (black arrows).**

Fig. 48.26 shows a portion of the umbilical cord at higher magnification. The amnioblasts appear as a simple epithelium (simple cuboidal here), and the mesenchyme is embryonic/fetal connective tissue with few extracellular fibers. Although the vessels are not well developed, the artery (red arrow) has more substantial smooth muscle than the vein (blue arrow).

Video 48.10 Umbilical cord at 5 months

Be able to identify:
— Umbilical cord
  • Amnioblasts
  • Mesenchyme
  • Umbilical vein
  • Umbilical arteries

https://www.thieme.de/de/q.htm?p=opn/tp/308390101/978-1-62623-414-7_c048_v010&t=video

Fig. 48.27 is a cross section of the umbilical cord at term. Note that the mesenchyme is more fibrous and the umbilical arteries (red arrows) and umbilical vein (blue arrow) are more developed than in the umbilical cord at 5 months.

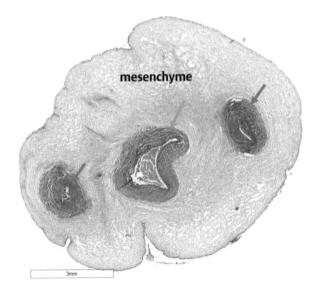

Fig. 48.27 **Umbilical cord at term, scanning magnification. The core of mesenchyme contains the developing umbilical vein (blue arrow) flanked by umbilical arteries (red arrows).**

Video 48.11 Umbilical cord at term

Be able to identify:
— Umbilical cord
  • Amnioblasts
  • Mesenchyme
  • Umbilical vein
  • Umbilical arteries

https://www.thieme.de/de/q.htm?p=opn/tp/308390101/978-1-62623-414-7_c048_v011&t=video

48.10 Chapter Review

The placenta and umbilical cord are designed to support nutrient and waste exchange between the mother and developing embryo and fetus. This structure is created from tissues of the fetus (amnion and villous chorion) and mother (maternal decidua basalis). The fetal side includes the amnion and chorion, which are loosely fused together. The amnion is composed of amnioblasts (amnion epithelial cells) and extraembryonic mesenchyme. The chorion is composed of extraembryonic mesenchyme and covered by cytotrophoblast and syncytiotrophoblast. Extensions of the chorion are villi, which extend into the intervillous space, which, in life, contains maternal blood. Like the chorion, villi have a core of mesenchyme with fetal blood vessels, covered by trophoblast cells. Villi elaborate during development to provide more efficient molecular exchange. This includes growth and branching, which increases surface area. In addition, the cytotrophoblast cells cease dividing and are not numerous. The syncytiotrophoblast cytoplasm thins, and its nuclei cluster to form syncytial knots. Fetal blood vessels move to the edge of the villi, and the basement membranes of endothelial cells fuse with the trophoblast basement membrane. Therefore, the barrier to molecular exchange consists only of fetal endothelial cell → fused basement membrane → syncytiotrophoblast. The cytotrophoblast cells have large, euchromatic nuclei and pale cytoplasm. The syncytiotrophoblast is much more active; the numerous organelles present imparts the cytoplasm of this multinuclear mass with more intense staining. Some villi extend to the decidual side of the placenta, where trophoblast cells stream from the villus and into the decidual tissue. Cytotrophoblast cells form a sheet, the cytotrophoblastic shell. Trophoblast cells and decidual cells become hormone-secreting and are recognized as large cells with large, euchromatic nuclei and abundant eosinophilic cytoplasm. Decidual cells in areas where implantation did not occur, the decidua parietalis, have a similar appearance. Highly eosinophilic extracellular material in the maternal decidua is called fibrinoid. The umbilical cord has a core of mesenchyme covered by amnioblasts (amniotic epithelial cells), in which the single umbilical vein and two umbilical arteries develop.

Questions and Answers

An online-only section of questions and answers accompanying this chapter is hosted on Thieme's MedOne Education site: https://medone-education.thieme.com. Use the code on the media page at the front of this book to gain access. An institutional license to the site is required to access these questions in an interactive format, and individual users are required to register for an individual account to track results.

Index

Note: *f* indicates a figure; *t*, a table.